Medical Robotics

Edited by
Vanja Bozovic

Medical Robotics

Edited by Vanja Bozovic

Republished by InTech

Janeza Trdine 9, 51000 Rijeka, Croatia

Additional hard copies can be obtained from orders@intechopen.com

Medical Robotics, Edited by Vanja Bozovic
p. cm.
ISBN 978-3-902613-18-9

For EU product safety concerns:
IN TECH d.o.o., Prolaz Marije Krucifikse Kozulić 3, 51000 Rijeka, Croatia,
info@intechopen.com or visit our website at intechopen.com.

Preface

The first generation of surgical robots are already being installed in a number of operating rooms around the world. Robotics is being introduced to medicine because it allows for unprecedented control and precision of surgical instruments in minimally invasive procedures. So far, robots have been used to position an endoscope, perform gallbladder surgery and correct gastroesophogeal reflux and heartburn. The ultimate goal of the robotic surgery field is to design a robot that can be used to perform closed-chest, beating-heart surgery. The use of robotics in surgery will expand over the next decades without any doubt.

Minimally Invasive Surgery (MIS) is a revolutionary approach in surgery. In MIS, the operation is performed with instruments and viewing equipment inserted into the body through small incisions created by the surgeon, in contrast to open surgery with large incisions. This minimizes surgical trauma and damage to healthy tissue, resulting in shorter patient recovery time.

The aim of this book is to provide an overview of the state-of-art, to present new ideas, original results and practical experiences in this expanding area.

Nevertheless, many chapters in the book concern advanced research on this growing area. The book provides critical analysis of clinical trials, assessment of the benefits and risks of the application of these technologies.

This book is certainly a small sample of the research activity on Medical Robotics going on around the globe as you read it, but it surely covers a good deal of what has been done in the field recently, and as such it works as a valuable source for researchers interested in the involved subjects, whether they are currently "medical roboticists" or not.

Editor
Dr. Vanja Bozovic
E-mail: vanjabozovic@gmail.com

Contents

1

The learning curve of robot-assisted laparoscopic surgery

E. Olthof[1], D. Nio[1] and W.A. Bemelman[2]
[1] *Department of Surgery, Spaarne Hospital, Hoofddorp,*
[2] *Department of Surgery, Academic Medical Center, Amsterdam*
The Netherlands

1. Introduction

Endoscopic surgery has proven to be beneficial to the patient with regard to reduction of hospital stay, postoperative pain and earlier return to daily activities. After its introduction, development of new instrumentation improved and facilitated endoscopic performance (Yohannes et al, 2002). Despite this development, laparoscopic procedures have been limited by fixed distances, restricted freedom of motion of the surgical instruments, impaired visualization and small working space (Sarle et al, 2004). With the introduction of surgical robotic systems an attempt was made to overcome these technical difficulties. Many conventional laparoscopic procedures have been duplicated with assistance of a surgical robotic system. Endoscopic cardiac procedures, that were not feasible before applying conventional laparoscopic techniques, are currently performed robotically-assisted. Several advantages of robotic surgery compared to conventional laparoscopy have been identified: additional degrees of freedom of motion, downscaling of movements, enhanced stability (both of visualization and surgical instrumentation), restoration of the eye-hand target axis, elimination of the fulcrum effect and improved ergonomics for the surgeon. These features are supposed to enhance surgical performance by improved accuracy, dexterity and visualization. Consequently, it can be expected that endoscopic surgical skills are more easily mastered and the learning curve is shortened. The learning curve can be defined as the amount of practice (in time or number of repetitions) necessary to achieve a consistency of a specified parameter. A time-action analysis, the time to complete a task, the number of actions required and the number of errors made, are parameters used to evaluate the learning curve for a specific task. In daily practice, other parameters viz. conversion rate, operating time, blood loss, morbidity and hospital stay are used to assess the learning curve for a specific procedure. Most advanced endoscopic procedures are characterized by a long learning curve. Learning curves are associated with prolonged operative times, increased patient morbidity and higher costs. These difficulties might delay further implementation of advanced endoscopic techniques. Although a surgical robotic system might impose as the ideal endoscopic instrument, most clinical studies have not shown benefit with regard to operative time compared to conventional endoscopy. The objective of this study is to systematically review the available literature to evaluate the impact of a surgical robotic system on the learning curve of endoscopic procedures compared to conventional endoscopy.

2. Methods

A computer-assisted search was performed in the medical databases Medline (from January 1966 to June 2007), Embase (from January 1988 to June 2007) and the Cochrane Database of Systematic Reviews, using a combination of the keywords "Learning curve, robot, telemanipulation and computer-assisted surgery". After identifying relevant titles, the abstracts of these studies were read to decide if the study was suitable. Two authors (EO and DN) independently read the abstracts. A manual search of reference lists of studies thus obtained was conducted for any relevant articles not found in the computerized search.

2.1 Criteria for inclusion

Clinical and experimental studies eligible for inclusion had to describe a learning curve for robot-assisted procedures. Articles in languages other than English, German or French were excluded. Articles, in which a summary of different procedures executed with the aid of a robotic surgical system was described, were excluded.

3. Results

In total 21 studies were identified. Most excluded studies were case reports, small series or reports of the author's experience with a variety of surgical procedures using a robotic system without evaluation of a learning curve. The search resulted in 10 experimental studies on laparoscopic skills. In general surgery, articles reporting a learning curve were mostly those describing robot-assisted cholecystectomy and robot-assisted antireflux surgery (fundoplication), respectively 7 and 4 studies. There were some incidental reports of other surgical procedures viz. gastric bypass (3) and aortoiliac surgery (1). Reports on other fields than general surgery as urology and cardiac surgery were not included for evaluation. As a result this review concentrates on the learning curve of robot-assisted standard experimental exercises, laparoscopic cholecystectomy and laparoscopic fundoplication.

4. Robot-assisted laparoscopic skills

Ten experimental studies described standardized exercises with either Zeus (4/10) or Da Vinci (6/10) robotic system. In all studies basic endoscopic tasks such as transferring beads/rings, rope passing, knot tying and suturing were reported. The drills were predominantly performed by laparoscopic novice participants sometimes compared with laparoscopic experienced surgeons. In 6 studies (Prasad et al, 2001; Yohannes et al, 2002; Maniar et al, 2004; Nio et al, 2005 ; Blavier et al, 2006; Heemskerk et al, 2007) the robotic learning curve (RLC) was compared to the manual learning curve (MLC). In most studies the learning curve was defined on the basis of 2 parameters; completion time and amount of errors, often given as a combined score. Results are shown in table 1. In most studies the initial performance using the robotic system was inferior to the conventional laparoscopy. Although a rapid improvement of robotic performance was observed, conventional laparoscopic performance was rarely equalled. In all but one study a significant improvement of outcome parameter after time was shown, which suggested a significant learning curve. Only one study (Heemskerk et al, 2007) showed a flat RLC from the beginning. Most novice participants showed an initial inferior performance in comparison to laparoscopic experienced participants. This resulted in a steeper early phase of their RLC.

When RLC and MLC were compared results were not conclusive. When steeper learning curves were described in either the robotic of conventional laparoscopic group, they were attributed to an initially worse performance.

	Robotic system	Skill	No. of repetitions	Participants LN/LE	Parameter	Learning curve
Yohannes	Da Vinci	Dexterity task Suturing/Knot-tying	5	4LN/4LE	Time	Yes
Prasad	Zeus	Bead transfer Rope pass	5	17LN/11LE	Calculated score (time + error) Precision score	Yes
Maniar	Zeus	Bead transfer Rope pass	15	20LN	Calculated score % improvement	Yes
Heemskerk	Da Vinci	Bead drop/transfer Needle cap Suturing	3	8LN	Time Accuracy	No
Blavier	Da Vinci	Passing needle through rings	6	10LN	Performance score Error score Ambidexterity score	Yes
Nio	Zeus	Suturing Knot-tying	20	1LN/1LE	Number of actions / stitch or knot	Yes
Chang	Zeus	Knot-tying	> 5 -14 h training	8?	Time Composite score	Yes
Hernandez	Da Vinci	Suturing	5	7N/6E	OSATS Time	Yes
Narazaki	Da Vinci	Pick and place Needle passing Suturing	4 weeks training*	7LN	Time (Travelling distance)	Yes
Ro	Da Vinci	5 drills	5-6	17 LN/2LE	Performance score (time+error)	LN :Yes LE : No

LN: laparoscopic naive, LE: laparoscopic experienced, OSATS: objective structured assessment of surgical skills
* 6 sessions of training

Table 1. Learning curve. Results of robotic skill studies

5. Robot-assisted laparoscopic cholecystectomy

Seven robot-assisted cholecystectomy studies describing the learning curve were identified. Four series were comparative studies (Perez et al, 2003; Guilianotti et al, 2003; Caratozollo et al, 2005; Heemskerk et al, 2005) and 3 series consisted of consecutive patient series

(Chitwood et al, 2001; Ruurda et al, 2002; Vidovszky et al, 2006). In 6 studies the Da Vinci was used, in only one the Zeus-AESOP robotic system. Laparoscopic experienced surgeons performed the laparoscopic cholecystectomy. The set-up time and operative time were used as the parameters for the learning curve. Four studies (Caratozollo et al, 2005, Vidovszky et al, 2006, Ruurda et al, 2002, Chitwood et al, 2001) showed a decrease of the robotic set-up time, but in only 2 studies this decrease was significant (Chitwood et al, 2001;Vidovszky et al, 2006). In one study robotic set-up time did not change in time (Heemskerk et al, 2005) and 2 studies did not report on the robotic set-up time (Perez et al, 2003, Giulianotti et al, 2003).

The operating time decreased in 3/7 studies (Perez et al, 2003, Giulianotti et al, 2003; Caratozzolo et al, 2005), of which 2 studies showed a significant decrease. All 3 studies reported that the mean robotic operative time at the end of the series was equal compared to manual laparoscopic cholecystectomy. One study mentioned that 20 operations were needed to complete the learning phase. (Guilianotti et al, 2003). No major intra-operative complications occurred. Conversion was necessary 7/219 times as a result of severe cholecystitis, poor visualization or obscure anatomy. The conversion rate was not higher in the robotic laparoscopic cholecystectomy. No study mentioned at which moment of the learning curve conversion was necessary. Three studies mentioned mechanical problems such as a malfunctioning/interfering of the robotic arms, which necessitated repositioning of the robotic arms and exchange of instruments (Caratozzolo et al, 2005; Vidovszky et al, 2006) and in one case detachment of the robotic instrument resulted in a minilaparotomy (Ruurda et al, 2002).

	Robotic system	No. of patients	Surgeon (LN/LE)	Parameter	Learning curve	Conversion
Caratozzolo	Zeus	29	2LE	Set-up time Operative time	Yes Yes	2/29
Heemskerk	Da Vinci	N=12*	1LE	Set-up time Operative time	No No	0/12
Vidovsky	Da Vinci	N=51	NR	Set-up time Operative time	Yes, significant No	3/51
Ruurda	Da Vinci	N=35	3LE	Set-up time Operative time	Yes No	1/35
Chitwood	Da Vinci	N=20	LE	Set-up time Operative time Combined time	Yes, significant No Yes, significant	0/20
Perez	Da Vinci	N=20	3 LE	Operative time	Yes, significant	0/20
Giulianotti	Da Vinci	N=52**	NR	Operative time	Yes, significant	1/52

LN: laparoscopic naive, LE: laparoscopic experienced, NR not reported
* Vs. historical robotic series;** 14 procedures were combined procedures (with fundoplication, hepatic and gastric resection)

Table 2. Learning curve of robot-assisted laparoscopic cholecystectomy

6. Robot-assisted anti-reflux surgery

Four fundoplication studies showed the learning curve of experienced surgeons all performed with Da Vinci. Only one study compared the RLC with the MLC (Morino et al, 2006). The decrease in set-up time and operative time was used to compare the mean results of the first and second part of the series to assess the learning curve. The set-up time, reported in 2 studies (Chitwood et al, 2001; Wykypiel et al 2003), decreased but not significantly. The operative time decreased in 3 studies. One study reported equivalence in operating time when compared with conventional laparoscopic fundoplication already after 2 procedures (Wykypiel et al 2003). Another study reported that 20 robotic procedures were necessary to complete the learning phase (Guilianotti et al, 2003). Two conversions due to operative complications, not related to the robotic system were reported. No mechanical problems were described. Results are shown in table 3.

	Robotic system	No. of patients	Surgeon LE/LN	Parameter	Learning curve	Conversion
Giulianotti	Da Vinci	N=49	NR	Operative time	Yes, significant	2/49
Chitwood	Da Vinci	N=14	LE	Set-up time Operative time	Yes, NS Yes, significant	NR
Wykypiel	Da Vinci	N=10	LE	Set-up time Operative time	Yes, significance nr Yes, significance nr	0/10
Morino	Da Vinci	N=25	LE	Operative time	No, significance nr	0/10*

LN: laparoscopic naive, LE: laparoscopic experienced, NR not reported, NS not significant
*1 conversion to manual laparoscopy

Table 3. Learning curve robot-assisted laparoscopic fundoplication

7. Discussion

Few reports on the learning curve of robotic surgery are available. Studies to compare robotic with conventional laparoscopic learning curves were even scarcer. To measure the learning curve of robotic surgical performance a diversity of parameters was used throughout most studies. These parameters were not always well defined. Furthermore, a great variety of practice/time was used to define an early or late experience phase of the learning curve. An experience bias was expected in most clinical series, because of prior laparoscopic experience of the participating surgeons. All these issues limit an objective evaluation of the learning curve of robotic surgery. However, although robotic systems are supposed to be "intuitive" in use, this technique showed to have a learning curve. This was most clearly demonstrated for laparoscopically inexperienced persons.

A long learning curve might prevent implementation of a new technology, but the most important feature of a new technology, despite its learning curve, should be its advantage for the patient or the surgeon. Does it result in a reduction of morbidity or mortality? Does it facilitate and enhance laparoscopic surgical performance? These important questions remain unanswered with the current data. Furthermore, the financial cost-benefit should also be considered (Heemskerk et al, 2005).

A learning curve consists of an initial steep phase in which performance increases rapidly. When the change in improvement slows down, the learning curve reaches a plateau phase, in which variability in performance is small. The number of repetitions in most reported experimental series are to low to reach the consistency which characterizes the end of the learning curve. Only the first and steepest part is evaluated, in which the most improvement is expected. However, in 9/10 studies a learning curve was described, with the majority of participants being laparoscopically naïve. When compared to laparoscopic experienced participants the RLC of the laparoscopic naïve persons was steeper, due to inferior performance at the beginning. This suggests more impact of a robot on laparoscopic naïve persons, whereas a laparoscopic experienced person quickly adapts to the advantages of operating robotically (fulcrum effect) and benefits of his prior laparoscopic experience.

In the clinical series more "repetitions" are performed. As for the robot-assisted laparoscopic cholecystectomy, in 3/7 studies no learning curve was described for the robotic operative time, although a learning curve for the robotic set-up time was seen in all reported studies. All 4 comparative studies described equal operative times for robotic assisted cholecystectomy with conventional laparoscopic cholecystectomy after 20-50 procedures. All procedures were done by experienced laparoscopic surgeons. Proficiency for a conventional laparoscopic cholecystectomy is reached after 30 procedures (Dagash et al, 2002).

Only in one out of the four studies no learning curve was observed for robot-assisted fundoplication operative time. Set-up time showed a learning curve in all studies. One study, which compared RLC and MLC of fundoplication reported equal operative times after only two robotic procedures. Proficiency of a conventional laparoscopic fundoplication is said to be reached after 28 procedures. The variability in operating time remains high for this procedure even in the late phase of surgical experience (Dagash et al. 2003).

Most advantage of a robotic system is expected in advanced or complicated operative procedures. A laparoscopic cholecystectomy might be too simple, since it does not necessitate fine and complex movements. It might not be the appropriate procedure to evaluate the robotic learning curve. Although a laparoscopic fundoplication asks for more skill, most advantage of a robotic system is expected only during suturing of the wrap, which is a small part of the total procedure. Total operative time is not an accurate parameter to evaluate performance and learning curve.

An expected learning curve for the robotic set-up time was found, but not quantified in most studies. However, the clinical importance of a small increment in total operative time due to robotic set-up time is low, especially when operative times are long.

The use of robotic systems in laparoscopic surgery does not obviate the learning curve. Application of this technology has its own learning curve with respect to set-up of the system and getting accustomed to the specific features of the robotic systems. The limited data suggest that this learning curve is comparable with conventional laparoscopic surgery. Laparoscopically naive surgeons might benefit more from the advantages of a robotic system such as 3-D visualization and the absence of the fulcrum effect. This results in a steeper first phase of the robotic learning curve. However, experienced laparoscopic surgeons benefit from their prior laparoscopic experience shortening the robotic learning curve when compared to novice surgeons.

8. Referenties

Ballantyne GH: Robotic surgery, telerobotic surgery, telepresence and telementoring; review of early clinical results. *Surg Endosc* 2002 July;16:1389-1402

Blavier A, Gaudissart Q, Cadiere G et al: Comparison of learning curves and skill transfer between classical and robotic laparoscopy according to the viewing conditions: implications for training. *Am J Surg* 2007, July; 194: 115-121

Caratozzolo E, Recordare A, Massani M, et al: Telerobotic-assited laparoscopic cholecystectomy: our experience on 29 patients; *J Hepatobiliary Pancreatic Surg* 2005; 12:163-166

Chang L, Satava RM, Pellegrini CA et al: Robotic surgery: identifying the learning curve through objective measurement of skill. *Surg Endosc* 2003, November; 17: 1744-1748

Chitwood WR, Nifong LW, Chapman W.H., et al: Robotic surgical training in an academic institution. *Ann Surg* 2001, October; 234:475-484; discussion 484-486

Dagash H, Chowdhury M, Pierro A. When can I be proficient in laparoscopic surgery? A systematic review of the evidence. *J Pediatr Surg* 2003, May;38:720-724

Giulianotti PC, Coratti A, Angelini M, et al: Robotics in general surgery:personal experience in a large community hospital. *Arch Surg* 2003, July; 138:777-784

Heemskerk J, van Dam R, van Gemert WG, et al: First results after introduction of the four-armed da Vinci surgical system in fully robotic laparoscopic cholecystectomy. *Dig Surg* 2005, February; 22: 426-431

Heemskerk J, van Gemert WG, de Vries J et al: Learning curves of robot-assisted laparoscopic surgery compared with conventional laparoscopic surgery: An experimental study evaluating skill acquisition of robot-assisted laparoscopic tasks compared with conventional laparoscopic tasks in inexperienced users. *Surg Laparosc EndoscPercutan Tech* 2007, June; 17 : 171-174

Hernandez JD, Bann SD, Munz Y, et al: Qualitative and quantitative analysis of the learning curve of a simulated task on the da Vinci system. *Surg Endosc* 2004, March; 18: 372-378

Maniar HS, Council ML, Prasad SM et al: Comparison of skill training with robotic systems and traditional endoscopy: Implications on training and adoption. *J Surg Res* 2005, May; 125: 23-29

Morino M, Peegrino L, Giaccone C, et al: Randomized clinical trial of robot-assisted versus laparoscopic Nissen fundoplication. *Br J Surg* 2006,May; 93:553-558

Narazaki K, Oleynikov D, Stergiou, et al: Robotic surgery training and performance: Identifying objective variables for quantifying the extent of proficiency. *Surg Endosc* 2006, January; 20: 96-103

Nio D, Bemelman WA, Balm R, et al: Laparoscopic vascular anastomoses: Does robotic (Zeus-Aesop) assistance help to overcome the learning curve? *Surg Endosc* 2005, August; 19: 1071-1076

Perez A, Zinner MJ, Ashley SW, et al: What is the value of telerobotic technology in gastrointestinal surgery? *Surg Endosc* 2003,May; 17:811-813

Prasad SM, Maniar HS, Soper NJ et al: The effect of robotic assistance on learning curves for basic laparoscopic skills. *Am J Surg* 2002, June; 183: 702-707

Ro CY, Toumpoulis IK, Ashton RC, et al: A novel drill set for the enhancement and assessment of robotic surgical performance. *Stud Health Technol Inform* 2005; 111:418-21

Ruurda JP, Broeders IA, Simmermacher RP, et al: Feasibility of robot-assisted laparoscopic surgery: an evaluation of 35 robot assisted laparoscopic cholecystectomies. *Surg Laparosc Endosc Percutan Tech* 2002, February; 12:41-45

Sarle R, Tewari A, Shirvastava A et al: Surgical Robotics and laparoscopic training drills. *J Endourol* 2004; 18: 63-67

Vidovszky TJ, Smith W, Ghosh J, et al: Robotic cholecystectomy: learning curve, advantages, and limitations. *J Surg Res 2006,*December; 136, 172-178

Wykypiel H, Wetscher GJ, Klaus A, et al: Robotic-assisted laparoscopic partial posterior fundolplication with the Da Vinci system: initial experiences and technical aspects. *Langenbecks Arch Surg* 2003, February; 387:411-416

Yohannes P, Rotariu P, Pinto P, et al: Comparison of robotic versus laparoscopic skills: is there a difference in the learning curve? *Urology* 2002, July; 60: 39-45

2

The Must-Have in Robotic Heart Surgery: Haptic Feedback

Eva U. Braun[1], Hermann Mayer[1, 2], Alois Knoll[2], Ruediger Lange[1] and Robert Bauernschmitt[1]
Technische Universität München
[1]German Heart Center Munich, Clinic for Cardiovascular Surgery,
[2]Fakultät für Informatik, Robotics and Embedded Systems, Technische Universität München
Germany

1. Introduction

The minimally invasive endoscopic surgery was introduced in the late 1980s in the abdominal surgery as revolutionary surgical technique (Voges et al., 1997). Surgeons no longer needed to physically place their hands within the body to perform an operation. In minimal invasive surgery, instruments and viewing equipments are inserted into the body through small incisions. Long manipulators are used to perform operations under manual guidance. This does not only minimize the collateral surgical trauma of an access incision but results also in quicker recovery.

In heart surgery the introduction of endoscopic techniques were promising, but not satisfying like the application of robots in other surgical disciplines (Bholat et al., 1999; Gutt et al., 2004; Mitsuishi et al., 2000). Complex cardiac surgery had to be performed by long instruments without tremor filter or adequate freedom of movement, so satisfactory results were missing. In heart surgery pure endoscopic techniques have not established since the demanded high precision in this speciality did not reached with endoscopic instruments only.

The promise of telemanipulated endoscopic assistance was to eliminate many of the beginning impediments, with the concurrent enhancements of motion scaling, tremor filtration, 3-dimensional vision and fulcrum effect. The surgeon could now operate with a surgical mechatronic assist system in a comfortable, dextrous and intuitive manner.

The solution for the initial problems was the implementation of telemanipulators that offer with the endoscopic instruments as much degrees of freedom in movement as the hand of the surgeon in conventional open surgery performing 6 degrees of freedom instead of four in conventional endoscopic instruments. Furthermore the telemanipulator had to dispose of 3D-optic and a filter of tremor (Suematsu & Del Nido, 2004). The new system has been a telesystem controlled remotely by the surgeon.

The implementation of totally endoscopic heart surgery was realised ten years later with the telemanipulator Da Vinci® (Intuitive Surgical, Inc., Sunnyvale, CA, USA) after introducing endoscopic surgery in abdominal surgery.

Nevertheless technical limitations still exist that limit the application in special heart diseases and surgical indications in expert medical centres only.

This telemanipulated technology is available for a minimal part of heart surgical patients only since the technical inconvenience of the system and the clumsy system is considerably limited in valve surgery, congenital heart surgery and a bigger part of bypass surgery.
The necessity of haptic feedback is discussed controversially by robotically working surgeons and haptic engineers (Bethea et al., 2004; Fager, 2004; Hu et al., 2004). The postulate, that the integration of a supplementary haptic channel in addition to the visual channel improves the quality of surgical work and enhances the immersion for the surgeon in a remote system, is not yet demonstrated and evidenced.
For virtual and artificial scenarios tactile sense and haptic feedback is an essential part (Darggahi & Najarian, 2004; Van Beers et al., 1999), but in the research of surgical telepresence for remote real scenarios the necessity of haptic feedback is still discussed very intensely. Several microsurgical telerobot systems are implemented by research groups all over the world (Cavusoglu et al., 2003; Garcia-Ruiz et al., 1997; Kwon 1998), but important questions and problems arising while operating are not answered and solved sufficiently. The breaking of surgical suture material and the damage of tissue are basic and unsolved problems in telemanipulated surgery. A further hypothesis is not yet explored: The especially high fatigue of the surgeon while and after robotic operations is caused in visual compensation of the skills and movements (Thompson et al., 1999). The basic solution seems to be the implementation of force feedback.
In our study haptic feedback is built up in the experimental setup of a surgical telemanipulator system (fig. 1) as technical modification (Schirmbeck et al., 2004 a; Bauernschmitt et al., 2005 a; Mayer et al, 2005), the application on surgical skills is analysed and evaluated (Schirmbeck et al., 2005 ; Bauernschmitt et al., 2005 b; Freyberger et al., 2005; Mayer et al., 2005).

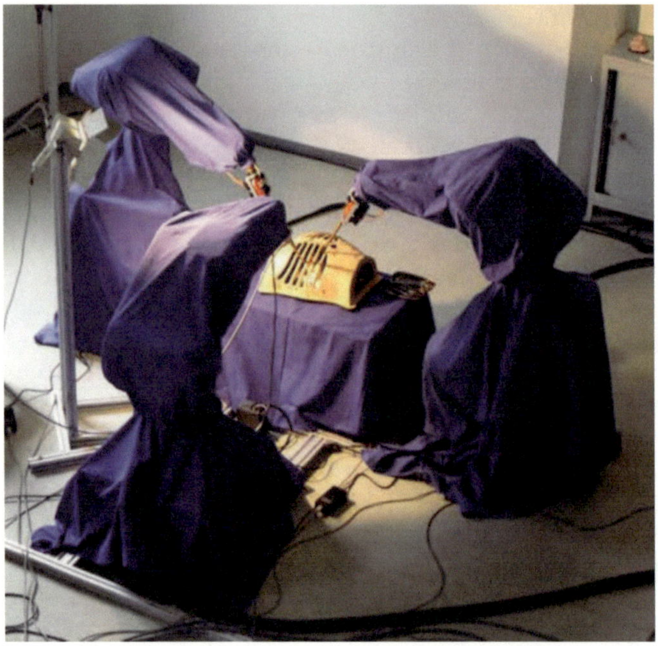

Figure 1. Surgical telemanipulator system: Two instruments and one 3-D camera

2. Methods

2.1 Robotic system for endoscopic heart surgery

We built up a telemanipulated surgical experimental platform with commercially available equivalent surgical instruments to present comparable conditions for the surgeons. The difference and advancement is our implementation of haptic feedback in the instruments and the new robotic system.

The setup comprises like typical systems for robotic surgery an operator-side master console for in-output and a patient-side robotic manipulator that directly interacts with the operating environment.

A bi-manual telemanipulator is built up not only capable performing delicate operations, but also capable of applying real-time image processing tools like coronary artery detection (Nagy et al., 2004), navigation features (Mayer et al., 2004) and autonomous procedures (Schirmbeck et al., 2004 b).

Telemanipulator system

The robotic system consists of two surgical manipulators, which are controlled by two PHANTOM® 1.5 input devices (SensAble Technologies, Inc., Woburn, MA, USA), and a third robot, which carries a stereoscopic camera (Richard Wolf GmbH, Knittlingen, Germany). Each manipulator is composed of a KUKA KR 6/2 robot (KUKA Roboter GmbH, Augsburg, Germany), that bears a surgical instrument of Intuitive Surgical®. The KUKA robot disposes of six degrees of freedom. The surgical instruments provide three degrees of freedom. Therefore each robotic arm has eight degrees of freedom which enables free surgical manipulation via trocar kinematics. A micro-gripper at the distal end of the shaft can be rotated and the adaptation of pitch and yaw angles is possible.

We developed an adapter to link the robotic arm with the instrument. For security reasons all flange adapters are equipped with magnetic security couplings. Those disengaged exercising forces exceed a certain level and might cause harm on instruments or tissue. All movable parts of the gripper are driven by steel wires. Their motion is controlled by four driving wheels at the proximal end of the instrument, one four each degree of freedom (two for yaw of the fingers). In order to control the instrument, we have flanged servos to each driving wheel by means of an Oldham coupling. This guarantees instrument movement free of jerk. The servo controllers are connected via serial lines to a multiport card. This redundancy renders the end effector possible to reach every position and orientation within the working space under restriction of trocar kinematics for surgical use.

Haptic instruments and haptic interface

We modified the instruments of the Da Vinci® telemanipulator system for measuring forces while executing surgical tasks (Bowersox et al., 1998). Since the shaft of the surgical instruments is made of carbon fibre, force sensors have to be very sensitive and reliable. Therefore strain gauge sensors are applied, which are employed for industrial force registration. The sensor gauges are applied at the distal end of the instrument's shaft near the gripper in order to display realistic forces during operation.

The strain gauge force sensors measure forces along two translational directions of the instrument's shaft. One full bridge of sensors is used for each direction. Forces are displayed to the user by means of two PHANTOM®, which act at the same time as input devices. The signals of the sensors are amplified and transmitted via CAN-bus to a PC system. Since reading of direct sensor is associated with noise a smoothing filter is applied in order to

stabilize the results. Position and orientation of the manipulators are controlled by the two PHANTOM® input devices.
The working space of approximately 20x25x40 cm provides enough space to perform surgical procedures. The user controls a stylus pen equipped with a switch that can be used to open and close the micro-grippers. The basic idea of minimally invasive surgery is that only small incisions have to be made into the surface of the patient's body. The translational movements of the instruments are essentially restricted by shifts and rotations about these fulcrums (trocar kinematics).
The most interesting feature of the employed PHANTOM® devices is their capability of displaying forces to the user. Forces are fed back by small servomotors incorporated in the device. They are used to steer the stylus pen in a certain direction. This creates the impression of occurring forces, while the user is holding the pen at a certain posture.

Optical system: 3D-endoscope and head mounted display

To enable proper telemanipulation a 3D-display (Falk et al., 2001) is indispensable providing a distinct vision of the region of interest. An additional robot is equipped with the stereo endoscopic camera.
This camera can also be moved by means of trocar kinematics as the instruments and can be actively controlled either by the operator or automatically track the instruments. Images taken from the stereo camera system can be displayed via three options, while time delay and least asynchrony in video have to be avoided (Thompson et al., 1999). One is a head mounted display (HMD) that is part of the input console. The second possibility is to alternately display left and right images on a Cathode Ray Tube- (CRT-) screen. In this case, the operator has to wear shutter glasses, which are triggered by the output on the screen. A third option is the projection of online-acquired polarized operation sequences on a silver screen with two video projectors. The projectors are equipped with polarising filters that are orthogonally arranged. Observers have to wear glasses with an appropriate polarisation for the corresponding eye.

2.2 Evaluation of force feedback

Human participants

The human subjects of this study included 25 surgeons divided in three groups within the Clinic for Cardiovascular Surgery in the German Heart Center Munich in different levels of surgical training and age (table 1).

	all participants n=25	**young surgeons** n=8	**experienced surgeons** n=12	**robotic surgeons** n=5
Surgical experience (years) mean value (sd)	6.1 (±7.4)	0.4 (±0.3)	11.5 (±7.6)	2.4 (±2.0)
Age (years) mean value (sd)	36 (±8)	29 (±7)	39 (±8)	39 (±5)

Table 1. Random sample of the human subjects for the evaluation of haptic feedback

One group of robotically working surgeons and two groups of surgeons without experience in robotic surgery (one group with conventionally experienced surgeons and one with young surgeons) were evaluated.

Every surgeon executed three surgical tasks three times under three different haptic levels (no haptic feedback, 1:1 real haptic feedback and 1:2 doubled force feedback). The order of the haptic conditions (type of task and haptic condition) were completely balanced to avoid learning effect and were double blinded.

Training skills

Before executing the main surgical tasks of the evaluation, the trainees got 15 minutes to get familiar with handling the robotic system.

First, soft coloured pellets had to be transferred from one cup and in a second next right to the first one. Second, a rubber band had to be threaded through five eyelets. In addition the surgeons got time to tie several knots to be prepared for the main tasks of the evaluation.

The surgical tasks

The study intended basic surgical and cardiac surgical procedures. Knot tying, breaking suture material and detection of arteriosclerosis had to be performed in a defined cycle with double blinding. These tasks imply at least basic knowledge in surgical principles. The participants dealt with three different levels of haptic feedback: no haptic, actually fed back forces and enhanced force feedback. During the entire experiment, the arising forces were recorded.

Breaking of suture material:

The breaking of suture material represents the amount of telepresence and immersion of the robotic system for the surgeons. The surgeons had to tension the thread until the supposed breaking point and had to mention this point before breaking. The difference of force between the supposed and the real breaking of a surgical thread was measured in Newton. The used surgical suture material Prolene® 6-0 (ETHICON Inc., Somerville, NJ, USA) is a common and frequently used non-absorbable thread made from Polypropylene in heart surgery.

Knot tying:

The human subjects had to tie surgical knots with two surgical instruments equipped with haptic feedback. The surgeons had ten minutes to perform precisely as much knots in alternate way (left and right taught knots) as possible. The total number of knots, the applied forces and the breakage of suture material while knot tying were recorded. The speed and course of motion and the coordination of the graspers were analysed.

In addition the trauma of the surrounding tissue has been rated while knot tying. Following parameters have been analysed: number of dents, holes, fissures and breaks of tissue. Furthermore, the number of outbreaks of knots and insufficient knots were counted.

The finished objects with the knotted tissue were analysed in completion to the rated variables of the video recording.

Detection of arteriosclerosis:

The surgeons had to detect possible stenosis with one haptic instrument in realistic arteries made from polymer precisely and at the same time rapidly.

The errors in detecting short, long or no stenosis in three arteries were counted. The applied forces while detecting were recorded in Newton and the time of detecting in seconds.

The critical flicker fusion frequency CFF

The critical flicker fusion frequency (CFF) is an individual part of the Wiener Testsystem (Schuhfried GmbH, Mödling, Austria) analysing the progression of fatigue during the evaluation (Wiemeyer, 2002). The CFF is regarded as an indicator for the central-nervous

function capacity, the activation level and the progression of fatigue during practical tasks (Johansson & Sandström, 2003).
The flicker fusion frequency has been identified between three blocks of tasks with the three different degrees of haptic levels (no haptic, 1:1 haptic and 1:2 haptic feedback).

3. Results

3.1 Surgical knot tying

Force feedback influences the application of forces significantly ($p<0,05$) in surgical knot tying. In increasing the force feedback the applied forces are reduced significantly ($p\leq 0,05$). The experience of the surgeons does not influence the amount of applied forces ($p>0,05$). Haptic feedback does not show any influence on the quality of surgical knot tying ($p=0,05$).

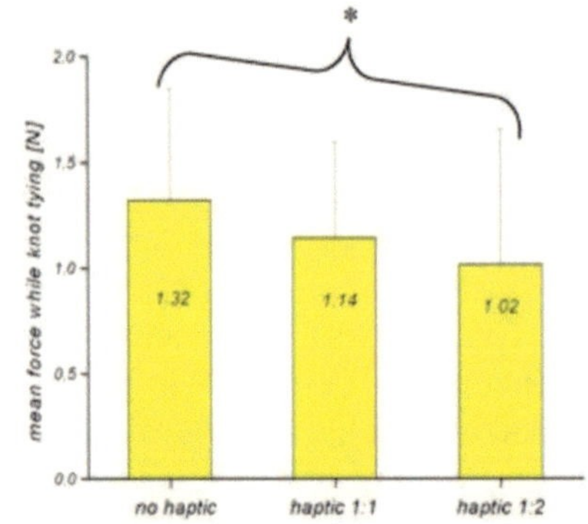

Figure 2. Forces while knot tying. With increasing haptic feedback the applied forces decrease significantly, *$p<0.05$

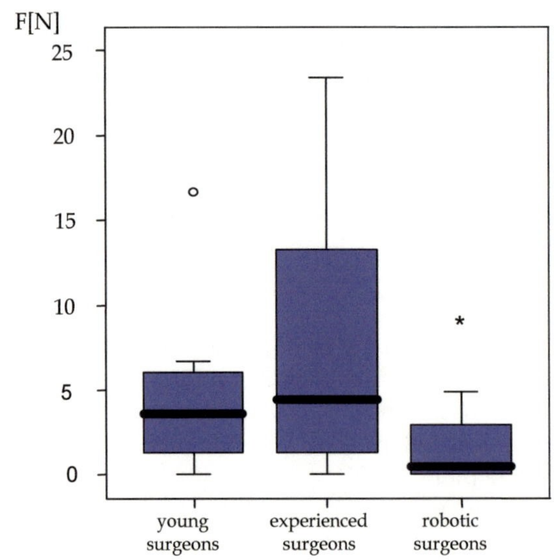

Figure 3. Robotic surgeons apply significantly less forces while knot tying with doubled force feedback, *$p< 0,05$

3.2 Breaking of suture material

The difference of forces was calculated where the thread was breaking supposed by the surgeon and the force where the thread was actually breaking. Haptic feedback showed a significant effect of the force difference ($p<0,05$). In increasing the haptic feedback the difference decreased ($p<0,05$), which signifies the precision of the estimated force when the thread was breaking and the high grade of telepresence of the telemanipulator system.

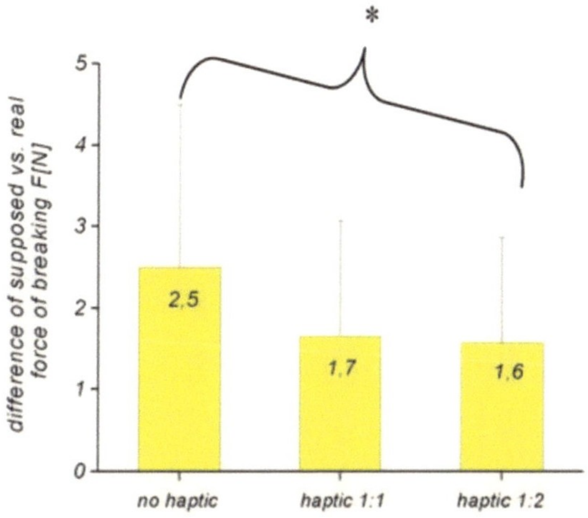

Figure 4. The difference of the supposed and the real force while breaking a surgical suture decreases significantly with haptic feedback, *$p<0.05$

3.3 Detection of stenosis

Haptic feedback influences significantly the amount of applied forces while detecting arteriosclerosis ($p<0,05$). In increasing the force feedback the applied forces decrease significantly ($p<0,05$). This effect is independent of the surgical experience ($p>0,05$).

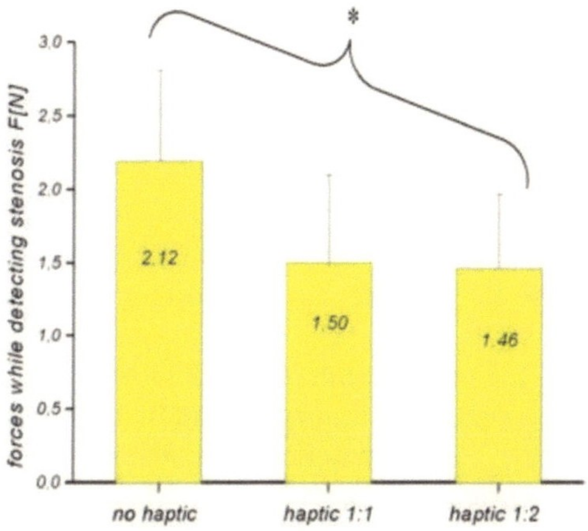

Figure 5. The applied forces decrease significantly (*$p<0.05$) with the increase of haptic feedback

3.4 Fatigue of the surgeons

The visual fatigue decreases significantly while operating with haptic feedback for young and conventionally experienced surgeons. Haptic feedback decreases the visual stress and fatigue ($p<0,05$).

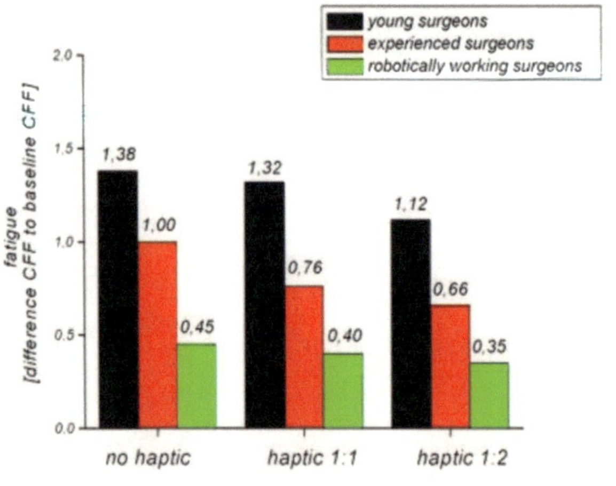

Figure 6. The critical flicker fusion frequency CFF: the visual fatigue decreases with increasing haptic feedback in young, experienced and robotic surgeons

4. Conclusion

Robots have a number of advantages over humans in performing routine manipulation tasks. Their accuracy and repeatability allow robots to succeed in the medical and surgical market. Some of the weaknesses in current robotic devices, such as substantial lack of haptic feedback and adaptability are to be highlighted. Currently it is not possible to "program" a robot to perform steps of a surgical operation autonomously. Nevertheless, some of these limitations do not prevent robots from being useful in the operating room; rather considerable human, technical and surgical input, guidance and advancement are needed. Surgical robots can be viewed as "extending and enhancing human capabilities" rather than replacing surgeons, in contrast to the example of industrial replacement of humans by robots.
Intuitive Surgical® intended to create with the Da Vinci® Surgical System a conception of a surgeon-robot interface so transparent to the surgeon that his set of skills can be used in a natural and instinctive manner. Its accurate visualisation is critical since visual cues are used to compensate for the loss of haptic feedback.
The haptic feedback is currently limited to interact with rigid structures, such as tool-on-tool collisions, not soft tissues. This requires the surgeon to rely on visual feedback in tasks such as suturing. Especially for fine suture material approaches began in research groups to analyse haptic feedback (Okamura, 2004; Kitagawa et al., 2005), but the way of the evaluating setup is not fulfilling the special medical interest for heart surgeons. The basic consideration in our work is to offer the heart surgeon an accessory sensory channel in addition to the visual channel not only to avoid breakage of surgical suture material and tissue, but also to decrease visual fatigue.

New applications of the technology are beginning to emerge as creative surgeons do their work (Marohn & Hanly, 2004; Maurin et al., 2004). Nevertheless, present-day robotic surgical systems have limitations that have slowed the widespread introduction and the continuation. One major problem is the lack of haptic (Czibik et al, 2002; Awad et al., 2002). A second major concern is the cumbersome and not versatile nature of the robotic system. It is quite easy to envision integrated imaging, navigation and enhanced sensory capabilities being available in the next generation of telesurgical systems (Howe & Matsuoka, 1999; Kennedy et al., 2002).
The goal of our experiments was to examine claims about necessity of force feedback for robot-assisted surgical procedures in cardiac surgery. We present a novel approach of a robotic system for minimally invasive and endoscopic surgery. The main purposes of the system are evaluation of force feedback and machine learning. The performance of certain surgical tasks like knot tying will profit from this feature. Experiments have shown that haptic feedback can be employed to prevent the surgeon from potentially harmful mistakes. Tension of thread material and tissue parts can be measured and displayed in order to restrict force application to tolerable amplitude. In addition, the collision of instruments can be detected and intercepted by the evaluation of real-time forces. Using multi-dimensional haptic styluses, forces are measured at the surgical instruments and fed back into the surgeon's hands.
In our experimental setup, the feel for different and morbidly changed tissues cannot be analysed sufficiently. The setup of the robots does not allow to suture for example anastomosis of arteries. Leak-proof stitches could be an excellent parameter for surgical quality. In addition, the amelioration of our visual display terminal is necessary.
The next generation of surgical experimental telemanipulator with haptic feedback, semi-autonomous capability and navigation tool is arising.
Future plans are the evaluation of real tissue to test the variable surgical quality with haptic feedback and the implementation of the results in this advanced surgical robotic system for the adoption in the operating room.
For the future clinical use the perfection is planned by improving the set-up of the instruments and by incorporating these results of the evaluation into the control software. A simulation environment is designed for modelling haptic interaction with a tissue model. This can be applied for offline evaluation of critical tasks. In our experimental set-up, we are able to demonstrate that the surgical procedure in robotic heart surgery is safer, quicker and gentler for the patient and more comfortable for the surgeon using force feedback.
Consequently, we require haptic feedback for surgical robotics to increase the safety of patients, to increase the ease of handling for the surgeon in a complex surgical environment, to relieve the surgeon's fatigue and to increase the number of indications for surgery and the variety of robotic applications for surgery.
Future surgical systems with integrated haptic feedback could be used to train young surgeons for exercising and teaching critical and difficult steps of surgical operations by the system as simulator.

5. References

Awad, H.; Wolf, R.K. & Gravlee, G.P. (2002). The future of robotic and cardiac surgery. *J Cardiothor Vasc An*, 2002;16(4):395-6

Bauernschmitt, R.; Schirmbeck, E.U.; Mayer, H.; Nagy, I.; Knoll, A.; Wessel, N.; Wildhirt, S.M. & Lange, R. (2005 a). Telemanipulator enhanced heart surgery: implementation of autonomous procedures, *Biomed Tech,* 2005, 50,*1(2):1260-1*

Bauernschmitt, R.; Schirmbeck, E.U.; Knoll, A.; Mayer, H.; Nagy, I.; Wessel, N.; Wildhirt, S.M. & Lange, R. (2005 b). Towards robotic heart surgery: Introduction of autonomous procedures into an experimental surgical telemanipulator system. *Int J Med Robot Comput Assisted Surg,* 2005,1(3):74-9

Bethea, B.T.; Okamura, A.M.; Kitagawa, M.; Fitton, T.P.; Cattaneo, S.M.; Gott, V.L.; Baumgartner, W.A. & Yuh, D.D (2004). Application of haptic feedback to robotic surgery. *J Laparoendosc Adv Surg Tech,* 2004;14(3):191-5

Bholat, O.S.; Haluck, R.S., Murray, W.B.; Gorman, P.J. & Krummel T.M.(1999). Tactile feedback is present during minimally invasive surgery. *J Am Coll Surgeons,* 1999;189(4):349-55

Bowersox, J.C.; Cordts, P.R. & LaPorta, A.J. (1998). Use of an intuitive telemanipulator system for remote trauma surgery: an experimental study. *J Am Coll Surg,* 1998;186:615–21

Cavusoglu, M.C.; Williams, W.; Tendick, F. & Sastry, S.S. (2003). Robotics for telesurgery: Second generation Berkeley/UCSF laparoscopic telesurgical workstation and looking towards the future applications. *Industrial Robot,* Special Issues on Medical Robotics, 2003;30(1):22-29

Czibik, G.; D´Ancona, G.; Donias, H.W. & Karamanoukian, H.L. (2002). Robotic cardiac surgery: Present and future applications. *J Cardiothor Vasc An,* 2002;16(4):495-501

Darggahi, J. & Najarian, S. (2004). Human tactile perception as a standard for artificial tactile sensing - a review. *Int J Med Robot Comput Assisted Surg,* 2004;1(1):23-35

Fager, P.J. (2004). The use of haptics in medical applications. *Int J Med Robot Comput Assisted Surg,* 2004;1(1):36-42

Falk, V.; Mintz, D.; Grunenfelder, J.; Fann, J.I. & Burdon, T.A. (2001). Influence of three-dimensional vision on surgical telemanipulator performance. *Surg Endosc,* 2001;15(11):1282-8

Freyberger, F.K.B.; Popp, M.M.; Färber, B.; Mayer, H. & Schirmbeck, E.U. (2005). Experimentelle Evaluation haptischer Rückmeldung eines robotergestützten Systems für minimal-invasive Herzchirurgie. Zustandserkennung und Systemgestaltung, *Fortschritt-Berichte VDI,* 2005, Vol. 19, ISBN 3-18-302222-2

Garcia-Ruiz, A.; Smedira, N.G.; Loop, F.D.; Hahn, J.F.; Miller, J.H.; Steiner, C.P. & Gagner, M. (1997). Robotic surgical instruments for dexterity enhancement in thoracoscopic coronary artery bypass graft. *J Laparoendosc Adv Surg Tech A,* 1997;7(5):277-83

Gutt, C.N.; Oniu, T.; Mehrabi, A.; Kashfi, A.; Schemmer, P. & Büchler, M.W. (2004). Robot-assisted abdominal surgery. *Brit J Surg,* 2004;91(11):1390-7

Howe, R.D. & Matsuoka, Y. (1999). Robotics for surgery. *Annual Review of Biomedical Engineering,* 1999;1:211-40

Hu, T.; Tholey, G.; Desai, J.P. & Castellanos, A.E. (2002). Evaluation of a laparoscopic grasper with force feedback. *Surg Endosc,*2002;18(5):863-7

Johansson, A. & Sandström, M. (2003). Sensitivity of the human visual system to amplitude modulated light. *Arbetslivsrapport* Nr. 2003:4. Arbetslivsinstitutet, National Institute for Working Life 2003. Umeå, Sweden

Kennedy, C.W.; Hu, T.; Desai, J.P.; Wechsler, A.S. & Kresh,. JY. (2002). A novel approach to robotic cardiac surgery using haptics and vision. *Cardiovascular Engineering,* 2002;2(1):15-22

Kitagawa, M.; Dokko, D.; Okamura, A.M. & Yuh, D.D. (2005). Effect of sensory substitution on suture-manipulation forces for robotic surgical systems. *J Thorac Cardiovasc Surg,* 2005;129(1):151-8

Kwon, D.-S.; Woo, K.Y.; Song, S.K.; Kim, W.S. & Cho, H.S. (1998). Microsurgical Telerobot System. *IEEE/RSJ International Conference on Intelligent Robots and Systems,* 1998;945-50

Marohn, C.M.R. & Hanly, C.E.J. (2004). Twenty-first century surgery using twenty-first century technology: surgical robotics. *Current Surgery,* 2004;61(5):466-73

Maurin, B.; Piccin, O.; Bayle, B.; Gangloff, J.; De Mathelin, M.; Soler, L. & Gangi, A. (2004). A New Robotic system for CT-guided percutaneous procedures with haptic feedback. *International Congress Series,* 2004;1268:515-20

Mayer, H.; Nagy, I.; Knoll, A.; Schirmbeck, E.U. & Bauernschmitt, R. (2004). Robotic system to evaluate force feedback in minimally invasive computer aided surgery. *ASME e-Proceedings of the International Design Engineering Technical Conferences & Computers and Information in Engineering Conference DETC/CIE,* 2004

Mayer, H.; Nagy, I.; Knoll, A.; Schirmbeck, E.U. & Bauernschmitt R. (2005). An experimental system for robotic heart surgery. *Proceedings of the 18th IEEE Symposium on Computer-Based Medical Systems CBMS, 2005*

Mitsuishi, M.; Tomisak, S.; Yoshidome, T.; Hashizume, H. & Fujiwara, K. (2000). Tele-micro surgery system with intelligent user interface. *IEEE International Conference on Robotics and Automation ICRA,* 2000;2:1607-14

Nagy, I.; Mayer, H.; Knoll, A.; Schirmbeck, E.U. & Bauernschmitt R. (2004). Real-time matching of angiographies with in situ heart image sequences. *IEEE Proceedings of the 17th IEEE Symposium on Computer-Based Medical Systems CBMS,* 2004;516-22

Okamura, A.M. (2004). Methods for haptic feedback in teleoperated robot-assisted surgery. *Industrial Robot: An International Journal,* 2004;31(6):499-508

Schirmbeck, E.U.; Nagy, I.; Mayer, H.; Knoll, A.; Lange, R. & Bauernschmitt, R. (2004 a). Automatic coronary artery detection on in situ heart images. *IEEE Proceedings of the 31st Annual Meeting of Computers in Cardiology CinC,* 2004, 85-788, ISBN 0-7803-8927-1, Chicago/IL, IEEE, Piscataway/NJ

Schirmbeck, E.U.; Nagy, I.; Mayer, H.; Knoll, A.; Lange, R. & Bauernschmitt, R. (2004 b). Evaluation of force feedback in minimally invasive robotic surgery. *Biomed Tech,* 2004;49,2:108-9

Schirmbeck, E.U.; Haßelbeck, C.; Mayer, H.; Nagy, I.; Knoll, A.; Freyberger, F.K.B.; Popp, M.M.; Lange. R. & Bauernschmitt, R. (2005). Evaluation of haptic in robotic heart surgery. *Proceedings of the 19th International Congress and Exhibition Computer Assisted Radiology and Surgery CARS,* 2005. International Congress Series, Elsevier. 730-734

Suematsu, Y. & Del Nido, P.J. (2004). Robotic pediatric cardiac surgery: Present and future perspectives. *Am J Surg,* 2004;188(4A):98S-103S

Thompson, J.; Ottensmeier, M. & Sheridan, T. (1999). Human factors in telesurgery: effects of time delay and asynchrony in video and control feedback with local manipulative assistance. *Telemed Journal,* 1999;5(2):129-37

Van Beers, R.J.; Sittig, A.C. & Van der Gon, J.J.D. (1999). Integration of proprioceptive and visual position-information: an experimentally supported model. *The American Physiological Society,* 1999;1355-64

Voges, U.; Holler, E.; Neisius, B.; Schurr, M. & Vollmer, T. (1997). Evaluation of ARTEMIS, the Advanced Robotics and Telemanipulator System for Minimally Invasive Surgery. *Proceedings International Advanced Robotics Programme IARP,* 1997;137-48

Wiemeyer, J. (2002). Flimmerverschmelzungsfrequenz und zentralnervöse Aktivierung. *Neurol Rehabil,* 2002;8(1):29-34

3

Robot-Assisted Epicardial Ultrasound for Coronary Artery Localization and Anastomosis Quality Assessment in Totally Endoscopic Coronary Bypass Surgery

Ricardo P.J. Budde, Cornelius Borst, Patricia F.A. Bakker and Paul F. Gründeman
Heart Lung Center Utrecht, University Medical Center Utrecht
The Netherlands

1. Introduction

Coronary artery bypass grafting (CABG) is a routine procedure, traditionally performed via median sternotomy access on the arrested heart with use of cardiopulmonary bypass (on-pump). It is the clinical gold standard for myocardial revascularization in patients with multivessel coronary heart disease but remains associated with significant morbidity and mortality (Borst & Gründeman, 1999).

Over the last 2 decades, minimally invasive approaches to CABG in the form of smaller incisions (Diegeler et al., 2002) and elimination of the heart lung machine (off-pump) (Borst et al., 1996) have been introduced to reduce surgical trauma and adverse effects of cardiopulmonary bypass, respectively. The introduction of robotic systems with 3D vision, tremor elimination and instruments with 7 degrees of freedom (mimicking the human wrist) has provided an important part of the technology that enables the ultimate form of minimally invasive CABG, namely off-pump totally endoscopic CABG (TECAB) (Loulmet et al., 1999; Falk et al., 2000a; Argenziano et al., 2006). TECAB (both on-pump and off-pump) remains a technically highly demanding procedure that is performed by only a selected number of surgeons worldwide. Major obstacles in TECAB include: creation of adequate working space, identification of the target vessel, exposure and stabilization of the coronary segment, anastomosis suturing and the evaluation of anatomosis quality.

High frequency (7.5 - 15 MHz) epicardial ultrasound (ECUS) is a non-invasive means to both locate and evaluate coronary arteries and assess the quality of the coronary anastomosis in open chest CABG (Suematsu et al., 2001; Haaverstad et al., 2002). In 2002, a 13 MHz epicardial ultrasound mini-transducer has become available that is small enough to pass a trocar and be handled by surgical robot systems (Budde et al., 2004a).

In this chapter we will summarize our previously published results of the endoscopic application of this ECUS mini-transducer to locate and assess target coronary arteries for bypass grafting as well as its use for quality assessment of the coronary anastomosis in a porcine model of robot-assisted closed-chest off-pump CABG (Budde et al., 2004a; Budde et al., 2004b; Gründeman et al., 2003).

2. Da Vinci robot system

The robot system has been described in detail before (Loulmet et al., 1999). In brief, the surgeon sits at the surgeon console where a three-dimensional image from the endoscope is projected. By manipulating instrument controllers, the surgeon controls the actions of the surgical end-effectors in the patient that reproduce the motion of the surgeon's hands. The endoscope position is also controlled using the instrument controllers. The end-effectors of the endoscopic instruments have 7 degrees of freedom that mimick the human wrist, "endowrist". The endoscopic camera and instruments are attached to the patient console that is positioned at the operating table.

3. TECAB

The first TECAB procedure was described by Loulmet et al. in 1999 (Loulmet et al., 1999). Since then several groups have explored and refined this approach (Falk et al., 2000a; Kappert et al., 2001; Subramanian et al., 2005) and the results of a multicenter trial have been published (Argenziano et al., 2006). The current experience demonstrates that the procedure is feasible, remains mainly limited to single and double vessel disease, is associated with technical difficulties in up to 50% of cases (Bonatti et al., 2006) and requires long operative times (approximately 6 hours for a single vessel case) (Argenziano et al., 2006).

4. Ultrasound equipment

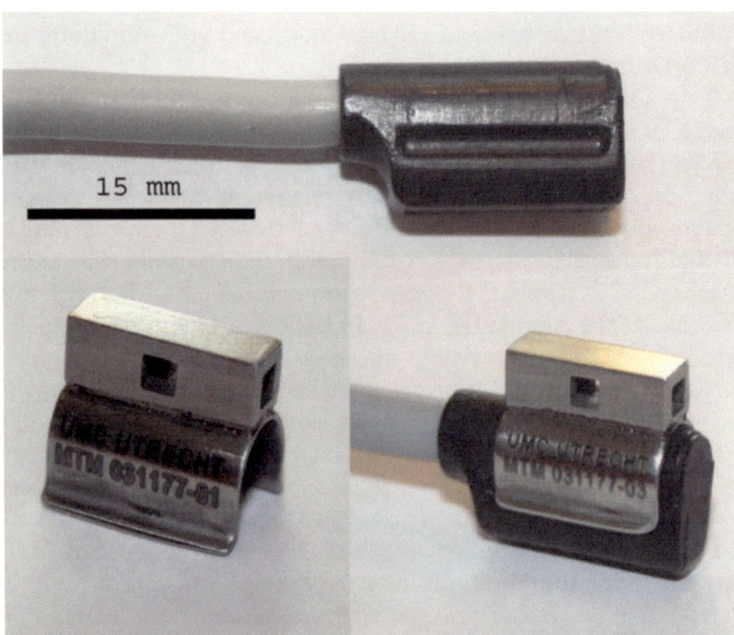

Figure 1. Thirteen MHz epicardial ultrasound mini-transducer (upper panel), custom made snap-on metal clip (left lower panel) and clip attached to mini-transducer (right lower panel). The clip is designed specifically for easy handling of the mini-transducer by the end-effectors of the robot instruments

A linear array ultrasound mini-transducer (Aloka, Tokyo, Japan) with an imaging frequency of up to 13 MHz has become available in 2002. It measures 15 mm in length, 6 mm in width and 9 mm in height, has an image scanwidth of 10 mm, an image depth of approximately 4 cm and offers both B-Mode and color-Doppler imaging (Figure 1). We used it in combination with an SSD 5000 Prosound ultrasound system (Aloka, Tokyo, Japan) for imaging. A custom made snap-on metal probe holder was developed by us to enable the end-effectors of the robot instruments to easily manipulate the mini-transducer inside the chest (Budde et al., 2004a).
The transducer is placed in a gel-filled protective cover which acts as a stand-off sleeve to facilitate scanning and improve image quality by limiting near-field artefacts. Furthermore, the sleeve acts as a sterile and current isolating barrier.
The ultrasound image is displayed picture-in-picture on the master console of the robot system. This provides the surgeon with the endoscopic and real-time ultrasound image simultaneously (Figure 2).

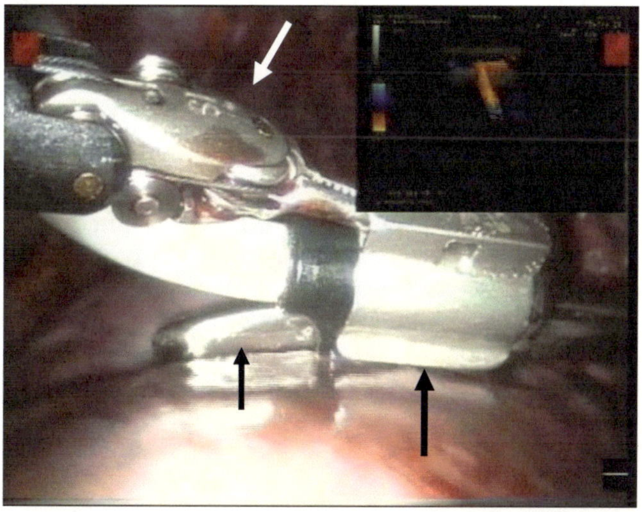

Figure 2. Surgeon's view on the master console of the robot system during scanning of the left anterior descending coronary artery in the porcine OPCAB model. The ultrasound mini-transducer (large black arrow) is positioned using the end effector of the robotic instrument (white arrow). The EndoOctopus suctionpod (small black arrow) is positioned on the epicardium behind the ultrasound transducer. The real-time ultrasound image is displayed as a picture-in-picture in the right upper hand corner which allows direct integration of the location of the probe and the visualized structures

5. Porcine off-pump TECAB model

We developed a porcine model of off-pump TECAB surgery (Gründeman et al., 2003). Pigs of 50-100 kg were anaesthetized and ports (5 or 6) for the instruments, camera and mini-transducer were placed on the left and right side of the thorax. Adaptations to the Octopus cardiac stabilizer (Borst et al. 1996; Gründeman et al. 2003) and Starfish cardiac positioner (Gründeman et al., 2003; Gründeman et al., 2004). were made for endoscopic use. To create additional working space inside the thorax, the sternum was lifted ventrally using a custom made sternum lift. In this model, by manipulation of the heart with the Endo-Starfish, access to all common target sites for CABG surgery can be obtained.

6. Coronary artery localization and assessment

In open chest CABG, the revascularization sites determined preoperatively on the angiogram are located intra-operatively by visual inspection and palpation. A thick layer of epicardial fibro-fatty tissue and/or an intramyocardial vessel course will render visual localization difficult.

In TECAB, in addition to the above mentioned difficulties, the limited overview, tangential angle of view and shift or lack of anatomical landmarks make the recognition of the anatomy by visual inspection even more difficult. Furthermore, the robot system lacks force feed back which prevents palpatory assessment of the target coronary artery. Failure to locate the left anterior descending artery (LAD) endoscopically resulted in intra-operative conversion to an open-chest procedure in up to 9% of patients undergoing TECAB (Kappert et al., 2001). In some cases, the diagonal branch of LAD or a coronary vein was mistakenly grafted instead of the LAD itself (Schachner et al., 2007).

7. Endoscopic vessel localization with ECUS

In the porcine TECAB model (n=8), we employed the ECUS mini-transducer to locate the common target arteries for bypass grafting (Budde et al., 2004a) The mini-transducer was introduced through a 15-mm port and was first manipulated over the anterior side of the heart in order to locate the LAD. Subsequently, the heart was lifted ventrally by the Endo-Starfish and the mini-transducer was manipulated over the posterior side of the heart to locate the third obtuse marginal (OM3) branch and the right posterior descending (RDP) coronary artery. The scanning procedure was performed both on the freely beating and partially stabilized heart. After localization of the vessel by ECUS, it was marked with a clip. Subsequently, the animal was terminated and the heart taken out to perform selective angiography of the left and right coronary arteries in order to determine the accuracy of ECUS localization.

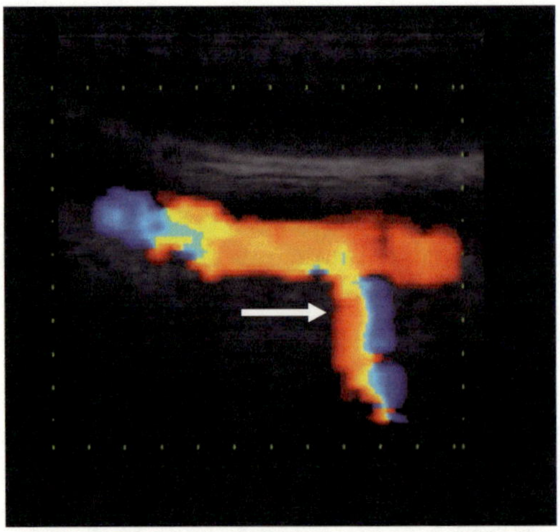

Figure 3. Longitudinal color-Doppler ultrasound image of the LAD with a septal perforator branch (arrow) scanned endoscopically

Localization required a median of 20 seconds (range: 12-25 seconds) for the LAD and 28 seconds (range 12-70 seconds) for the RDP on the freely beating heart. A subsequent scout scan in the up and downstream direction to evaluate the artery required 70 seconds (60-96 seconds) for the LAD and 51 seconds (18-104 seconds) for the RDP. After partial stabilization, the OM3 was located within 16 seconds (5-60 seconds) and assessed in 52 seconds (21-90 seconds). Side branches were easily seen (Figure 3). Overall, 23 out of 24 arteries were successfully located. One OM3 branch turned out to be a diagonal branch. The coronary anatomy, however, in this particular pig was somewhat unusual (diagonals extending prominently to the left lateral side of the heart).

Falk (Falk et al., 2000b) demonstrated feasibility of vessel assessment as well using a different ultrasound system in a canine TECAB model.

8. Anastomosis quality assessment

Even with a robot, endoscopic anastomotic suturing is difficult and technically challenging due to one or more of the following factors: motion of the target area, blood obscuring the arteriotomy edge, suboptimal angle of view, absence of force feedback on the telemanipulation systems and lack of an assistant to present the graft. The number of suture errors is reflected by the high number of intra-operative anastomotic failures in TECAB (11%, on the arrested heart) (Schachner et al., 2007). Intra-operative anastomosis quality assessment allows for direct graft revision in case of suboptimal results.

A number of techniques for anastomosis quality assessment have been described in open-chest CABG (Balacumaraswami & Taggert, 2007), but most can not be used in an endoscopic approach due to the large size of the imaging camera or potential risk for graft damage. Angiography is used but is invasive and the equipment is not available in most operating rooms. Furthermore, imaging time may be excessive (up to 110 minutes) (Schachner et al., 2007). and the intra-operative findings may be difficult to interpret (Hol et al., 2002).

ECUS is a promising technique for anastomotic quality assessment in open chest CABG and the advent of a mini-transducer has opened the possibility for its endoscopic use as well.

9. Endoscopic anastomosis quality assessment with ECUS

To evaluate the ability of the ECUS mini-transducer to assess anastomotic quality in TECAB, we constructed a total of 16 internal mammary artery (IMA) to LAD anastomoses in the porcine TECAB model. Eight of the anastomoses were constructed to be fully patent and the other 8 with an intended construction error (suture cross-over, in which the suture is interlocked in the middle of the anastomotic orifice). After endoscopic stabilization, the anastomosis was properly visualized endoscopically in both longitudinal and transverse directions by manipulating the mini-transducer over the anastomosis. Imaging required approximately 3 minutes per anastomosis.

The ultrasound images were stored and the still images of the anastomosis were scored perfectly off-line as correct (Figure 4) or incorrect (Figure 5) by 2 blinded observers in all 16 cases.

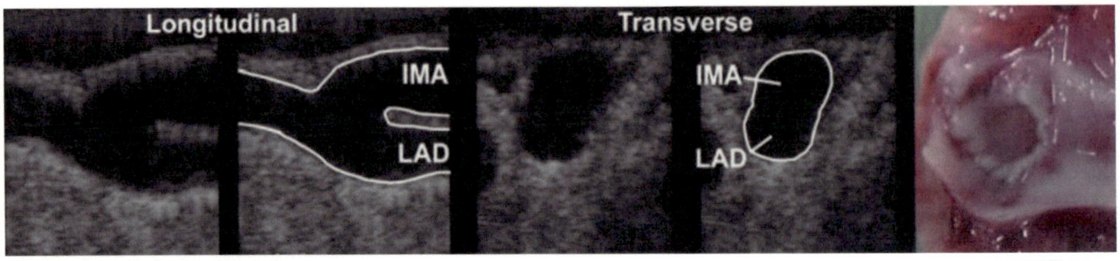

Figure 4. Longitudinal and transverse ultrasound images of a correct anastomosis with corresponding macroscopic view of the anastomotic orifice after incision of the posterior wall of the LAD. (Reprinted with permission from Budde R. et al, Robot-assisted 13 MHz epicardial ultrasound for endoscopic quality assessment of coronary anastomoses. Interactive Cardiovascular and Thoracic Surgery 2004;3:616-20)

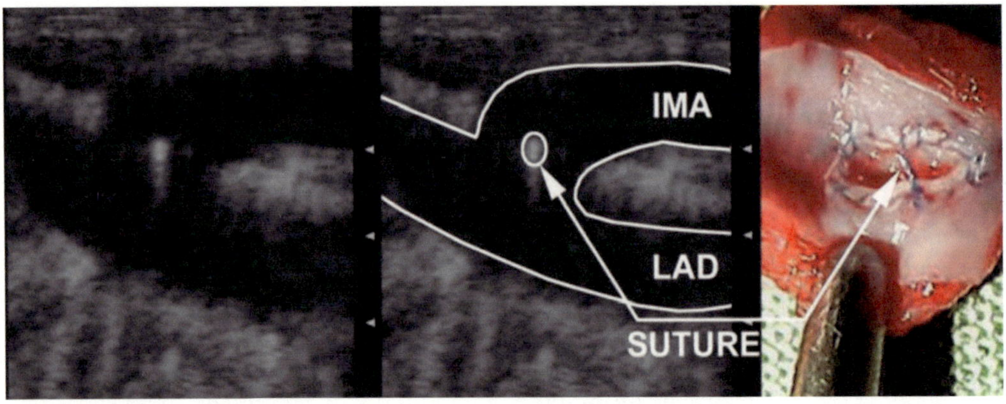

Figure 5. Longitudinal ultrasound image of an incorrect anastomosis with suture cross-over with corresponding macroscopic view of the anastomotic orifice after incision of the posterior wall of the LAD. Arrow indicates overcrossing suture. (Reprinted with permission from Budde R. et al, Robot-assisted 13 MHz epicardial ultrasound for endoscopic quality assessment of coronary anastomoses. Interactive Cardiovascular and Thoracic Surgery 2004;3:616-20)

9. Future of TECAB

The future of TECAB remains to be determined. Currently, routine multivessel TECAB seems still too challenging. Hybrid approaches, however, in which the left internal mammary artery is anastomosed to the LAD endoscopically and the other coronary arteries are treated by percutaneous transluminal coronary angioplasty with stent placement are being explored (Katz et al., 2006).

Coronary connectors may advance TECAB as well by providing a means to facilitate anastomosis construction and omit the tedious suturing process (Falk et al., 2003). ECUS can be used for size matching and quality assessment of some of the connectors (Budde et al., 2005).

10. Conclusions

Epicardial ultrasound can successfully locate and assess the coronary arteries and assess anastomotic quality in the porcine TECAB model within a few minutes. It therefore is a promising tool to help advance TECAB, but clinical confirmation of the experimental results remains to be established.

11. References

Argenziano, M.; Katz, M.; Bonatti, J.; et al. (2006). Results of the prospective multicenter trial of robotically assisted totally endoscopic coronary artery bypass grafting. *Ann Thorac Surg*,81,5,1666-1674.

Balacumaraswami, L. & Taggart, D. (2007). Intraoperative imaging techniques to assess coronary artery bypass graft patency. *Ann Thorac Surg*, 83,6,2251-2257.

Bonatti, J.; Schachner, T.; Bonaros, N.; et al. (2006). Technical challenges in totally endoscopic robotic coronary artery bypass grafting. *J Thorac Cardiovasc Surg*, 131,1,146-153.

Borst, C.; Jansen, E.; Tulleken, C.; et al. (1996). Coronary artery bypass grafting without cardiopulmonary bypass and without interruption of native coronary flow using a novel anastomosis site restraining device ("Octopus"). *J Am Coll Cardiol*,27,6,1356-1364.

Borst, C. & Gründeman, P. (1999). Minimally invasive coronary artery bypass grafting: an experimental perspective. *Circulation*,99,11,1400-1403.

Budde, R.; Meijer, R.; Bakker, P.; et al. (2004a). Endoscopic localization and assessment of coronary arteries by 13 MHz epicardial ultrasound. *Ann Thorac Surg*,77,5,1586-1592.

Budde, R.; Dessing, T.; Meijer, R.; et al. (2004b). Robot-assisted 13 MHz epicardial ultrasound for endoscopic quality assessment of coronary anastomoses. *Interact CardioVasc Thorac Surg*,3,616-620.

Budde, R.; Suyker, W.; Suyker, P.; et al. (2005). Quality assessment of distal S(2)AS connector anastomosis by 13 MHz epicardial ultrasound. *Eur J Cardiothorac Surg*,28,6,833-837.

Diegeler, A.; Thiele, H.; Falk, V.; et al. (2002). Comparison of stenting with minimally invasive bypass surgery for stenosis of the left anterior descending coronary artery. *N Engl J Med*,347,8,561-566.

Falk V.; Diegler, A.; Walther T. et al . (2000a). Total endoscopic off-pump coronary artery bypass grafting. *Heart Surg Forum*,3,1,29-31.

Falk, V.; Fann, J.; Grunenfelder, J.; Burdon, T. (2000b). Endoscopic Doppler for detecting vessels in closed chest bypass grafting. *Heart Surg Forum*,3,4,331-333.

Falk, V.; Walther, T.; Stein, H.; et al. (2003). Facilitated endoscopic beating heart coronary artery bypass grafting using a magnetic coupling device. *J Thorac Cardiovasc Surg*, 126,5,1575-1579.

Gründeman, P.; Budde, R.; Mansvelt Beck, H.; et al. (2003). Endoscopic exposure and stabilization of posterior and inferior branches using the endo-starfish cardiac positioner and the endo-octopus stabilizer for closed-chest beating heart multivessel CABG: hemodynamic changes in the pig. *Circulation*,108, Suppl II,II34-II38.

Gründeman, P.; Verlaan, C.; van Boven, W.; Borst, C. (2004). Ninety-degree anterior cardiac displacement in off-pump coronary artery bypass grafting: the Starfish cardiac positioner preserves stroke volume and arterial pressure. *Ann Thorac Surg*,78,2,679-684.

Haaverstad, R.; Vitale, N.; Williams, R.; Fraser, A. (2002). Epicardial colour-Doppler scanning of coronary artery stenoses and graft anastomoses. *Scand Cardiovasc J*,36,2,95-99.

Hol, P.; Fosse, E.; Lundblad, R.; et al. (2002). The importance of intraoperative angiographic findings for predicting long-term patency in coronary artery bypass operations. *Ann Thorac Surg*,73,3,813-818.

Kappert, U.; Schneider, J.; Cichon, R.; et al. (2001). Development of robotic enhanced endoscopic surgery for the treatment of coronary artery disease. *Circulation*,104,12,I102-I107.

Katz, M.; van Praet, F.; de Canniere, D.; et al. (2006). Integrated coronary revascularization: percutaneous coronary intervention plus robotic totally endoscopic coronary artery bypass. *Circulation*,114,I473-I476.

Loulmet, D.; Carpentier, A.; D'Attellis, N.; et al. (1999). Endoscopic coronary artery bypass grafting with the aid of robotic assisted instruments. *J Thorac Cardiovasc Surg*,118,1,:4-10.

Schachner, T.; Feuchtner, G.; Bonatti, J.; et al. (2007). Evaluation of robotic coronary surgery with intraoperative graft angiography and postoperative multislice computed tomography. *Ann Thorac Surg*,83,4,1361-1367.

Subramanian, V.; Patel, N.; Patel, N.; Loulmet, D. (2005). Robotic assisted multivessel minimally invasive direct coronary artery bypass with port-access stabilization and cardiac positioning: paving the way for outpatient coronary surgery? *Ann Thorac Surg*,79,5,1590-1596.

Suematsu, Y.; Takamoto, S.; Ohtsuka, T. (2001). Intraoperative echocardiographic imaging of coronary arteries and graft anastomoses during coronary artery bypass grafting without cardiopulmonary bypass. *J Thorac Cardiovasc Surg*,122,6,1147-1154.

4

Image Guided Robotic Systems for Focal Ultrasound Based Surgical Applications

Sunita Chauhan
School of Mechanical & Aerospace Engineering, Nanyang Technological University
Singapore

1. Introduction

Surgical resection remains the mainstay for conventional treatment of cancers/tumors. Normally, a margin area surrounding the cancer is removed to minimize relapse. However, due to the need for large access wounds for excising deep-seated abnormalities, traditional open surgery is associated with several operative and post-operative complications resulting into high morbidity and mortality rates. Many patients are not good candidates for resection. Minimally Invasive Surgery (MIS), though introduced in the earlier part of the 20th century, started to gain wide clinical acceptance during the 1980s. In MIS, also known as key-hole surgery, the affected area is laparoscopically or, endoscopically resected under visual guidance. In these applications, specialized tools and devices are used that can be inserted through constrained access holes while the surgeon views the operative filed through the video images reproduced at the surgeon's console. Hand-eye coordination using indirect means (2D imaging) presents a challenge to the clinical users for precise visual and tactile feedback and thus involves a steep learning curve. Minimally invasive procedures offer several advantages over open, conventional surgery, notably shorter length of stay, decreased analgesic requirements, shorter recovery time, decreased post-operative complications, and in some cases a lower morbidity rate as well. Surgery, either in an open or key-hole mode, is usually followed by adjuvant and non-invasive procedures, such as radiotherapy and chemotherapy, particularly when the neoplastic growth is stage-II and beyond.

Minimally invasive and non-invasive ablation procedures (thermal-ablation/cryoablation/chamical ablation) in the management of cancers for deep-seated abnormalities are available using various modalities, for instance, radio-frequency, ultrasound, microwaves etc. (Giovannini and Seitz 1994; Crews et al 1997; Kennedy et al 2003). In thermo-therapeutic techniques, heat diffusion to sites adjacent to the target is common due to extended periods of exposure and convection by blood perfusion (Lang et al 1999). Achieving temperature control at desired levels is very difficult. Therapeutic techniques such as radiation therapy, chemotherapy, hyperthermia may be effective only in early stages. Such therapies are given either alone or in appropriate combination (Ando et al 2003; Soo et al 2005). For instance, cellular membrane permeability (and thus the efficiency) of chemotherapy is increased if hyperthermia is induced prior to or, along with drug infusion. For completely non-invasive interventions, the use of High Intensity Focused Ultrasound (HIFU), alternatively known as

Focal Ultrasound Surgery (FUS), is gaining importance in the recent years (Madersbacher et al 1993; Hynynen et al 2001; Chauhan et al 2001; Uchida et al 2002; Kennedy et al 2003). This modality has shown promising clinical evidence, particularly in the field of urology and oncology and as the technique and instrumentation is evolving, the application base is further broadening.

Advanced manipulation by the use of robotic technology and computational tools can be used in pre-planning, registration, and navigation of surgical devices based on the image data. Thanks to the availability of noninvasive imaging techniques, such as computed tomography (CT), magnetic resonance imaging (MRI) and functional MRI, positron emitted tomograpgy (PET) ultrasonography etc., which can provide digitized images for precise location and function of diseased areas. Robotic assistance provides several benefits such as higher accuracy, precision and repeatability in positioning surgical tools and maneuvering controlled trajectories (Ballantyne 2002; Davies et al 1999, Cleary and Nguyen 2002; Mack 2001). Other systems include minimally invasive repetitive orthopaedic tasks, percutaneous needle puncture, soft tissue biopsy and surgery as well as non-invasive radiosurgery. The representative examples include master-slave robotic system - Da Vinci system (Intuitive Surgical, Inc. USA), orthopaedic surgery systems - ROBODOC (Integrated Surgical Systems, Inc. USA), CASPAR (ortoMAQUET GmbH, Germany), Active constraint robotic devices (Acrobot Company Ltd, UK) and radiosurgery system - Cyberknife (Accuray Inc. USA) (Bodner et al 2004; Davies et al 2005; Taylor and Stoianovici 2003).

In this chapter, system overview and salient features of a range of image-guided robotic systems for non-invasive applications using FUS, devised by the Biomechatronics group, Robotics Research Center at our University, are described. These robotic systems, named FUSBOTs (acronym for **F**ocal **U**ltrasound **S**urgery ro**BOTs**) are developed for several clinical applications such as breast surgery (superscript BS: FUSBOT-^{BS}), urological surgery (FUSBOT^{US}) and neuro-surgery (FUSBOT^{NS}). The chapter is organised into four main sections: introduction, methods and means, system overview followed by discussions/conclusions.

2. Methods and Means

2.1 The modality: HIFU

HIFU is emerging as a potential non-invasive modality for thermally induced ablation of deep-seated abnormalities because of its unique ability in non-invasively targeting deep-seated tissue volumes. Focused ultrasound surgery prevents the risk of ionization as prevalent in other non-invasive modalities such as LASER, microwave and X-ray – based ablations. Ultrasound waves are mechanical waves that can propagate through biological tissues and can be brought to a tight focus. The physical mechanisms responsible for therapeutic effects of ultrasound are both thermal and mechanical stress. Tissue ablation due to HIFU is primarily effected by conversion of mechanical energy of an ultrasound wave into heat energy at its focal point. A temperature range of 60-80°C is achieved and the thermal effect could lead to immediate coagulative necrosis within the focal zone (an irreversible damage due to protein denaturation, protein synthesis inhibition, chemical bond disintegration in DNA /RNA molecules and other associated mechanisms). The temperature elevation produced in the focal region of the targeted beam produces immediate cytotoxity with a very sharp boundary between dead and live cells at its contour; the damaged region is called a *lesion*.

The targeted beam shape in FUS can be evaluated by modelling the ultrasonic field in front of the transducers (Porges 1972; Kinsler and Fry 1982). When ultrasound energy propagates through a biological medium, a part of it is absorbed and gets converted into heat. For a plane wave of intensity I_0, travelling in a medium with amplitude absorption-coefficient, α, the rate at which heat is generated Q, is given by:

$$Q = 2.\alpha.I_0 \tag{1}$$

This heat energy is responsible for various reversible or irreversible biological changes depending upon the irradiation parameters. For precise computation of temperature, the following Bio-heat equation is used to determine the spatial distribution of temperature in the tissues (Pennes 1948)-

$$\rho.c.\partial T/\partial t = \nabla.k\nabla T + q - Q_p + Q_m \tag{2}$$

where, ρ is the density (kg/m^3), c is the specific heat (J/Kg·K), k is the thermal conductivity (W/m·K), T is the temperature (°C), q is the heat source (W/m^3), Q_p is the perfusion heat loss (W/m^3), and Q_m is the metabolic heat generation (W/m^3). The exposure duration is kept very small (on the order of 1-10s) as compared to hyperthermia (10-40 min). The problems posed by heat diffusion due to blood perfusion are, therefore, less significant.

2.2 Prevalent HIFU Applicators

The common types of HIFU applicators include spherically focused transducers (also called focused bowls) and electronic phased arrays. Either type can be used in various modes: extracorporeal, intracavitary or, directly placed near the target site using minimally invasive techniques. Ultrasound frequencies on the order of 1-4 MHz and transducers with apertures upto 10 cm in diameter are reported in the literature. The dosage and treatment planning require the ability to model the system to predict exposure outcomes. The calculations for modeling the acoustic field of a spherical radiator at a single frequency have been suggested by many researchers, who derived a two-dimensional field model based upon the Huygen's principle and the Fresnel-Kirchhoff diffraction theory (Goodman 1968). The acoustic intensity, I, at any arbitrary point P in the field at a distance r from the source and time t is given by the following relation:

$$I = (A/\rho c m^2)\left\langle \sum_m \sqrt{\frac{2\lambda}{\pi r}}.e^{i(wt-kr)} \right\rangle^2 \tag{4}$$

where, λ is the wavelength of acoustic waves, ω is the angular frequency, k is the wave number, ρ is the density and c is the velocity of acoustic waves in the medium, m represents the number of probes and A is an arbitrary constant. However, fixed focus, large aperture bowl shaped transducers present several limitations such as reduced flexibility in beam positioning, ineffective coupling, large treatment duration and presence of off-focal hot-spots in the intervening tissue while scanning the beam to cover the target region. In order to obviate some of these problems, the use of multiple transducers have been proposed (Chauhan et al, 2001; Davies et al 1999; Haecker et al 2005), which are positioned to form a confocal region. The participating probes being smaller than the conventional HIFU probes have lower energy in the off-focal areas. The spatial configurations of these probes with respect to each other and with respect to the target tissue were studied by developing 2-D and 3-D numerical models and verified in *in vitro* and *ex vivo* tests. The selected beam-characteristics for a trio of HIFU probes (aperture 25.4 mm; Frequency 2 MHz) are reproduced in table 1 (Chauhan et al 2001).

Probe configuration	Axial spread (mm)	Axial intensity (I_f/I_o)	Radial spread (mm)	Radial intensity (I_f/I_o)
$C0(\theta = 0°)$	38.0	490	2.0	485
$C1(\theta = 23°)$	7.0	1150	1.5	820
$C2(\theta = 32°)$	13.0	825	3.0	945
$C3(\theta = 45°)$	23.0	750	2.5	780
$C4(\theta = 60°)$	20.0	704	3.5	780
$C5(\theta = 75°)$	25.0	490	2.0	670
$C6(\theta = 90°)$	Not well defined	650	Not well defined	585

Table 1. Selected beam characteristics for various spatial configurations of multiple probes

The computer simulations help in treatment planning for dosage levels and optimum range of inter-probe distances and angles of orientation (defining size and shape and intensity in the superimposed foci) as suited to a specific application. The 3-D model, by analogy with optical field theory, uses the Fresnel-Kirchoff's diffraction theory to evaluate the pressure amplitude at any location in front of the transducer by taking a double integral over the entire surface of the source:

$$p = \frac{i\rho ck}{2\pi} U_o \int_0^a R \left(\int_0^{2\pi} \frac{e^{i(\omega t - kr)}}{r} d\phi \right) dR \tag{5}$$

where, U_0 is the peak amplitude at the transducer face, a is the radius of the transducer, R is the radial location on the transducer face, ϕ is the angular location on the transducer face and other symbols have their usual meanings as described earlier.

Phased array transducers use the same basic acoustic principles as acoustic lenses that focus a sound beam. Variable delays are applied across the transducer aperture. The delays are electronically controlled and can be changed instantaneously to focus the beam in different regions. Phased arrays can be used for electronically steering the beam over the area of interest without mechanically moving the transducer, and thus provide more flexibility in the shape and size of the resulting lesions and various focal patterns can be planned. However, the inherent disadvantages include increased complexity of scanning electronics (particularly for large arrays), higher cost of transducers and scanners, formation of interference zones which may produce pseudo foci beyond the actual focal regions, large number of elements and hence greater complexity in treatment control. With improvement in array technology, both linear and 2-D arrays are now available which can provide high-quality HIFU applicators.

In the past over a decade, various HIFU devices and systems were made commercially available. A FUS device called Sonablate 200™ (Focal Surgery Inc. of Indianapolis Milpitas, CA) was developed for the treatment of Benign Prostatic Hyperplasia (BPH) and prostate cancers. Other systems targeted for BPH and cancer treatment are Ablatherm™ and Ablatherm^R (Technomed International, France; EDAP TMS S.A., France). Magnetic Resonance Image (MRI) guided HIFU surgery system ExAblate® 2000 (Insightec Ltd., Israel) is FDA approved for the treatment of uterine fibroids. It utilizes MRI to visualize treatment planning and monitoring in real time. Model JC Haifu focused ultrasound based tumor therapeutic System by Chonqing Haifu technology company, China, is used for clinical ablation of solid tumors.

3. An Overview of Robotic FUS Systems

As mentioned earlier, we devised a series of robotic systems called FUSBOTs (Focused Ultrasound Surgery Robots) in our laboratory for facilitating automated image-guided focal ultrasound procedures to treat cancers/tumors in various parts of the human body (Chauhan 2002; Chauhan et al 2004; Chauhan et al 2007). The operation of the ablative system requires appropriate positioning of HIFU transducer(s) in a pre-arranged spatial configuration. Single as well as multiple probe approaches are used for deploying HIFU energy in the specified targets. The lesion created by a single exposure in HIFU based ablation is often smaller than the desired target region. The confocal region of the probes is thus required to be mechanically scanned over the region of interest. For FUSBOTs, the robotic manipulator design, and thus kinematics and dynamics of mechanical configuration, are based on specific application. The common features include: image guidance using diagnostic ultrasound, surgical feedback and interactive & supervisory control by the surgeon. Once the surgical protocol is decided in the pre-planning phase, the robots accurately position the HIFU transducer(s) at specified locations such that the focus (or, the con-focal region in case of multiple probes) is coincident with the planned lesion position on a given 2D image. Before proceeding for the overview of individual systems, first some common features of FUSBOTs are discussed.

3.1 Image Guided Robotic Surgery

Various radiological techniques such as CT, MRI, PET, ultrasound etc. are available today to study the anatomy and functionality of human body for either diagnostic purposes and/or surgical update during a procedure. In systems involving image guided surgery (IGS), the operative procedure is planned and effected by continuous acquisition and update of real-time images. These images are registered to the operative field or, region of interest (ROI) and are presented to the surgeon on a monitor/display which can help in guiding and manupulating the surgical tools in intended position (Weese et al 1997; Ballantyne et al 2002; Cleary and Nguyen 2002; Chauhan 2002). IGS systems are a leading indication, for instance, in locating tumours/cancers while planning for surgical resection or biopsy. To track patient's position, intra-operative position sensing and tracking devices are often used in Computer Assisted Surgery (CAS). Such devices are useful for precisely localizing (position and orientation) surgical tools with either external or, impregnated markers or, rigid anatomical structures proximal to the ROI. The principle of information acquisition is governed by the type of sensor(s) used in the intervention. In certain cases, where pre-operative imaging modality differs from the real-time imaging modality, multi-modality registration is required to locate abnormalities. The use of augmented reality, by superimposing graphical overlays of internal anatomy on a surgeon's view of the patient helps in guiding through a surgical intervention.

IGS is vastly adopted in robotic surgery wherein the robot coordinates are mapped to the on-line images and end-effectors are geometrically linked to surgical work-space. For image guided surgical robots, the target and surgical protocol is pre-defined by the surgeon based on pre-operative and/or interventional data. The correlation of data along with coordinate transformation helps in guiding surgical tools through specified trajectories to the target. The imaging data is usually integrated in a graphical user display (GUI). Through visual localization, GUI allows interactive planning and coordination of user-guided and/or automated surgical tools in the target site. Since most of the imaging modalities provide images in digitized format, it is accurate and efficient to register the medical image to the patient using robots for subsequent manipulation. Robotic/mechatronic assistance and imaging guidance yields higher accuracy, precision, reliability and repeatability in manipulating surgical instruments in desired locations.

3.2 Image Guided, Surgical Feedback Sub-system

In order to make FUS clinically acceptable as a treatment modality, the availability of lesion positioning and feedback during HIFU exposure are crucial. It is highly desirable that some means should be devised for measurement and control of thermal dosage in order to adjudge the efficacy of FUS systems. Clinical evidence supports that MRI can provide reliable, on-line temperature feedback during HIFU exposure (Hynynen et al 2001; Kopelman et al 2006). However, the energy application system integrated with MRI, besides bringing high costs to the treatment procedure, also involve compatibility of the ultrasound source with high magnetic fields and restricted scanning to reach intended targets.

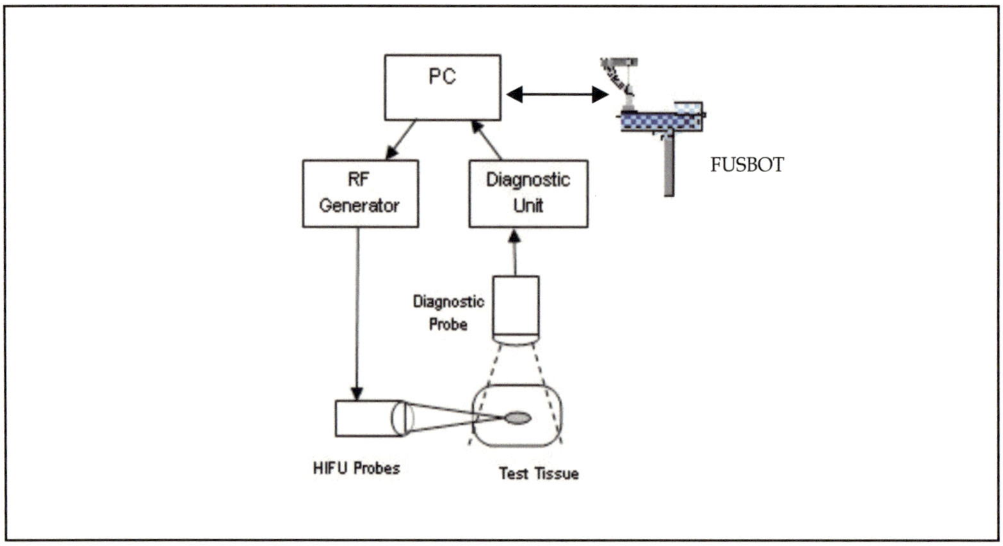

Figure 1. System schematic diagram - experimental set-up

Precise monitoring of variations in physical parameters of the tissue interacting with the incident modality, such as velocity of propagation, absorption and attenuation properties of the external energy etc., can provide vital information in discerning overall success of the treatment (Chauhan et al 1990; Chauhan et al 2007). We developed image guided surgical feedback sub-system with the goal of tracking the lesion position and monitoring the ablation procedure by recording thermal map on-line. Both of these crucial parameters are correlated and fused with the real-time ultrasound imaging. A sensory sub-system integrates robotic sensors for proximity and reach with diagnostic ultrasound through a central processor as shown in figure 1. A temperature dependent parameter, such as velocity of the incident beam (amplitude and phase-shift of the echo) is recorded before and after the exposure for building a thermal map. Temperature data is experimentally calibrated with the help of bead thermistors impregnated at the target sites. The control software for system operation is written in Visual C++. Probe positioning mechanisms and scanning of the focal region in the desired target is done using dedicated manipulator systems as will be presented in the following sub-sections. The dimensions and range of motions of FUSBOTs correspond to human anthropomorphic data.

3.3 FUSBOT^{BS}: The Breast Surgery Robotic FUS System

The robotic system, FUSBOT^{BS} was developed in order to mechanically scan and ablate a specified target in human breast. The lastest version of custom designed robotic system for this application has 5-DOFs (3 for positioning, 1 orientation of end-effector and 1 for imaging) in order to guide an end-effector through a pre-determined and image-guided trajectory (figure 2). The end-effector comprises a purpose built jig for mounting the HIFU transducer(s) and it operates in a degassed water tank. HIFU probes are positioned such that the focal zone (of single probe) or, joint focus (of multiple probes) overlap within the affected target area. Fragmentation of energy into multiple low energy beams help in minimizing hot spots in overlying structures.

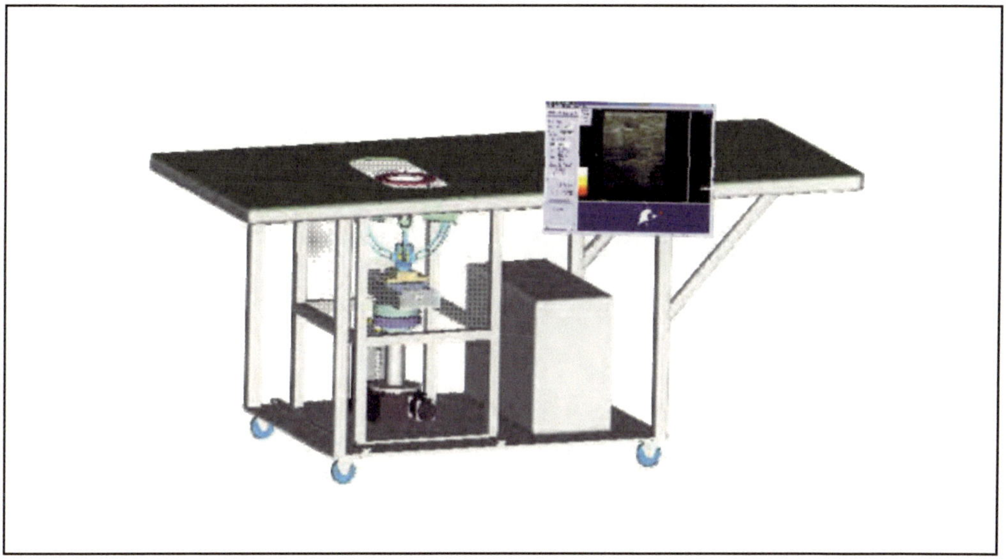

Figure 2. FUSBOT system for Breast Surgery and trans-abdominal route applications

For a target tumor area larger in size than the focal zone of the beam, the HIFU probe(s) need to sweep the entire volume of the lesion in 3D. The probe manipulation modules and robotic work-envelope encompass the human torso region and thus are capable in reaching and treating cancers/tumors other than the breast, such as through acoustic windows in trans-abdominal and supra-pubic routes. The specific area of interest can be reached by using a sliding window opening at the top of the water-tank. At present the end-point accuracy of this system is tested to be within ± 0.2 mm. Various laboratory trials in tissue *in vitro* and *ex vivo* using the system validate its excellent precision and repeatability.

3.4 FUSBOT^{US}: The Urological Surgery Robotic FUS System

The changeable end-effectors in FUSBOT^{BS} system (as described in the previous section) can allow surgery through trans-abdominal route to reach urological organs. The purpose of contriving the FUSBOT^{US} system (superscript US=> Urological Surgery), however, was to enhance the flexibility to deliver multi-probe, multi-route access to remote and disparate organs for two main reasons: 1. to produce adequate dosage in the selective overlapping focal zone while keeping low dosage exposure in individual beam paths 2. in order to gain better access to areas which may not be reached by any one route alone due either to deterioration of beam convergence along a long path or, due to inhibited (bone/air) access window. The system schematics and GUI layout are shown in figure 3.

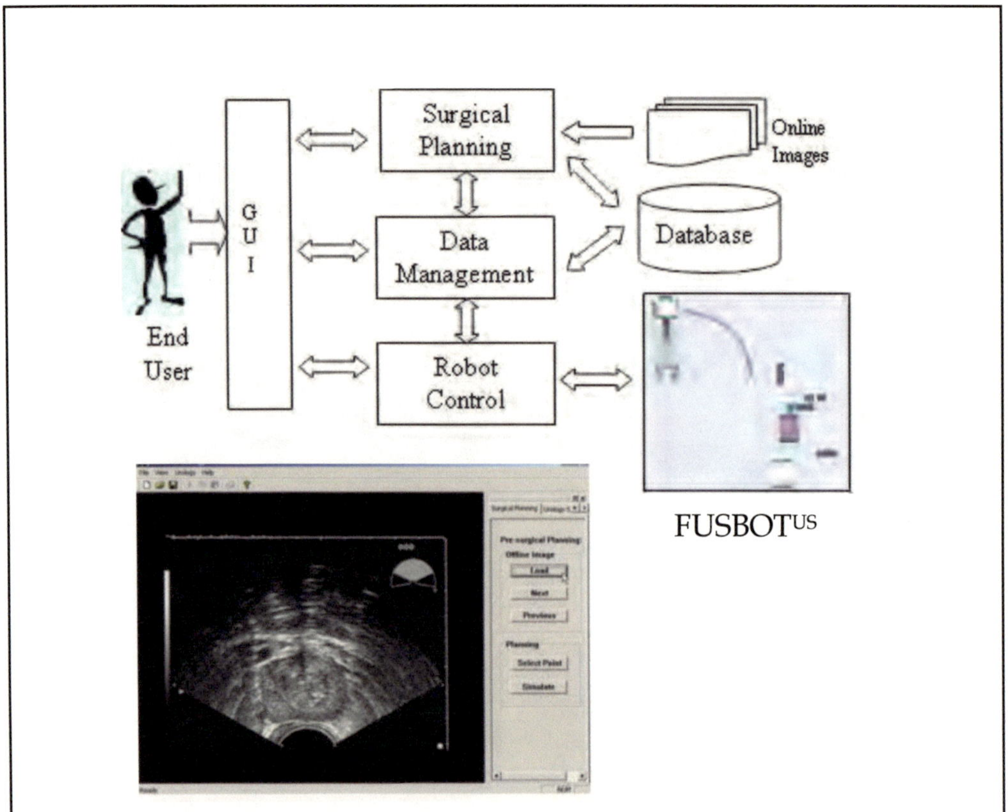

Figure 3. FUSBOT ^{US}: Urological Surgery System - Software structure of control module; Graphical User Interface

A modular approach is adopted for safety reasons. The main components of the system include: Probe manipulation modules each of which are equipped with 3-degrees of freedom; a base harness registered to the operating table, Graphical User Interface and image control. HIFU dosage delivery is controlled separately so as to avoid any interference with the manipulation system. Similar to the previous system, the treatment is planned using image guided (diagnostic ultrasound) interface, which employs image coordinate transfer to the robotic manipulator with respect to the patient coordinates for a selective dosage delivery .

3.5 FUSBOT^{NS}: The Neuro-Surgery Robotic FUS System

The present version of neuro-surgical system is developed for both single and multi-probe *in situ* approach for surgery of deep-seated targets of the brain through a precise craniotomy. The desired craniotomy is performed using Neurobot system with an integrated precision Hexapod system (a Skull base drilling system developed at MAE under our previous project, led by Prof. Teo MY). The accuracy of this system is within ± 0.1 mm. An optical tracking system, OPTOTRAK®, tracks the displacements of infrared markers placed both on the hexapod mobile platform and on the patient. A detailed atlas of the brain can be developed using pre-operative MRI scans to help the neurosurgeons in precisely calculating 3D volume of the region of interest during pre-planning phase.

In the ablative approach using HIFU, the target site is registered to an extended end-effector, called HIFU-effector, at the Neurobot system through an appropriate couplant bellow to the *dura mater* with a provision for attaching changeable end-effectors for a surgical drill unit (as used for creating craniotomy). This module is rigidly coupled on the Hexapod and is actuated with the 7th DOF of the robot, thus maintaining the original accuracy and registration (figure 4).

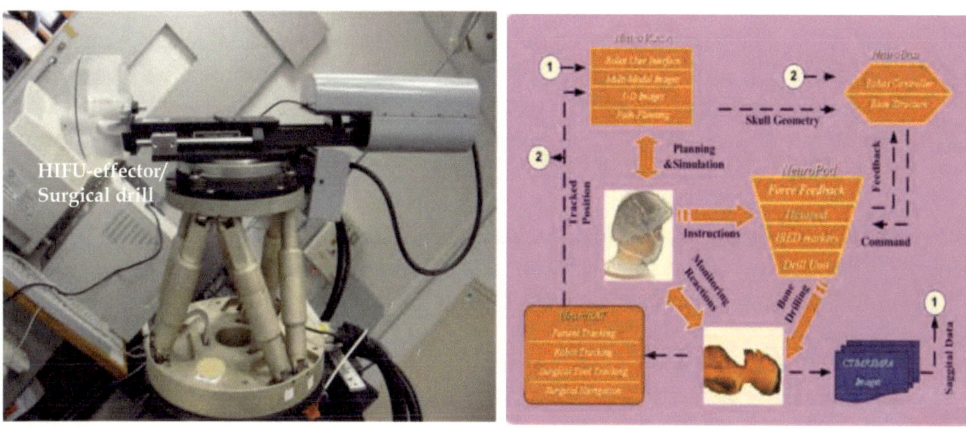

Figure 4. The Neurobot base mounted with a HIFU-effector; various planning modules of Neurobot

4. Conclusive Remarks

A brief overview of a series of novel surgical robotic systems dedicated to FUS applications of various parts/organs of the human body was discussed in this paper. The range of benefits reaped in other medical procedures by the use of robotic technology should be extended to non-invasive ablative procedures, which share extended problems of image guidance, precise targeting and control. Besides automated scanning using multi-probe HIFU technique, control algorithms for on-line feedback information such as lesion tracking and temperature mapping using diagnostic ultrasound are implemented in FUSBOTs. The power levels sufficient for creating a lesion result in a change in tissue reflective characteristics and affect echo amplitude. Our preliminary test results in excised porcine adipose tissue establish the feasibility of this technique under varying dosage protocols. In these tests, a lesion detected by the algorithms correlated well within the macroscopic position as found after resection. The maximum positioning error was found to be within 0.5mm in the lateral dimension. Future work would include integration of HIFU dosage control sub-system with the image/data fusion in order to update computed dosage on-line. Further tests would also be desirable in tissue *in vivo*.

5. Acknowledgements

The author would like to thankfully acknowledge the funding support from Agency for Science, Technology and Research, A*STAR, Singapore and Ministry of Education, Singapore. Many thanks also go to collaborators at NTU and clinical collaborators at Klinikum Mannheim, University of Heidelberg, Germany and NNI, Singapore, . The assistance from students and staff at the robotic research center, in helping to implement the concepts presented here, is highly appreciated.

6. References

Ando, N.; (2003), Iizuka, T., Ide, H., Ishida, K., Shinoda, M., Nishimaki, T., Takiyama, W., Watanabe, H., Isono, K., Aoyama, N., Makuuchi, H., Tanaka, O., Yamana, H., Ikeuchi, S., Kabuto, T., Nagai, K., Shimada, Y., Kinjo, Y., Fukuda, H. (2003), Surgery plus chemotherapy compared with surgery alone for localized squamous cell carcinoma of the thoracic esophagus: a Japan Clinical Oncology Group Study--JCOG9204, *J Clin Oncol.* Vol. 21, No. 24, Dec. 2003, 4592-4596.

Ballantyne, G.H.; (2002), Robotic surgery, telerobotic surgery, telepresence, and telementoring, *Surgical Endoscopy*, Vol. 16, No. 10, Oct. 2002, 1389-1402

Bodner, J.; (2004) Wykypiel, H., Wetscher, G., Schmid, T., First experiences with the da VinciTM operating robot in thoracic surgery, *Eur J Cardiothorac Surg* Vol. 25, 2004, 844-851.

Chauhan, S.; (1990), Singh, V.R., Chakarvarti, S.K., Non-Invasive Measurement Of Temperature In Biological Media Under Ultrasonic Irradiation, *J. Acoust. Soc. India*, Vol. 18, No. 3&4, 1990, 273-276.

Chauhan, S.; (2001), Lowe, M.J.S, Davies, B.L., A multiple focused probe approach for HIFU based Surgery, *Journal of Ultrasonics (Medicine and Biology)*, UK, Vol.39, No.1, 2001, 33-44.

Chauhan, S.; (2002), A Mechatronic System for Non Invasive Treatment of the Breast Tissue, In: *Mechatronics and Machine Vision: current Practice*, 2002, 359-366, Research Studies Press Ltd., UK.

Chauhan, S., Teo, M.Y., Teo, W. (2004), Robotic System for Ablation of Deep-seated Skull Base Cancers - A Feasibility Study, *Proceedings of the 34th International MATADOR Conference,* Manchester, UK, July 2004, UK.

Chauhan, S.; (2007), Amir, H., Chen, G., On-line interpretation and dynamic compensation for focal ultrasound based image-guided robotic surgery, *International Journal of Computer Assisted Radiology and Surgery*, Vol. 2, No. 1, June, 2007, 191-203.

Cleary, K.; Nguyen, C. (2002), State of the art in surgical robotics: Clinical applications and technology challenges, *Computer Aided Surgery*, Vol. 6, No. 6, April 2002, 312 – 328

Crews, K.A.; (1997), Kuhn, J.A., McCarty, T.M., Fisher, T.L., Goldstein, R.M., Preskitt, J.Y., Cryosurgical ablation of hepatic tumors, *Am. J. Surg*. Vol. 174, No.6, Dec. 1997, 617-618.

Davies, B.L; (1999), Chauhan, S., Lowe, M.J.S., A Robotic Approach to HIFU Based Neurosurgery. *Lecture Notes in Computer Science*, Springer Verlag, October, 1999, 386-396.

Davies, B.; (2005), Harris, S., Jakopec, M., Rodriguez, F., Gomes, P., Cobb, J. (2005), Robotic Clinical Trials of Uni-condylar Arthroplasty, *Int. Jl Medical Robotics and Computer Aided Surgery*,. Vol. 2, No. 4, 2005, 20-28.

Fujimoto, S.; (1990), Shrestha, R.D., Kokubun, M., Kobayashi, K., Kiuchi, S., Konno, C., Takahashi, M., Ohta, M., Koike, S., Okui, K., Kitsukawa, Y., Mizutani, M., Chikenji, T. (1990). Clinical Outcome of Intraperitoneal Hyperthermic perfusion Combined with Surgery for Gastric Cancer with peritoneal Dissemination or Serosal Invasion, *Jpn J Gastroenterol Surg*, Vol. 23, No. 9, Sep. 1990, 2209-2214.

Giovannini, M.; (1994), Seitz, J.F.: Ultrasound-guided percutaneous alcohol injection of small liver metastases. *Cancer,* Vol.73, No. 2, Jan. 1994, 294-297.

Goodman, J.W. (1968), Introduction To Fourier Optics, Mcgraw Hill, New York.

Häcker, A.; (2005) Peters, T., Michel, M.S., Hildenbrand, R., Alken, P., Marlinghaus, E., Köhrmann, K.U., Chauhan, S., Multiple Hifu-Probes For Kidney Tissue Ablation, *Journal of Endourology*, Vol. 19 , No. 8, 2005, 1036-1040.

Hynynen, K.; (2001), Pomeroy, O., Smith, D.N., Huber, P.E., McDannold, N.J., Kettenbach, J., Baum, J., Singer, S. and Jolesz, F.A. (2001) MR Imaging-guided focused ultrasound surgery of fibroadenomas in the breast: A feasibility study, *Radiology*, Vol. 219, 2001, 176–185.

Kennedy, J .E.; (2003), ter Haar, G. R., and Cranston, D, (2003), High intensity focused ultrasound: surgery of the future?, *The British Journal of Radiology*, Vol. 76, 2003, 590–599.

Kinsler, L.E., Fry, A.R. (1982), Fundamentals Of Acoustics, John Wily & Sons Inc., New York.

Kopelman, D.; (2006), Inbar Y., Hanannel, A., Freundlich, D., Castel, D., Perel, A., Greenfeld, A., Salamon, T., Sareli, M., Valeanu, A., Papa, M. (2006), Magnetic resonance-guided focused ultrasound surgery (MRgFUS): ablation of liver tissue in a porcine model, *Eur J Radiol*, Vol. 59, No.2, Aug 2006, 157-162.

Lang, L.; (1999), Erdmann, B., Seebass, M. (1999), Impact of nonlinear heat transfer on temperature control in regional hyperthermia, *IEEE Trans. Biomedical Engrg*. Vol. 46, No. 9, 1999, 1129-1138.

Mack, M.J.; (2001), Minimally Invasive and Robotic Surgery, *The Journal of the American Medical Association*, Vol. 285, No.5, Feb 2001, 568-572.

Madersbacher S.; (1993), Kratzik C., Szabo N., Susani M., Vingers L., Marberger M., Tissue ablation in benign prostatic hyperplasia with high-intensity focused ultrasound. *Eur Urol,* Vol. 23, No. 1, 1993, 39–43.

Pennes, H.H.; (1948), Analysis of tissue and arterial blood temperatures in the resting human forearm, *J. Appl. Phys*. Vol. 1, 1948, 93-122.

Porges, G.(1979), Applied Acoustics, Academic Press, London.

Soo, K.C.; (2005), Tan, E.,H., Wee, J., Lim, J., Tai, B.C., Khoo, M.L., Goh, C., Leong, S.S., Tan, T., Fong, K.W., Lu, P., See, A. and Machin, D. (2005), Surgery and adjuvant radiotherapy vs concurrent chemoradiotherapy in stage III/IV nonmetastatic squamous cell head and neck cancer: a randomised comparison, *British Journal of Cancer*, Vol. 93, July 2005, 279-286.

Taylor, R.H.; (2003), Stoianovici, D., (2003), Medical robotics in computer-integrated surgery, *IEEE Transactions on Robotics and Automation*, Vol. 19, No. 5, Oct. 2003, 765-781

Uchida, T.; (2002), Sanghvi, N.T., Gardner, T.A., Koch, M.O., Ishii, D., Minei, S., Satoh, T., Hyodo, T., Irie A., Baba S. (2002), Transrectal High Intensity Focused Ultrasound for Treatment of Patients with Stage T1b-2N0M0 Localized Prostate Cancer: A Preliminary Report, *Urology*, Vol. 59, No. 3, 2002, 394-399.

Weese, J.; (1997), Penney, G.P., Desmedt, P., Buzug, T.M. , Hill, D.L.G., Hawkes, D.J. (1997), Voxel-based 2-D/3-D registration of fluoroscopy images and CT scans for image-guided surgery, *IEEE Transactions on Information Technology in Biomedicine*, Vol. 1, No. 4, Dec. 1997, 284-293.

5

Robotic Applications in Neurosurgery

M. Sam Eljamel, MBBCh, MD, FRCSIr, FRCSEd, FRCS(SN), FABI
Department of Neurosurgery, The University of Dundee, Scotland
United Kingdom

1. Introduction

Recent advances in neuro-imaging and stereotactic and computer technology gave birth to minimally invasive keyhole surgery to the extent that the scale of neurosurgical procedures, demanded by patients, will soon be so small that it will not be within the capability of the most gifted and skilled neurosurgeons of today. Neurosurgical robotics is the natural progression in this field. Furthermore, the economic advantages, increased precision and improved quality in industrial applications of robotics have stimulated robotic applications in neurosurgery. These neurosurgical robots have significant manipulative advantages over neurosurgeons; neuro-robots are reliable to perform the same procedure over and over, again and again without tiresomeness, variation or boredom. They possess near absolute geometric accuracy and are impervious to biohazards and hostile environments and can work through very narrow and long surgical corridors most suited for surgery on the brain, which is an organ uniquely suited for robotic applications; it is symmetrically confined within a rigid container, the skull, and the brain can be easily damaged by even the smallest excursions of surgical instruments. Robots can also see around corners that are beyond the line of sight of the neurosurgeons during operations and in a way, robots extend the visual and manual dexterity of neurosurgeons beyond their limits.

Several ergometric studies during surgery were reported (Berguer, 1999) that have demonstrated substantial muscle fatigue occurring during procedures related to procedure duration and the angle of surgical instruments. Over the last two decades several systems were developed for use in neurosurgery; some of these neuro-robots have been used in clinical practice while others have not been near a patient because of safety and ethical concerns. Among those robots which were used included the PUMA 200 (Kwoh et al., 1985 and Drake et al., 1991), the Minerva robot from the University of Lausanne in Swtizerland (Burckhart et al., 1995), the NeuroMate from Integrated Surgical Systems (Benabid et al., 1987 & 1998), the MRI compatible robot developed in Japan (Masamune et al., 1995), the Evolution 1 (Universal Robotics Systems, Schwerin, Germany), the CyberKnife (Accuracy Inc, Sunnyvale, CA), the RoboSim neurosurgery simulator (Radstzky & Radolph, 2001), the neuroArm (Louw et al., 2004), the PathFinder (Eljamel, 2006) and lastly the SpineAssist (Shoham et al., 2007). Robots were also integrated within current neurosurgical tools such as the microscope, the SurgiScope stereotactic system (Elkta AB, Stockholm, Sweeden) and the MKM microscope system (Carl Zeiss Inc, Oberkochen, Germany).

2. History of Robotics in Neurosurgery

Neurosurgical robotics had a long gestation period spanning over two decades. The main reason for this long period of development is the stringent regulation of health and safety. In contrast, industrial robots leaped into production very quickly because they can be isolated from human contact in a cage or a highly secure environment; neurosurgical robots on the other hand are designed to interact with surgeons and perform or assist the surgeon to perform complex surgical procedures on alive but anaesthetised patients. Hence, the evolution of neurosurgical robotics was slow as follows.

- **The Unimation PUMA 200** (Advances Research & Robotics, Oxford, CT):

A standard industrial robot (PUMA 200) was used to hold a stereotactic biopsy needle in a 52-year-old man on a CT scanner table, the target was identified on the CT images and the robot was used to orient a guide tube through which a needle was inserted (Kwoh et al., 1985). Localization of the target was achieved by using the Brown-Roberts-Wells (BRW) stereotactic frame localization plates and the head was secured to the CT scanner table using the stereotactic frame reference ring. It is a programmable, computer-controlled, versatile robot that was designed to perform highly accurate, delicate work, yet it was rigid enough to provide stable trajectory. It was a safe robot, designed to work with humans and its joints were equipped with spring-applied, solenoid-released brakes that automatically clamped should any mechanical or electrical defect occur. It has 6 degrees of freedom; movements are executed by DC servomotors; tracking is achieved by optical encoders and it can be used in passive or active programmable modes. It has an accuracy of 2mm and repeatability of 0.05mm. It uses the Brown-Roberts-Wells stereotactic frame for registration and CT scan for imaging. The use of the cumbersome stereotactic frame is a constraint and as such its accuracy and performance are similar to the frame, it has an advantage over the frame in those tedious calculations and manual adjustments were automatically executed by the robot. It was used as a retractor during resection of thalamic astrocytomas (Drake et al., 1991) (Figure 1).

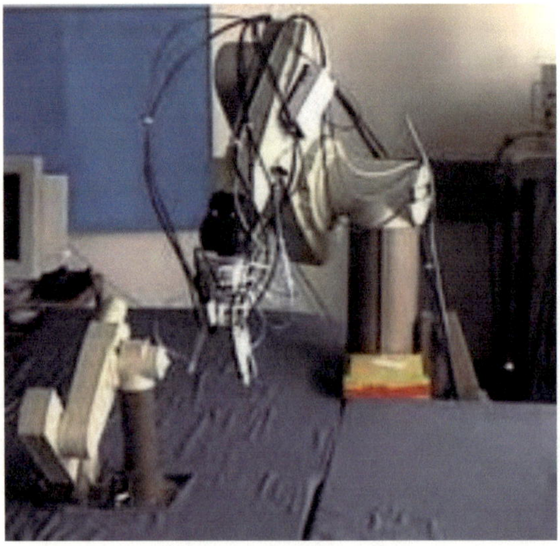

Figure 1. The PUMA Robot (Courtesy Helge Ritter, Bielefeld University, Germany)

- **The Minerva System** (University of Lausanne, Switzerland):

The Minerva system was designed to perform within 5 degrees of freedom. It had two linear axes (vertical and lateral), two rotary axes (moving in a horizontal and vertical planes), and a linear axis (to move the tool to and from the patient's head). The robot is mounted on a horizontal carrier which moves on rails. A stereotactic frame, the Brown-Roberts-Wells (BRW) reference frame, is attached to the robot gantry and coupled to the motorized CT table by two ball-and-socket joints arranged in series. The system was used for two operations on patients in September 1993 at the CHUV Hospital in Switzerland, but the project has since been discontinued. The problems with this project were the limited degrees of freedom, the robot was unwieldy and located within the CT scanner making the environment not ideal for performing neurosurgical procedures and diagnostic imaging. It did not get rid of the cumbersome stereotactic frame and as such it did not offer performance advantage compared to the frame. It was fixed to the scanner making the procedure longer and was not cost-effective as the CT scan suite was unusable for other diagnostic scans during the procedure.

- **Evolution 1** (Universal Robotics Systems, Schwerin, Germany):

This robot was designed for both brain and spinal applications and has 6 degrees of freedom. It is a hexapod robot based on parallel actuator configuration to provide a high degree of accuracy and high payload capacity for drilling applications such, as drilling in the spinal pedicles, and more laterally was used to steer a neuroendoscope (Zimmermann et al., 2002).

- **An MRI compatible robot** (Masamune et al., 1995, Chenzie & Miller, 2001, DiMaio et al., 2006):

This robotic system was devolped by Harvard Medical School in collaboration with Mechanical Engineering Laboratory, AIST, MITI (Tsukuba, Japan). It has 5 degrees of freedom and is MRI compatible. It works with intraoperative MRI system (Signa SP/1, General Electric, Milwaukee, WI) and it has non-magnetic ultrasonic motors based on parallel configuration. It consists of a three-degree-of-freedom Cartesian positioning stage and a two-degree-of-freedom orienting mechanism, and is mounted above the surgeon's head in the open MRI magnet. Two long rigid arms reach into the surgical space and form a parallel linkage for manipulating an acrylic needle holder or guide. The five motion stages are driven by ultrasonic motors (Shinsei USR-60N) attached to lead screws, and motion is measured by optical encoders with 10μm resolution (Encoder Technology, Cottonwood, AZ). A flashpoint sensor is attached to the needle holder to provide independent redundant encoding. This robot has been integrated with a software planning interface (built into the 3D Slicer), and a tracking and control system for percutaneous interventions in the prostate under MR-guidance. The surgeon interacts with the planning interface in order to specify a set of desired needle trajectories, based on anatomical structures and lesions observed in the patient's MR images. All image-space coordinates are computed and used to automatically position the needle guide, thus avoiding the limitations of the traditional fixed template guide. Once the needle holder is in position, the robot remains stationary while the surgeon manually inserts the needle through the guide and into the tissue, with real-time imaging for monitoring progress. The disadvantage of this device is its dependence on intraoperative MRI scan and MRI compatible instruments. Whilst it is beyond the reach of most centres worldwide today, it may become part of MRI technology in the future as more and more surgery is performed at the time of diagnosis.

- **The NeuroMate Robot** (Integrated Surgical Systems, Davis, California, USA):

It is commercially available and FDA approved and evolved from the work of Benabid's group in Gernoble University, France. It has 6 degrees of freedom, incorporates CT, MRI and angiographic neuroimages. It was used in conjunction with a stereotactic frame to position a cannula or probe for biopsy or targeting deep brain structures. It is a six-axis robot for neurosurgical applications. The original system was subsequently redesigned to fulfil specific stereotactic requirements and particular attention was paid to safety issues. To carry out a procedure by the NeuroMate, the robot must know where it is located relative to the patient's anatomy. This is typically done using a calibration cage, which is placed on the end-effecter of the robot around the patient's head. This cage looks like an open cubic box and the four sides are each implanted with nine X-ray opaque beads, the positions of which have been precisely measured. Two X-rays are taken which show the position of these beads along with the fiducial markers of the patient's frame. In the newer versions of this robot, an ultrasonic-based registration is performed using the reference markers shown in Figure 2. This information is used to determine the transformation matrix between the robot and the patient. The defined trajectory is used to command the robot to position a mechanical guide, which is aligned with this trajectory. The robot is then fixed in this position and the physician uses this guide to introduce the surgical tool such as a drill, probe or electrode (Figure 2).

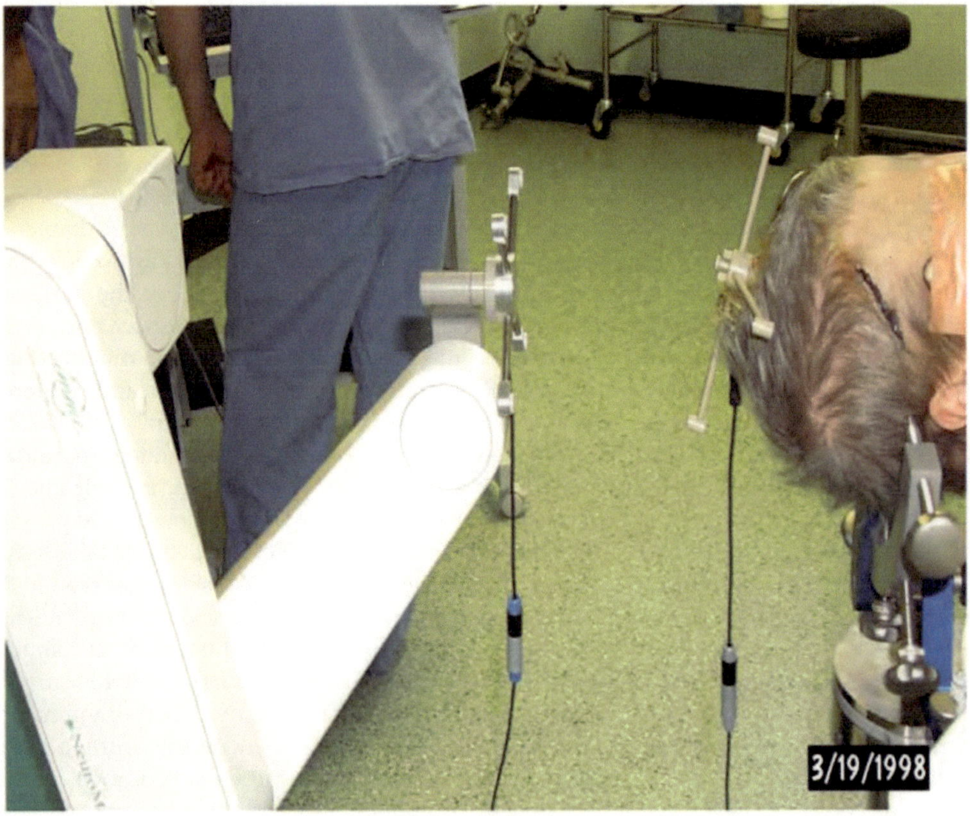

Figure 2. The NeuroMate robot during registration (courtesy TRK Varma, Liverpool)

- **The CyberKnife** (Accuracy Inc, Sunnyvale, CA):

It was designed for frameless stereotactic radiosurgery and its accuracy compares well to localization errors in contemporary frame-based systems. The unique targeting capability of the CyberKnife's multi-jointed robotic arm uses a guidance system to track the location of tumours in real-time and automatically adjusts its focus to a patient's respirations to deliver high-level radiation with pinpoint accuracy. This enables access to previously unreachable tumours with faster, safer, and more comfortable treatments. The CyberKnife is an example of a robotic system delivering treatment that the surgeon cannot do (Figure 3).

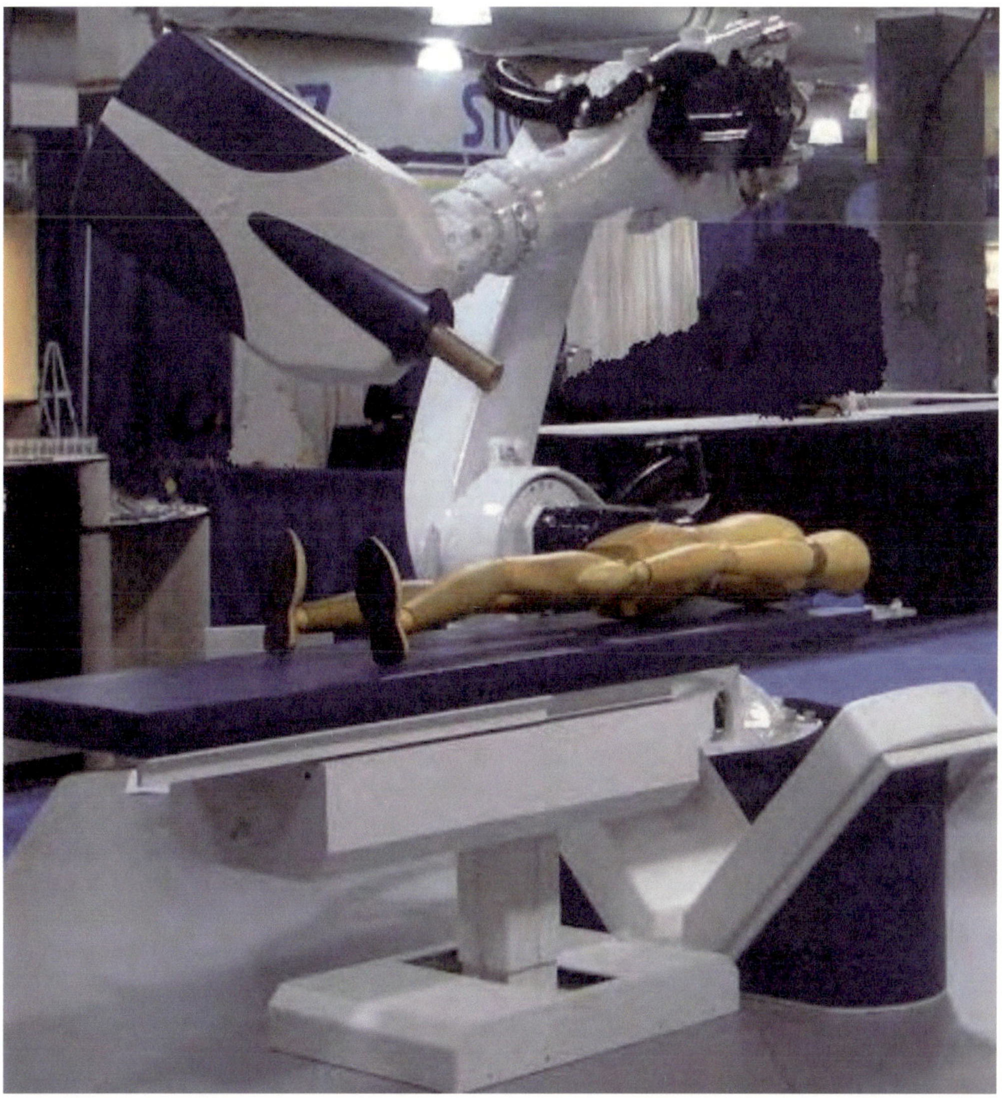

Figure 3. The CyberKnife

The CyberKnife radiosurgical system is being used as a minimally invasive alternative to traditional surgery in a variety of clinical areas in neurosurgery as well as other disciplines. It offers an effective treatment option for patients who cannot undergo traditional open surgery or whose lesions are inaccessible with traditional surgical approaches. Residual tumours left after partial resection may also be treated. It has also been used as a boost to standard radiation therapy and to treat failed surgery or radiotherapy. For intracranial conditions, the CyberKnife system has been used to radiosurgically treat a variety of tumours such as residual small skull base menigiomas, small acoustic schwanomas (Sakamoto et al., 2005), small pituitary adenomas, and small metastases (Young et al., 2005) as well as other abnormalities such as small arteriovenous malformations (AVMs) and intractable pain such as in Trigeminal Neuralgia (Massaudi et al., 2005). With the Synchrony™ motion tracking system, tumours in organs moving with respiration such as the lung (Brown et al., 2005), the pancreas (Goodman & Koong, 2005), the liver and the kidney can be successfully targeted. Other tumours based in more rigid body anatomy, where minimal motion is expected, may be tracked via rigidly implanted markers including those in the spine and the prostate (Medbery et al., 2005). The CyberKnife system's range of applications is limited only by the imagination of clinicians who currently have, or will eventually have access to this technology. To date, more than 10,000 patients have benefited from the revolutionary concept of marrying robotics to image-guided radiosurgery. Scientific presentations and publications on the clinical applications of the CyberKnife are numerous - including intracranial (Young et al., 2005), spine (Gerszten et al., 2005), paediatric (Giller et al., 2005), prostate (Medbery et al., 2005), pancreas (Goodman & Koong, 2005), kidney and lung (Brown et al., 2005).

- The RoboSim Neurosurgery Simulator (Radstzky A & Radolph M, 2001):

This robotic neurosurgical simulator consists of a workstation and a robotic arm (NeuRobot). The MRI image data-set is transferred into the system and the surgical target, its coordinates and planning trajectories are programmed. It was developed as part of the Roboscope project for minimally invasive neurosurgical procedures. Minimally invasive neurosurgery is mainly of importance for treatment of diseases in the central area of the brain, which is accessible to the surgeon only by transgression of healthy normal brain tissue, such as hydrocephalus due to cystic brain tumors and ventricular tumours.

As we enter the 21st century, real-time simulation of surgical procedures is becoming the norm in neurosurgical practice. The RoboSim is a robotic platform for surgical simulation and planning minimally invasive and complex neurosurgical procedures. Another important aspect of neurosurgery is the training of junior surgeons on how to anatomically orient them while operating within the miniaturised operating field of minimally invasive procedures. Image-guided simulation of the procedure will then allow the control of accessibility of the diseased area along the pre-planned trajectory.

- **The neuroArm** (Louw et al., 2004):

The neuroArm is an MRI-compatible, ambidextrous robot. Its dextrous components are two image-guided manipulators with end-effectors that mimic human hands and are capable of interfacing with new microsurgical tools. It has tremor filters that eliminate unwanted hand tremors seen under the microscope. It consists of a surgeon-machine interface and multiple surgical displays. The interface consists of two hand controllers which hold tools. It has 8 degrees of freedom for each arm, payload of 0.5 Kg, a force of 10 N, tip-speed of 0.5-

5mm/sec and submillimetric positional accuracy. It has optical and force sensors and can work continuously for more than 10 hours.

- **The PathFinder** (Prosurgics, UK):

The PathFinder is a neurorobotic system that is portable with a very stable base which can be wheeled in and out of the operating room. The robotic arm can rotate in a horizontal plane 90 degrees to the left or right. The base fixes to the surgical space by an attachment to the Mayfield head clamp. The proximal arm articulates with the next arm that moves in a vertical plane that articulates with the third arm which again moves in a vertical plane. The most distal arm holds the end-effecter, which can rotate 360 degrees and flexes/extends by 180 degrees. The combined movements at all these joints give the PathFinder 6 degrees of freedom. The PathFinder differs from other neurosurgical robots in that it does not require X-rays, ultrasound or mechanical means to locate the surgical field; instead it depends on identifying reflectors attached to the patient's head using a camera system integrated in its head (Figure 4).

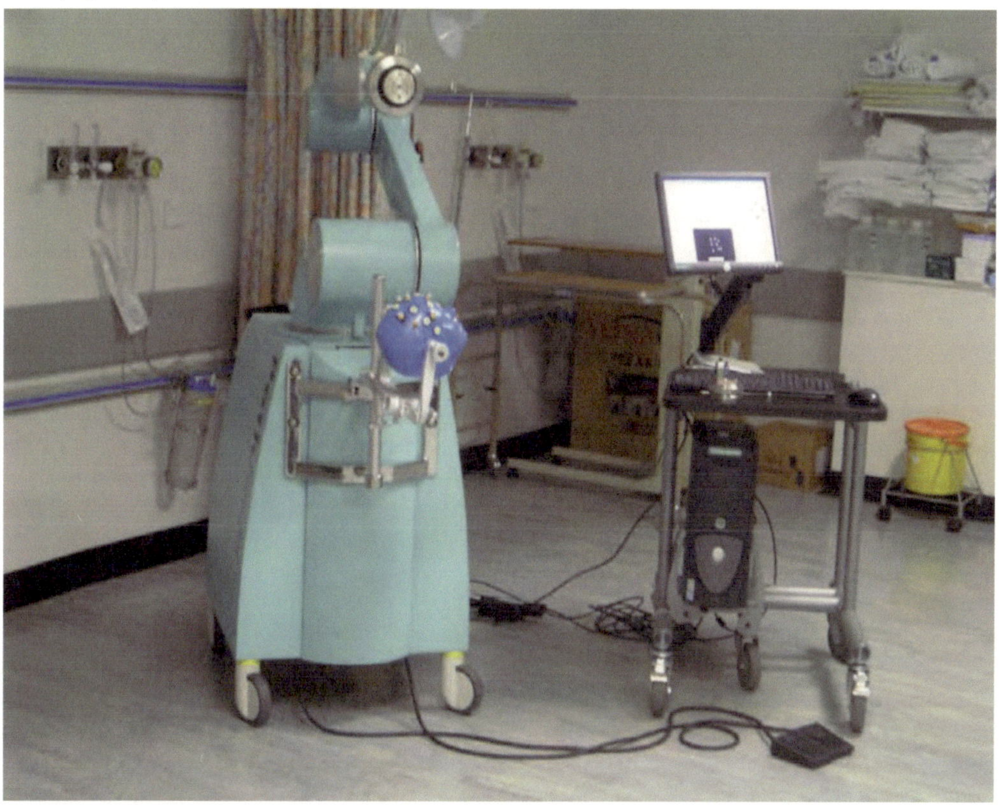

Figure 4. The PathFinder neurosurgical robotic system

The robot is driven by Windows® based task program and planning software. The planning software and PathFinder robot detect the fiducial markers automatically with a maximum accepted registration error of 1.25 mm. The tool holder is attached to the PathFinder's end-effecter. The predefined path is used to command the PathFinder to align its instrument holder to the planned trajectory. Once the instrument holder is aligned to the trajectory, the robot locks in position and instruments can then be passed to the predetermined depth such as probes, electrodes or catheters (Figure 5).

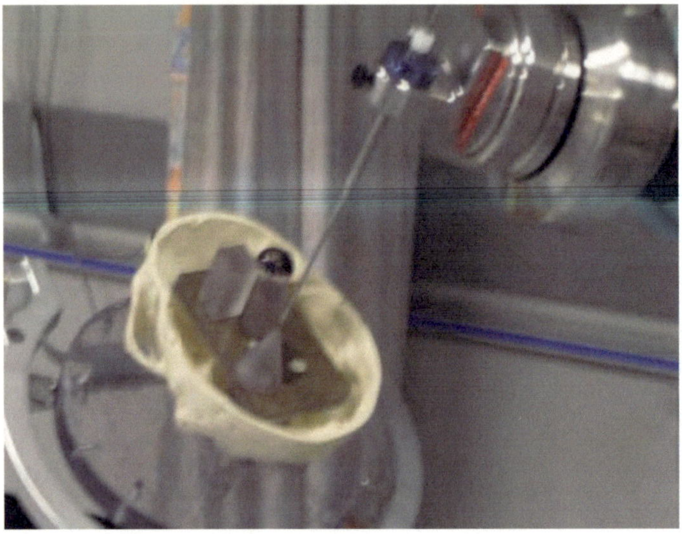

Figure 5. The instrument holder of the PathFinder

- **SmartAssist®** (Mazor Surgical Technologies, Caesarea, Israel):

This miniature robotic system was designed to overcome the need to rigidly immobilise the surgical field during robotic application. This robot achieved this by fixing the robot directly to the bony element of the surgical field. This concept was clinically used in spinal pedicle screw fixation using the SpineAssist robotic system (Shoham et al., 2007). The system consists of the miniature robot that aligns the end effectors with 6 degrees of freedom and a workstation that runs graphic user interface software and performs image manipulation, planning, registration, kinematic calculations and real-time robot control. Once the system was assembled and intraoperative registration using intraoperative fluoroscopy was performed, the plan for each pedicle screw is executed by the robot and the surgeon manually drills the pilot drill-hole and passes K-wire in the desired position. The SpineAssist is an automated pointing robot that gives the surgeon full control.

3. Pre-clinical Work

Our plan was to develop the PathFinder (Prosurgics, UK) (Figure 4) to achieve stereotactic accuracy better than the stereotactic frame with the flexibility and user-friendly features of frameless image guidance systems. Therefore we assembled two of the best available stereotactic frames around, the Cosman-Roberts-Wells (CRW) stereotactic frame (Radionics, MA, USA) (Figure 6), the Zamorano-Dujovny (ZD) stereotactic frame (Fischer-Leibinger, Freiberg, Germany) (Figure 7), and one of the best frameless stereotactic image guidance systems, Stealth Station image guidance system (Medtronic, Sofarmor Danek, Memphis, TN, USA) (Figure 8). The CRW frame localisation technique involved fixing the frame base ring to the skull, the CT localiser with its 9 rods was fixed to the frame ring and CT was obtained in an axial plane at zero angle and calculation of the target co-ordinates was obtained using frame specific software. On the other hand, the ZD frame ring was also attached to the skull and the ZD localiser, U-version, was used and CT scan was obtained at zero angle and the coordinates were calculated using ZD frame specific software. The Stealth Station is an image guidance system using optical tracking technology to track the surgical field position, the surgical tools and the surgical microscope.

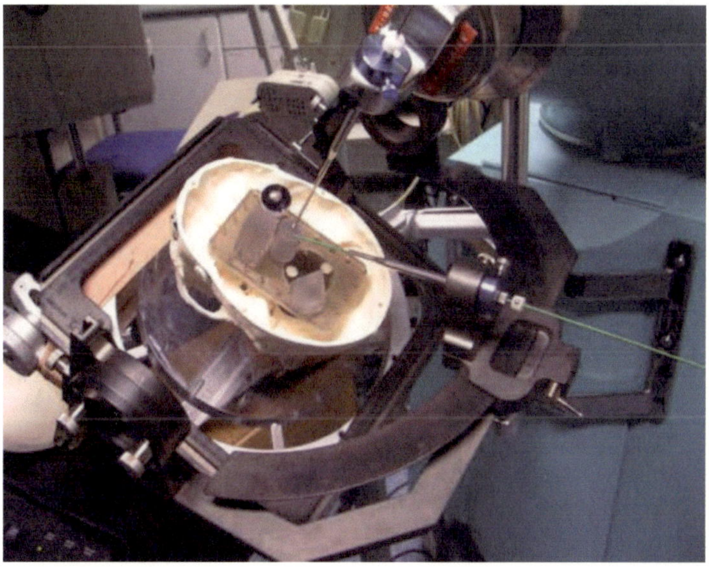

Figure 6. A photograph of the human head phantom and the CRW frame in position and the robotic system pointing to the same target from different trajectories

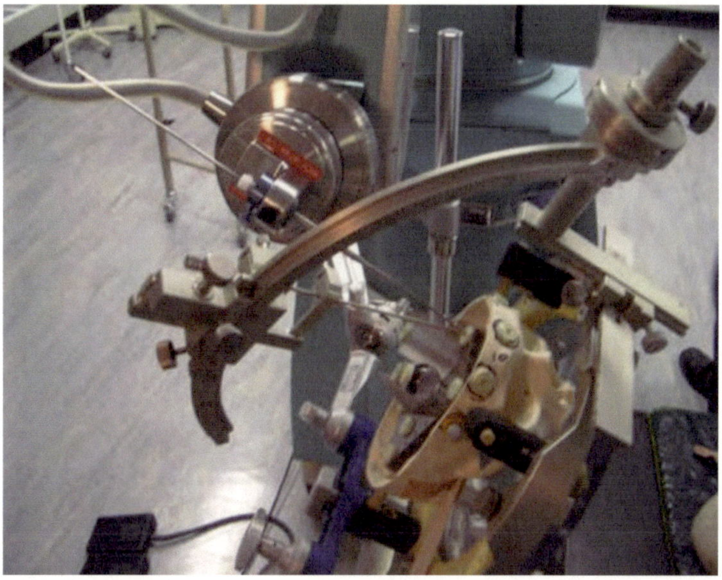

Figure 7. A photograph of the human head phantom with ZD frame in position and the robot pointing to the same target

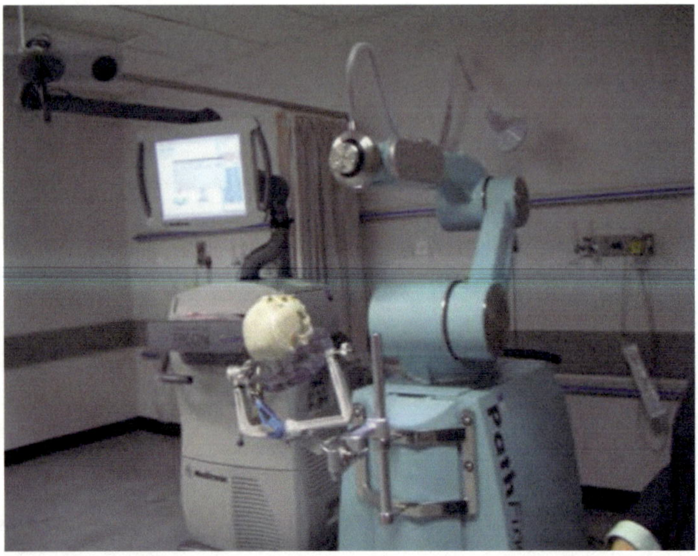

Figure 8. A photograph of the Stealth Station and PathFinder during experiment

- **Methods:**

We performed several experiments using a replica of the human head (phantom). The surface markings of the phantom were an exact match to the human skull and the inside was fitted with easily recognisable targets at different depths from the skull vault mimicking the basal ganglia locations. The phantom was fitted with 10 surface and 9 internal targets (Figure 9 a & b).

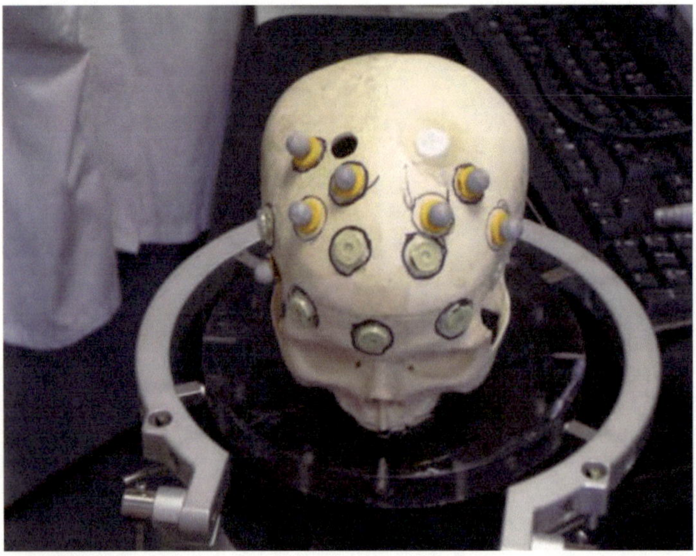

Figure 9 a. A photograph of the human head phantom with surface targets (buttons) and robotic fiducials (reflective balls)

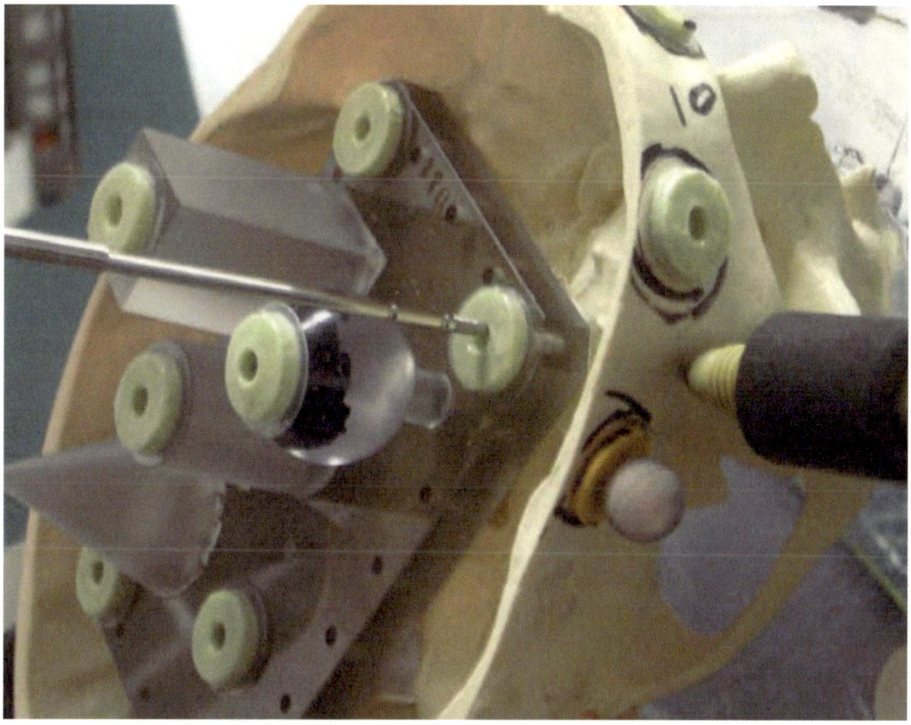

Figure 9 b. A photograph of the human head phantom with depth targets

In addition, 8 robot specific surface fiducials were fitted for robotic registration (Fig 9a). The skull was scanned using helical CT scanner at zero angle and 1 mm slice thickness twice; once with the ZD frame localiser attached and once with the CRW localiser attached. The images were transferred into Frame Link software to calculate the X, Y and Z co-ordinates of each of the 19 targets for each of the two stereotactic frames. The targets were then approached by each frame whenever possible. The same images were imported into robot specific software and the same targets were chosen in a robotic plan. The robotic planning software identified the registration markers automatically. The robot was connected to the skull through its attachment to the Mayfield head fixator. The robot performed its automatic registration by a camera embedded in its head by taking three sets of two images at different angles of the reflective robotic specific surface fiducials. We set the maximum acceptable registration error at 1.25 mm. Targeting was automated by using a foot pedal and once the instrument holder was aligned a probe was passed to manually to reach the target (Figure 6, 7, 9b). The same experiment was repeated using the Stealth Station image guidance system.

- **Steps of the procedure:**
  - Fiducials and markers:

Before neuro-imaging, PathFinder specific fiducials are fixed to the surface of the surgical field. These fiducials are impregnated with radio-opaque material so that they can be easily seen on CT and picked up by the planning software. They are also coated with reflective material so that the robotic camera can easily pick them up (Figure 9a). It is important that these fiducials are placed at a reasonable distance from each other (5 cm) and placed in a non-symmetrical fashion to make it easy for the registration process. They should also be spread around the surgical volume. These fiducials can be fixed to the skin using double sided adhesive tape or alternatively a registration plate can be rigidly attached to the skull (Figure 10).

- Image acquisition:

The registration process is heavily dependant on CT images; these should be acquired at zero angle in an axial plane at 1-3 mm slice thickness. MRI scan should also be obtained in an axial plane at zero angle with no spacing. Although the best sequence is volumetric MPRage, T1 or T2 axial sequences could also be used.

- Preoperative planning:

The surgeon imports the image data-sets into the planning software. The software automatically builds sagittal, coronal and 3D reconstructions of the primary axial images. The CT data-set is used to recognise the fiducials and either the CT or MRI images could be used to plan the target and entry points of the trajectory. The CT and MRI data-sets are merged to provide the final plan. The surgeon can then rehearse the plan and get a visual feedback before the surgery and can change the planned trajectories to avoid any critical structures (Figures 12 & 13).

- Robot set up:

The PathFinder robot is positioned either at right angle (opposite to the surgical side) or at an acute angle parallel to the patient. This position provides the maximum degrees of freedom for the robot and the surgeon and keeps the robot out of the way when it is not in use. The robot is attached to the head via a rigid fixing arm attaching to the Mayfield head clamp. The robot is connected to the computer and switched on. Once it is ready to receive commands from the workstation, the robot task controller software is executed.

- Quality assurance:

The first quality check in the PathFinder is the robot self-test to establish that the workstation and the robot communicate to each other. The system then asks the surgeon to load the surgical plan. The second quality check is confirmation that the surgical plan loaded is in fact that the one was intended by the surgeon. The final quality check deals with the accuracy of the system starting with the registration accuracy and then the application accuracy on the surface.

- Registration:

The robot performs registration on command from the workstation and a foot-pedal press. The registration is achieved by taking and analysing three sets of photographic images of the fiducials. The maximum registration error is 1.25 mm. The system displays a registration error at the end of the registration process. The most common reasons of registration failure are: bright light in the room, some of the fiducials were invisible, fiducial images were superimposed on each other or fiducials were covered by hair. The system displays an image of the fiducials during each registration steps and paying attention to these images often make it easier to resolve any failed registration. If the registration process fails, it can be repeated after paying attention to the cause of failure.

- Plan execution:

Once the registration process is complete, executable surgical trajectories are displayed and can be tested by the surgeon. The tool length can be changed and the entry point can also be fine tuned from within the task controller. The surgeon then prepares the surgical field and drapes the robot and the patient. The surgeon manually performs the entry burr hole or craniotomy, then aligns the robot for the planned trajectories and manually advances the surgical tool to the target.

- **Results:**

When the robotic system was compared to the golden standard of stereotaxy, the stereotactic frame, the robot was successful in approaching 17 out of 19 targets (89.5%). To reach the remaining two it was necessary to change the position of the robot in relation to the phantom axis, without the need for re-scanning or re-planning. On the other hand, both the CRW & ZD frames failed to reach points above certain depth due to the fact that the frame ring in both frames was positioned at a low level in the phantom, primarily to avoid distorting the artificial skull by the frame-ring fixation mechanism. Each frame however, was able to reach 4 targets out of 19 (21.1%). When the targets were possible, the robot, the CRW and the ZD systems were very accurate (0.5 mm in the Robot and 0.98 mm in the Frames) (Table 1).

Device	Robot System		CRW frame		ZD Frame	
Target / result	No.	%	No.	%	No.	%
Superficial	8/10	80	0/10	0	0/10	0
Deep targets	9/9	100	4/9	44.4	4/9	44.4
Overall result	17/19	89.5	4/19	21.1	4/17	21.1
Accuracy in mm	0.5		0.98		0.98	

Table 1. Comparison of the PathFinder neurosurgical robotic system and the CRW and ZD stereotactic frames using CT scan and a Phantom human head

The clear advantages of the robotic system over the frames in these experiments were avoidance of cumbersome frame ring, ability to target multiple areas in the same plan, avoidance of manual adjustments of the coordinates, coverage of all the surgical field with no limitations imposed by frame ring fixation primary position and flexibility to change the plan without the need for rescanning, as well as changing the position of the robot in relation to the phantom head without the need for rescanning or replanning.

When the robotic system was compared to frameless stereotactic system, the Stealth Station, the robotic system outperformed the Stealth Station in accuracy, precision and repeatability (Table 2). The accuracy remained the same irrespective of the target location, while the frameless image guidance system accuracy was good near the surface of the phantom but deteriorated as the target moved backwards and deeper (Table 2).

The system	Robotic system	Frameless image guidance
Accuracy	0.44 mm	1.96 mm
Surface accuracy	0.44 mm	1 mm
Deep anterior	0.44 mm	1-2 mm
Deep middle	0.44 mm	2-3 mm
Deep posterior	0.44 mm	3-4.4 mm

Table 2. Comparison of the PathFinder neurosurgical robotic system and the Stealth Station image guidance system using CT scan and a Phantom human head

From these experiments, we found that the robotic system provided the accuracy, precision and repeatability of the stereotactic frame and the flexibility of the frameless system.
While these experiments demonstrated that the robotic system outperformed both existing stereotactic systems in use, there is still the possibility that the robot will not perform in the clinical setting because skin markers do move during and after scanning. Therefore, we designed a registration plate that can be fixed to the patient's skull via three microscrews. The plate can then be removed and reapplied at will, allowing scanning and planning to be divorced from the registration and the operation in time and place. (Figure 10)

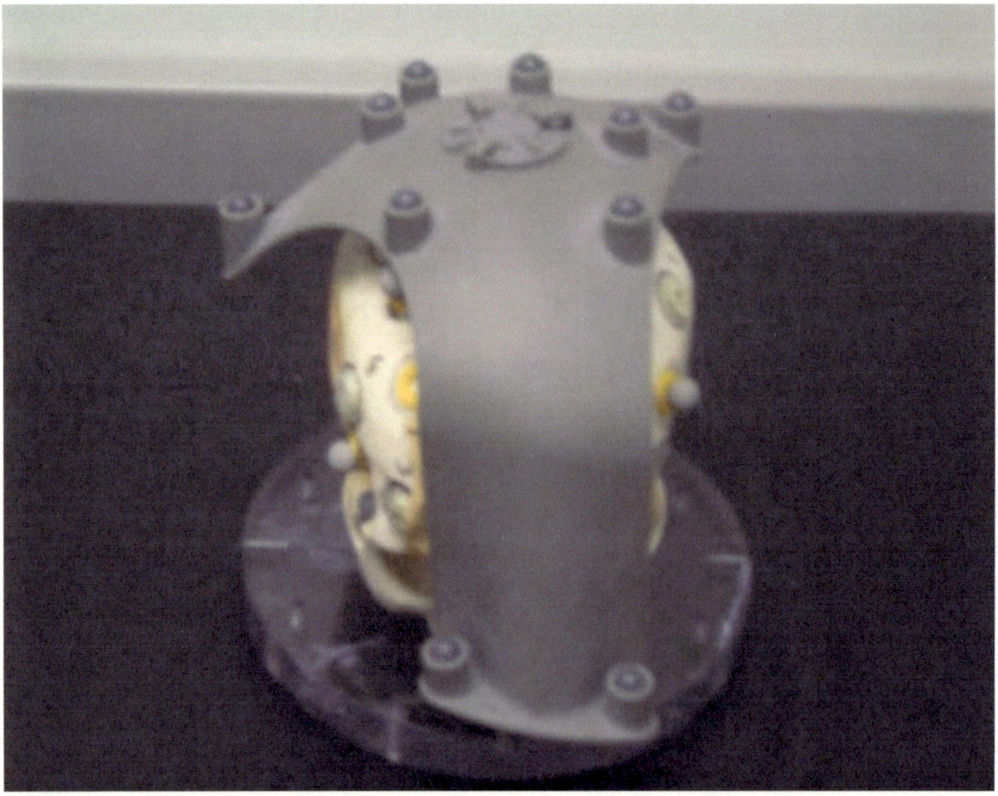

Figure 10. A photograph of the relocatable registration plate

We have encountered several problems during development. Bright fluorescence operating room lights may interfere with the registration process, therefore theatre lights are not switched on till after registration. Power failure during a procedure can lead to loss of registration, therefore a rechargeable battery was fitted which can keep the Robot and workstation going, and finally the axis of the patient in relation to the robot is important as the best position was to place the robot at an angle of 20-30 degrees.

4. Clinical Applications

The human brain is uniquely suited for robotics applications because it is contained in a rigid structure, the skull, and the slightest intrusion of surgical tools can produce devastating, irreversible and potentially fatal complications. The robotic system is useful in the following ways:

- **Planning:**

The robotic systems of today come with robust image processing and planning software, which can segment CT and MRI images, merge these imaging modalities and display the output in axial, coronal, sagittal, 3D and probe eye views. The surgeon can gain significant insight in the pathology under consideration, enhancing his/her understanding of the anatomical relationships of the lesion to the surrounding brain and external landmarks allowing planning trajectories that avoid critical structures taking the shortest and safest route. Furthermore, the planning software allows surgeons to rehearse their surgical trajectories modifying them if felt necessary before embarking on the procedure. It provides an excellent teaching tool for trainees and residents (Figure 11).

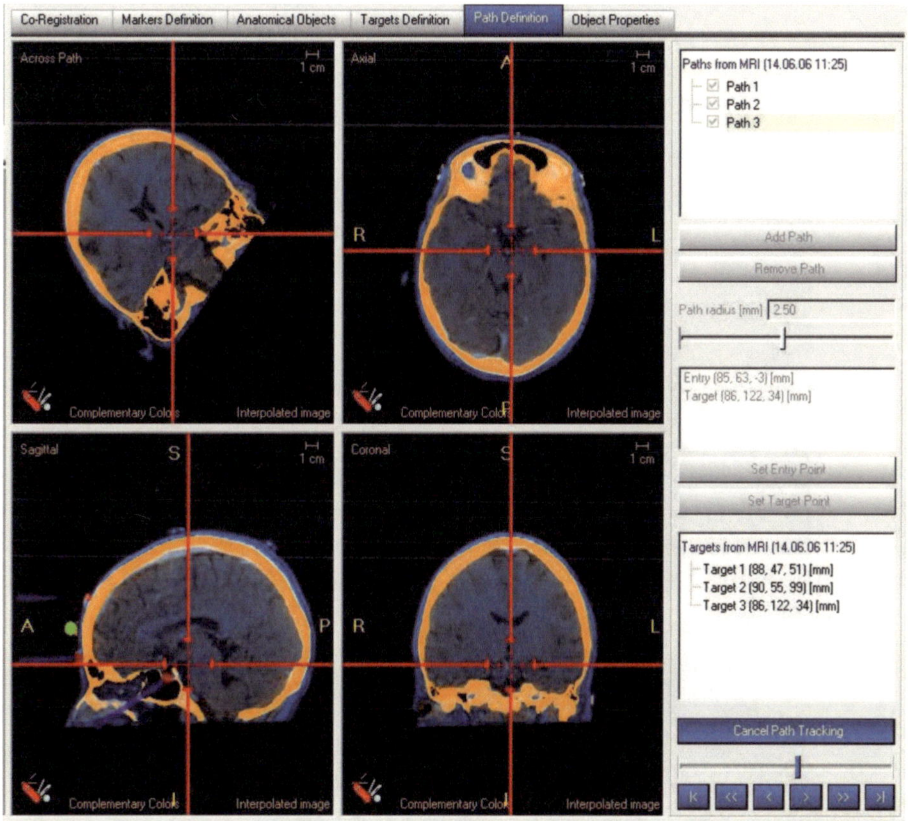

Figure 11. A robotic platform for planning, planning and rehearsing trajectory is very simple

- **Assist in performing stereotactic procedures:**

The advantages of using a robotic system to assist in performing almost all stereotactic procedures are automation of target coordinates, transformation to the tip of the robotic instrument in a moment without the tedious calculations of the X, Y & Z coordinates, transforming and adjusting these coordinates to the aiming arc of the stereotactic frame and the flexibility to perform multiple targeting, multiple trajectories and multiple plans without the tedious and time-consuming steps of fixing the frame reference ring to the patient's head, rescanning, recalculating and readjusting the aiming frame-arc. It was clear that robotic systems would be faster, more automated, more flexible, more reliable, and more accurate. The neurosurgical robots can be used in the following applications.

- Intracranial tumours:

Intracranial tumours are suitable applications for robotics in neurosurgery because they often require stereotactic biopsy which can be performed elegantly by the robotic system. The advantage for using the robot in this area is the ability to perform accurately multiple biopsies to obtain the exact pathological classification of the tumour rather than getting a piece of necrotic centre. The robotic system could be used to plan and insert interstitial radiotherapy, victor therapy or photodynamic therapy. Furthermore, the robotic system would be an ideal tool to plan and execute the plan to excise a tumour by placing a fence around the tumour margins before opening the skull (Figure 12).

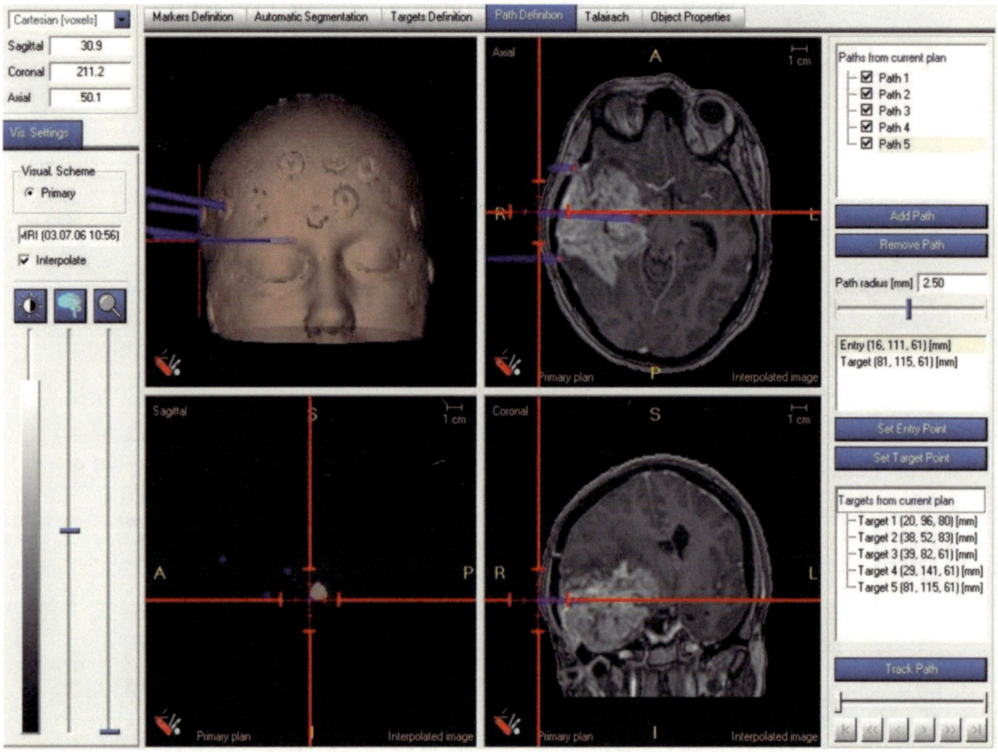

Figure 12. A fencing robotic plan for Glioblastoma multiforme

- Intracranial abscess:

The management of intracranial abscess is drainage, which can be performed using freehand needle aspiration or more appropriately using a stereotactic aspiration. The tendency in common practice is to use freehand aspiration because to put a stereotactic frame is often thought to be cumbersome. However, a flexible robotic system would be an ideal precise way to aspirate such abscess to obtain the micro-organism and drain the pus as the main therapeutic procedure.

- Deep brain stimulation:

Deep brain stimulation is widely used in practice to treat advanced Parkinson's disease, Benign Essential tremor, rubral tremor of Multiple Sclerosis, dystonia, obsessive compulsive disorders and treatment refractory depression. These procedures require the accuracy of the stereotactic frame and neurophysiological monitoring using micro-electrode recordings or macrostimulation and measurement of impedance. The robotic system would be an ideal planning and execution system for performing these procedures precisely. It would be used for the anatomical planning to target the subthalamic nucleus in Parkinson's disease, the Globus pallidus internal in dystonia, the ventral intermediate nucleus of the thalamus for tremor control, the anterior capsule in obsessive compulsive disorders or the cingulum in treatment refractory depression (Figure 13).

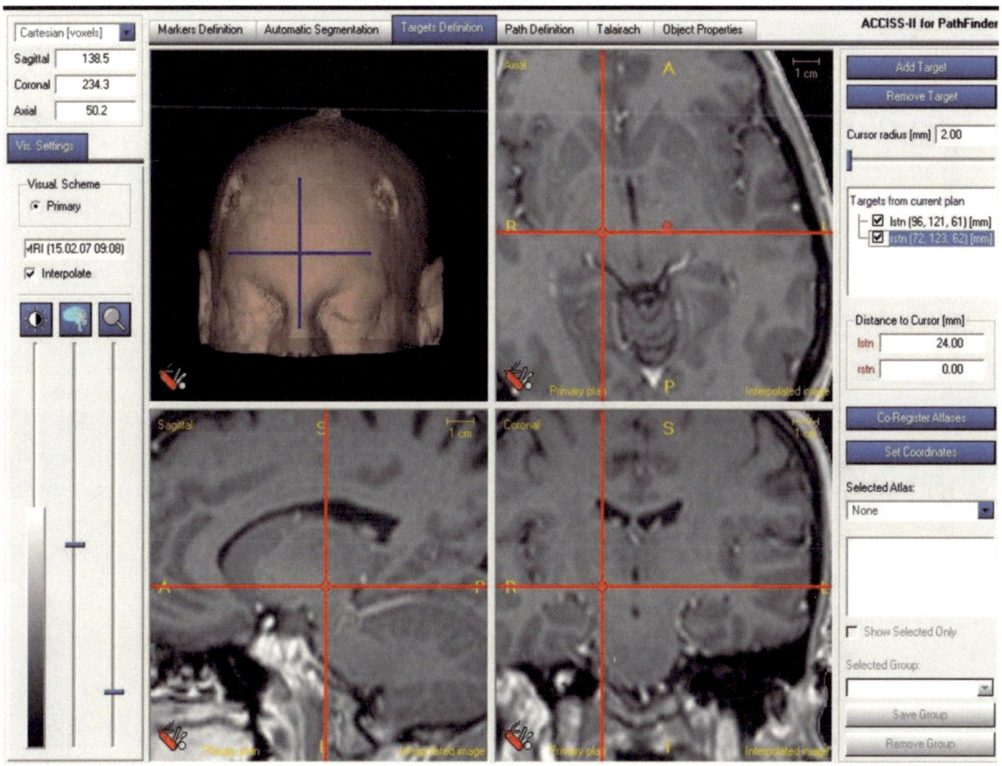

Figure 13. A robotic plan for DBS placement or lesion generation in the left subthalamic nucleus

- Intracranial lesion generation:

Intracranial lesions are less commonly used nowadays in neurosurgery as the neurostimulation technology provides the same clinical efficacy of lesions with a lesser risk. However, lesions in one side of the pallidum, thalamus, internal capsule or the cingulum still have a place in the management of functional disorders of the brain. Their precise planning and execution requires the accuracy of the stereotactic frame and the flexibility of image guidance. Precise accuracy and flexibility are the characteristics of the robotic system and therefore it would be an ideal system to execute these lesions (Figure 12).

- Epilepsy surgery:

Temporal lobe surgery is a cost-effective treatment for drug resistant temporal lobe epilepsy (Alarcon et al., 2006 and Kelemen et al., 2006). Its success is dependant on pre and intra-operative localisation of the epileptogenic focus and the surgery is facilitated by early identification of the temporal horn. To locate precisely the temporal horn and the epilepsy focus we explored the use of a neurosurgical robot. We found that the robotic system was very useful in inserting depth electrodes precisely to localise the seizure focus and was very helpful to identify the temporal horn early on, shortening the procedure (Figure 14) (Eljamel, 2006).

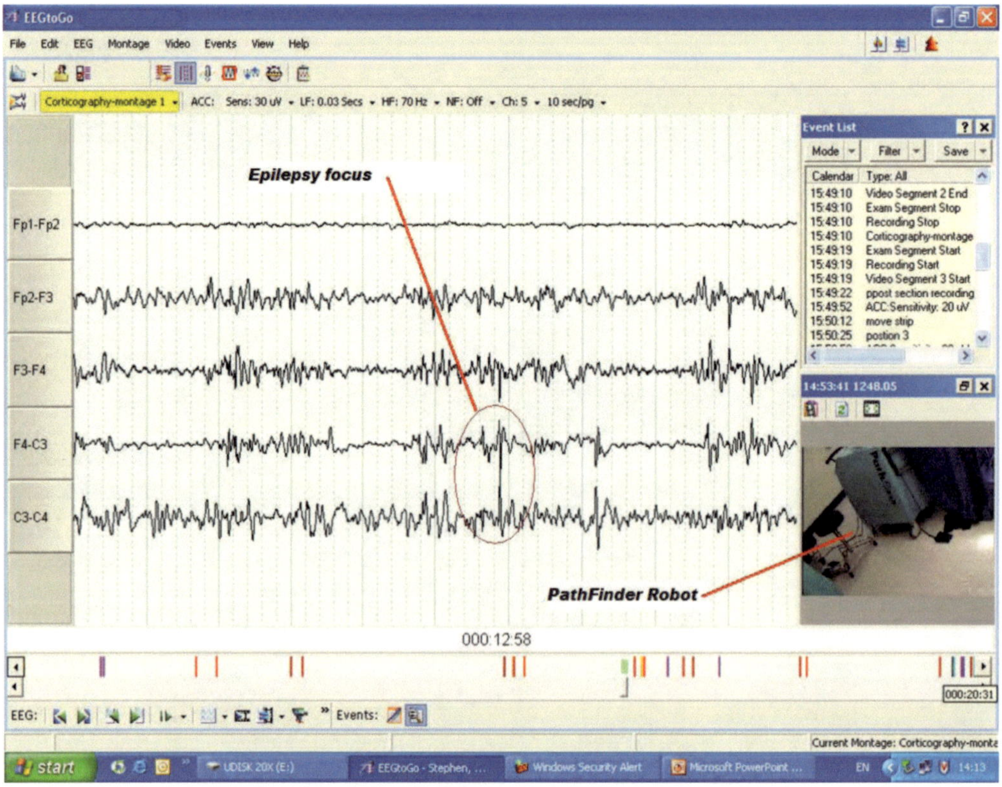

Figure 14. Intraoperative corticography for epilepsy focus localisation, notice the PathFinder in the right bottom corner where it was used to insert depth electrodes and insert a catheter in the temporal horn of the lateral ventricle during medial temporal lobectomy for temporal lobe refractory epilepsy

- Intracranial vascular lesions:

Intracranial arteriovenous malformation (AVM) and intracerebral haematomas can be treated using the robotic system. The system could be used to localise the AVM and planning of the surgery, while in spontaneous haematoma the robot could be used to aspirate the blood clot precisely.

- Hydrocephalus and intracranial cysts:

The robotics system is ideally suited for draining intracranial cysts. A colloid cyst which lies within the third ventricle and can cause hydrocephalus can be drained using the robot. Pineal body cysts and other cysts of the third ventricle can also be drained this way. Craniopharyngioma is another tumour that can present with large cysts and other tumour cysts (Figure 15) and can also be drained using the robotic system. The robot can also be used to place shunt tubing into any of the aforementioned cystic lesions or hydrocephalus. These intracystic catheters can then be connected to a valve to shunt the fluid away to a suitable absorption cavity such as the peritoneum in hydrocephalus or the catheter can be connected to a subcutaneous reservoir for future aspirations or instillation of therapeutic agents in the case of tumour cysts.

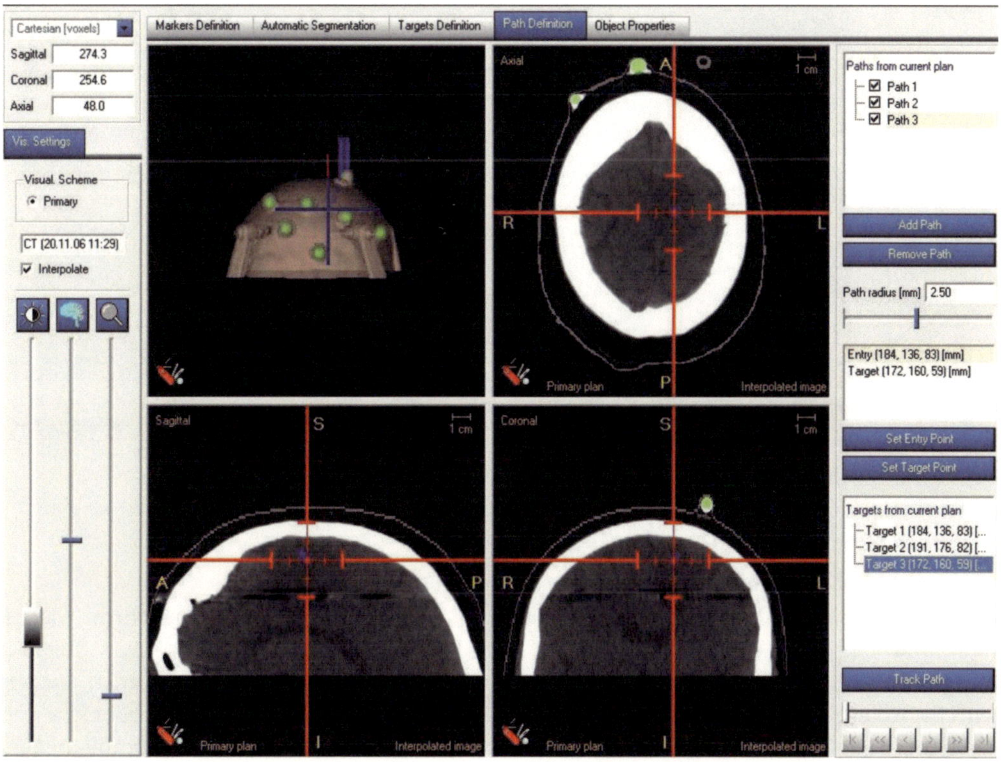

Figure 15. A robotic plan for drainage and biopsy of left frontal lobe cyst

- Head trauma:

In head trauma, the lateral ventricles are often very small and cannot be drained effectively using freehand methods, a robotic system will be an ideal tool to insert very precisely an external ventricular drain when required to drain cerebrospinal fluid (CSF) and control the raised intracranial pressure in these critical patients.

- Pituitary lesions:

Pituitary lesions, including simple cysts, pituitary abscess and Rathke cleft cysts, can be drained using the robot via the trans-nasal - transsphenoidal route (Figure 16). Furthermore pituitary ablation using chemicals, such as alcohol, can be performed.

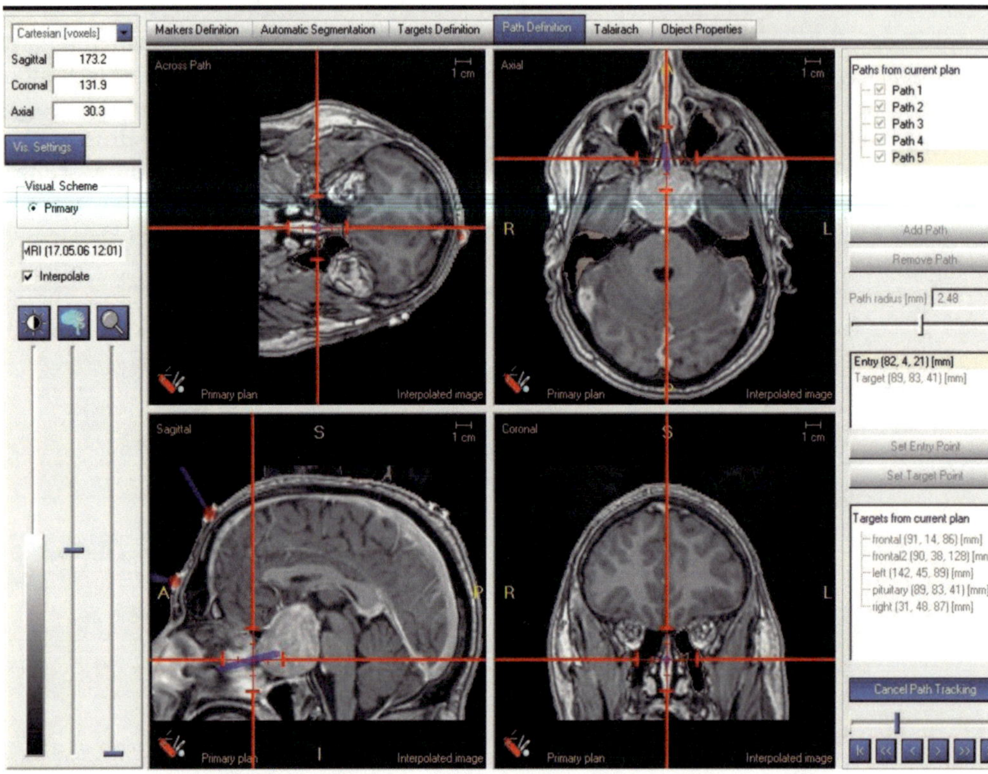

Figure 16. A robotic plan for reaching a pituitary lesion through the transnasal-transsphenoidal route for either aspirating a pituitary abscess, pituitary cyst, Rathke cleft cyst or injecting a chemical to ablate the pituitary gland

- Spinal surgery:

There are potential spinal applications in spinal surgery to perform needle aspiration/biopsy of spinal pathology or to align trajectories for pedicle screw fixation, lateral mass plating or C1/2 fixation. The principles are the same as intracranial surgery with the exception that each vertebral level had to be registered in turn or the robotic system needed to be integrated with fluoroscopy, which can be easily achieved. An example of such robotic application is the SpineAssist® (Shoham et al., 2007).

- Cranial and body radiotherapy:

The CyberKinfe is an excellent example of cranial and body radiotherapy application of robotics, allowing a high tumour irradiation dose with minimal normal tissue exposure to the harmful radiation as discussed earlier in this chapter. Furthermore, the robotic system could be used to insert radioisotope implants or intraoperative radiosurgery machines such as the Photoelectrone radiosurgery system 400 (Figure 17 and 18). The advantage of robotic systems in this modality of therapy is the precision, the speed at which therapy can be delivered and the ability of the system to deliver therapy remotely in a radiation shielded environment without the risk of radiation to the surgeon or other staff looking after the patient.

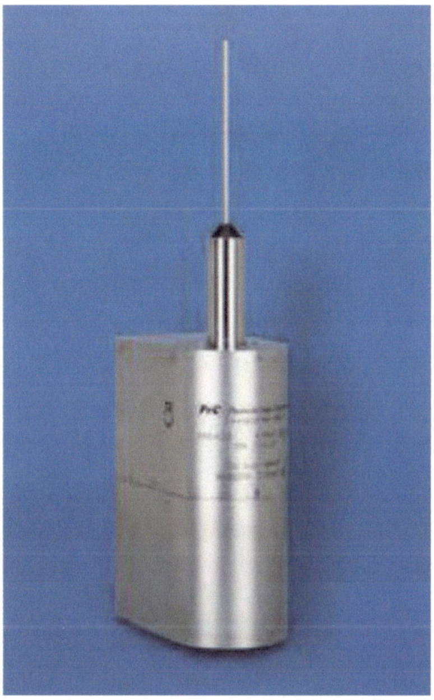

Figure 17. Intraoperative Photoelectron radiotherapy system (PRS400) which can fit nicely in the Pathfinder robot. The robot could perform a stereotactic biopsy followed by radiosurgery

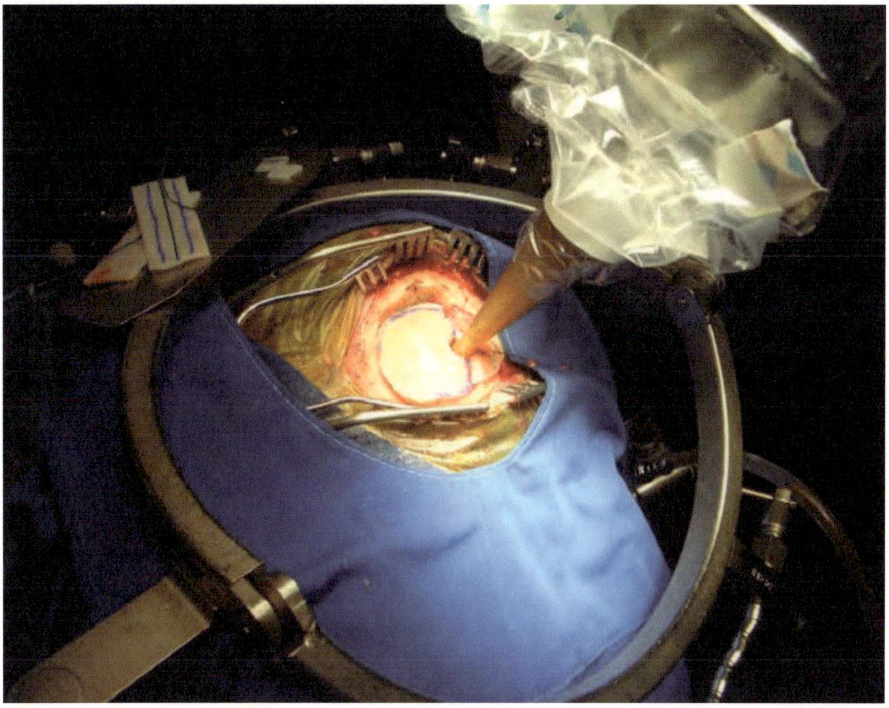

Figure 19. Intraoperative radiotherapy of a malignant brain tumour using the Photoelectron radiotherapy system (PRS400)

- Futuristic therapies:

The robotic system is an ideal tool to implant micro-catheters in deep structures of the brain to deliver missing or deficient neurotransmitters or growth factors such as glial derived neurotrophic factor (GDNF) to promote neuro-regeneration (Gill et al., 2003). It would be also an ideal delivery system for neurotansplantation (Ourednik & Ourednik, 2004) and victor and gene therapy (Alavi & Eck, 2001). Although these modalities of therapy are still in their infancy at present, it is only a matter of time before they will be used on a large scale to treat neuro-degenerative diseases such as Parkinson's disease and Alzheimer's disease.

5. The Future of Robotics in Neurosurgery

The future of robotics in neurosurgery is bright and it is not going to be long before each neurosurgical operating room, each neuro CT scanner and each neuro MRI scanner will be integrated with a robotic system. This inevitable progression is natural as we move along the path from image-guided minimally invasive surgery to a technology driven nano surgery. The scale of neurosurgical procedures in the future is going to be so small that neurosurgeons will not be able to deliver them without the assistance of robotics. The amount of collateral damage acceptable by patients in the future is going to be none that current technology and human performance would not be able to guarantee without the use of robotics. Patients in the future will be asking a different question from what present patients are asking: it is not going to be "who is the surgeon?" but who is the surgeon's assistant?

Robotics in the future will incorporate new technology that will make it possible for these systems to analyse tissue composition by combining imaging, biochemical and biological markers of these tissues to deliver specific treatment and repair any abnormal tissue damage. One example of such futuristic application which can be integrated in robotics is the NASA smart probe project which utilises neural network and fuzzy logic algorithms to integrate data from multiple sensors in real-time for tissue identification (Andrews et al., 2006).

6. References

Alarcón G, Valentín A, Watt C, Selway RB, Lacruz ME, Elwes RDC, Jarosz JM, Honavar M, Brunhuber, F Mullatti N, Bodi I, Salinas M, Binnie CD, Polkey CP. (2006). Is it worth pursuing surgery for epilepsy in patients with normal neuroimaging? *J Neuro Neurosurg Psych* 77: 474- 480.

Alavi JB, Eck SL. (2001). Gene therapy for high grade gliomas. *Expert Opin Biolog Ther.* 1: 239- 252.

Andrews R, Mah R, Papasin R, Guerrero M, DaSilva L. (2006) The NASA Smart Probe Project for real-time tissue identification; poential application in neurosurgery, In: *Minimally Invasive Neurosurgery and Multidisciplinary Neurotraumatology* , Kanno, Tetso(Ed.), p 212-215, Springer, 978-4-431-28551-9, Japan.

Benabid AL, Cinquin P, Lavalle S, Le Bas JF, Demongest J, de Rougemont J. (1987). Computer-driven robot for stereotactic surgery connected to CT scan and magnetic resonance imaging; technological design and preliminary results. *Appl Neurophysiol* 50: 153- 154.

Benabid AL, Hoffmann D, Ashraf A, Koadse A, Esteve F, La Bas JK. (1998) Robotics in neurosurgery; current status and future aspects. *Chirurgie* 123:25-31.

Berguer R.(1999). Surgery and ergometrics. *Arch Surg* 134: 1011- 16.

Brown MJ, Perman M, Wu X, Yang J, Schwade JG. (2005). Image-guided robotic stereotactic radiosurgery for treatment of lung cancer, In: *Robotic Radiosurgery, Volume I,* Mould RF, Bucholz RD, Gagnon GJ, Gerszten PC, Kresl JJ, Levendag PC, Schlz RA, (Eds), p 255 - 268, The CyberKnife Society Press, 0-9731241-3, Sunnyvale, CA.

Burckhart CW, Flury P, Glauser D. (1995). Stereotactic Brain Surgery *IEEE Engineering in Medicine and Biology* 14: 314- 317.

Chenzie K, Miller K. (2001). Towards MRI guided surgical manipulator. *Med Sci Monit* 7: 163- 173.

DiMaio SP, Pieper S, Chinzei K, Hata N, Balogh E, Fichtinger G, Tempany CM, Kikinis R. (2006). Robot-assisted needle placement in open-MRI: system architecture, integration and validation. *Studies Health Technol. Informatics* 119:12 6–131.

Drake JM, Joy M, Goldenberg A, Kreindler D. (1991). Computer and robot assisted resection of thalamic astrocytomas in children. *Neurosurgery* 29: 27- 29.

Eljamel MS .(2006). Robotic application in epilepsy surgery. *Int J Med Robotics Comp Ass Surgery* 2: 233- 237.

Gerszten PC, Burton SA, Ozhasogla C, Vogel WJ, Quinn AE. (2005). CyberKnife radiosurgery: single fraction treatment for spinal tumors, In: *Robotic Radiosurgery, Volume I,* Mould RF, Bucholz RD, Gagnon GJ, Gerszten PC, Kresl JJ, Levendag PC, Schlz RA, (Eds), p 171 - 186, The CyberKnife Society Press, 0-9731241-3, Sunnyvale, CA.

Gill S, Patel NK, Hotton GR, O'Sullivan K, McCarter R, Bunnage M, Brooks DJ, Svendsen CN, Heywood P. (2003). Direct Brain Infusion of Glial Cell Line Derived Neurotrophic Factor in Parkinson's disease. Nature medicine, 9:589-595.

Giller CA, Berger BD, Delp JL, Bowers DC. (2005). CyberKnife radiosurgery for children with malignant central nervous system tumors, In: *Robotic Radiosurgery, Volume I,* Mould RF, Bucholz RD, Gagnon GJ, Gerszten PC, Kresl JJ, Levendag PC, Schlz RA, (Eds), p 133 - 146, The CyberKnife Society Press, 0-9731241-3, Sunnyvale, CA.

Goodman KA, Koong AC. (2005). CyberKnife radiosurgery for pancreatic cancer, In: *Robotic Radiosurgery, Volume I,* Mould RF, Bucholz RD, Gagnon GJ, Gerszten PC, Kresl JJ, Levendag PC, Schlz RA, (Eds), p 301 - 314, The CyberKnife Society Press, 0-9731241-3, Sunnyvale, CA.

Kelemen A. Barsi P. Eross L. Vajda J. Czirjak S. Borbely C. Rasonyi G. Halasz P.(2006). Long-term outcome after temporal lobe surgery--prediction of late worsening of seizure control. *Seizure.* 15: 49- 55.

Kwoh YS, Hou J, Jonckheere GA, Hayah S. (1988). A Robot with improved absolute positioning accuracy got CT- guided stereotactic brain surgery. *IEEE Trans Biomed Eng* 55:153-160.

Louw DF, Fielding T, McBeth PB, Gregoris D, Newhook P,. Sutherland GR. (2004). Surgical robotics: a review and neurosurgical pro-. totype development. *Neurosurgery* 54: 525- 534.

Masamune K, Kobayashi E, Masutani Y. (1995). Development of an MRI comatible needle insertion manipulator for stereotactic neurosurgery. *J Image Guided Surgery* 1: 242-248.

Massaudi F, Chenery SG, Cherlow J, Danmore S, Chehabi HH. (2005). CyberKnife clinical outcome in trigeminal neuralgia, In: *Robotic Radiosurgery, Volume I*, Mould RF, Bucholz RD, Gagnon GJ, Gerszten PC, Kresl JJ, Levendag PC, Schlz RA, (Eds), p 117- 123, The CyberKnife Society Press, 0-9731241-3, Sunnyvale, CA.

Medbery CA, Young MM, Morrison AE, Archer JS, D'Souza MF, Parry C. (2005). CyberKnife monotherapy in prostate cancer, In: *Robotic Radiosurgery, Volume I*, Mould RF, Bucholz RD, Gagnon GJ, Gerszten PC, Kresl JJ, Levendag PC, Schlz RA, (Eds), p 325 - 332, The CyberKnife Society Press, 0-9731241-3, Sunnyvale, CA.

Ourednik V, Ourednik J. (2004). Multifaceted dialogue between graft and host in neurotransplantation. *J Neuroscience Res,* 76: 193- 204.

Radstzky A, Radolph M. (2001). Simulating tumor removal in neurosurgery. *Int J Med Inf* 64: 461- 472.

Sakamoto G, Sinclair J, Gibbs C, Adler JR, Chang SD. (2005). Stereotactic radiosurgery for acoustic neuroma using the CyberKnife, In: *Robotic Radiosurgery, Volume I*, Mould RF, Bucholz RD, Gagnon GJ, Gerszten PC, Kresl JJ, Levendag PC, Schlz RA, (Eds), p 125 - 132, The CyberKnife Society Press, 0-9731241-3, Sunnyvale, CA.

Shoham M, Lieberman H, Benzel EC, Togawa D, Zehavi E, Zilberstein B, Roffman M, Bruskin A, Fridlander A, Joskowicz L, Brink-Danan S, Knollier N. (2007). Robotic assisted spinal surgery – from concept to clinical practice. *Computer Aided Surgery* 12; 105- 115.

Young MM, Medbery CA, Morrison AE, Gumerlock MK, White B, Angles C, Reynolds WE, D'Souza MF, Parry C, Harriet V. (2005). Stereotactic radiosurgery in brain metasteses from non-small cell lung cancer, comparison of Gamma Knife and CyberKnife, In: *Robotic Radiosurgery, Volume I*, Mould RF, Bucholz RD, Gagnon GJ, Gerszten PC, Kresl JJ, Levendag PC, Schlz RA, (Eds), p 97- 107, The CyberKnife Society Press, 0-9731241-3, Sunnyvale, CA.

Zimmermann M, Krishnan R, Raabe A, Seifert V. (2002). Robot-assisted navigated neuroendoscopy. *Neurosurgery* 51: 1446 - 1451.

6

Autonomous Virtual Mobile Robot for the Exploration of 3D Medical Images

Luca Ferrarini, Hans Olofsen, Johan H.C. Reiber and Faiza Admiraal-Behloul
Leiden University Medical Center – Department of Radiology, Division of Image Processing
The Netherlands

1. Introduction

Imaging techniques, such as Magnetic Resonance Imaging (MRI) and Computerized Tomography (CT), can provide nowadays high-resolution volumetric representations of the inner human body. Thus, non-invasive visualization and analysis of organs' structures and functions have become increasingly more important in medical research and clinical practice. Nevertheless, any thorough examination involves massive amount of images, and a manual exploration is simply a prohibitive and time-consuming task. Consequently, several (semi-) automatic tools have been developed to support physicians, including the detection of regions of interest, structural and functional analyses, and data-driven visualization techniques for data exploration. Virtual endoscopy is a highly intuitive and non-invasive approach to the analysis of structures with tubular topology (e.g., blood vessels, airways, colons, cochleae, etc.): different implementations are available, and the majority of them rely on the detection of the central path of the tubular structure.

Several methods have been presented in the literature for central line extraction, based on distance maps and minimal path search (Truyen et al., 2001; Haigron et al., 2004), skeletons (Kirali et al., 2004), and wave-propagation (Marquering et al., 2005). The different approaches present some limitations: methods based on wave-propagation need to control the wave's front to avoid leaking outside the lumen; skeleton-based approaches often require post-processing steps such as pruning of the skeleton, smoothing and closing of the final path, etc.; finally, methods based on depth-maps are usually computationally heavy and therefore difficult to apply in daily clinical practice. The most desirable properties of a virtual endoscopy system are a smooth and unique trajectory through the structure, quantitative analysis of well-defined properties (e.g., radius estimation, detection of anomalies, etc.), and real time interaction (when required by the user); finally, a virtual endoscopy system should be as general as possible, allowing for the exploration of different organs of similar topology.

In this chapter, we present a new approach to central line detection and virtual endoscopy, based on Autonomous Virtual Mobile Robots (AVMRs). Mobile robots have already proved helpful in several situations in which direct human intervention is either impossible or highly dangerous: blasting operations, oceanographic explorations, space missions, etc.

Small robots provided with cameras have also been used in medical applications (Rentschler et al., 2006). The literature on mobile robot navigation is copious: for a more extensive bibliography, the reader is referred to Ng & Trivedi, 1998, and Braunstingl et al., 1995. Most of the literature on real mobile robot deals with planar exploration, thus with a 2-dimensional (2D) navigation problem. In a previous work (Admiraal-Behloul et al., 2004), we already proved that a 2D virtual mobile robot could successfully be trained to detect the myocardium contour in MR short axis images of the heart. We extended that idea to a 3D non-holonomic autonomous virtual mobile robot, which can explore 3D virtual reconstructions (MRI volumetric data) of tubular structures. The central path extracted by the robot is always unique (i.e. no further pruning is required); moreover, by applying non-holonomic constraints one can guarantee a smooth solution for the final path. The AVMR is provided with three modules: a sensory system to perceive the surroundings, a virtual camera to provide real-time internal views, and a trajectory planner to navigate in the environment, maintaining a central position with respect to the tube. Two kinds of navigation modules are presented: a 3D neuro-fuzzy controller (NFC) (based on the 2D solution presented by Ng & Trivedi, 1998), and a distance-map based approach for branch detection. A thorough validation on challenging synthetic environments was performed to prove the robustness of our approach; moreover, we applied our method on several medical datasets, showing how AVMRs can elegantly overcome some critical issues in central path detection and improve virtual endoscopy.

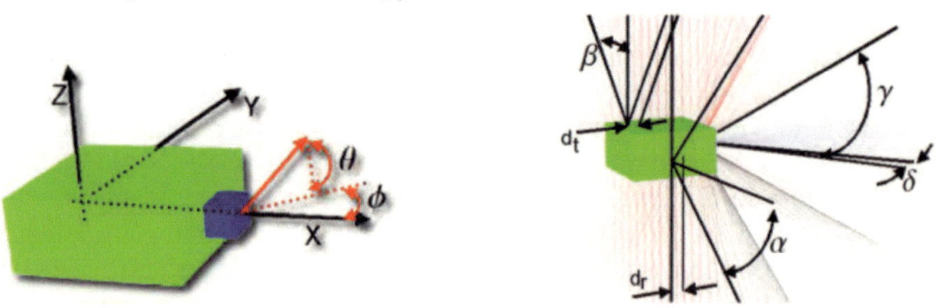

a b

Figure 1. (a) Local coordinate system of the mobile robot and steering vector: the desiderd direction is fully described by two angels in the local system. (b) Sensory system of the AVMR: frontal sensors are described by two angles, γ and δ; lateral sensors are described by an angle α and a relative distance d_r (β and d_t for top and down sensors)

2. Method

One can think of the AVMR as a flying object fully characterized by geometrical properties, kinematics constraints, and a trajectory planner. Aim of the AVMR is to move through a tubular structure keeping a central position: in order to accomplish that, a *sensory module,* based on virtual range sensors, senses the surrounding and feeds the results back to the *trajectory planner*. Depending on the particular navigation technique, the AVMR evaluates the desired direction for its next step: the feasibility of such a step is tested by the *Kinematics and Feasibility* module, and the actual new direction is assessed in according with the kinematics constraints. The modular design of the AVMR makes it possible to easily add new functionalities to the robot, as we will see in the section 5 (as future work).

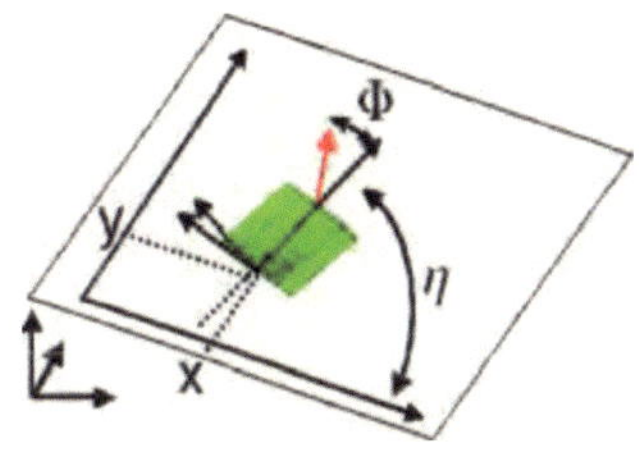

Figure 2. Three dimensional nonholonomic constraints: the AVMR moves following 2D nonholonomic constraints, applied at each step on a well-defined plane (see eq. 1, 2, and 3)

2.1 The geometrical properties of the AVMR

The geometry of the AVMR is fully characterized by few parameters: its length L, its width W, and its thickness T (see Fig. 1.a). A steering system is located at the front of the robot (indicating the direction for the next step); considering a local coordinate system fixed on the AVMR, the steering vector is described by two angles, ϕ and θ, on the xy and xz local planes.

The *sensory system* is formed by virtual range sensors located all around the robot (see Fig. 1.b): each sensor is fully described by two angles in the local coordinate system, and is represented as a line which propagates through the virtual environment until a certain condition is matched: if we call *lumen* the inner part of the tubular structure the AVMR has to explore, then the stopping criteria for a sensor will be the detection of lumen's boundaries[1].

Finally, the AVMR is provided with a virtual camera orientated along the local x axis of the robot: 3D rendering techniques are used to generate real-time internal views of the explored structure.

2.2 The 3D non-holonomic kinematics and feasibility test

The information retrieved by the *sensory* module is fed to the *trajectory planner* module (presented in the next section): the output is a desired direction in 3D which keeps the robot's position and orientation aligned to the structure. The angles ϕ and θ, describing the steering vector, are constrained to guarantee smooth movements: $\phi \in [\phi_{min}, \phi_{max}]$, $\theta \in [\theta_{min}, \theta_{max}]$. During an offline phase, these intervals are discretized, and minimum corridors are estimated for each direction: when a disered direction is given to the robot, the AVMR looks for the closest descrete solution (i.e. corridor), and compares the sensory information with the prior-knowledge of minimum corridor space previously learnt. If the available distances returned by the sensors are not sufficiently safe (to avoid obstacle collision), a more suitable corridor is chosen.

---

[1] In this work, we present different kinds of datasets: synthetic environments were generated as binary volumes; medical datasets were either pre-segmented (thus, converted in binary volumes), or used in their original gray values: in this case, prior-knowledge and local adjustments of the lumen intensity distribution are needed to detect the boundaries during the exploration. A detailed explanation on intensity estimation is not in the scope of this article: it is sufficient to say that even when gray value images are considered, from the robot point of view all goes down to a binary representation of the environment.

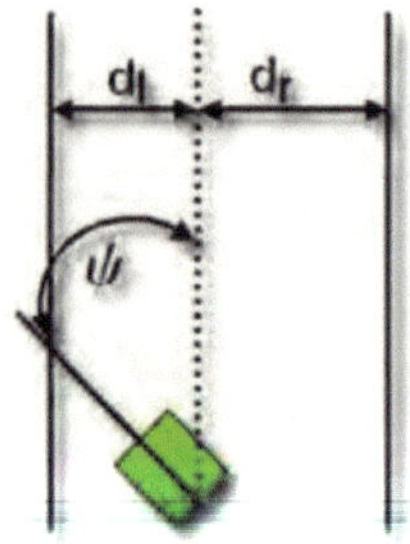

Figure 3. The AVMR estimates its position and orientation relative to the tube by using its range sensors: the three dimensional problem is split into two two-dimensional problems on local planes

Once a feasible corridor (i.e., direction) has been found, the AVMR has to move one step in that direction, respecting the non-holonomic constraints. In 2D, the formulae for non-holonomic movements are well known (see Fig. 2): considering the robot's position (x^t,y^t), the speed v, the desired direction Φ, and the current orientation η, the new position and orientation at *t+1* are given by:

$$x^{t+1} = x^t + v\cos(\Phi)\cos(\eta)\Delta t, \tag{1}$$

$$y^{t+1} = y^t + v\cos(\Phi)\sin(\eta)\Delta t, \tag{2}$$

$$\eta^{t+1} = \eta^t + \frac{v}{L}\sin(\Phi)\Delta t. \tag{3}$$

In order to apply these formulae in 3D, one needs to define a new 2D plane at each step of the robot (see Fig. 2), identified by the local x axis and the steering vector. A new local coordinate system is defined on the plane, with the new x axis along the AVMR's x axis and the origin located in the origin of the robot's coordinate system (in Fig. 2, the coordinate system is drawn in a different position just to simplify the representation): the previous equations are then simplified, since η^t always equals 0 and (x^t,y^t) always equals (0,0).

2.3 Trajectory Planner

The *trajectory planner* developed for the AVMR is based on a neuro-fuzzy controller. The aim of the controller is to keep the AVMR in a centered position and aligned orientation with respect to the tubular structure. A 2D neuro-fuzzy controller for real robot navigation was introduced by Ng & Trivedi, 1998. We extended their approach to 3D by splitting the three-dimensional navigation problem into two two-dimensional problems: one on the local *xy* plane, and one on the local *xz* plane. By using its range sensors, the AVMR estimates its position and orientation (related to the structure) on both planes: this information is fed into two independent neuro-fuzzy controllers which provide back the desired directions (ϕ, θ for the local *xy* and *xz* planes respectively) the AVMR should take to maintain a central position and orientation. We summarize the procedure for the local *xy* plane only.

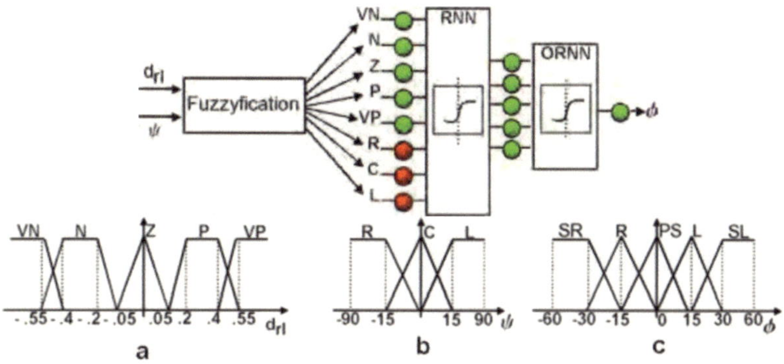

Figure 4. (*top*) General scheme for the NFC: the input variables are fuzzyfied before being fed to the RNN neural network. The fuzzy output membership functions are defuzzyfied by the ORNN neural network. (*bottom*) Membership functions for position (a), orientation (b), and desired output angle (c)

The sensors of the AVMR, depending on their orientation with respect to the local coordinate system, contribute to the evaluation of the AVMR's distance from either the left or right wall (see Fig. 3): d_l and d_r. These two distances are normalized into a single measurement:

$$d_{rl} = \frac{d_r - d_l}{d_r + d_l}, \tag{4}$$

with d_{rl} = -1, when the AVMR is close to the right wall, and 1 when close to the left wall. The orientation of the robot ψ is evaluated by using only its lateral sensors (see Fig. 3). The d_{rl} and ψ variables are finally given to a neuro-fuzzy system, whose scheme is shown in Fig. 4. The input variables are first fuzzyfied using the membership functions shown in Figures 4.a 4.b. Subsequently a first neural network (RNN, Rule Neural Network) is used to map the 8 fuzzy values onto 5 membership functions corresponding to output categories (Fig. 4.c). Finally, a second neural network (ORNN, Output Refinement Neural Network) is used to defuzzyfy its input into a single crisp value: the desired steering angle ϕ on the xy plane. When the same procedure is applied to the local xz plane, the desired steering angle θ is obtained: the combination of ϕ and θ gives the desired direction in 3D. For more details on the training and implementation of the neuro-fuzzy controller, the reader is referred to Ferrarini et al., 2005, and Ng & Trivedi, 1998.

3. Validation in Synthetic Environments

The performances of the mobile robot were thoroughly validated. Several synthetic environments were created, and the AVMR was asked to detect their central lines: at each step, the error from the ideal path was evaluated. A statistical analysis was performed over 50 runs through each synthetic environment. Straight corridors, u-shaped corridors, and s-shaped corridors were created for the tests. The robustness of the AVMR was tested adding noise to the environments: surface locations were randomly removed creating holes. Using the straight tube, we also tested the effects of changing radii on the final performances. In Fig. 5, some of the synthetic environments are shown. In structures without noise, the

AVMR could detect the central line with an average error of about 6% of the diameter. The error increased to 9% of the diameter when noise was introduced: the amount of randomly removed surface ranged from 20% to 80% of the total surface. A more complete overview of the AVMR's performances can be found in Ferrarini et al., 2005.

Figure 5. Synthetic environments used for the validation: (*left*) example of straight tube with changing radius; (*center*) u-shaped tube; (*right*) close-up on random noise in u-shaped tube: the central path is also visible

4. Application to Medical Datasets

The AVMR was applied to the exploration of different medical datasets: a colon, a carotid artery, and 8 cochleae. These organs differ substantially, both topologically and geometrically: nevertheless, only few parameters of the AVMR needed to be tuned in order to have a successful exploration of the environments. The colon dataset had an anisotropic resolution of 2.9x2.9x1 mm^3, and the colon's length was approximately 1.3 m; the cochleae were scanned post-mortem with micro-CT: they presented an isotropic resolution of 0.07 mm, a total length of about 30 mm, and a diameter changing from 2 mm down to 0.5 mm; finally, the CT dataset of the carotid artery was acquired with a resolution of 0.23x0.23x0.6 mm^3, and presented changes in diameter due to stenosis and normal anatomical variations.
The AVMR could successfully explore all the environments: the only application-dependent parameters were the AVMR's dimensions and speed, and the angle constraints on the maximum steering angle (smooth constraint). While exploring the datasets, internal view were available in real-time to the end user. Results are shown in Fig. 6. The central paths obtained for the 8 cochleae were compared to manually delineated central lines: the AVMR differed in average for less than 4% of the total length.

5. Latest developments and Future Work

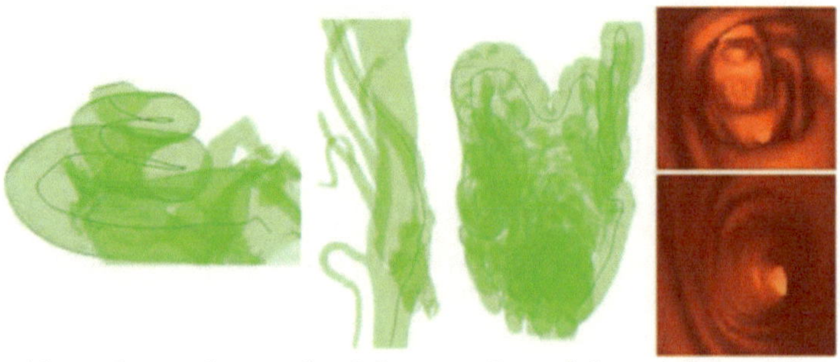

Figure 6. Central lines detected in medical datasets. From left to right: cochlea, carotid artery, colon, and two internal views of the colon obtained with the virtual camera

The virtual mobile robot, as presented in the previous sections, represents a first attempt of merging together the fields of autonomous mobile robots and virtual endoscopy to improve the exploration of medical datasets. Although the first results look very promising, several other modules can be added to the AVMR to improve its performances. In this section, we briefly introduce some of them, and present preliminary results.

5.1 Radius Estimation

The local estimation of the radius along the strcture is important in several medical applications: in carotid arteries, sudden changes in the diameter might indicate aneurysims or stenosis; in clinical pre-operative images of the cochlea, local measurements of the diameter might help planning the surgery and choosing the proper implants (Postnov et al., 2006). We have equiped the robot with a module for radius estimation: at each step during the exploration, lateral sensors collect a cylindrical cloud of surface points; subsequently, an efficient Hough transform (Rabbani & v.d. Heuvel, 2005) is used to fit a cylinder to the cloud of points. The local x direction of the robot is chosen as fixed axis for the cylinder, and the radius is optimized. Preliminary results are shown in Fig. 7 for the carotid artery.

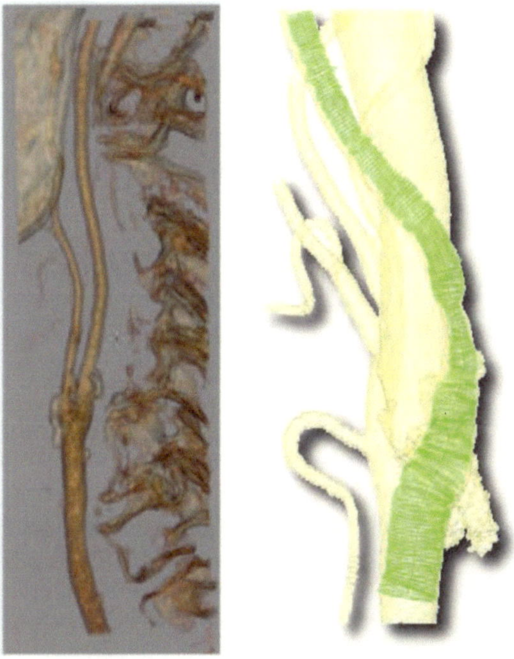

Figure 7. (*Left*) Volume rendering of a carotid artery (CT scan); (*Right*) Local radii estimated by the AVMR

5.2 Navigation based on Distance Maps (branch detection)

One of the characterstics of the neurofuzzy controller is that it does not check for multiple branches along the way: it is designed to keep a central line in tubes of fixed topology. This approach is useful when the topology of the structure is known in advance, like with the cochlea: prior knowledge on the absence of bifurcations makes the method more roboust to noise. Nevertheless, there are cases in which the topology of the structure is not fixed, nor known a priori: in the carotid arteries, the vessel splits into two branches (changing topology); brain vessels present several bifurcations which are not easily modelable beforehand. New navigation modules can be designed to deal with these situations, and the approach we investigated is based on distance maps: while moving through the structure, the AVMR uses the frontal sensors to build up a 2D view of the environment; two dimensional Hough transforms can then be used to identify blobs in the distance maps which correspond to potential corridors in the environment (Fig. 8.a). Prior knoweldge can still be incorporated as the maximum number of branches the AVRM can find along the way. Once a branch is detected, the AVMR clones itself, and the two AVMRs can continue the exploration in parallel. Preliminary results have been obtained both in a binary dataset of brain vessels and in a gray-value dataset of a carotid artery (see Fig. 9.b and 9.c).

6. Discussion and Conclusions

The use of an autonomous virtual mobile robot for the exploration of 3D medical datasets represents the main novelty of this work. Most of the critical issues in central line detection can be elegantly overcome by using an AVMR: the detected path is always unique, connected, and smooth. Moreover, a virtual camera located on the AVMR provides internal views in real-time, allowing intuitive interaction during the exploration.

The important contribution of prior-knowledge in medical image analysis has been shown in previous studies (Passat et al., 2006; Hassouna et al., 2006). The AVMR can easily integrate prior-information in different ways: proper geometrical and kinematics constraints can guide the robot through specific corridors, limit the curvature angles, and reduce the sensitivity to noise. Moreover, global knowledge can be included in the system at a higher level: the second neural network proposed by Ng & Trivedi, 1998 (ORNN) is used, in the current implementation, simply to defuzzyfy the output membership functions; had this to be the only goal, the use of a mathematical formula would be sufficient. Nevertheless, a neural network can be trained for far more complicate tasks: an expert clinician could guide the robot through different environments, and the ORNN could learn a more appropriate mapping for a given application.

The performances of the AVMR were tested on synthetic environments: results showed good accuracy for central line detection, even when substantial noise was added to the structures. When applied to binary and grey-value medical datasets, the AVMR proved to be highly adaptable: by tuning few parameters (i.e., dimensions, speed, and maximum steering angles), the AVMR could successfully explore different environments, such as colons, carotid arteries, and cochleae. The central paths for colon and carotid artery were validated visually, while the measurements of the 8 micro-CT cochleae were compared with manually delineated central paths. The detection of the central line is an important step towards a quantitative analysis of complex anatomical structures: nevertheless, more quantitative information should be extracted by the AVMR: some preliminary results on radius estimation were presented. The module for radius estimation was applied to the exploration of the cochlea and carotid artery: the preliminary results showed on one hand the potential of such approach, and on the other hand some limitations due to noise in the dataset. Finally, different navigation modules are needed for the exploration of complex structures: we have shown preliminary results, based on distance maps, in which the AVMR could successfully detect branches in carotid arteries and brain vessels, clone itself, and continue the exploration in parallel.

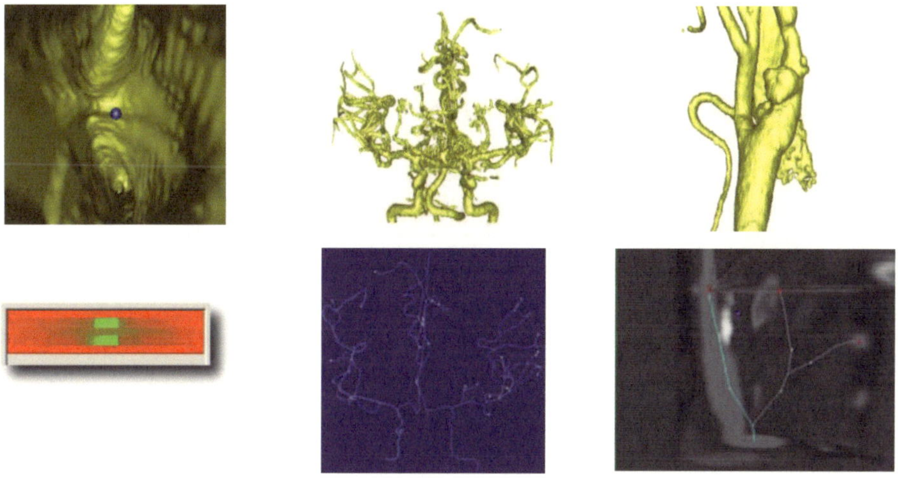

a b c

Figure. 8. (a) Internal 2D view (*top*) reconstructed by the AVMR: the two branches are seen as green blobs in the 2D panel (*bottom*); (b) brain vessels: binary volume (*top*) and central paths detected by the AVMRs (*bottom*); (c) carotid artery: binary volume and close-up to three AVMRs exploring different branches

In conclusion, we have presented an integrated approach to virtual endoscopy: autonomous virtual mobile robots, artificial intelligence techniques, and image processing tools are merged together to provide a robust, efficient, and adaptable solution for three dimensional virtual exploration of medical images.

7. Acknowledgments

The work described in this chapter was supported by the Technology Foundation STW (project number LNN. 6122), and by Medis medical imaging systems bv, Leiden, The Netherlands (www.medis.nl).

8. References

Admiraal-Behloul, F., Lelieveldt, B., Ferrarini, L., Olofsen, H., van der Geest, R. & Reiber, J. (2004). A virtual exploring mobile robot for left ventricle contour tracking, *Proceedings of IJCNN (vol. 1)*, Budapest, Hungary, pp. 333-338.

Braunstingl, R., Sanza, P. & EzkerraJ. (1995). Fuzzy logic wall following of a mobile robot based on the concept of general perception. *Proceedings of the 7th International conference on Advanced Robotics (ICAR)*, Sant Feliu de Guixols, Spain, pp. 367-376.

Ferrarini, L., Olofsen, H., Reiber, J. & Admiraal-Behloul, F. (2005). A neurofuzzy controller for 3D Virtual Centered Navigation in Medical Images of Tubular Structures, *Proceedings in International Conference on Artificial Neural Network (ICANN)*, LNCS 3697, Warsaw, Poland, pp. 371-376

Haigron, P., Bellemare, M., Acorsa, O., Goksu, C., Kulik, C., Rioual, K. & Luca, A. (2004). Depth-map-based scene analysis for active in virtual angioscopy. *IEEE Trans. Med. Imaging*, 23(11), 1380-1390.

Hassouna, M., Farag, A., Hushek, S. & Moriarty, T. (2006). Cerebrovascular segmentation from TOF using stochastic models. *Medical Image Analysis*, 20, 2-18.

Kiraly, A., Helferty J., Hoffman, E., McLennan, G. & Higgins, W. (2004). Three-dimensional path planning for virtual bronchoscopy. *IEEE Trans. Med. Imaging*, 23(11), 1365-1379.

Marquering, H., Dijkstra, P., de Koning, P., Stoel, B. & Reiber, J. (2005). Towards quantitative analysis of coronary cta. *The International Journal of Cardiovascular Imaging*, 21, 73-84.

Ng, K. & Trivedi, M. (1998). A Neuro-fuzzy controller for mobile robot navigation and mutlirobot convoying. *IEEE Trans. on Systems, Man, and Cybernetics - part B*, 28(6), 829-840.

Passat, N., Ronse, C., Baruthio, J., Armspach, J. & Maillot, C. (2006). Magnetic resonance angiography: from anatomical knowledge modeling to vessel segmentation. *Medical Image Analysis*, 10, 259-274.

Postnov, A., Zarowski, Z., de Clerk, N., Vanpoucke, F., Offeciers, F., van Dyck, D. & Peeters, S. (2006). High resolution micro-CT scanning as an innovatory tool for evaluation of the surgical positioning of cochlear implant electrodes. *Acta Oto-laryngologica*, 126, 467-474.

Rabbani, T. & v.d. Heuvel, F. (2005). Efficient Hough transform for automatic detection of cylinder in point clouds, *Proceedings of ISPRS WG III/3 III/4 V3 Workshop – Laser scanning*, Enschede, The Netherlands.

Rentschler, M., Dumpert, J., Platt, S., Ahmed, S., Farritor, S. & Oleynikov, D. (2006). Mobile in vivo camera robots provide sole visual feedback for abdominal exploration and cholecystectomy. *Surg. Endoscopy*, 20, 135-138.

Truyen, R., Deschamps, T. & Cohen, L. (2001). Clinical evaluation of an automatic path tracker for virtual colonoscopy, *Proceedings of Medical Image Computing and Computer-Assisted Intervention (MICCAI)*, Utrecht, The Netherlands, October 2001.

7

Robotic Foregut Surgery

Daniel T. McKenna, M.D. and Jon C. Gould, M.D., FACS
University of Wisconsin School of Medicine and Public Health,
Department of Surgery
United States of America

1. Introduction

Laparoscopy and minimally invasive operative techniques revolutionized abdominal surgery, beginning with the first laparoscopic cholecystectomy in 1987 (Mouret, 1996). Patients, surgeons, and industry alike have promoted the application of these techniques to a wide range of procedures. Smaller incisions and less abdominal wall trauma contribute to improved cosmesis, shorter hospitalizations, less pain, and quicker recovery than is observed following open procedures. Laparoscopic techniques have been widely adopted in a variety of foregut procedures. The laparoscope has allowed surgeons to visualize areas that are more difficult to see in standard open procedures such as the gastroesophageal junction or the diaphragmatic hiatus. These factors have contributed to a population-based rate of antireflux surgery that more than doubled in the United States between 1990 and 1997 (Finalyson, *et* al, 2003).

Several limitations inherent to a laparoscopic approach have prevented its widespread use in some areas of general surgery. The visualization during laparoscopic surgery is typically two-dimensional and limited by camera operator fatigue and abrupt movements. There is diminished tactile feedback, and complex maneuvers are difficult secondary to fixed trocar position and non-articulated instruments. In addition, the length of the instruments amplifies one's natural tremor at the tip of the instrument. During a standard laparoscopic procedure, surgeons frequently must stand in ergonomically awkward positions for extended periods of time.

Surgical robots, or computer-assisted telemanipulators as they are more properly described, allow the surgeon to overcome many of these limitations. Ergonomics are improved as the surgeon sits at a console remote from the patient and manipulates controls for the surgical instruments. The computer eliminates tremor and scales all motions to a selected degree. This allows for very fine and precise movements of the surgical instruments. Since the robotic instruments are multi-articulated and capable of a full range of motion, complex maneuvers are possible. These articulated instruments provide movements similar to the human arm and hand. In addition, high-definition, three-dimensional visualization provides image detail and depth superior to that of a standard laparoscopic system. The camera is manipulated by a robotic arm controlled by the operating surgeon. These features translate to certain advantages during complex foregut procedures when compared to a standard laparoscopic approach.

2. Surgical Robotic Systems

The AESOP system was the first robotic device approved for clinical use by the Food and Drug Administration (FDA) in 1994. The acronym AESOP stands for *A*utomated *E*ndoscopic *S*ystem for *O*ptimal *P*ositioning. This device was developed with research funding from the Pentagon's Defense Advanced Research Projects Agency (DARPA) program. AESOP holds the laparoscope steady without wandering, distraction, or fatigue. The laparoscope and AESOP can be redirected manually by the surgeon. Initially, AESOP functioned via a foot switch or hand control, but eventually voice activated manipulation became standard. AESOP connects to the side of any standard operating table and can accept any rigid laparoscope. While solo surgeon procedures are facilitated with this system, AESOP moves much more slowly than a skilled assistant, which contributed to its limited use by surgeons. The Zeus robotic surgical system was FDA approved for use in abdominal operations in the United States in 2001. Zeus utilized the AESOP system for camera navigation along with two additional multi-articulated robotic arms. Zeus is no longer commercially available. At the time of this writing, the da Vinci robotic surgical system (Intuitive Surgical, Sunnyvale, CA, USA) is the only FDA approved and commercially available robotic system. Da Vinci has received FDA approval for a wide variety of applications including cardiac, thoracic, gynecologic, urologic, and abdominal procedures. This system consists of an operating console, a patient-side cart, and a tower for the insufflator and video electronics. The surgeon sits at the operating console remote from the patient, but usually within the same room. The surgeon's head rests on the console where a high definition, three-dimensional stereoscopic images is displayed. While in this position, the surgeon is able to manipulate the camera and two or three robotic arms in a more natural and ergonomic position than is often possible during standard laparoscopy. The surgeon can toggle manual controls between the camera and any two of the 3 additional arms. The da Vinci's surgical instruments are designed to mimic the dexterity of the human wrist with a full seven degrees of freedom. This provides greater control when performing fine tissue dissection or complex technical procedures when compared to a standard rigid laparoscopic instrument.
There are several limitations to the da Vinci surgical system. The surgeon is provided with essentially no haptic or tactile feedback. Visual cues are necessary to judge tissue tension during dissection or suturing. The da Vinci system is capable of generating a tremendous amount of force, which can be particularly dangerous when movements are made outside of the visual field. The patient side cart and console are large and occupy a lot of floor space in the operating room. The size of the patient side cart limits access by additional personnel (i.e., anesthesiology, circulating nurses) during the procedure to the patient. Once the robot is engaged to the cannulas, the table or patient cannot be repositioned without disengaging the robot. The da Vinci system is also quite expensive and requires specialized instruments with a limited number of uses controlled by the computer. This has been a major factor preventing the wide-spread dissemination of this technology in operating rooms throughout the world.

3. Antireflux Surgery

Laparoscopic antireflux procedures require an advanced set of surgical skills. A surgeon must be adept at fine dissection and suturing. Nissen fundoplication was among the first procedures to be performed robotically. The first two cases of robotic fundoplication were reported by Guy Bernard Cadiere in 1999 (Cadiere, *et* al, 1999). A subsequent prospective randomized trial by Cadiere and colleagues included 21 patients to undergo either a robotic or a laparoscopic Nissen fundoplication. While patients in each study group had similar blood loss, length of stay, and perioperative morbidity, mean operative time was significantly increased (72 vs. 52 minutes; $p<0.01$) in the robotic patients. The authors commented on some difficulties with instrument manipulation and decreased visualization during the robotic cases. These procedures were performed on an earlier version of the da Vinci robotic system known as Mona (Cadiere, *et al*, 2001).

Melvin's group performed a prospective, non-randomized comparative trial of robotic versus standard laparoscopic Nissen fundoplication. Outcomes for the first 20 robotic fundoplications were compared with a group of twenty consecutive laparoscopic fundoplications. On average, the robotic cases took 45 minutes longer. Clinical outcomes, assessed at follow-up by a survey, were similar in the two groups (Melvin, *et al*, 2002). Morino randomized 50 consecutive patients to either robotic or a standard laparoscopic Nissen fundoplication. Total operative time and skin-to-skin time were significantly shorter for conventional laparoscopy. These authors examined the 'learning curve' for robotic cases and determined that there was no difference in the operative time for the first ten and final ten robotic procedures. These surgeons felt that the increased operative time was secondary to robot set-up time, more difficult trocar positioning, and increased time taken to suture the wrap. The cost of the robotic procedure was significantly higher than that for standard laparoscopic fundoplication (euros 3151 vs. euros 1527; $p<0.001$). There were no differences in outcomes based on clinical, endoscopic, or functional assessment (Morino, *et al*, 2006).

Nakadi performed a prospective randomized study to compare the benefits and costs associated with laparoscopic and robot-assisted Nissen fundoplication in 20 patients. Robot-assisted Nissen fundoplication was associated with longer operative times and higher costs compared to the laparoscopic approach. Increased cost for the robot-assisted cases was related to many causes ranging from the initial investment and maintenance, to nursing costs, to the costs for the specialized robotic instrumentation with a limited number of uses (Nakadi, *et al*, 2006).

Several other authors have examined the issue of the impact of a robotic-assisted approach on operative times for fundoplication. Lehnert demonstrated that performing the robotic Thal fundoplication in children took a significantly longer amount of time (Lehnert, *et al*, 2006). When the times were further analyzed, it was clear that time for setup of the robot was significantly longer (20.8±7.5 vs. 34.6±9.2 minutes, $p< 0.05$), but that the actual time to completion of the fundoplication was significantly shorter (30.8 ±8.7 vs. 20.2±5.3 minutes, $p<0.05$). Recently, Muller-Stich and colleagues reported the results of their prospective randomized trial including 40 patients to undergo either conventional laparoscopic fundoplication or a robotic-assisted fundoplication. Contrary to what was observed in several previous trials, the total operative time was shorter for robotic-assisted compared to laparoscopic fundoplications (88 vs. 102 min; p = 0.033). Robotic cases in this series took longer to set-up (23 vs. 20 min; p = 0.050) but involved a shorter effective operating time (65 vs. 82 min; p = 0.006). Outcomes were similar for each technique, but costs were significantly higher for robotic cases (euro 3244 vs. euro 2743, p = 0.003). These investigators concluded that in experienced hands, robotic Nissen fundoplications can be performed faster than conventional laparoscopic fundoplications, but that given the increased cost and equivalent outcomes, laparoscopy should be the preferred choice (Muller-Stich, *et al*, 2007).

Currently, the literature suggests that the robotic-assisted antireflux surgery is as safe and effective as a traditional laparoscopic approach. Computer-assisted fundoplications may be associated with an increased operative time and a higher cost than a traditional laparoscopic approach. At the current level of technology, computer-assisted antireflux surgery does not appear to offer major clinical advantages to patients with skilled and experienced laparoscopic surgeons.

4. Heller Myotomy

Achalasia is a relatively rare condition which can lead to dysphagia and other symptoms related to impaired esophageal emptying. Laparoscopic Heller myotomy has become a standard treatment option for achalasia and has been demonstrated to be effective in greater than 90% of patients. Occasionally, during the course of a myotomy, mucosal perforation occurs. The incidence of mucosal perforations is approximately 5% (Finley, *et al*, 2001). If recognized at the time of the procedure, it is unlikely that the outcome will be affected by this perforation. However, a perforation does require time and advanced laparoscopic suturing skills to repair. Theoretically, robotic surgical system offer several advantages over traditional laparoscopic Heller myotomy. Three-dimensional imaging and more precise and complex movements may contribute to a decreased incidence of mucosal perforation, and if one should occur, robotic systems may facilitate precise mucosal reapproximation and secure repair.

A multi-institutional retrospective study published in 2005 demonstrated that the mean operative time for robotic-assisted Heller myotomy and partial fundoplication was 140.5 minutes in a series of 104 patients. This operative time decreased from 162.6 minutes to 113.5 minutes when the time periods of 2000-2002 and 2003-2004 were compared (p=0.0001). In this study, there were no esophageal mucosal perforations. (Melvin, *et al.*, 2005).

In a prospective, non-randomized study of 121 patients comparing laparoscopic to robotic-assisted Heller myotomy, Horgan demonstrated that operative time was significantly longer in the robotic group (141 vs. 122 minutes, p<0.05). Perhaps demonstrating the effect of the 'learning curve', in the last 30 cases, there was no difference in the operative times between the two groups (108 vs. 104 minutes, p= NS). There were no mucosal perforations in the robotic group compared to 16% rate in the laparoscopic group (p<0.01) Successful relief of symptoms was 90% at 22 months and did not vary based on study group (Horgan, 2005). A recent case series demonstrated similar findings in regards to mucosal perforation rates for robotic myotomy. When comparing 19 robotic myotomies with 51 laparoscopic myotomies, the mucosal perforation rate was 0% for robotic compared to 7.8% for laparoscopic myotomy (Iqbal, *et al*, 2006). Galvani and colleagues found that of 54 patients undergoing robotic Heller myotomy between September 2002 and February 2004, the average operative time was 162 minutes, there were no mucosal perforations, and 93% of patients had symptomatic relief at 17 months follow-up (Galvani, *et al*, 2006).

Based on the results of these published studies, it would appear that robotic-assisted Heller myotomy is safe and effective. Robotic technology may help to decrease the rate of esophageal mucosal perforations. Presumably, this relates to the superior three-dimensional visualization and more complex and precise maneuvers possible with computer-assisted surgical systems.

5. Bariatric Surgery

Morbid obesity is becoming an increasingly prevalent condition world wide. In the United States, obesity is the second leading cause of preventable death (Ogden *et* al, 2002). Many significant medical conditions are associated with obesity including hypertension, diabetes mellitus, heart disease, sleep apnea, osteoarthritis, and hyperlipidemia among others. Bariatric surgery has been demonstrated to lead to significant and durable weight loss, with an improvement or resolution of these obesity-related medical conditions in many cases. Minimally invasive bariatric surgery has several significant advantages when compared to the open approach including a decrease in wound infections, hernias, pulmonary complications, and a shorter hospital stay (Ngyun *et* al, 2001). Laparoscopic bariatric surgery is a complex procedure with a steep learning curve. Computer-assisted surgical devices may be useful tools for these difficult procedures.

Jacobsen demonstrated the advantages of robotic-assisted gastric bypass in 2003. An informal survey of 11 surgeons performing robotic-assisted gastric bypass was conducted. In 107 cases, no anastomotic leaks were reported. The surgeons found this technology useful for several reasons. The three-dimensional view, instruments with articulating 'wrists', and motion-scaling facilitated the construction of a hand-sewn gastrojejunostomy. Several surgeons to respond to this survey felt that this fact may have allowed for the construction of a smaller gastric pouch than is possible with a traditional stapled gastrojejunostomy. Another perceived advantage was that the stiffer robotic instruments did not bend like a conventional laparoscopic instrument might during minimally invasive gastric bypass in especially obese patients with a very thick abdominal wall. Operative times were longer for robotic-assisted procedures compared to traditional open or laparoscopic techniques in the experience of the surgeons to complete this survey (Jacobsen, *et* al, 2003).

Ali and colleagues reported their experience with 50 robotic-assisted laparoscopic Roux-en-Y gastric bypasses (RYGB). In this series, the robotic system was used only for the construction of the gastrojejunostomy using robotic suturing techniques. The remaining portions of the procedures in this series were performed using conventional laparoscopic and stapling techniques. The robot setup time and total operative time decreased as the authors gained experience. Two complications were observed including one anastomotic leak repaired at the time of the original operation, and a gastrojejunostomy stenosis. (Ali, *et al*, 2005).

Docking the patient side robotic cart and setting up this device takes time. With experience, surgical teams have demonstrated that this robot set-up time can be minimized. While robot set-up is a time commitment not required for a case performed using standard laparoscopic techniques, some authors have demonstrated that overall operative times can be decreased for certain procedures when performed robotically. Presumably, this is related to the superior maneuverability and dexterity of robotic surgical instruments. One thought is that this may facilitate and simplify the performance of complex tasks such as suturing. Mohr and colleagues compared their operative times and perioperative complication rates for their first ten totally robotic RYGB cases with a retrospective matched sample of ten patients undergoing RYGB using conventional laparoscopic techniques. The median surgical time (169 vs. 208 minutes; p = 0.03) and median operative time divided by body mass index (BMI) (3.8 vs. 5.0; p = 0.04) were significantly lower for the totally robotic procedures (Mohr, *et al*, 2005). This same group also reported a retrospective review of the operative times and complication rates for their first 75 totally robotic RYGB procedures.

Results were compared between three minimally invasive surgery fellows in order to determine the 'learning curve' for totally robotic RYGB. Each laparoscopic fellow reached a five case running average metric of 3.5 min/BMI by 6th, 7th, and 9th case, with a learning curve of 10-15 cases. This was significantly faster than that of laparoscopic RYGB where the authors averaged 3.7 min/BMI for their first 100 cases, 2.9 min/BMI for their second 200 cases. The authors of this study conclude that totally robotic RYGB is superior to laparoscopic RYGB and that is associated with a faster learning curve (Mohr, *et al*, 2006).
Sanchez and colleagues randomized a new laparoscopic surgery fellow's first 50 cases to either laparoscopic or totally robotic. While there was no differences in age, gender, co-morbidities, complication rates, or length of stay; the mean operating time was significantly shorter for the robotic group (130.8 versus 149.4 minutes; $p = 0.02$). Additionally, they demonstrated a significant difference in minutes per BMI (2.94 versus 3.47 min/BMI; $p = 0.02$). The largest difference was in patients with a BMI > 43 kg/m^2, for whom the difference in procedure time was 29.6 minutes (123.5 minutes for robotic versus 153.2 minutes for laparoscopic; $p = 0.009$), with a significant difference in minutes per BMI (2.49 versus 3.24 min/BMI; $p = 0.009$) (Sanchez, *et al*, 2005).
Robotic performance of bariatric procedures including adjustable gastric banding and biliopancreatic diversion has also been reported. During the course of placing an adjustable gastric band, multiple gastro-gastric sutures are placed in the anterior, proximal gastric wall. This can be quite technically challenging due to poor visualization and ergonomic conditions in some patients. Horgan and colleagues reported operative outcomes for 32 robot-assisted adjustable gastric band placements. Robotic gastric band placement had a lower complication rate and a similar length of stay as gastric bands placed with conventional laparoscopy. Operative times were greater for robotic-assisted cases. These surgeons felt that the robotic system was especially useful in the super obese patient population who can often have a very thick abdominal wall. (Moser and Horgan, 2004). The biliopancreatic diversion is a technically challenging laparoscopic procedure which can require quite a bit of suturing. Sudan and colleagues recently published their experience with robotic biliopancreatic diversion. In a series of 47 patients , the mean operative time was 514 min (range, 370-931 min). The median operative time for the last 10 patients was 379 min (range, 370-582 min). All anastomosis in these cases were performed using robotic suturing techniques. Three patients underwent conversion to open surgery, and four patients experienced postoperative leaks with no mortality (Sudan, *et al*, 2007). Robotic surgical systems with their improved ergonomics and multi-articulated instruments seem ideally suited to very long procedures requiring lots of suturing such as these cases.
The relevant literature suggests that robotic-assisted bariatric surgery is feasible and safe. It is possible that robotic surgical systems may help to shorten the learning curve for surgeons just getting started in minimally invasive bariatric surgery. For experienced surgical teams, it is also possible that these systems may help to decrease operative times, particularly for cases where a lot of suturing is required. Surgery in patients with an elevated BMI or very thick abdominal walls may also be more easily accomplished. Further research and experience is necessary to determine the exact role of robotics in bariatric surgery.

6. Esophagectomy

Esophagectomy is a procedure that can have a high morbidity and mortality rate. Although the optimal surgical approach to esophagectomy remains controversial, the two most frequent approaches within the United States are transhiatal and transthoracic. Minimally invasive surgical approaches to esophagectomy have been reported. These involve laparoscopic and thoracoscopic techniques. Horgan and colleagues reported their initial experience with a case of robotically assisted transhiatal esophagectomy in 2003. The total operative time was 246 minutes and the patient lost less than 50mL of blood. There were no major perioperative complications. It was believed that the three-dimensional image and the articulating wrists allowed them to perform a nearly bloodless dissection of the esophagus. In addition, they found that they could mobilize the esophagus beyond the level of the carina through a trans-abdominal robotic approach. These surgeons felt that this was due to the fact that the robotic instruments are 7.5 cm longer than standard laparoscopic instruments. A thoracoscopic approach to complete esophageal dissection and mobilization was avoided in this case (Horgan, *et al*, 2003).

Gutt and colleagues recently reported their experience with a robotic-assisted trans-hiatal esophagectomy in a patient who had lower esophageal cancer and was a high medical risk for surgery. Esophageal resection and reconstruction was possible without intraoperative incident and with minimal blood loss (Gutt, *et* al, 2006). Van Hillegersberg and colleagues reported their initial experience with robot-assisted thoracoscopic esophagectomy (RTE) with mediastinal lymphadenectomy. Twenty-one consecutive patients with esophageal cancer who underwent RTE with the da Vinci robotic system were evaluated. A total of 18 (86%) procedures were completed thoracoscopically. Robot-assisted thoracoscopic esophagectomy was found to be feasible and safe (van Hillegersberg, 2006).

Recently, Kernstine and colleagues detailed their initial experience with totally robotic esophagectomy with a three field lymphadenectomy. A total of 14 patients with a median age of 64 years underwent esophagectomy using the da Vinci robot. Group 1 consisted of the first three patients in the series, whose surgery was robotically-assisted in the thoracic portion only (robotically assisted esophagectomy). Group 2, the next three patients, had robotically assisted thoracic esophagectomy plus thoracic duct ligation and a laparoscopic abdominal portion with creation of a gastric conduit. Group 3, the last eight patients, underwent completely robotic esophagectomy. It was noted that the total operating room time was 11.1 +/- 0.8 h (range, 11.3-13.2 h), with a console time of 5.0 +/- 0.5 h (range, 4.8-5.8 h). The estimated blood loss was 400 +/- 300 ml (range, 200-950 ml). In this initial series, the operating room time was quite long. The console time or surgical robotic time of 4.9 h was similar to the transhiatal operative time of 4.2 h and less than the operating time of 7 h for the open three-field approach. The authors estimate that the robot docking, neck exposure, feeding tube placement, and esophagogastric anastomosis requires 1.5 h, the resultant true surgical time is estimated to be 6.4 h (4.9 +1.5 h), which leaves nearly 5 h of non-surgical time. To minimize the operating room time and improve efficiency, they felt several steps needed to be taken. These steps include the development of a focused robotic operating team, the use of an experienced surgical assistant and anesthesiologist, precise initial port placement and minimizing the frequency of robotic instrument changes (Kernstire, *et al*, 2007).

While experience with this technique is limited, it appears to be safe. Robotic instruments that are long and multi-articulated may facilitate the completion of minimally invasive esophagectomy to a greater degree than conventional rigid laparoscopic instruments. Further research and clinical experience in this area will be necessary to answer these questions.

7. Future Applications

The future of robotics in foregut surgery seems to be bright. Remote telesurgery is a concept where the surgeon manipulating the robotic controls is separated by a distance from the patient. Marescaux and colleagues performed the first transatlantic robotic procedure in 2001(Marecaux et al., 2001). They successfully removed the gallbladder of a woman in France from New York. Surgeons from McMaster University in Hamilton, Ontario and North Bay General Hospital 400 km north of Hamilton have established a robotic telesurgical service. Twenty-two procedures were performed including 13 fundoplications, 4 sigmoid resections, 3 right hemicolectomies, and 2 hernia repairs (Anvari, 2007). One of the major limiting factors, and a safety issue, relates to signal latency. Latency is the time between when the robotic master controllers are maneuvered, and when the remote robotic arm itself moves. In the experience with remote telesurgery, Anvari observed that a latency of greater than 200 msec required excessive and distracting compensation by the operating surgeon. In the future, with the development of larger and faster signal transfer capabilities, latency will be reduced and telesurgery may become more common. The technology is not the only issue that will need to be addressed before telerobotic foregut surgery becomes commonplace. Many legal and ethical dilemmas arise and will need to be considered carefully.

In vivo robots are miniature, self-propelled devices that can be placed into body cavities to perform certain tasks. At the University of Nebraska, investigators have successfully deployed small robots trans-gastrically into the peritoneal cavity to navigate, visualize, and to grasp or manipulate tissue. (Rentschler and Oleynikov, 2007). These miniature robots are currently in the early stages of development, but hold great promise for the future. Some day, foregut surgery without incisions may be facilitated by these miniature robotic devices deployed from a natural orifice.

Robotic surgical systems of the future may be integrated with sophisticated imaging systems. Preoperative and intraoperative radiographs may help guide a surgeon, or possibly even allow the robotic surgical system to perform parts of selected procedures autonomously.

8. Conclusion

Robotic-assisted foregut surgery is an evolving field with an exciting future. There are many potential advantages to robotic foregut surgery when compared to the conventional laparoscopic approach. The magnified, 3-dimensional image allows for a better view of the operative field and may facilitate the identification and dissection of anatomy. The full range of motion, tremor filtration, and motion scaling afforded by the robotic surgical system can enhance a surgeon's skill, possibly leading to better clinical outcomes and less fatigue. As demonstrated, these relatively new techniques may provide a clinical advantage to surgeons performing esophagectomy, esophageal myotomies, or bariatric procedures. In addition, robotic assistance may in the future allow expert laparoscopic surgeons to assist on procedures performed in remote settings. As robotic technology evolves and disseminates to more operating rooms, it is likely that robotic foregut surgery will become more common.

9. References

Ali MR, Bhaskerrao B, Wolfe BM. (2005). Robot-assisted laparoscopic Roux-en-Y gastric bypass. *Surgical Endoscopy;* Apr;19(4):468-472.

Anvari M. (2007). Remote telepresence surgery: the Canadian experience. *Surgical Endoscopy;* Apr; 21(4):537-41.

Cadiere GB, Himpens J, Vertruyen M, Bruyns J, Fourtanier G. (1999). Nissen fundoplication done by remotely controlled robotic technique. *Annales de Chirurgie;* 53(2): 137-141.

Cadiere GB, Himpens J, Vertruyen M, Bruyns J, Germay O, Lehman G, Izizaw R. (2001). Evaluation of telesurgical NISSEN fundoplication. *Surgical Endoscopy;*Sep;15(9):918-23.

Finlayson SR, Laycock WS, Birkmeyer JD. (2003). National trends in utilization and outcomes of antireflux surgery. *Surgical Endoscopy;* Jun;17(6): 864-867.

Finley RJ, Clifton JC, Stewart KC, Graham AJ, Worsley DF. (2001). Laparoscopic Heller myotomy improves esophageal emptying and the symptoms of achalasia. *Archives of Surgery;* Aug; 136(8): 892-896.

Galvani C, Gorodner MV, Moser F, Baptista M, Donahue P, Horgan S. Laparoscopic Heller myotomy for achalasia facilitated by robotic assistance. (2006). *Surgical Endoscopy;* Jul; 20(7): 1105-12.

Gutt CN, Bintintan VV, Koninger J, Muller-Stich BP, Reiter M, Buchler MW. (2006) Robotic-assisted transhiatal esophagectomy. *Langenbecks Archives of Surgery.* Aug;391(4):428-34.

Horgan S, Berger RA, Elli EF, Espat NJ. Robotic-assisted minimally invasive transhiatal esophagectomy. (2003). *American Surgeon;* Jul; 69(7): 624-626.

Horgan S, Galvani C, Gorodner MV, Omelanczuck P, Ell F, Moser F, Durand L, Caracoche M, Nefa J, Bustos S, Donahue P, Ferraina P. Robotic-assisted Heller myotomy versus laparoscopic Heller myotomy for the treatment of esophageal achalasia: multicenter study. (2005). *Journal of Gastrointestinal Surgery;* Nov;9(8): 1020-1029.

Iqbal A, Haider M, Desai K, Garg N, Kavan J, Mittal S, Filipi CJ. Technique and follow-up of minimally invasive Heller myotomy for achalasia. (2006). *Surgical Endoscopy;* Mar; 20(3): 394-401.

Jacobsen G, Berger R, Horgan S. The role of robotic surgery in morbid obesity. (2003). *Journal of laparoendoscopic & advanced surgical techniques;* Aug; 13(4): 279-283.

Kernstine KH, DeArmond DT, Shamoun DM, Campos JH. The first series of completely robotic esophagectomies with three-field lymphadenectomy: initial experience. (2007). *Surgical Endoscopy;* Jun 26: Epub ahead of print.

Lehnert M, Richter B, Beyer PA, Heller K. A prospective study comparing operative time in conventional laparoscopic and robotically assisted Thal semifundoplication in children. (2006). *Journal of Pediatric Surgery;* Aug;41(8):1392-1396.

Marescaux J, Leroy J, Gagner M, Rubino F, Mutter D, Vix M, Butner SE, Smith MK. Transatlantic robot-assisted telesurgery. (2001). *Nature;* Sep 27; 413(6854):379-380.

Melvin WS, Needleman BJ, Krause KR, Schneider C, Ellison EC. Computer-enhanced versus standard laparoscopic antireflux surgery. (2002). *Journal of Gastrointestinal Surgery;* Jan-Feb; 6(1):11-15.

Melvin WS, Dundon JM, Talamini M, Horgan S. Computer-enhanced robotic telesurgery minimizes esophageal perforation during Heller myotomy. (2005). *Surgery;* Oct; 138(4): 553-8.

Mohr CJ, Nadzam GS, Curet MJ. Totally robotic Roux-en-Y gastric bypass. (2005). *Archives of Surgery*; Aug; 140(8): 779-786.

Mohr CJ, Nadzam GS, Alami RS, Sanchez BR, Curet MJ. Totally robotic laparoscopic Roux-en-Y Gastric bypass: results from 75 patients. (2006). *Obesity Surgery*; Jun;16(6):690-6;.

Morino M, Pellegrino L, Giaccone C, Garrone C, Rebecchi F. Randomized clinical trial of robot-assisted versus laparoscopic Nissen Fundoplication. (2006) *British Journal of Surgery*;. May;93(5):553-558.

Moser F, Horgan S. Robotically assisted bariatric surgery. (2004). *American Journal of Surgery*; Oct; 188 (4a suppl): 38S-44S.

Mouret P. How I developed laparoscopic cholecystectomy. (1996). *Annals of the Academy of Medicine, Singapore*; Sep; 25(5): 744-747.

Müller-Stich BP, Reiter MA, Wente MN, Bintintan VV, Köninger J, Büchler MW, Gutt CN. Robot-assisted versus conventional laparoscopic fundoplication: short-term outcome of a pilot randomized controlled trial. (2007). *Surgical Endoscopy*; Mar 13: epub ahead of print.

Nakadi IE, Melot C, Closset J, DeMoor V, Betroune K, Feron P, Lingier P, Gelin M. Evaluation of da Vinci Nissen fundoplication clinical results and cost minimization. (2006). *World Journal of Surgery*; Jun;30(6):1050-1054.

Nguyen NT, Goldman C, Rosenquist CJ, Arango A, Cole CJ, Lee SJ, Wolfe BM. Laparoscopic versus open gastric bypass: a randomized study of outcomes, quality of life, and costs. (2001). *Ann Surg*; Sept; 234(3):279-289.

Ogden CL, Flegal KM, Carroll MD, Johnson CL. Prevalence and trends in overweight among US children and adolescents, 1999-2000. (2002) *JAMA*; Oct; 288(14):1728-1732

Rentschler ME, Oleynikov D. Recent in vivo surgical robot and mechanism developments. (2007). *Surgical Endoscopy*; May 19; epub ahead of print.

Sanchez BR, Mohr CJ, Morton JM, Safadi BY, Alami RS, Curet MJ. Comparison of totally robotic laparoscopic Roux-en-Y gastric bypass and traditional laparoscopic Roux-en-Y gastric bypass. (2005). *Surgery for obesity and related diseases : official journal of the American Society for Bariatric Surgery*; Nov-Dec;1(6):549-554.

Sudan R, Puri V, Sudan D. Robotically assisted biliary pancreatic diversion with a duodenal switch: a new technique. (2007) *Surgical Endoscopy*; 21(5): 729-33.

van Hillegersberg R, Boone J, Draaisma WA, Broeders IA, Giezeman MJ, Rinkes IH. First experience with robot-assisted thoracoscopic esophagolymphadenectomy for esophageal cancer. (2006) *Surgical Endoscopy*; Sep; 20(9): 1435-1439.

8

Robotic Long Bone Fracture Reduction

A. E. Graham[1], S. Q. Xie[1], K. C. Aw[1], W. L. Xu[2] and S. Mukherjee[3]
[1]*The University of Auckland,* [2]*Massey University,* [3]*Palmerston North Hospital*
New Zealand

1. Introduction

Medical robotics is still a relatively new field with researchers and companies all adopting various styles and techniques to solve the challenges faced. This chapter outlines one unique approach to the development of a medical robot for the reduction of broken femurs.

Fractures are common injuries, for example in adults over the age of 65 it is reported that 87% of falls results in a fracture (Canale & Campbell, 2003). This has lead to the development of focused trauma centers having the capability to quickly diagnose and respond with the appropriate treatment action and expertise. However, orthopedics as a discipline is relatively conservative with a large scope for improvement. Often techniques used are controversial and experience of the surgeon is limited as training is difficult. Historically the main drivers for improvements in the tools and methods used have been the large number of injuries during world wars. Development focus was on life and limb preservation while the technology has remained relatively constant. Now there is an opportunity with the increased advancement of technology to look at the processes and overcome problems that previously could not be addressed.

Orthopedics has been identified as particularly suitable for robotic applications as bones are relatively rigid structures and imaging techniques allow a computer to locate and register the location of bones. This has lead to the implementation of new medical robotic technologies such as ISS Robodoc for total hip replacement (Kazanzides et al., 1992.) and Acrobot for knee replacement (Jakopec et al., 2003). These systems are commercially available and have been successful in improving the accuracy and overall outcome of surgery.

Investigation into long bone fracture reduction in particular has received attention by several groups. Gösling et al. (2005) and Westphal et al. (2006) developed a joystick tele-operated system using a serial robot and carried out preliminary user studies. They showed that the robotic system can achieve precise alignment and reduce intra-operative imaging. Maeda et al. (2005) and Warisawa et al. (2004) also used a serial robot and examined three control modes of manual jogging, power assist and automatic. Graham et al. (2006) previously described a conceptual fracture reduction system including procedure planning assistance and a parallel robot mechanism for reduction, this work is a further development of that.

In previous research work many problems are only partially understood and/or solved. For example radiation exposure, fatigue and problems in pre-operative planning remain. To properly determine the needs and focus direction of research it is useful to form the framework in Fig. 1. From this figure the main stakeholders are presented as system recipients, users and designers typically representing patients, surgeons and researchers respectively. Each of these stakeholders has different areas for improvements and these can be determined by considering drivers from both the hospital and technology. There are three main outcomes or goals established for fracture reduction; these are 1) to improve the knowledge of fracture reduction surgery 2) to improve the process used to reduce the fracture and 3) to improve the outcome of fracture reduction. From the figure these have respective technology drivers of databases, interfaces and robotics. Combined they produce a matrix of challenges to be solved and are discussed in the following paragraphs.

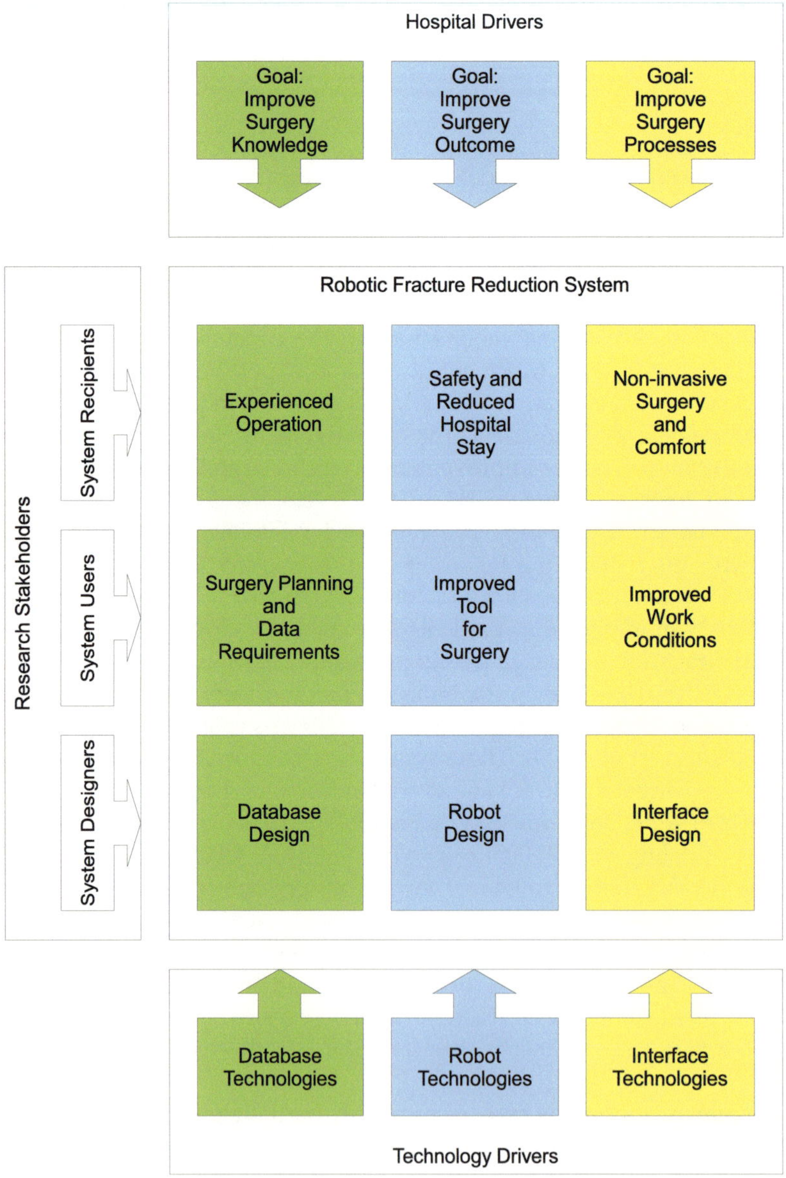

Figure 1. System stakeholders and drivers

If the needs of the recipients or patients are considered from Fig. 1. aims are to provide an experienced surgeon, maintain or increase the level of safety, reduce the length of hospital stays while providing non-invasive surgery and maintaining comfort. Currently training of new surgical staff for reduction procedures is difficult. Research has been undertaken to improve surgeon training and resource use through simulation (Sourina et al., 2007), however there still exists controversy around which existing solutions to apply. The result is that often long bone reductions are carried out by people with only a few previous examples to draw experience from. This leads to a discussion around surgery practices and outcomes which are not tracked in a concise and available format so it is difficult to see what is improving over time or to make comparisons between methods. Warisawa et al. (2004) and Graham et al. (2006) both suggested the need for gentle reduction. This has the potential to reduce trauma especially for elderly as the current manual reduction provides limited information about the internal problems that could be occurring. Gentle reduction also can lower the discomfort and pain experienced by the patient from the perineal post positioned between the groin to provide counter force for reduction. Replacing the manual control with a robotic device does raise safety questions for the patient and to solve this mechanical fuses have been used (Warisawa et al., 2004; Masamune et al., 2001) along with monitoring force in various forms to slow or prevent action (Davies et al. 2000; Ho et al., 1995; Taylor et al., 1994; Paul et al., 1992). Robot patient registration should be non-invasive and avoid the use of fiducials which can lead to patient discomfort (Howe & Matsuoka, 1999; Cinquin et al. 1995).

Referring back to Fig. 1. again from the perspective of system users or the surgeon it is seen that there is a desire to improve the planning of surgery, have access to the correct data when needed and a better tool for carrying out the actual reduction. This needs to be addressed in a way that improves the existing problems with the operating room (OR) work environment. Planning surgery takes time requiring a physical examination and pre-operative x-rays which are difficult to interpret and visualize in a 3 dimensional (3-D) format. The outcome of the plan is generally based on hands-on experience and text book knowledge of the surgeon. The plan for reduction is currently executed with a manual reduction table and fluoroscope machine. Reduction can be problematic and statistics from Germany report 4111 patients are required to undergo corrective surgery from malrotation alone, requiring at lest 7 additional days stay in hospital (Gösling et al., 2005). This can be attributed in part to the reduction table which is limiting in the degrees of freedom (DoF) and obtainable accuracies combined with mental strain from reconstructing images in 3-D. The manual traction interface to carry out the operation requires the surgeon to exert forces to counteract reduction which have been reported between 201 and 411 Newtons (Maeda et al., 2005; Gösling et al., 2006) and can lead to physical fatigue. Radiation reduction is a contributing motivator for a number of medical robotic research projects (Loser & Navab, 2000; Stoianovici et al., 2003; Cleary et al., 2002). In long bone reduction the same applies where the close proximity to the fluoroscope machine can have harmful effects on the surgeons health or effectively limit the number of operations they can carry out per year without an appropriate distancing tool (Skjeldal & Backe, 1987). Finally a concern for the broader user is resource (such as floor space and budgets) in the operating room which is usually limited and new developments in long bone reduction should appropriately consider this limitation in the design.

To address the problems listed in the previous two paragraphs this research has taken steps towards developing the driving technologies. Driving technologies are those that provide solutions to the needs of users and recipients, ultimately achieving the three driving factors from the hospital. Specifically the robot technologies for a parallel fracture reduction device are being designed and prototyped. This will provide a new smart tool for the user addressing the issue of radiation exposure, physical fatigue and manipulation accuracies. It will also remain compact and integrate with existing hospital technologies. The underlying modeling and analysis is carried out to produce a tool for robot control development and identify appropriate data to be stored as a database to aid treatment planning pre-operatively and inter-operatively. Interface technologies allowing interaction between the user and robot are being developed for effective surgery to take place. The methods used to develop these technologies are discussed in section 2. This is followed description of the results obtained to date in section 3 and a discussion on what has been achieved in section 4. Finally section 5 presents the future work to be done.

2. Methods

This section provides details on the methods and tools used to develop the solutions to the driving technologies. This consists of the interface which includes visualizing the fracture, planning assistance and human-robot-interaction. The physical robot and control design methods are given followed by the database method, describing what is stored and the motivation behind it.

2.1 Interface: Visualization of the Fracture

The main problem to be addressed here is the visualization of the fracture. This has an impact on both the surgery process and also the method to perform pre-operative planning. Visualization is concerned with taking fluoroscopy images and presenting them to the surgeon in a useful form that can be easily interpreted. This is achieved by providing a 3-D view to the surgeon generated from only a small number of fluoroscope images that can be manipulated in real time. Fluoroscope images are used as opposed to detailed computer tomography (CT) often seen in medical robotics applications (Jakopec et al. 2003; Joskowicz et al. 1998; Kazanzides, 1992) as they are less resource intensive for the hospital, can be obtained inter-operatively and is the same imaging technology currently used for reduction. Previously concepts of fluoroscopy servoing have been presented using specially designed needles although for some applications it is found that the level of detail contained in an image is not sufficient (Cleary et al., 2002; Cleary et al., 2003; Loser & Navab, 2000). Other applications have aimed at using fluoroscope images to register nail insertion with pre-operative CT scans during closed medullary nailing in long bone surgery (Joskowicz et al., 1998) and similarly use the images obtained of the nail for robot guidance (Wang et al., 2004). The proposed approach in this research is to have a stored number of generic structures or bones and take a minimum number of fluoroscope images to match the appropriate model. Initial investigation into implementing matching of 2-Dimensional (2-D) images has been undertaken however the limiting contrast and soft tissue obstruction in fluoroscopy images still needs to be overcome. Currently the surgeon is required to manually match 22 points in two consecutive images (Rensburg et al., 2005).

After matching the femur, a 3-D view is displayed. This has the option to view the femur, fibula, tibia, sacrum, hip, patella, visible muscle and muscle attachment lines. 3-D models currently used are finite element meshes derived for the widely used Visible Human dataset and are stored in the generic WRL file format, also known as VRML (virtual reality modeling language).

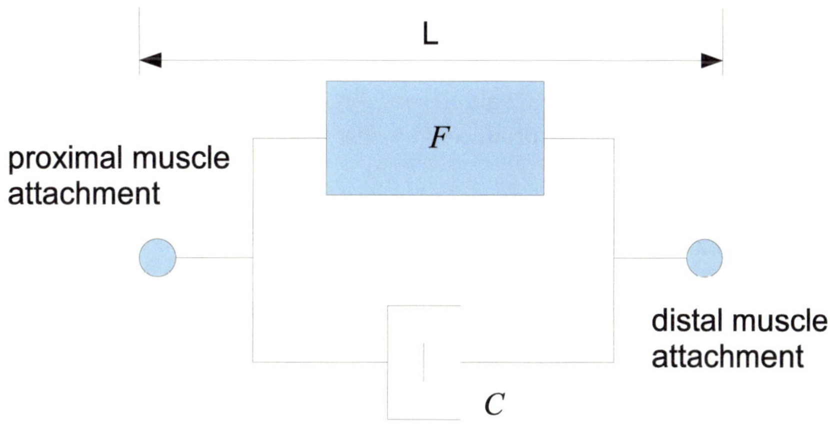

Figure 2. Structure of the Hill muscle model

2.2 Interface: Planning Assistance

To assist the surgeon in planning the operation a model is developed to estimate the expected force of each muscle. This will provide information intra-operatively about the expected internal state of the fracture and assist by presenting a planned reduction path based on minimal force exertion and position. The model also has further use in creating and understanding robot requirements and developing control of the robot mechanism as presented in section 2.4. In order to create the model the attachment location of visible muscle on the bone mesh is obtained for each muscle. The well established Hill type muscle model (Winters & Stark, 1985; Winters & Stark, 1988; Friederich & Brand, 1990) as in Fig. 2. is then used to determine the force by each muscle as given in Eqn. 1.

$$F = \frac{F_{\max}}{e^{sh} - 1}\left(s^{sh\,\Delta L / \Delta L_{\max}} - 1\right) \tag{1}$$

where

$$F_{\max} = 0.5\ MPa\ A_{pcs} = 0.5\ MPa\left[m/(2\rho y)\right]\sin(2\alpha) \tag{2}$$

$$sh = 1.5 + 3 \times smf \tag{3}$$

and F is the force generated by the equivalent muscle spring element in Fig. 2., sh is a shape parameter, ΔL is the muscle extension, A_{pcs} is the physiological cross sectional area, m is the muscle mass, y is the thickness, ρ is the muscle density, α is the muscle pennation angle, smf is the percentage of slow muscle fibers and MPa is Mega Pascal's. The spring element is modeled in parallel with a dash-pot having damping ratio, c

The muscle models combined with the moving geometry of the distal fragment during reduction result in a system of equations in generalized coordinate q . This can be written in a state space form as Eqn. 4.

$$M_b(q)\ddot{q} + C_b(q,\dot{q})\dot{q} + G_b(q) = F_b + R_b \tag{4}$$

where $M_b(q)$ is the mass matrix, $C_b(q,\dot{q})$ are the velocity terms, $G_b(q)$ terms due to gravity, F_b and R_b are the force produced by the muscles and external reaction force respectively.

2.3 Interface: Human-Robot-Interaction

The interface presented to the surgeon to control the robot plays an important role in the success of implementation. Robot psychologists suggest humans are increasingly accepting robots as co-workers and partners in tasks as opposed to a mechanical tool to be commanded (Libin & Libin, 2004). Incorporating a user into the control is done in one of four ways; by direct, supervisory, collaborative, or shared control (Bruemmer et al., 2005; Shen et al., 2004). These are typically discussed in relation to navigation through tele-operation of robotics, here they are applied to medical robotics. In direct or manual control the user directly commands what to do for all movement. For supervisory control the robot is still treated as a slave where the user makes higher level changes to the state of the controllers and monitors the status. Under collaborative control the user becomes a resource to the robot where both the robot and human share dialog to overcome difficulties. Lastly shared control puts the human as a virtual presence in the system and can result in more autonomy. Although there are many other definitions for control schemes such as adjustable autonomy (Goodrich et al., 2007), tele-operation with safeguard (Krotkov et al., 1996) and control with active constraint (Ho et al., 1995), the previously mentioned terminology will be used as they cover the range of implementations. Most robotic applications use a form of supervisory control where the robot will enact human commands with various levels of autonomy depending on the complexity of the task. Fong et al. (2006; 2003; 2001) have made many contributions on collaborative control which treats the robot as a partner and communication occurs through a set of semantic dialogues. Shared control is not suitable for long bone fracture reduction, however would find uses in applications such as heart surgery where sharing the operation tasks and decisions could allow treatment of a beating heart. Trusting the robot is important for a medical robot application. By allowing the robot to take initiatives and decide when not to follow user instruction and suggest improvements to users decision trust is gained. There will also be an increase in both safety and the outcome. To achieve this a collaborative control approach is used. Under the collaborative control scheme conversation needs to occur between the robot and human. Previously the authors have suggested the use of technologies such as voice or augmented reality to bring human qualities to the robot and allow the surgeons attention to remain on the operation (Graham et al., 2006). Such dialogue could include "I have planned a reduction path would you like to make corrections?", "ready to begin reduction, shall I proceed?" or "Force higher than expected, should I continue reduction?". This takes the best aspects of supervisory control with the robot following a plan specified by user understanding but allows the robot to make situation critical decisions.

2.4 Robot Design: Physical Description

The work envelop requirements and accuracies have been derived from consultation with OR staff and are given in Table 1, where x, y, z are defined as in Fig. 3. and θ, ϕ, φ are rotations about the axes respectively. The requirements reflect a desire to have 6 DoF when manipulating the fracture back into correct anatomical alignment. The unit needs to be compact so it doesn't take up too much valuable OR floor space and can be moved easily if needed. Remote operation should be allowed to move the surgeon away from the source of radiation exposure. The device should also have fail safe features to prevent unnecessary harm to the patient on an internal or external failure such as loss of power. As shown in Fig. 3. the current manual device has 3 DoF to globally locate the position of the leg, these are in region a_1 consisting of joints θ_1, d_1 and d_2. Region a_2 provides an additional 3 DoF used when performing the reduction.

Parameter	Range (mm/deg)	Accuracy (mm/deg)
x	± 100	< 1
y	± 100	< 1
z	± 150	< 1
θ	± 10	< 1
ϕ	± 10	< 1
φ	± 30	< 1

Table 1. Workspace requirements for fracture reduction

To replace the manual device a robotic parallel mechanism is selected. A computer model of the design is shown in Fig. 4. comprising of 6 powered links in parallel joining a base and top plate. The parallel structure can provide 6 DoF to correct the translation and malrotation and has a number of benefits over similar featured serial mechanisms. There is a high payload to weight ratio and a low moving mass meaning the device can be relatively small while still being able to counteract the deforming forces from muscles. Multiple closed loop chains increase stiffness and the linear actuators used often have a high gear ratio preventing any back driving. This adds to safety if there is a failure during the operation because the robot pose will remain held. Accuracy is high as error is averaged over the parallel links rather than accumulated as in a serial mechanism. A restricted work volume increases safety in an error state where the links cannot extend large amounts. Although this restricts the overall motion by maintaining the passive joints in region a_1 from Fig. 3. the motion is more than sufficient. Similar approaches where a global localization system is used for a smaller, inherently safer devices can be seen in (Loser & Navab, 2000; Davies et al. 2000; Stoianovici et al. 2003; Cleary et al. 2002).

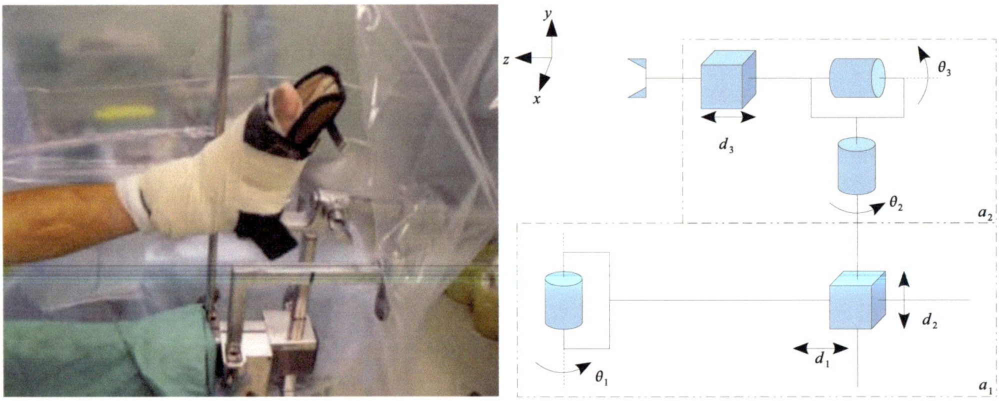

a) b)

Figure 3. Existing manual reduction device attached to patients foot a) the actual manual device b) manual DoF diagram

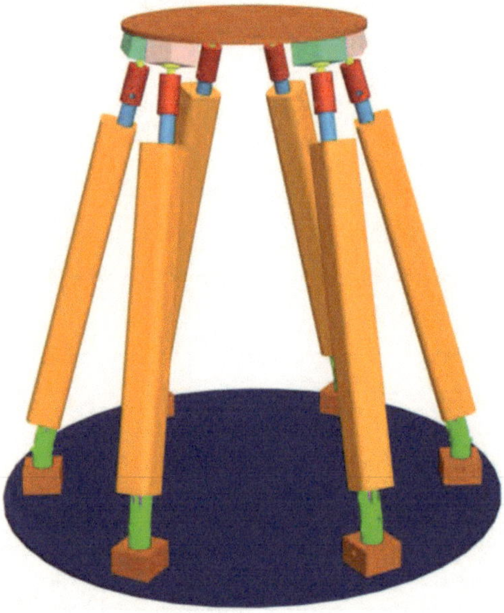

Figure 4. CAD model of parallel mechanism

2.4 Robot Design: Control

The requirement for control of position and force for the robot is currently not well understood. Efforts have been made to determine the maximum forces involved by Maeda et al. (2005) and Gösling et al. (2006). They have both used different methods to measure forces experimentally and have provided useful data however, results suffer from a number of shortcomings. External events influence the force measured either from muscle activation, friction, or additional measured force components from the techniques used. Modeling and simulation offers an alternative to the limitations of *in vivo* results and has been used widely in other applications such as determining the passive force the jaw (Curtis et al., 1999; Peck et al., 2002).

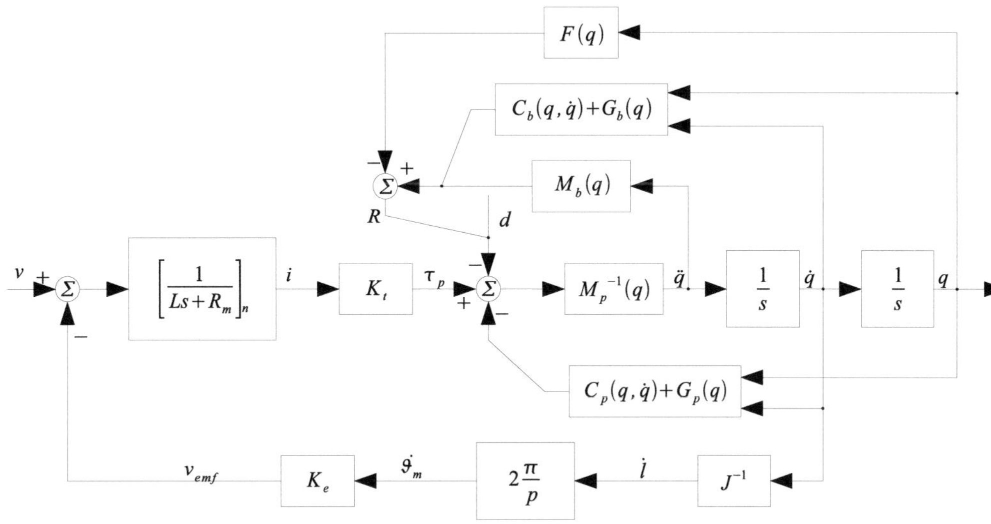

Figure 5. System diagram of the parallel robot and fractured bone

To construct a model for developing control strategies the simulated fracture force Eqn. 4. in section 2.2 is combined with a simulated parallel platform. Modeling of a parallel platform is well understood and examples of kinematics and dynamics can be found in work by Harib & Srinivasan (2003) or Guo & Li (2006). The model used in this research incorporates dynamics of the platform, link dynamics and actuator electrical and mechanical dynamics. The resulting equation is also presented in the form

$$M_p(q)\ddot{q} + C_p(q,\dot{q})\dot{q} + G_p(q) = \tau_p - d \tag{5}$$

where

$$\tau_p = K_t i \tag{6}$$

$$L\frac{di}{dt} + R_m i + K_e \dot{\vartheta}_m = v \tag{7}$$

and τ_p are the actuating forces for each link, d an external disturbance, K_t motor torque constant, i the current, L motor armature inductance, R_m motor armature resistance, K_e back emf, $\dot{\vartheta}_m$ motor angular velocity, and v the voltage applied.

The complete system is shown in Fig. 5. where the external reaction force from the fractured bone is treated as a disturbance.

The parallel robot should achieve reduction with a low force as well as position accuracy to prevent damage to soft tissue while achieving best possible union. Considering the main control tasks involve pulling and twisting the leg to comply with the environment there is an intrinsic requirement for controlling force as well as position. To enable this a force sensor is attached between the plate of the parallel robot and the end-effector interacting with the patient measuring the three orthogonal axes. This will also serve as a safety device if forces become larger than a threshold value. This will be achieved by providing the correct level of perception and cognition as part of the collaborative control.

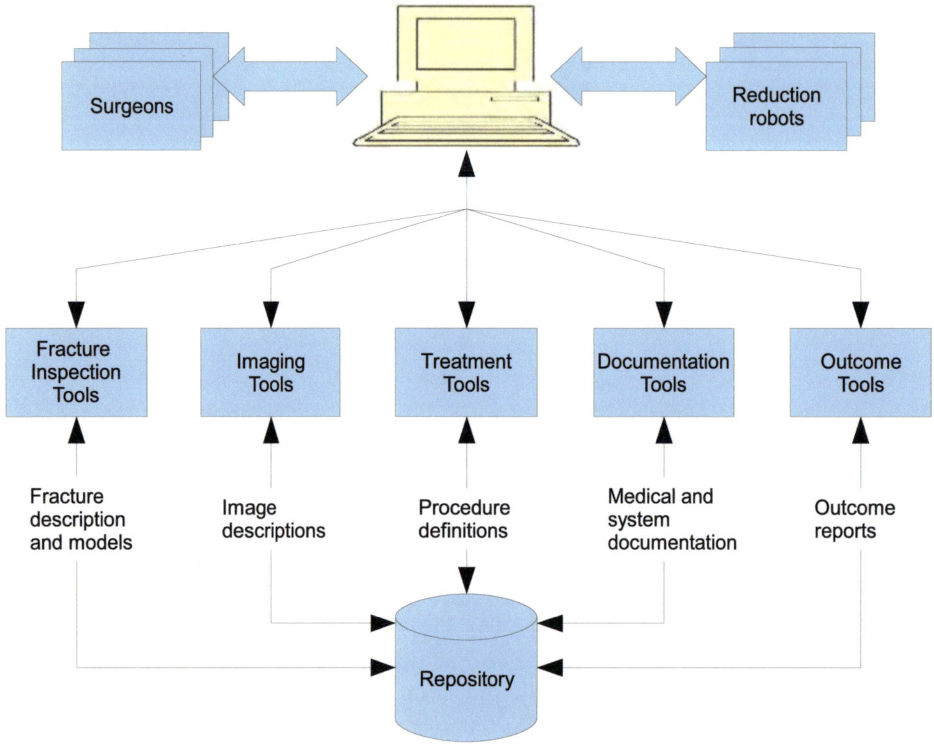

Figure 6. Database for a medical robotic system used to reduce fractured bones

2.3 Database Support

A database is used to track surgery performance. Typically true success of operations may not be known for a period of time measured by years, so improvements and new techniques are slow to propagate through. With operations performed in the digital domain many aspects of the surgery can be stored and tracked, potentially leading to the development of metrics that can be assessed. This may allow evaluation of good or bad outcomes or even indicate the appropriate corrective action much quicker. The database should also act as a supporting technology for pre-operative planning and inter-operative surgery and help bring greater expertise to the surgeon and patient through wide distribution of knowledge and experience. Data stored here would include the generic models of bones, muscle data, and tools that can be used during the surgical process.

Fig. 6. shows how such a system could work with multiple surgeons performing multiple operations with the fracture reduction robot. These are interfaced through a computer to a single global repository where the data is stored. Fracture descriptions, models, image descriptions, procedure definitions, medical and system documentation and outcome reports can be stored within the repository and updated each time the surgeon and robot takes the appropriate action. Storing the data will help build the tools used for all future fracture inspections, lead to enhancement in imaging and accurate treatment with a high rate of successful outcomes. Documentation tools on the same system provide quick and uniform access to searchable information saving time through reading distributed text books. Overtime this could potentially build to be a very useful resource and help to identify the metrics to better assess the surgical procedure.

3. Results

In this section the results that have been achieved to date are presented. These are from modeling and visualization of the geometric bones to display to the surgeon and investigate the fracture as well as the expected force generated. The prototype robotic platform is presented along with the setup to mimic the fracture reduction environment. Lastly the initial results from processing fluoroscopy x-ray images are given.

3.1 Modeling and Visualization

The modeled bones (Fig. 7.) are used to view the lower extremity, allowing rotation, and zooming. The user can select which bones to view from the sacrum, hip, femur, tibia, fibula, patella as well as which muscles to show if desired. Similarly a fracture can be created and explored. The user also has the option of displaying which muscles will have an influence on the force required to achieve reduction (Fig. 8.). These are displayed as lines from the muscle insertion locations. The location of muscles, parameters that define their force generation and the size of the bones may be changed as the user desires.

The force during a reduction may be found from any pose of the distal fragment by Eqn. 4. and calculated during the movement of the fragment. For example the reduction force under constant velocity has a maximum force of -352 N (Fig. 9.) from an initial displacement of 20,-40,40 *mm* in x, y and z respectively with no malrotation.

3.2 Prototype Device

The prototype device (Fig. 10.) consists of a 6 DoF parallel platform mechanism and reduction table. The platform is mounted horizontally and attaches to the manual DoF part of the reduction table. In this example a foot holster is used to attach the platform to the recipients leg and perform reduction. Alternatively the robot may be attached directly to the femur with a pin through the femur head. The user can currently control the trajectory of the parallel platform from a work station located away from the fractured bone. The specified trajectory consists of a number of discrete points which are processed by a 6 axis control card and amplified to the move the platforms 6 individual ball screw actuators. Optical encoders on each actuator provide position feedback for closed loop control of the trajectory.

3.3 3-D Bone Reconstruction

To determine the pose of the distal fragment consecutive images are joined together by the user to create a panorama of images showing the bone in lateral and anteroposterior (AP) views. The translation is then found by the user selecting 22 common points (Fig. 11.). These points are typically located around the perimeter of the bone similar to where the surgeon would usually inspect during surgery. Points are selected by a point and click method and accuracy depends on the average error of selected locations. Malroation is computed by comparing the fractured bone with a healthy bone image and a best fit match is found. This is a statistical method to give the most likely orientation.

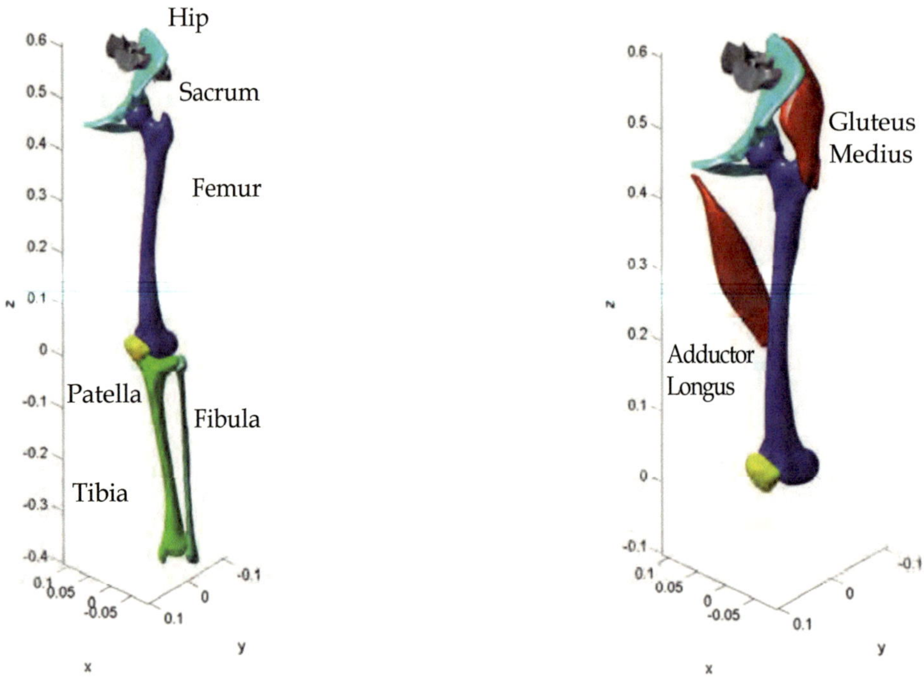

Figure 7. Investigating lower extremity, with and without visible muscle

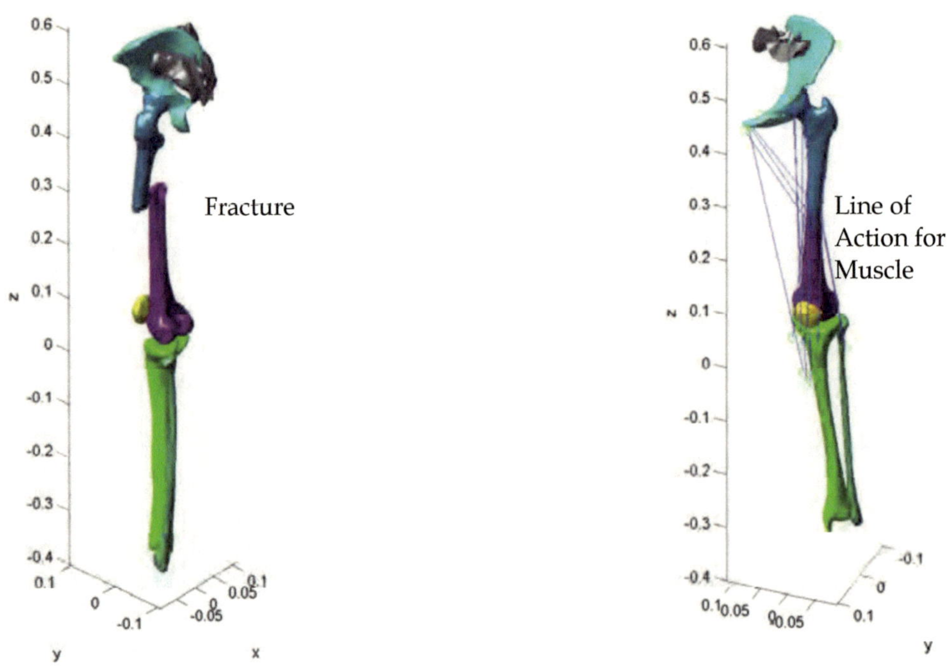

Figure 8. Investigating lower extremity when fractured and force causing muscles

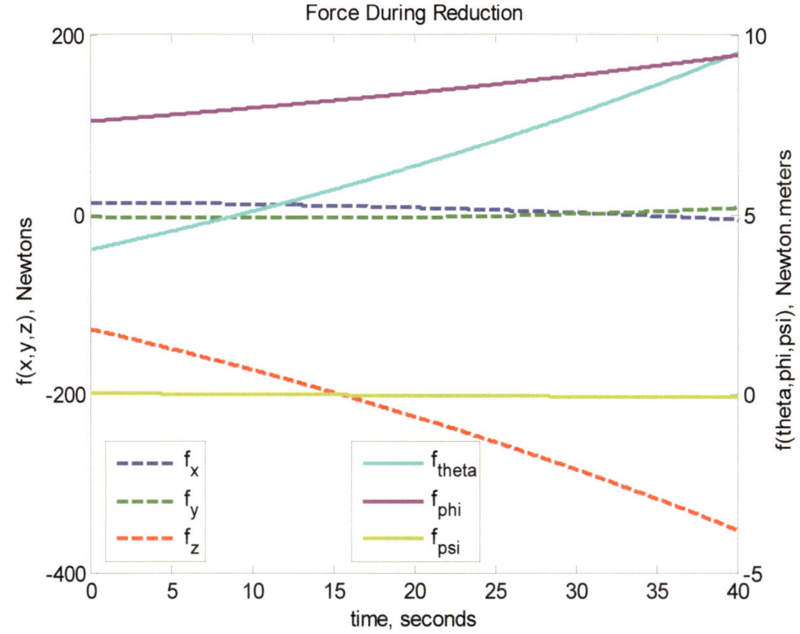

Figure 9. Simulated force during reduction

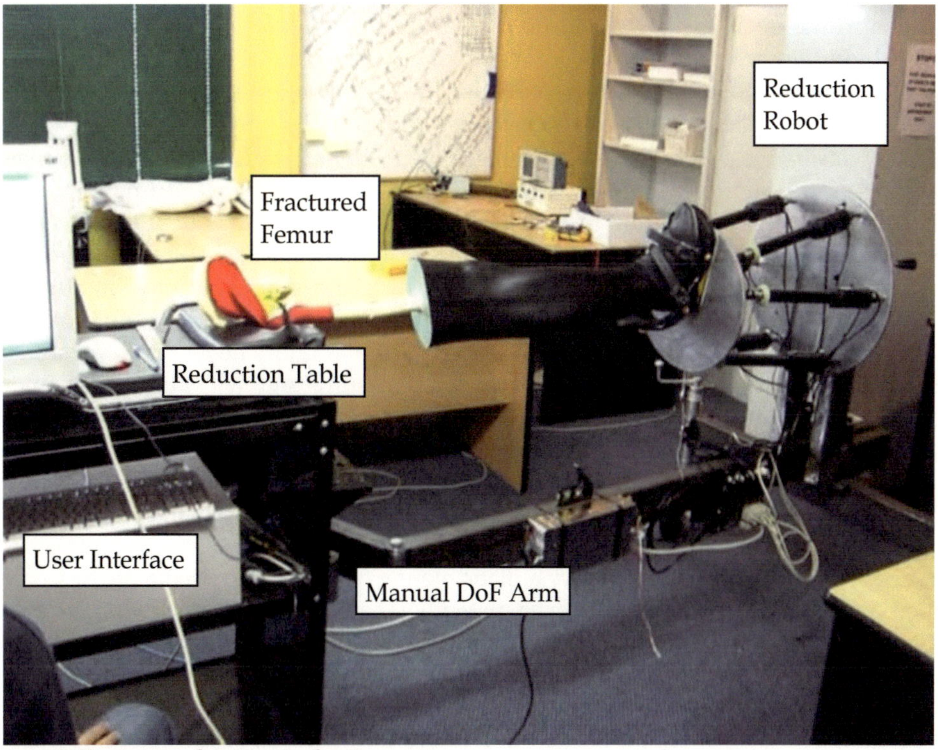

Figure 10. Prototype fracture reduction setup

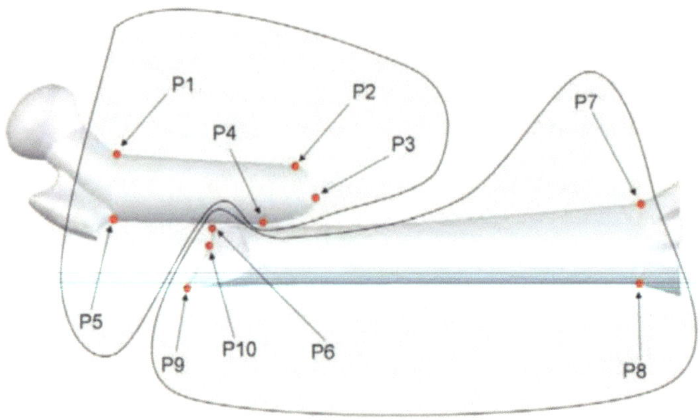

Figure 11. Selecting points in AP view

4. Discussion

This research into a medical robot for realigning fractured bones aims to develop the interface, robot, and database technologies to improve the working situation for users and outcome for recipients.

Compared with other approaches to fracture reduction, the system being developed here has a number of novel features. The geometric modeling has been effective in allowing a surgeon to visualize the fractured bone and has not been reported elsewhere for fracture reduction to the authors knowledge. By displaying the images to users in this form any mental strain they would face from reconstructing images can be removed. In addition to this, modeling of the forces during reduction has provided a means to determine the requirement for a robotic device. Previously *in vivo* results had been presented (Maeda et al., 2005; Gösling et al., 2006), however these were limited and suffered from problems associated with taking measurement from living humans. The developed model provides results similar to those measured by Gösling and can be seen to validate these results. This provides a force requirement for the robot to at lest exert around 400 Newton's of force.

The force model also allows the reduction to be planned and verified in 3-D while inspecting the position and expected forces involved. The combined models of bone, force and that of the parallel platform provides a mechanism to rapidly develop control strategies initially without the need for *in vivo* or phantom testing and will aid in achieving an algorithm design that provides both position accuracy and gentle reduction force. The model itself does also have limitations though. The interface between the platform and leg is assumed rigid which is not strictly true for the use of a foot holster, but if the reduction technique consisting of a pin through the femur is used this becomes more valid. Also the parameters used to develop the model are based on those of averaged cadavers taken from literature so force requirements of very athletic, young or old people need to be treated with caution. Values can be adjusted, however currently what these are is unknown. The parallel design of the robot is inherently safer than a serial mechanism and still allows the user to be distant from the fluoroscopy machine preventing the harmful radiation exposure. Although the use of parallel mechanism in the general medical robotics is not new (Jakopec et al., 2003; Brandt et al., 1999) its application to fracture reduction is. As a replacement for the existing manual traction device and using legacy imaging technology it integrates into the current procedure. This saves the hospital resources spent on a completely new system. Matching of x-ray images to determine the pose of the fractured bone means there can be a reduction in the overall number of images. The images provide a transformation for the modeled distal fragment to the correct initial pose. This is good for the recipient reducing their radiation exposure. However the problem of processing the fluoroscopy x-ray images still needs to be properly solved.

The technologies that are still in development from the methods proposed also offer a lot of potential. In particular the control scheme to gently reduce fractures as part of a collaborative control scheme. Most medical robotics use force only as a monitored component for safety purposes. There are a few applications such as the active constraint (Ho et al., 1995) and for skin harvesting (Dombre et al., 2003) which have incorporated force into the core control however much work is left to be done here to allow safe and compliant interaction between man and machine. For the proposed scheme here it has been suggested that treating the robot as a partner is important rather than a tool. This has potential to increase acceptance which has been problematic in the field so far (Howe & Matsuoka, 1999). To achieve this the collaborative control schema will be used.

Databases are well understood, what has been described here is a method of storing the information from surgery in the digital domain over time. It is hoped that this will help spread the knowledge of what processes work and identify trends both good and bad that will ultimately lead to greater patient care.

With an increased capacity to control the reduction of the fracture and visualize the operation patients can expect fast, quality treatment. Errors in correcting malrotation can be overcome and patients can expect shorter stays in hospital while surgeons experience increases by distributing knowledge and they see an improved working environment.

This chapter has identified the problems with the existing fracture reduction method to three main stakeholders. It has then gone on to discuss a method for development of a robot for long bone fracture reduction that will address the problems each stakeholder has and presented the results obtained to date.

5. Future Research

Future work will be undertaken to continue to develop the driving technologies. In particular development of the control of the robotic device and the interface to surgeon. Control is currently only by position, and it is intended to expand this to include a form of force control. The robot will also be given the ability to interpret the data from its sensors and make decisions based on that data. A phantom study is planned to assess the effectiveness of the developed control strategy using artificial bones.

Much work still needs to be done into the processing of fluoroscopy images to determine if it is viable to use these for registration and obtaining the pose of the fracture segments. Even with the manual matching of images the accuracy needs to be achieved to less than 1 *mm* so the robot position requirements can be achieved.

6. References

Brandt, G.; Zimolong, A.; Carrat, L.; Merloz, P.; Staudte, H. W.; Lavallee, S.; Radermacher, K. & Rau, G. (1999). CRIGOS: a compact robot for image-guided orthopedic surgery, *IEEE Transactions on Information Technology in Biomedicine* 3(4), 252-260.

Bruemmer, D. J.; Few, D. A.; Boring, R. L.; Marble, J. L.; Walton, M. C. & Nielsen, C. W. (2005). Shared Understanding for Collaborative Control, *IEEE Transactions on Systems, Man, and Cybernetics-Part A: Systems and Humans*, Vol. 35, No. 4, 494-504.

Canale, S. T. & Campbell, W. C. (2003). *Campbells operative orthopaedics*, Vol. 3, Mosby, St. Louis.

Cinquin, P.; Bainville, E.; Barbe, C.; Bittar, E.; Bouchard, V.; l. Bricault; Champleboux, G.; Chenin, M.; Chevalier, L.; Delnondedieu, Y.; Desbat, L.; Dessenne, V.; Hamadeh, A.; Henry, D.; Laieb, N.; lavallee, S.; Lefebvre, J.M.; Leitner, F.; Menguy, Y.; Padieu, F.; Peria, 0.; Poyet, A.; Promayon, M.; Rouault, S.; Sautot, P.; Troccaz, J. & Vassal, P. (1995). Computer Assisted Medical Interventions: Passive and semi-active aids, *IEEE Engineering in Medicine and Biology Magazine*, Vol. 14, No. 3, 254-263.

Curtis, D. A.; Plesh, O.; Hannam, A. G.; Sharma, A. & Curtis, T. A. (1999). Modeling of jaw biomechanics in the reconstructed mandibulectomy patient. *Journal of Prosthetic Dentistry*, Vol. 81, No. 2, 167-173.

Cleary, K.; Clifford, M.; Stoianovici, D.; Freedman, M.; Mun, S. K. & VanceWatson (2002). Technology Improvements for Image-Guided and Minimally Invasive Spine Procedures, *IEEE Transaction on Information Technology in Biomedicine*, Vol. 6, No. 4, 249-261.

Cleary, K.; Ibanez, L.; Navab, N.; Stoianovici, D.; Patriciu, A. & Corral, G. (2003). Segmentation of surgical needles for fluoroscopy servoing using the insight software toolkit (ITK), *Proceedings of the 25th Annual lnternational Conference of the IEEE EMBS*, pp. 698-701.

Davies, B.; Starkie, S.; Harris, S. J.; Agterhuis, E.; Paul, V. & Auer, L. M. (2000). Neurobot: a special-purpose robot for neurosurgery, *International Conference on Robotics and Automation*, Vol. 4, 4103-4108.

Dombre, E.; Duchemin, G.; Poignet, P. & Pierrot, F. (2003). Dermarob: A safe robot for reconstructive surgery, *IEEE Transactions on Robotics and Automation*. Vol. 19, No. 5, 876-884.

Fong, T.; Grange, S.; Thorpe, C. & Baur, C. (2001). Multi-robot remote driving with collaborative control, *Proceedings 10th IEEE International Workshop on Robot-Human Interactive Collaboration*, pp. 237-242.

Fong, T.; Thorpe, C. & Baur, C. (2003). Robot, asker of questions. *Robotics and Autonomous Systems*, Vol. 42, 235–243.

Fong, T.; Scholtz, J.; Shah, J. A.; Fluckiger, L.; Kunz, C.; Lees, D.; Schreiner, J.; Siegel, M.; Hiatt, L. M.; Nourbakhsh, I.; Simmons, R.; Ambrose, R.; Burridge, R.; Antonishek, B.; Bugajska, M.; Schultz, A. & Trafton, J. G. (2006). A preliminary study of peer-to-peer human-robot interaction, *Proceedings of the IEEE Conference on Systems, Man, and Cybernetics*.

Friederich, J. A. & Brand, R. A. (1989). Muscle fiber architecture in the human lower limb. *Department of Orthopaedic Surgery Biomechanics Laboratory Technical report*, The University of Iowa, Iowa.

Goodrich, M. A.; McLain, T. W.; Anderson, J. D.; Sun, J. & Crandall, J. W. (2007). Managing autonomy in robot teams: observations from four experiments, *Proceeding of the ACM/IEEE international conference on Human-robot interaction*, pp. 25-32.

Gösling, T.; Westphal, R.; Hüfner, T.; Faulstich, J.; Kfuri Jr., M.; Wahl, M. & Krettek, C. (2005). Robot-assisted fracture reduction: A preliminary study in the femur shaft. *Medical and Biological Engineering and Computing*, Vol. 43 No. 1, 115-120.

Gösling, T.; Westphal, R.; Faülstich, J.; Sommer, K.; Wahl, F.; Krettek, C. & Hufner, T. (2006). Forces and Torques during Fracture Reduction: Intraoperative Measurements in the Femur. *Journal of Orthopaedic Research*, Vol. 24 No. 3, 333-338.

Graham, A. E.; Xie, S. Q.; Aw., K. C.; Xu, W. L. & Mukherjee, S. (2006). Design of a Parallel Long Bone Fracture Reduction Robot with Planning Treatment Tool, *Proceedings of the 2006 IEEE/RSJ International Conference on Intelligent Robots and Systems*, pp. 1255-1260.

Guo, H. B. & Li, H. R. (2006), Dynamic analysis and simulation of a six degree of freedom Stewart platform manipulator, *Proceedings of the Institution pf Mechanical Engineers*, 61 - 72.

Harib, K. & Srinivasan, K. (2003), Kinematic and dynamic analysis of Stewart platform-based machine tool structures. *Robotica*, Vol. 21, 541-554.

Ho, S. C.; Hibberd, R. D. & Davies, B. L. (1995). Robot assisted knee surgery. *IEEE Engineering in Medicine and Biology Magazine*, Vol. 14, No. 3, 292-300.

Howe, R. D. & Matsuoka, Y. (1999). Robotics for surgery. *Annual Review of Biomedical Engineering*, Vol. 1, 211-40.

Jakopec, M.; Rodriguez y Baena, F.; Harris, S. J.; Gomes, P.; Cobb, J. & Davies, B. L. (2003). The hands-on orthopaedic robot "acrobot": Early clinical trials of total knee replacement surgery. *IEEE Transactions on Robotics and Automation*, Vol. 19, No. 5, 902-911.

Joskowicz, L.; Milgrom, C.; Simkin, A.; Tockus, L. & Yaniv, Z. (1998). FRACAS: a system for computer-aided image-guided long bone fracture surgery. *Computer Aided Surgery*, Vol. 3, No.6, 271-288.

Kazanzides, P.; Zuhars, J.; Mittelstadt, B.; Williamson, B.; Cain, P.; Smith, F.; Rose, L. & Musits, B. (1992). Architecture of a surgical robot, *IEEE International Conference on Systems, Man, and Cybernetics*, Vol. 2, 1624-1629.

Krotkov, E.; Simmons, R.; Cozman, F. & Koenig, S. (1996). Safeguarded Teleoperation for Lunar Rovers: From Human Factors to Field Trials, *Proceedings of the IEEE Workshop on Planetary Rover Technology and Systems*.

Libin, A. V. & Libin, E. V. (2004). Person-robot interactions from the robopsychologists' point of view: the robotic psychology and robotherapy approach, *Proceedings of the IEEE*, Vol. 92, No. 11, 1789-1803.

Loser, M. H. & Navab, N. (2000). A new robotic system for visually controlled percutaneous interventions under CT fluoroscopy, In: *Medical Image Computing and Computer-Assisted Intervention – MICCAI 2000*, Springer Berlin, Heidelberg, pp. 887-896.

Maeda, Y.; Tamura, Y.; Saito, M.; Yamamoto, T.; Yonenobu, K.; Warisawa, S.; Mitsuishi, M. & Sugano, N. (2005). Measurement of traction load and torque transferred to the lower extremity during simulated fracture reduction. *International Congress Series* 1281, 674-679.

Masamune, K.; Fichtinger, G.; Patriciu, A.; Susil, R. C.; Taylor, H. R.; Kavoussi, L. R.; Andreson, J. H.; Sakuma, I.; Dohi, T. & Stoianovici, D. (2001). System for Robotically Assisted Percutaneous Procedures with Computer Tomography Guidance. *Computer Aided Surgery*, Vol. 6, 370-383.

Paul, H. A.; Bargar, W. L.; Mittlestadt, B.; Kazanzides, P.; Musits, B.; Zuhars, J.; Cain, P. W.; Williamson, B. & Smith, F. G. (1992). Robotic execution of a surgical plan, *IEEE International Conference on Systems, Man and Cybernetics*, Vol. 2, 1621-1623.

Peck, C. C., Sooch, A. S. & Hannam A. G. (2002). Forces resisting jaw displacement in relaxed humans: a predominantly viscous phenomenon. *Journal of Oral Rehabilitation*, Vol. 29, No. 2, 151-160.

Rendsburg, M.; Xu, W. & Mukherjee, S. (2005). Surgeon-instructed, Image-guided and Robot-assisted Long Bone Fractures Reduction, *1st International Conference on Sensing Technology*, pp. 78-84.

Shen, J.; Ibanze-Guzman, J.; Ng, T. C. & Chew, B. S. (2004). A Collaborative-Shared Control System With Safe Obstacle Avoidance Capability, *Proceeding of the 2004 IEEE Conference on Robotics, Automation and Mechatronics*, pp. 119-123.

Skjeldal, S. & Backe, S. (1987). Interlocking medullary nails - Radiation doses in distal targeting. *Archives of Orthopaedic Trauma Surgery*, Vol. 106, 179-181.

Sourina, O.; Sourin, A. & Sen, H. T. (2007). Orthopedic Surgery Training Simulation. *Journal of Mechanics in Medicine and Biology*, Vol. 7, No. 1, 37–53.

Stoianovici, D.; Cleary, K.; Patriciu, A.; Mazilu, D.; Stanimir, A.; Craciunoiu, N.; Watson, V. & Kavoussi, L. (2003). AcuBot: a robot for radiological interventions. *IEEE Transactions on Robotics and Automation,* Vol. 19, No. 5, 927-930.

Taylor, R. H.; Mittelstadt, B. D.; Paul, H. A.; Hanson, W.; Kazanzides, P.; Zuhars, J. F.; Williamson, B.; Musits, B. L.; Glassman, E. & Bargar, W. L. (1994). An image-directed robotic system for precise orthopaedic surgery. *IEEE Transactions on Robotics and Automation*, Vol. 10, No. 3, 261-275.

Wang, T.; Liu, W. & Hu, L. (1992). BPOR: a fluoroscopy-based robot navigating system for distal locking of intramedullary nails, *Proceedings of 2004 IEEE/RSJ International Conference on Intelligenl Robots and Systems*, pp. 3321-3326.

Warisawa, S.; Ishizuka, T.; Mitsuishi, M.; Sugano, N.; Yonenobu, K. & Nakazawa, T. (2004). Development of a femur fracture reduction robot, *Proceedings of the 2004 IEEE International Conference on Robotics & Automation*, pp. 3999-4004.

Westphal, R.; Gösling, T.; Oszwald, M.; Bredow, J.; Klepzig, D.; Winkelbach, S.; Hüfner, T.; Krettek, C. & Wahl, F. (2006). 3D Robot Assisted Fracture Reduction. *Proceedings of 10th International Symposium on Experimental Robotics.*

Winters, J. & Stark, L. (1985). Analysis of fundamental movement patterns through the use of indepth antagonistic muscle models. *IEEE Transactions on Biomedical Engineering.*, Vol. 32, 826-839.

Winters, J. M. & Stack, L. (1988). Estimated mechanical properties of synergistic muscle involved in movements of a variety of human joints. *Journal of Biomechanics*, Vol. 21, 1027–1041.

Non-Invasive Estimates of Local Field Potentials for Brain-Computer Interfaces: Theoretical derivation and comparison with direct intracranial recordings

Rolando Grave de Peralta Menendez and Sara L. Gonzalez Andino
Electrical Neuroimaging Group. ***Department of Clinical Neurosciences****, Geneva University Hospitals Switzerland*

1. Introduction

Recent experiments have shown the possibility to use the brain electrical activity to directly control the movement of robots or prosthetic devices in real time. As such, it is particularly relevant as an aid for paralyzed humans, although it also opens up new possibilities in human-robot interaction for able-bodied people. Such neuroprostheses can be invasive or non-invasive, depending on how the brain signals are recorded.

Initial demonstrations of the feasibility of controlling complex neuroprostheses have relied on the invasive approach using intracranial electrodes implanted in the brain of monkeys (Wessberg *et al.*, 2000; Meeker *et al.*, 2002; Serruya *et al.*, 2002; Taylor *et al.*, 2002; Carmena *et al.*, 2003; Mehring *et al.*, 2003). In these experiments, one or more array of microelectrodes records the extracellular activity of single neurons (their spiking rate) in different areas of the cortex related to planning and execution of movements—motor, premotor and posterior parietal cortex. From the real-time analysis of the activity of the neuronal population, it has been possible to predict either the animal's movement intention (Meeker *et al.*, 2002; Mehring *et al.*, 2003) or the monkey's hand trajectory (Wessberg *et al.*, 2000; Taylor *et al.*, 2002; Carmena *et al.*, 2003), and to drive a computer cursor to desired targets (Serruya *et al.*, 2002; Taylor *et al.*, 2002). Thus, in principle, invasive approaches could provide a more natural and flexible control of neuroprostheses, However, for humans, non-invasive methods are preferable because of ethical concerns and medical risks.

Non-invasive approaches mainly use scalp electroencephalogram (EEG) signals and their main disadvantage is that these signals represent the noisy spatiotemporal overlapping of activity arising from very diverse brain regions. As a consequence, current EEG-based brain-actuated devices are limited by a low channel capacity and are considered too slow for controlling rapid and complex sequences of movements. This is probably why so far control tasks based on human EEG have been limited to simple exercises such as moving a computer cursor to the corners of the screen (Wolpaw and McFarland, 1994) or opening a hand orthosis (Pfurtscheller and Neuper, 2001) or need to resort to intelligent robotics (Millan et al 2004) to attain an acceptable control performance. It is not surprising that some people still believe that only invasive approaches will provide natural and flexible control of robots (Nicolelis, 2001; Donoghue, 2002). The rationale is that surgically implanted arrays of electrodes will be required to properly record the brain signals because the non-invasive scalp-recordings with the EEG lack spatial resolution.

However, recent advances in EEG analysis techniques have shown that the sources of the electric activity in the brain can be estimated from the surface signals with relatively high spatial accuracy (6-9mm). This resolution compares with the resolution provided by the methods used to detect activation in functional magnetic resonance imaging (fMRI) using 1.5/3 Tesla machines. Note that this is very different to the resolution of the anatomical images provided by the MRI. Aiming at combining the benefits of both approaches, we propose to rely on the non-invasive estimation of local field potentials (eLFP) in the whole human brain from the scalp measured EEG data using a recently developed distributed linear inverse solution termed ELECTRA (Grave de Peralta Menendez *et al.*, 2000). The use of linear inversion procedures yields an on-line implementation of the method, a key aspect for real-time applications.

The development of a brain interface based on ELECTRA—i.e., non-invasive estimates of LFP— would allow for methods identical to those used for EEG-based brain interfaces but with the advantage of targeting the activity at specific brain areas. In this respect our approach aims to parallel the invasive approaches described before that directly feeds intracranial signals into the classification stage of the brain interface, except that we calculate these intracranial signals from the surface EEG data. An additional advantage of our approach over scalp EEG is that the latter represents the noisy spatio-temporal overlapping of activity arising from very diverse brain regions; i.e., a single scalp electrode picks up and mixes the temporal activity of myriads of neurons at very different brain areas. Consequently, temporal and spectral features, which are probably specific to different parallel processes arising at different brain areas, are intermixed on the same recording. For example, an electrode placed on the frontal midline picks up and mix activity related to different motor areas known to have different functional roles such as the primary motor cortex, supplementary motor areas, anterior cingulate cortex, and motor cingulate areas.

In addition, the proposed approach bears two main advantages over invasive approaches. Firstly, it avoids any ethical concern and the medical risks associated to intracranial electrocorticographic recordings in humans. Secondly, the quality of the signals directly recorded on the brain deteriorates over time requiring new surgical interventions and implants in order to keep the functionality of the device.

In this chapter we describe in detail the theoretical framework needed for the non invasive estimation of Local field potentials, the rationale for its application and compare these estimates with the raw EEG (used to estimate the eLFP). To shed some light on the question of the feasibility of non-invasive brain interfaces to reproduce the prediction properties of the invasive systems, we compare the classification results of eLFP non invasively estimated from the EEG with intracranial recordings (IR) during a visuo-motor task.

2. Theoretical and practical aspects of LFP estimation

2.1 From the sources to the scalp fields

Brain function is investigated at two different scales: 1) A microscopic level encompassing the activity of a single or few neurons studied by means of single or multiunit recordings and 2) A macroscopic level reflecting the activity of larger neuronal ensembles recorded by either intracranial local field potentials in patients or animals or by scalp-recorded electric and magnetic fields.

At the origin of all these measurements are identical neural phenomena. During cell activation, large quantities of positive and negative ions cross the cell membrane, moving from the intracellular to the extracellular fluid, and vice versa. For all practical purposes, this ion movement is equivalent to a current flow, and it is responsible for all the recorded neurophysiological signals. The name used to refer to these microscopic currents varies somewhat. Within the modeling community, they are referred to as impressed currents while most neurophysiological researchers term them active currents. Active or impressed are terms used to differentiate these currents from the passive (also termed return or volume) currents that manifest as the electrical response of the media to compensate for charge accumulation at specific sites driven by the active currents.

At the microscopic level the redistributions in extracellular ionic charge due to neuronal transmembrane current flows generate extracellular volume currents throughout the head. These microscopic volume currents, in turn set up field potential gradients that follow Ohm's law and are proportional both to the magnitude of the local currents and to the tissue conductivity. As such, they are termed ohmic currents.

For axonal and cardiac tissue several comparisons of the relative field strength from both impressed and volume currents at the microscopic level show only the latter to be significant (see Plonsey, 1982 and references therein). Consequently, at the macroscopic level observable by Local Field Potentials, electroencephalography (EEG), and magnetoencephalography (MEG), the primary currents are dominated by the microscopic volume currents and can therefore be modeled as ohmic currents. Macroscopic passive volume currents, result from the gross conductivity changes associated to the existence of different compartments in the head, that is, brain, cerebrospinal fluid, skull and scalp.

Importantly, since macroscopic primary sources are dominated by the microscopic volume currents, then the primary currents perceived by EEG and MEG are ohmic. The mathematical implication is that they can be modeled as irrotational currents (Grave de Peralta Menendez et al. 2000).

2.2 Theoretical aspects of LFP computation

The formal relationship between intra-cerebral currents and scalp-measured fields can be derived from Maxwell equations that describe the propagation of electromagnetic fields within arbitrary volume conductor models, i.e.:

$$\nabla \circ \mathbf{E} = \rho / \varepsilon \qquad (1')$$

$$\nabla \times \mathbf{E} = -\partial \mathbf{B} / \partial t \qquad (2')$$

$$\nabla \circ \mathbf{B} = 0 \qquad (3')$$

$$\nabla \times \mathbf{B} = \mu(\mathbf{J} + \varepsilon \partial \mathbf{E} / \partial t) \qquad (4')$$

where **E** and **B** are the electric and magnetic fields, **J** is the total current density vector, ε and μ stand for physical properties of the media, and ρ is a (charge or current) density.

Equations (2') and (4') indicate that time varying electric and magnetic fields are interrelated. However, since the range of frequencies (Plonsey and Heppner 1967) associated with

electromagnetic fields in vivo-media is usually less than 1000 Hz, it is possible to suppress the contribution of the temporal terms. This is referred to as the quasi-static approach and implies that the capacitive and inductive effects produced by the temporal variations of the electric field **E** and the magnetic field **B** (see 2′ and 4') are irrelevant. The practical consequence of the quasi-static approach is that electric and magnetic fields recorded at the scalp are instantaneously reflecting the underlying neural processes and thus, electromagnetic processes taking place in the past are irrelevant for the present measurements. No evidence against this approximation has been reported so far.
This quasi-stationary assumption, allows for the separate modeling of the electromagnetic fields, i.e., the electric field is not dependent upon temporal variations of the magnetic field and vice versa:

$$\nabla \circ \mathbf{E} = \rho / \varepsilon \tag{1}$$

$$\nabla \times \mathbf{E} = 0 \Leftrightarrow \mathbf{E} = -\nabla \mathbf{V} \tag{2}$$

$$\nabla \circ \mathbf{B} = 0 \Leftrightarrow \mathbf{B} = \nabla \times A \tag{3}$$

$$\nabla \times \mathbf{B} = \mu \mathbf{J} \Rightarrow \nabla \circ \mathbf{J} = 0 \tag{4}$$

The total current emerging in biological tissue can be split into two terms: a primary and neurophysiologically driven current (J_p), and the volume or secondary current (σ**E**, i.e. $\mathbf{J} = J_p + \sigma\mathbf{E}$). From equation (4) derives that the divergence of total current (**J**) is zero, which when combined with previous current decomposition, and equation (2) yields Poisson's equation for the electric potential field:

$$\nabla \circ (\sigma \nabla V) = \nabla \circ J_p \tag{5}$$

This equation establishes that the actual generators of potential V are determined by the sources and the sinks obtained from the divergence of the primary current. This is mathematically identical to the Laplacian of the intracranial fields or the current source density (CSD).
Denoting by Q the brain region and using the Green function ψ associated to the solution of (5) we can rewrite it as a (first kind) Fredholm linear integral equation:

$$V(s) = -\int_Q \nabla \circ J_p(r) \psi(s,r) dQ \tag{6}$$

Designating the (vector) lead field by $L(s,r) = \nabla_r \psi(s,r)$ and noting that the primary current source distribution is bounded to the brain, it results the standard formulation of the neuro-electromagnetic inverse problem:

$$V(s) = \int_Q L(s,r) \bullet J_p(r) dr \tag{7}$$

denoting the relationship between the data measured at the external point, *V(s)*, and the superposition of the contribution of the unknown current source density distribution J_p at locations r inside the brain (Grave de Peralta Menendez, et al. 2004; Greenblatt 1993; M. Hämäläinen 1993; Sarvas 1987). The symbol "•" denotes the scalar or the vector product for the electric or magnetic case respectively. For the derivation of the magnetic lead field see Grave de Peralta Menendez et al. 2004.
Several (theoretical) source models have been used to solve equation (7) and thus to describe the sources of the electromagnetic activity of the brain, e.g., dipoles, monopoles, current density vector. Without entering into a formal discussion about the plausibility of these mathematical models, it is important to note that except for currents, none of these theoretical source models actually exists within the brain nor is any physically measurable. Instead, real measurements are the result of quantifiable potentials at different "measurable" levels. At the microscopic (neuron) level, this is the membrane potential. At the macroscopic (region) level, this is the local field potential (LFP). Through volume conduction, the effect of these potentials arrives at the scalp where they are measured as the Electroencephalogram (EEG). It is then natural to question whether potentials inside the brain can be related to and thus computed from potentials measured at the scalp.
A positive answer to this question can be given if we notice that, as discussed in previous section, macroscopic primary sources, i.e. the generators of the EEG, are dominated by microscopic secondary (volume) currents or in Plonsey words (Plonsey 1982) that "the fields measured do not even arise from J_p [the current source density vector field] but rather from secondary sources only. These secondary sources, in turn, depend on both the electrical field and the interfaces, and hence are related to divergence of J_p and the geometry". This kind of source corresponds to a potential distribution inside the brain.
A definitive theoretical argument can be obtained if we note that, according to the Helmholtz theorem, the current density vector field can be written as the sum of a solenoidal vector field plus an irrotational vector field plus the gradient of a harmonic function. That is,

$$J_p = J_s + J_i + J_h \tag{8}$$

where $J_h = \nabla\Omega$ with Ω harmonic in the brain region and $\nabla \circ J_s \equiv \nabla x J_i \equiv \nabla^2\Omega \equiv 0$. Here zero denotes the neutral for the addition of functions of each space.
Substitution of decomposition (8) in equation (6) yields:

$$V(s) = -\int_Q \nabla \circ J_s(r)\psi(s,r)dQ - \int_Q \nabla \circ J_i(r)\psi(s,r)dQ - \int_Q \nabla^2\Omega(r)\psi(s,r)dQ \tag{9}$$

Based on Green identities, it follows that only the second integral, corresponding to the irrotational current contributes to the measured potentials (EEG). In mathematical parlance, it means that the EEG generators fulfill:

$$\nabla x J_p = 0 \Leftrightarrow J_p = \nabla \varphi \tag{10}$$

where φ is a potential field within the brain. Assuming piece-wise constant conductivities σ, substitution of (10) into Poisson's equation (5) shows that φ has the same sources and sinks as the EEG potential V, i.e.:

$$\sigma \nabla \circ (\nabla V) = \nabla \circ (\nabla \varphi) \tag{11}$$

Note that, plotting the modulus of the estimated primary current obtained by solving (7), which we would note has thus far been the common procedure used to depict inverse solutions results, does not reflect the actual generators. Instead, the actual generators are determined by the sources and the sinks obtained from the Laplacian of potential field φ or $\nabla \circ J_p$ (the divergence of the primary current density vector).

The irrotational source model corresponds to the solution of the following equation

$$V(s) = \int_Q \nabla \varphi(r') \circ \nabla \psi(s,r') dQ = \int_Q \nabla \circ J_p(r') \psi(s,r') dQ \tag{12}$$

with respect to one of the following magnitudes: 1) The estimation of an irrotational current density vector $J_p = \nabla \varphi$ with the vector lead field $L = \nabla \psi$. 2) The estimation of a scalar field, the current source density (CSD), $\nabla \circ J_p = I$ with the scalar lead field ψ. 3) The estimation of a scalar field, the potential distribution φ in Q with a transformed scalar lead field $\nabla \psi \circ \nabla$.

Using the vector lead field, the third alternative relating the potential distribution inside the brain with the potential distribution on the scalp (EEG) can be written as:

$$V(s) = \int_Q L(s,r') \circ \nabla \varphi(r') dQ \tag{13}$$

In real conditions, neither the measurements nor the lead field functions are known for arbitrary surface/brain locations, but rather only at restricted discrete sites. Thus, it is reasonable to introduce a discrete formalism where the integral equation in (13) is approximated by a discrete sum, which leads to the following underdetermined system of linear equations:

$$\mathrm{v=Lf} \tag{14}$$

Vectors **v** and **f** and matrix **L** represent the discretization of the continuous functions, i.e., $\mathbf{v_k}=V(s_k)$ for k=1 to Numbers of sensors, $\mathbf{f_m}=\mathbf{f}(r_m)$ for m=1 to Number of solution points, and $\mathbf{L}_{km}=w_{km}\,\mathbf{L}(s_k,r_m)\circ\nabla$ and w_{km} are the quadrature weights.

Unfortunately, the restriction of the source model is not enough to ensure a unique solution to equations (13)-(14). For that reason, additional information (independent of the measured data) should be included in the solution. In principle, any mathematical method proposed for the solution of ill-posed problems can be considered. For reviews see (Menke 1989; Tikhonov and Arsenin 1977). While there is a wide range of solutions, we would like to caution the reader about the selection of a method based on figures of merit obtained from the localization of single sources, such as the so-called "zero dipole localization" or "location bias". We have previously demonstrated that these measures are neither necessary nor sufficient for assessing the performance of inverse solutions (Grave de Peralta Menendez and Gonzalez Andino 2000; Grave de Peralta-Menendez and Gonzalez-Andino 1998).

Since our goal of additional information is to better imitate the behavior of real sources in the head, we prefer to use additional information derived from biophysical laws. Therefore, we copy the spatial structure of a well- known potential field generated by an irrotational (dipolar) source, i.e., (Grave de Peralta Menendez, et al. 2004):

$$\phi(r) = M.\frac{r-r'}{\left|r-r'\right|^3} = \frac{\left|M\right|\cos\theta}{\left|r-r'\right|^2} \qquad (15)$$

expressing that the potential field at given point r depends upon the activity at another brain site r' according to a square inverse law. While this law relates one solution point with all the others, in our current implementation (see next section) we use only neighborhoods with no more than 26 points. This range is enough to compute the local autoregressive average (LAURA) regularization operator (Grave de Peralta Menendez, et al. 2001, 2004). We would note that this is not the same exponent we use for vector fields where we consider a cubic inverse distance instead.

In summary, the main advantages of the irrotational source model are:

1. Reduction of the number of unknowns. Since we need to estimate only a scalar field instead of a vector field, the number of unknowns is reduced three-fold. Given that the ratio between the number of unknowns and the number of sensors is a measure of uncertainty, we can say that the inverse problem with irrotational sources (13) is better determined than the unrestricted (arbitrary current density vector) estimation problem (7). In practice this results in images with rather detailed patterns (see Grave de Peralta Menendez, et al. 2000 for examples of visual evoked potentials).
2. The use of a scalar magnitude facilitates the inclusion of additional *a priori* information from other modalities of images (e.g., fMRI, PET, SPECT) brain images and reduces the computational load. In addition, post-processing of the single time series associated to each solution point might be easier than the analysis of three time series of the current density vector model.
3. Unquestionable constraints. The existence of irrotational sources is a condition necessary and sufficient for the existence of EEG. More simply, EEG recorded at the scalp surface is due to, and only due to, the presence of irrotational sources inside the brain. This constraint is independent of the data.
4. Experimentally verifiable model. Although defined up to a sign change, the potential distribution produced by this source model can be directly compared with intracranial measures (e.g. spectrum, energy, etc) derived from them. Related to this point, these estimated LFPs could also be compared with similar measurements from other species.

2.3 Practical aspects of LFP computation

The general solution of equation (14) can be obtained as the solution of the following variational problem (Grave de Peralta-Menendez and Gonzalez-Andino 1998; Menke 1989):

$$\min\ (\mathbf{Lf}-\mathbf{v})^t\mathbf{W}_v(\mathbf{Lf}-\mathbf{v})+\lambda^2(\mathbf{f}-\mathbf{f}_p)^t\mathbf{W}_f(\mathbf{f}-\mathbf{f}_p) \quad (16)$$

Where $\mathbf{W}_V$ and $\mathbf{W}_f$ are symmetric (semi) positive definite matrices representing the (pseudo) metrics associated with the measurement space and the source space, respectively. Vector $\mathbf{f}_p$ denotes any available *a priori* value of the unknown, e.g., from other varieties of brain functional images. The regularization parameter is denoted by λ. Independently of the rank of **L**, the solution to (16) is unique if and only if the null spaces of $\mathbf{W}_f$ and $\mathbf{L}^t\mathbf{W}_V\mathbf{L}$ intersect trivially, i.e., $\mathrm{Ker}(\mathbf{W}_f)\cap\mathrm{Ker}(\mathbf{L}^t\mathbf{W}_V\mathbf{L})$ is the empty set. In this case, the estimated solution vector **f** can be obtained using the change of variable $\mathrm{f}=\mathrm{f}_p+\mathbf{h}$ and solving the resulting problem for **h**, i.e.:

$$\mathbf{f}=\mathbf{f}_p+[\mathbf{L}^t\mathbf{W}_v\mathbf{L}+\lambda^2\mathbf{W}_f]^{-1}\mathbf{L}^t\mathbf{W}_v[\mathbf{v}-\mathbf{Lf}_p]=\mathbf{f}_p+\mathbf{G}[\mathbf{v}-\mathbf{Lf}_p] \quad (17)$$

If and only if matrices $\mathbf{W}_f$ and $\mathbf{W}_V$ are positive and definite, equation (17) is equivalent to:

$$\mathbf{f}=\mathbf{f}_p+\mathbf{W}_f^{-1}\mathbf{L}^t[\mathbf{L}\mathbf{W}_f^{-1}\mathbf{L}^t+\lambda^2\mathbf{W}_v^{-1}]^{-1}[\mathbf{v}-\mathbf{Lf}_p]=\mathbf{f}_p+\mathbf{G}[\mathbf{v}-\mathbf{Lf}_p] \quad (18)$$

The latter equation might be used when the same head model is used with several electrode configurations. Storing the inverse of the metric $\mathbf{W}_f$ and $\mathbf{W}_V$, we can repeatedly use equation (18) that only requires the inversion of a matrix of size equal to the number of sensors.

The definition of the metric matrices and the a priori vector $\mathbf{f}_p$ vary according to the data available. For example, when dealing with average event-related potentials or another EEG window we could define $\mathbf{W}_V$ as the inverse of the covariance matrix. If we use all the single trials of one experiment, we can build a covariance matrix for each time point. In the following, we will assume that we have no information about matrix $\mathbf{W}_V$ and vector $\mathbf{f}_p$. That is, we will use $\mathbf{W}_V$ =Identity and $\mathbf{f}_p$=0.

To compute the metric of the source space, consider the auxiliary matrix A associated to the autoregressive averages with coefficients according to the square inverse law (equation 15):

$$A_{ii}=\frac{N}{N_i}\sum_{k\subset V_i}d_{ki}^{-2}\ ,\ A_{ik}=-d_{ki}^{-2} \quad (19)$$

Where V_i denotes the vicinity of each solution point, defined as the hexaedron centered at the point and comprising at most N=26 neighbors. N_k is the number of neighbors of point k and d_{ki} stands for the Euclidean distance from point k to point i.

Then, we can define the metric of the source space as:

$$\mathbf{W}_f=\mathrm{A}^t\mathrm{A} \quad (20)$$

For the computation of the regularization parameter we use the generalized cross validation method as described in (Davies 1992), i.e., we look for the value of λ that minimizes the following expression:

$$\frac{\frac{1}{N}\left\|\{\mathbf{I}-R(\lambda)\}\mathbf{v}\right\|^{2}}{\left[\frac{1}{N}Trace[\mathbf{I}-R(\boldsymbol{\lambda})]\right]^{2}} \tag{21}$$

where $\mathbf{R}(\lambda)$ is the influence matrix, also called the data resolution matrix (Menke 1989), defined as the product of the lead field matrix and the inverse matrix. That is, $\mathbf{R}(\lambda)=\mathbf{L}^*\mathbf{G}(\lambda)$ and $\mathbf{G}(\lambda)$ is the inverse defined by equations (17) or (18) for a particular value of λ.

In summary, the computation of LFPs comprises the following steps:

1. Compute the scalar lead field matrix (equation 14) of your head model as the product of the vector lead field matrix times the gradient operator matrix.
2. Compute the metric of the source space as described in equations (19) and (20). Select the metric on the data space according the information available as well as the a priori source value $\mathbf{f}_p$.
3. Compute the inverse defined by equations (16) or (17) using a regularization parameter obtained by minimizing equation (20).

To obtain local field potentials, apply the inverse matrix **G** to your data.

Finally note that, in all derivations in equations 14-21, we assumed that the lead field matrix **L** and the data **v** have the same electrical reference (e.g. reference electrode). If it is not the case, you can pre-multiply both, the lead field and the EEG data, by the centering matrix that transforms column vectors to common average reference vectors (i.e. zero sum vectors).

3. Comparison of EEG, eLFP and IR in real experimental conditions

3.1 Experiment and data recording

We recorded scalp EEG data and intracranial data in 4 subjects and two patients performing a simple visuo-motor reaction time task. Subjects were asked to fixate a central cross that also served as a warning signal and to respond as fast as possible with the right or left index finger to visual stimuli appearing 3-4 s following the onset of the cross. Stimuli were presented for 60 ms in random order either in the left visual field (LVF) or in the right visual field (RVF) (4° horizontal eccentricity). Reaction times (RT) to stimuli were measured using an external device. Subjects had to give manual responses independent of stimulus location (simple RT task) with only the left or the right hand, in two separate blocks. Each block consisted of 120 trials and was preceded by a training session. The position of the head was stabilized by means of a head and chin rest and the hand of the subjects rested over the response device throughout the experiment.

EEG recording: The electroencephalogram (EEG) was continuously monitored at 500 Hz during the whole experiment from 125 scalp electrodes (Electric Geodesic Inc. system, USA). Recordings were done using a cephalic reference placed at the vertex. Off-line processing of the data consisted of (1) Transformation of the EEG data to the common average reference, (2) rigorous rejection of trials contaminated by ocular or movement artifacts through careful visual inspection, and (3) bad channel selection and interpolation. Fourteen electrodes from the lowest circle on the electrode array, i.e., closest to neck and eyes, were excluded a posteriori because of their likeliness to pick up muscular artifacts. A final configuration of 111 electrodes was used for all the analysis.

eLFP estimation: EEG recordings obtained from previous step were transformed into Local Field potential estimates (eLFP) using the inverse matrix associated to the irrotational source model (ELECTRA) described in previous sections. This yielded LFP estimates for 4024 brain "electrodes" distributed all over the gray matter of a realistic head model.

Intracranial recording: Two patients that underwent intracranial recordings (IR) for presurgical epilepsy evaluation performed the same visuo-motor reaction time task as used in the healthy subjects. IR were recorded at 200 Hz from subdural electrodes covering motor cortex and parietal and temporal areas of one hemisphere. The covering of motor areas was assessed by direct electrical cortical stimulation. The local ethical committee approved the experiments, and written informed consent was obtained in all cases.

3.2 Data analysis methods

Analysis window: For the analysis of the 111 EEG channels and the 4024 eLFP estimated channels, we selected a stimulus-locked time window of duration equal to the subject's fastest response. This period was chosen because it is very unlikely to be contaminated by electromyographic activity as this period precedes the actual movement onset for each single trial. Since the IC recordings are unlikely to be contaminated by electromyographic activity, the duration of the analysis window was selected as the mean reaction time (what could favor this modality).

Features extraction: For each data set, the power spectral density (PSD) was computed for all electrodes and single trials during the analysis window using a multitaper method with seven sleepian data tapers. All computations were done in Matlab. For the healthy subjects, the whole analysis covered the frequency range from 0 to 250 Hz, i.e. half of the frequency sampling, while for patients it was limited to the 0 to 100 Hz range, defined by the frequency sampling set to 200 Hz.

Classification details: For all modalities (i.e. EEG, eLFP and IC) the whole data set was divided in two halves. The first half was used as a learning set and the second one as the test set. Classification was based on the linear OSU-SVM and the performance was evaluated with the leave-one-out method on the test set using the features selected on the learning set. Leave-one-out (LOO) cross-validation is a special case of the cross-validation technique used to estimate the predictive accuracy of a classifier. Given n trials available in the test set, a classifier is trained on (n-1) trials, and then is tested on the trial that was left out. This process is repeated n times until every trial in the test set, has been included once as a cross-validation instance. The results are averaged across the n trials to estimate the classifier's prediction performance.

Discriminative Power (DP): The DP reflects the separation between the left and right hand responses in terms of their power spectral density (PSD) for each individual frequency and each electrode. It is graded between 0 and 100, with zero representing complete overlap between both PSD distributions (no discrimination between movements is possible) and 100 representing the perfect separation between them. The DP provides an estimate of how many trials can be unambiguously classified as pertaining to right or left movements on the basis of a single feature. This measure provides an estimate of the percentage of true

positives that can be obtained classifying with each single feature given that the number of false positive is set to zero. For a detailed description see (Gonzalez Andino et al. 2006)
Feature selection: Features were selected according to their DP on the learning set. That is, for each data set the best 150 features, with highest DP, were selected from all possible electrodes and frequencies over the trials on the learning set.

3.3 Data analysis results

The results obtained for the 4 normal subjects and the two patients are summarized in table 1. As a figure of merit we used the percentage of correct classification (CC%) computed from the leave one out results on the test set. Healthy subjects are referred as S1 to S4 and the two patients by P1 and P2.

Subject	EEG or IC electrodes	eLFP estimated from EEG
P1	91	--------
P2	94	--------
S1	97	98
S2	91	93
S3	85	91
S4	97	99

Table 1. Classification results for the two patients (P1 and P2) and the four healthy subjects (S1-S4) for the direct measurements (EEG or IC) or eLFP estimated from the EEG

4. Discussion and Conclusions

This chapter shows that there is a mathematical relationship between potentials measured at the scalp (EEG) and a scalar field inside the brain. This scalar field is a potential field for the current source density vector sharing the same sources and sinks of the intracranial potential measured inside the brain volume. The estimation of this potential field is mathematically equivalent to the use of the irrotational source model of ELECTRA inverse solution and for that reason it is denoted as eLFP. Extensive theoretical and practical elements needed to understand and implement the estimation of eLFP are also included.
The simulations presented shed some light on the basic questions that can arise in front of these estimates, i.e., how much information can be obtained from the eLFP in comparison with the EEG used for their to estimation and in comparison with invasive intracranial recordings.
As described in Table I, the range of CC (in %) values observed for the eLFP estimated from the EEG in healthy subjects (91-98) are not lower than the CC values (91 and 94) obtained from invasive recordings in two patients. This could be because intracranial electrodes are not located to optimize classification but to study the neurological conditions of the patients. However, it could be also an evidence for the use of the non-invasive method proposed to guide the positioning of intracranial electrodes. Further investigation will be needed to confirm that.

From a theoretical point of view it is not surprising that eLFP performs better than EEG if we consider all the elements included in their estimation and not available "per se" on the scalp EEG data. Clear examples are the information about the geometry and the conductivities included in the lead field, the irrotational property of the source model (ELECTRA) and the spatial structure induced by the regularization operator (LAURA). Nevertheless, we would note that the eLFP results reported here are just slightly better than the EEG for the same task. In fact we have found using a larger set of experimental conditions (unpublished data) that for some simple tasks, as the self paced finger tapping or the reaction time task discussed here, the use of the EEG or the eLFP yield very similar results. In contrast, for more complex tasks (e.g. cognitive processing of words or emotional images or the determination of the hand movement direction) the eLFP produces systematically much better results than the EEG and still comparable with the intracranial recordings (Grave de Peralta Menendez et al. 2005, and Grave de Peralta Menendez and Gonzalez Andino 2006). For other applications to the so called "mind reading" problem or prediction of response speed based on non invasive eLFP see Gonzalez Andino et al. 2005 and 2007.

As for a conclusion we can say that as shown by the experimental results, this non-invasively estimated field (eLFP) performs, for the classification task discussed here, better than the EEG and at least as well as the IR obtained with invasive methods. This suggests that eLFP is a worthy alternative to explore that might be considered as a safe and efficient alternative for the development of direct non invasive BCIs.

5. Acknowledgments

This work has been supported by the Swiss National Science Foundation Grant IM2.MI on Brain Machines Interfaces and the European IST Program FET Projects FP6-003758 (MAIA) and FP6-IST-027140 (BACS). This paper only reflects the authors' views and funding agencies are not liable for any use that may be made of the information contained herein.

6. References

Carmena JM, Lebedev MA, Crist RE, O'Doherty JE, Santucci DM, Dimitrov DF, Patil PG, Henriquez CS, Nicolelis MAL (2003) Learning to control a brain-machine interface for reaching and grasping by primates. *PloS Biol* 1:193–208

Davies AR. Optimality in Regularization. In: *Pike ER*, editor. Malvern Physcs Series; 1992; Cape Cod, USA. Adam Hilger, Bristol, Philadelphia, New York. p 393-410.

Donoghue J (2002) Connecting cortex to machines: Recent advances in brain interfaces. *Nature Neurosci Supp* 5:1085–1088

Gonzalez Andino SL, Michel, CM, Thut G, Landis T and Grave de Peralta Menende R (2005) Prediction of response speed by anticipatory high-frequency (gamma band) oscillations in the human brain *Hum Brain Mapp*, vol. 24, pp. 50-8

Gonzalez SL, Grave de Peralta Menendez R, Thut G, Millan JR, Morier P, and Landis T (2006) Very high frequency oscillations (VHFO) as a predictor of movement intentions, *Neuroimage*, vol. 32, pp. 170-9

Gonzalez Andino SL, Grave de Peralta Menendez R, Khateb A., Pegna, AJ, Thut, G, Landis T (2007) A glimpse into your vision *Human Brain Mapping* 28:614–624

Grave de Peralta-Menendez R, Gonzalez-Andino SL. (1998): A critical analysis of linear inverse solutions to the neuroelectromagnetic inverse problem. *IEEE Transactions on Biomedical Engineering*, Vol. 45,(4, April):440-48.

Grave de Peralta Menendez R, Gonzalez Andino SL, Morand S, Michel CM, Landis T (2000) Imaging the electrical activity of the brain: ELECTRA. *Human Brain Mapping* 9:1–12

Grave de Peralta Menendez R, Gonzalez Andino SL. (2000): Discussing the capabilities of Laplacian Minimization. *Brain Topogr* 13(2):97-104.

Grave de Peralta Menendez R, Gonzalez Andino S, Lantz G, Michel CM, Landis T. (2001): Noninvasive localization of electromagnetic epileptic activity. I. Method descriptions and simulations. *Brain Topogr.* 14(2):131-137.

Grave de Peralta Menendez R, Murray MM, Michel CM, Martuzzi R, Gonzalez Andino SL. (2004): Electrical neuroimaging based on biophysical constraints. *NeuroImage* 21(2):527-539.

Grave de Peralta Menendez ,R. Gonzalez Andino, S. Khateb A. Pegna, A. Thut, G. Landis, T (2005) About the information content of Local field potentials non invasively estimated from the EEG. *ISBET meeting*, Bern, Switzerland

Grave de Peralta Menendez ,R. Gonzalez Andino SL (2006). Noninvasive estimation of Local Field potentials: Single trial single subject analysis of emotional data. *EMOTION workshop*, Geneva, Switzerland

Greenblatt RE. (1993): Probabilistic reconstruction of multiple sources in the bioelectromagnetic inverse problem. *Inverse Problems* 9:271-284.

M. Hämäläinen RH, R. Ilmoniemi, J. Knuutila, and O. V. Lounasmaa. (1993): Magnetoencephalography: theory, instrumentation, and applications to noninvasive studies of the working human brain. *Rev. Mod. Phys.* 65:413:497.

Meeker D, Cao S, Burdick JW, Andersen RA (2002) Rapid plasticity in the parietal reach region demonstrated with a brain-computer interface. *2002 Abstract Viewer/Planner,* Program No. 257.7.2002, Society for Neuroscience

Mehring C, Rickert J, Vaadia E, Cardoso de Oliveira S, Aerten A, Rotter S (2003) Inference of hand movements from local field potentials in the monkey motor cortex. *Nature Neurosci* 6:1253–1254

Menke W. 1989. Geophysical Data Analysis: Discrete Inverse Theory (Revised Edition). New York: Academic Press, Inc.

Millán J del R, Renkens F, Mouriño J, Gerstner W (2004) Non-invasive brain-actuated control of a mobile robot by human EEG. *IEEE Trans Biomed Eng* 51:1026–1033

Nicolelis MAL (2001) Actions from thoughts. *Nature* 409:403–407

Pfurtscheller G, Neuper C (2001) Motor imagery and direct brain-computer communication. *Proc IEEE* 89:1123–1134

Plonsey R. (1982): The nature of sources of bioelectric and biomagnetic fields. *Biophys J* 39(3):309-12.

Plonsey R, Heppner DB. (1967): Considerations of quasi-stationarity in electrophysiological systems. *Bull Math Biophys* 29(4):657-64.

Sarvas J. (1987): Basic mathematical and electromagnetic concepts of the biomagnetic inverse problem. *Phys Med Biol* 32(1):11-22.

Serruya MD, Hatsopoulos NG, Paninski L, Fellows MR, Donoghue J (2002) Instant neural control of a movement signal. *Nature* 416:141–142

Taylor DM, Helms Tillery SI, Schwartz AB (2002) Direct cortical control of 3D neuroprosthetic devices. *Science* 296:1829–1832

Tikhonov AN, Arsenin VY. 1977. Solutions of Ill-Posed Problems. New York: John Wiley.

Wessberg J, Stambaugh CR, Kralik JD, Beck PD, Laubach M, Chapin JK, Kim J, Biggs SJ, Srinivassan MA, Nicolelis MAL (2000) Real-time prediction of hand trajectory by ensembles of cortical neurons in primates. *Nature* 408:361–365

Wolpaw JR, McFarland DJ (1994) Multichannel EEG-based brain-computer communication. Electroenceph. Clin. *Neurophysiol* 90:444–449

10

Motion Tracking for Minimally Invasive Robotic Surgery

Martin Groeger, Klaus Arbter and Gerd Hirzinger
Institute of Robotics and Mechatronics, German Aerospace Center
Germany

1. Introduction

Minimally invasive surgery is a modern surgical technique in which the instruments are inserted into the patient through small incisions. An endoscopic camera provides the view to the site of surgery inside the patient. While the patient benefits from strongly reduced tissue traumatisation, the surgeon has to cope with a number of disadvantages. These drawbacks arise from the fact that, in contrast to open surgery, direct contact and view to the field of surgery are lost in minimally invasive scenarios. A sophisticated robotic system can compensate for the increased demands posed to the surgeon and provide assistance for the complicated tasks.

To enable the robotic system to provide particular assistance by partly autonomous tasks e.g. by guiding the surgeon to a preoperatively planned situs or by moving the camera along the changing focus of surgery, the knowledge of intraoperative changes inside the patient becomes important.

Two main types of targets can be identified in endoscopic video images, which are instruments and organs. Depending on these types different strategies for motion tracking become advantageous.

Tracking of image motion from endoscopic video images can be based solely on structure information provided by the object itself or can involve artifical landmarks to aid the tracking process. In the first case, the use of natural landmarks refers to the fact that the genuine structure of the target is used to find reference positions which can be tracked. This can involve intensity or feature based tracking strategies. In the second case of artifical landmarks, markers with a special geometry or colour can be used. This enables particular tracking strategies, making use of the distinctive property of these markers.

This chapter describes different motion tracking strategies used to accomplish the task of motion detection in minimally invasive surgical environments. Two example scenario are provided for which two different motion tracking strategies have been successfully implemented. Both are partly autonomous task scenarios, providing automated camera guidance for laparoscopic surgery and motion compensation of the beating heart.

2. Motion tracking and visual servoing

Visual motion tracking is dealt with here, i.e. tracking of motion from video images. This enables the use of the video endoscope for tracking, as used in minimally invasive surgery

(MIS). Other tracking strategies with special markers and sensors, e.g. optical tracking (e.g. by ARTtrack) or magnetic tracking (e.g. by NDI), which they are hard to be applied in minimally invasive surgery, are not covered.

2.1 Motion tracking

Visual tracking deals with objects of varying positions in a sequence of images. The challenge is to determine the image configuration of the target region of an object as it moves through the field of view of a camera (Hager & Belhumeur, 1998). The task of visual tracking is to solve the temporal correspondence problem, which is to match target regions on successive frames of an image stream.

Tracking involves particular difficulties due to variability in the following parameters:

1. Target pose and deformation: the object can change its position and orientation, and its image can also be deformed, eg. when viewed from different perspectives.
2. Illumination: pixel intensities may change significantly as the scene or parts of it are exposed to different lighting conditions.
3. Partial or full occlusion: the object may vanish from the scene or be partially occluded by other objects.

Tracking strategies Two different tracking strategies can be distinguished: tracking based on image features and tracking of complete regions or patterns in an image. Feature-based tracking requires the extraction of features, which yields robustness against changes of global illumination. But image features may be sparse, which requires additional constraints for the tracking process (Hager & Belhumeur, 1998). While region-based tracking saves the cost of feature extraction, it is burdened with a relatively high computational expense to find the best matching pattern in subsequent images. Direct operation on image intensities requires illumination compensation but has the advantage of using all intensity information available.

Tracking targets The target of tracking, to be detected and followed in a sequence of images, can be a particular image pattern of the object of interest with a distinctive structure. This distinctive structure implies a sufficient contrast in intensity and uniqueness to avoid losing the target in favor of a similar object in the image. Since these criteria may be difficult to fulfill in some environments, it can be advantegeous to aid tracking by the use of so-called *artificial landmarks.* These artificial landmarks are designed with a unique and distinctive structure or colour and are put on the object to be tracked. While this kind of tracking is often referred as being based on artficial landmarks, the other case, in which no additional markers are placed on the object of interest to aid the tracking process can be denoted as tracking based on *natural landmarks.* In this way, natural landmarks refer to prominent parts of the target object in the image. The use of natural landmarks is especially attractive when objects such as organ surfaces are tracked, where artificial landmarks would be difficult to fix. Artificial landmarks often involve a tracking approach, in which image features are extracted which relate to these landmarks. For the case of natural landmarks, the choice between a region- and a feature-based tracking strategy depends on the property of the scene and the target object.

2.2 Tracking of surgical instruments (rigid objects)

In principle, tracking surgical instruments seems much easier than of deformable objects such as organ surfaces, since the tracking targets are rigid. The rigidity property combined with the fact that the geometry of the objects is known enables the use of a predefined target model. Also, the application of artificial landmarks is much easier, as e.g. colour markers as in (Wei et al., 1997) or (Tonet et al., 2007). However, in the case of surgical instruments with direct contact to human tissue, particular medical requirements such as the biocompatibility and the sterilisability of the artificial markers have to be met (Wintermantel & Ha, 2001).

Most approaches for instrument tracking can be categorised into the two main classes of colour-based strategies and approaches without colour which mainly rely on a geometric model of the instrument.

The use of *colour markers* is particularly attractive, if the environment occupies only a limited range of colour, as is the case for the situs in laparoscopic surgery, which makes the design of a unique colour marker possible (Wei et al., 1997). Similarly, in a more recent publication (Tonet et al., 2007), a colour strip at the distal part of the instrument shaft is used to facilitate segmentation for the localisation of endoscopic instruments. As shown in (Wei et al., 1997) the use of an appropriate colour marker can yield a robust solution for the tracking of surgical instruments.

The approach in (Doignon et al., 2006) does without the aid of artificial markers but uses region-based colour segmentation to distinguish the achromatic surgical instrument from the image background (Doignon et al., 2004) to initiate the search for region seeds. Based on this a special pose algorithm for cylindrically shaped instruments is used to localise the instrument, which can regarded as the second class of model-based approaches.

Doing without the aid of colour information leads to approaches which base their tracking strategy on the geometry of the instrument. These approaches often involve the extraction of edge images of the scene including the instrument, as shown in Fig. 2. As this example shows, this brings along a lot of difficulties to distinguish the instrument from its surroundings. Therefore, these approaches tend to be time consuming and prone to errors, which means that robustness is hard to achieve. A common strategy to detect the instrument without the aid of colour is to use the Hough transform, e.g. in (Voros et al., 2006).

2.3 Tracking of organs (deformable objects)

The particular difficulty with tracking the motion of deformable objects arises from that fact that, in contrast to rigid objects such as surgical instruments, the shape of the object itself changes. Moreover, in the case of organs, an appropriate and precise motion model is hard to estimate and is nonlinear in general (Mclnerney & Terzopoulos, 1996). Tracking deformable objects often involves the estimation of deformation in a particular image area, e.g. to extract face motions (Black & Yacoob, 1995) or to track surfaces in volume data sets of the beating heart (Bardinet et al., 1996; Mclnerney & Terzopoulos, 1995).

However, if the temporal resolution of the image stream is sufficiently high, such that changes between two subsequent images are small, approximating the deformation by a rigid motion model (consisting of e.g. translation! and rotation) is often sufficient, as investigated in (Shi & Tomasi, 1994). This enables local structures of deformable objects to be tracked efficiently.

Fixing artificial markers to deformable objects is difficult, in particular in the case of organ surfaces. Therefore, tracking approaches based on natural landmarks are advantageous, which often involve a region-based strategy.

A region-based approach designed to enable robust motion tracking of the beating heart surface using natural landmarks (Groger et al., 2002) is described in more detail below in a scenario to compensate motion of the beating heart by a robotic system (5).

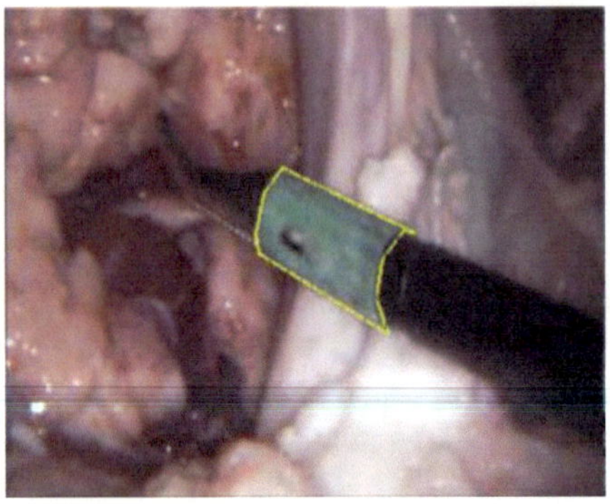

Figure 1. Laparoscopic instrument with colour marker (DLR)

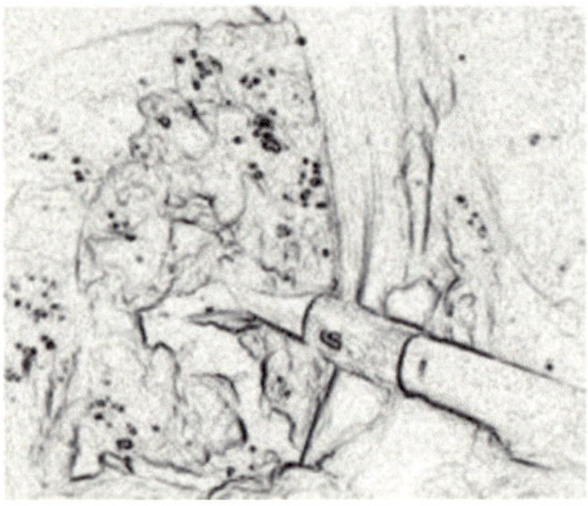

Figure 2. Edge image of laparoscopic instrument with colour marker

2.4 Visual servoing

"Visual servoing" in robotics denotes the control of an end effector in a control loop closed by imaging sensors. This requires the estimation and tracking of position and orientation of objects in the three-dimensional space, based on camera images (Corke, 1993; Hutchinson et al., 1996). Visual servoing involves the use of methods from realtime image processing, from visual tracking, and from robot control theory.

Many existing systems for visual servoing are based on artifical landmarks, which are mounted to the object of interest. However, this often increases the effort to set up the system or is hard to achieve, as e.g. with tracking of deformable objects such as organs. A region-based approach, which does not need any particular kind landmarks is described in (Hager & Belhumeur, 1998). This tracking system is successfully applied in a system for robust hand-eye coordination based on images of a stereo camera (Hager, 1997).

The use of stereo imaging from a stereo endoscope enables to estimate the three-dimensional position of the target, which is necessary for visual servoing tasks in 3D environments.

Two visual servoing scenarios for minimally invasive surgery are presented below. The automated la-paroscope guidance system enables a robot to automatically adjust the camera position to the current field of surgery (section 4). It is based on tracking a rigid object (surgical instrument) with aid of an artificial landmark (colour marker) mounted on it. The second scenario of motion compensation of the beating heart applies a region-based strategy with natural landmarks to track the motion of a deformable surface (the heart). Robust tracking of the heart, combined with a sophisticated robotic system enables to compensate the motion of the beating heart during surgery (section 5).

3. Minimally invasive robotic surgery

3.1 Minimally invasive surgery

Minimally invasive surgery only requires small incisions into the patient body. These incisions are used too introduce endoscopic instruments into the patient body, and also to insert an endoscopic camera, which provides a view of the site of surgery surgery inside the patient. In contrast to open surgery, minimally invasive surgery minimises trauma for the patient, decreases the loss of blood, speeds up patient convalescence, and reduces the time of the patient in the hospital.

While minimally invasive surgery brings along clear benefits for the patient, the surgeon is faces strongly increased demands, especially since direct contact to the field of surgery is lost. A sophisticated robotic system can compensate for the increased demands posed to the surgeon and provide assistance for the complicated tasks.

3.2 Robotic support for invasive robotic surgery

Surgical robots have been developed for a variety of specific applications, as summarised in (Taylor & Stoianovici, 2003). Most early first uses of robots in surgery occurred in neurosurgery (Y. S. Kwoh & et al., 1988), but the field soon expanded to other disciplines such as orthopaedics (Taylor et al., 1989,1994; Kazanzides et al., 1995) and laparoscopy (Sackier & Wang, 1996).

The use of robots allows to increase the accuracy of surgical interventions, as shown by early robotic systems in neurosurgery (Y. S. Kwoh & et al., 1988) and orthopaedics (Mittelstadt et al., 1996; Bargar et al., 1998). In minimally invasive surgery the drawbacks caused by loss of direct access to the field of surgery can be compensated by the aid of robotic systems, combined with techniques from the field of telepresence. Cartesian central, e.g., overcomes the the so-called "chopstick effect" when performing surgery through small incisions (Ortmaier & Hirzinger, 2000). Combined with increased dexterity of specially designed instruments (Rubier et al., 2005) this enables the surgeon to lead the instruments similar to in open surgery and to regain the dexterity as in open surgery. Force feedback (Preusche et al., 2001) together with specially designed sensorised instruments (Kubler et al., 2005) enables the surgeon to feel forces occurring at the tip of the instrument during surgery. Moreover, the use of stereo endoscopes enable a three-dimensional view to the field of surgery and as in open surgery. Different techniques of 3D display devices, such as head-mounted displays (HMDs) or a stereo console as in the daVinci system (Guthart & Salisbury, 2000).

The combination of preoperative planing with the surgical intervention enables intra operative support for the surgeon by medical robots, such as the guidance of instruments (Ortmaier et al., 2001).

3.3 Visual servoing for robots in medicine

Visual servoing closes the control loop between imaging sensors and robot control. It enables to perform partly autonomous tasks, depending on the current situation in the field of surgery.

Examples for autonomous robot functions are tasks to supervise the working room or the automated guidance of the camera in laparoscopy (Wei et al., 1997). Different scenarios, in particular from soft tissue surgery are the guidance of the robot end effector to particular positions, in relation to given tissue structure, e.g. to hold a lighting source or tissue parts, or the autonomous movement of the robot end effector to particular positions, as e.g. in liver biopsy.

Moreover, one can think of compensating the motions of organs, such that the relative configuration and distance between instrument and organ surface remains constant. Thus, the organ is stabilised virtually. In this case, however, it is also necessary to integrate the video image provided to the surgery into the motion compensation procedure and to maintain overall consistence of motion compensation.

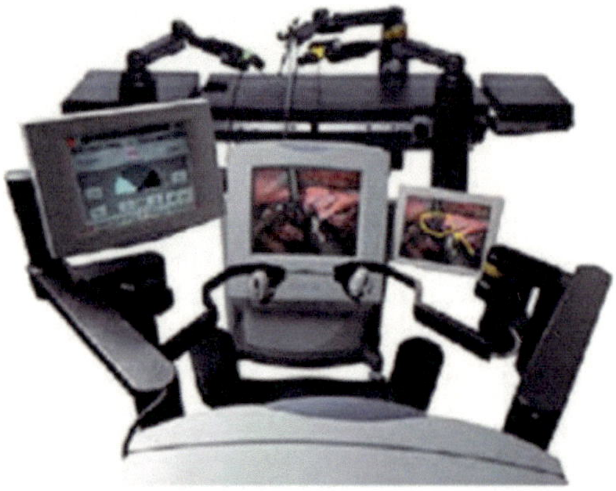

Figure 3. ZEUS robotic system by Computer Motion Inc

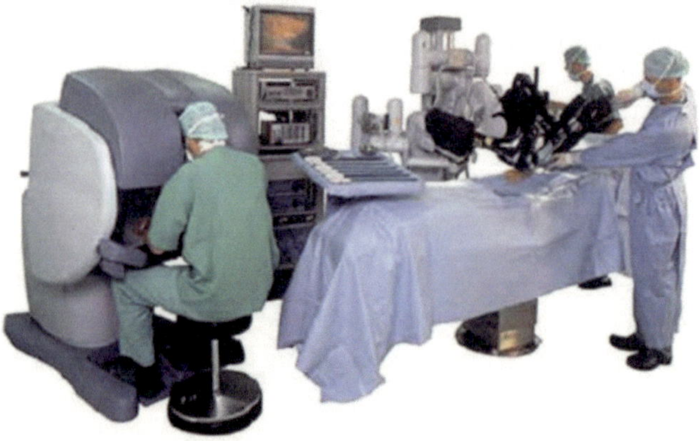

Figure 4. DaVinci robotic system by Intuitive Surgical Inc

3.4 Robotic systems for minimally invasive surgery

Many robotic systems that have been applied to surgery are based on industrial robots, as e.g. the *Robodoc* system for for hip surgery (Kazanzides et al., 1995; Taylor et al., 1994; Bargar et al., 1998), and are therefore large, heavy and hardly flexible. Other robotic systems, specially desgined to be applied for surgery, such as the *ZEUS* system ((Sackier & Wang,

1996), Fig. 3) by Computer Motion Inc. (Goleta, CA, USA; now: Intuitive Surgical Inc.) and the *daVinci* system ((Guthart & Salisbury, 2000), Fig. 4) by Intuitive Surgical Inc. (Cupertino, CA, USA) are much more flexible and light-weight. These systems are sufficient for laparoscopic assistance tasks such as the automated guidance of a laparoscope to provide the surgeon with a view of operating field. This is shown in the first example scenario below (section 4).

These robotic systems, however, lack the high degree of precision needed for orthopaedic surgery and additionally the high dynamics required for following the motion of the beating heart (section 5). The newly developed KineMedic surgical robot was specially designed to account for these increased demands, providing both light-weight and flexibility and the required high dynamics and precision.

The design of the KineMedic robot is based on the method of soft robotics pursued at the Institute of Robotics and Mechatronics, DLR, which leads to robotic systems such as the DLR light-weight robot (Hirzinger et al., 2001), which are light-weight, flexible and modular, and still maintain a high degree of dynamics and accuracy. Based on these techniques, the newly designed KineMedic robot has been developed as a joint partnership of DLR and BrainLab AG (Heimstetten, Germany), focussing on the demands of surgery (Ortmaier et al., 2006).

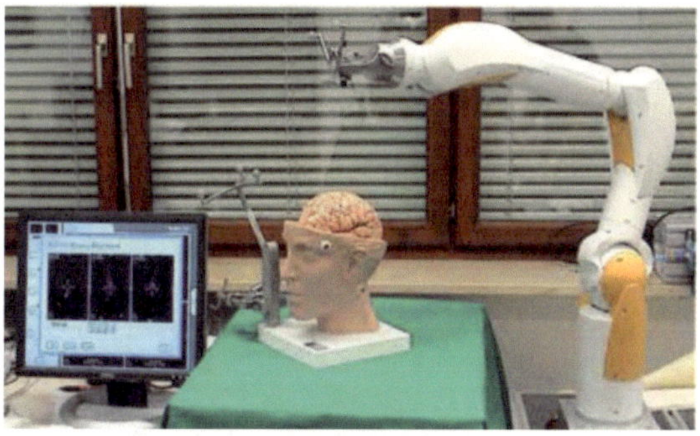

Figure 5. DLR-KineMedic medical robot arm

The KineMedic surgical robot (see prototype in Fig. 5) consists of sophisticated light-weight robotic arms, which reach a payload of 3 kg at a dead weight of only 10 kg. The redundant design of the robotic arm with seven joints enables, using null-space motion, to reconfigure the position of the robot, while the position and orientation of the instrument remains in the same position. With force-torque sensors, implemented in addition to the redundant design of the robot, the reconfiguration of the position can be performed in an intuitive way by touching and pushing the robot into the desired direction. Furthermore, the redundancy can be used to implement an arm control system which avoids collisions, which enables a more flexible setup in the operating room. Since the robot is built in light-weight design, it can be mounted or removed easily by a surgeon or nurse during a surgical intervention. This reduces mounting times in the operating room. For minimally invasive surgery usually two of these robot arms are used to manipulate surgical instruments, while a third arm moves the endoscope. An example of such a scenario is is presented in Fig. 6. The KineMedic robot arm is controlled at a rate of 3 Hz and has a high relative positioning accuracy. This way, the robot provides the dynamics required for following the motion of the beating heart.

The new KineMedic robot shows significant improvements on the medical robots avaible so far and enables highly demanding scenarios such as compensation the motion of the beating heart.

4. Automated laparoscope guidance

In laparoscopic surgery, the surgeon no longer has direct visual control of the operation area, and a camera assistant who maneuvers the laparoscope is necessary. Problems of cooperation between the two individuals naturally arise, and a robotic assistant which automatically controls the laparoscope can offer a highly reliable alternative to this situation. In this section a autonomous laparoscopic guidance system for laparoscopic surgery is described, developed at the DLR's robotics lab and thoroughly tested at MRIC (Department of Surgery at the Klinikum rechts der Isar (MRIC) of the Technical University of Munich) (Wei et al., 1997; Omote et al., 1999).

A robot holds the laparoscope and directs it to the operative field by means of image processing techniques. The method is based on colour coded instruments. The system originally operated at a maximum rate of 17 Hz for stereo-laparoscopes and 34 Hz for mono-laparoscopes (Wei et al., 1997). It now easily runs on a standard PC in realtime for stereo-laparoscopic images delivered at a framerate of 25 Hz. For mono-laparoscopes, tracking only in lateral directions (left/right and up/down) is enabled, but for stereo-laparoscopes tracking in the longitudinal direction (in/out), too.

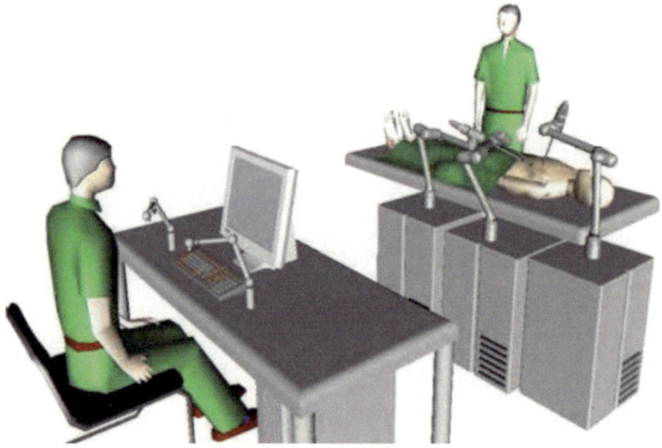

Figure 6. DLR scenario for minimally invasive robotic surgery

During the initial period of clinical evaluation 20 laparoscopic cholecystectomies have been performed and compared with those using human camera control. The longer set-up time was finally compensated by a shorter operation time. The frequency of camera correction caused by the surgeon as well as the frequency of lens cleaning was much less than with human control. The smoothness of motion was much better with the robot than with human assistants. Subjective assessments by the surgeon revealed that the robot performed better than the human assistant in a significant majority of cases.

4.1 Introduction

Laparoscopic surgery is minimally invasive, which offers the advantages of reduced pain, shorter hospital stay, and quicker convalescence for the patients. Unlike open surgery, laparoscopic surgery needs only several small incisions in the abdominal wall to introduce instruments such as scalpels, scissors, and a laparoscopic camera, such that the surgeon can operate by just looking at the camera images displayed on a monitor screen. While in open surgery vision and action are centered on the surgeon, he loses direct visual control in laparoscopic surgery. Another person, the camera assistant, has to point the laparoscope to the desired field of vision. The surgeon has to give instructions as to where the scope should be focused, and the camera assistant has to follow them. This naturally gives rise to problems of cooperation between the surgeon and the camera assistant. A certain amount of the assistant's experience and a mutual surgeon-assistant understanding are necessary, but usually difficult to obtain. The surgeon frequently has to give the commands to move the laparoscope onto the desired area of view. This gives him an additional task, detracting his attention from his main area of concentration. The laparoscopic image may become unstable in a long operation due to fatigue of the camera assistant.

To deal with these problems, several robotic assistance systems have been developed (Hurteau et al., 1994), (Taylor et al., 1995), (Sackier & Wang, 1996) to provide more precise positioning and stable images. For a more comprehensive review of robotic systems in other surgeries see (Taylor et al., 1994), (Troccaz, 1994), (Moran, 1993), and (Taylor & Stoianovici, 2003). Investigations indicate that the use of robots in surgery reduces personnel costs while almost maintaining the same operation time (Turner, 1995). A surgical robot may be controlled either by an assistant using a remote controller or by the surgeon himself using a foot pedal (Computer Motion Inc., 1994). Voice control seemed to be another attractive alternative, as it was available with the AESOP3000 medical robot arm (by Computer Motion Inc., Goleta CA, USA).

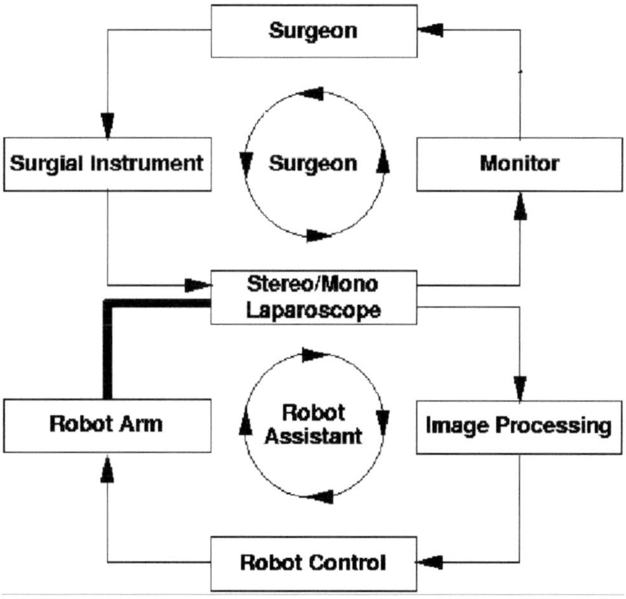

Figure 7. The structure of image-based robot-assisted minimally invasive surgery

To avoid the need for another assistant and to free the surgeon from the control task, an autonomous system that automatically servoes the laparoscope is highly desirable. The basic structure of an image based system is shown in Fig. 7. The surgeon handles the surgical instruments dependent on his observations on a monitor where the laparoscopic image is displayed, as usual in minimally invasive surgery. But instead of a human, the laparoscope is held by a robot arm which is controlled via an image processing system in order to track the surgical instrument smoothly. The use of the laparoscope as a sensor for the tracking system sounds attractive, because no extra sensor is needed, but it's hard to obtain reliable control signals under realistic clinical conditions and safety requirements. The dominant problems for image processing are ambiguous image structures, occlusions by blood, organs or other instruments, smoke caused by electro-dissection, and the need of (quasi-)real-time image processing. With respect to the slow robot motions during a surgery, an image processing rate of about ten frames per second (10 Hz) is considered to be enough, but is a lower limit to maintain the impression of smooth motion.

Several researchers have tried to use image processing techniques to track the instrument such that it is always centered in the visual image. Lee, *et al,* (Lee et al., 1994) used the colour signatures of the image to segment the instrument. Since the instrument and background often possess the same colour components, much post-processing, such as shape analysis, has to be done to remove false segmentations and to extract the position of the instrument in the image. No real-time implementation was reported in, (Lee et al., 1994), and it is not known whether the complexities of their shape analysis may allow implementations applicable to surgical operations. Casals, *et al.* (Casals et al., 1995), used patterned marks on the instrument to facilitate image segmentation by searching for the presumed structure in the contour image. The method was reported to operate at a rate of 5 Hz for a mono-laparoscope using customised image processing hardware. Since both the methods in (Lee et al., 1994) and (Casals et al., 1995) rely on the existence of a preassumed shape or structure, they may fail if the camera is to near to the instrument, or if the instrument is partially occluded by organs or contaminated by blood. In both cases, the preassumed shape may not be present. Taylor, *et al.* (Taylor et al., 1995), used multi-resolution image correlation to track an anatomical structure specified by the surgeon with an instrument-mounted joystick that controlled a cursor on the video display. A problem with this method might be that the anatomical structure deforms and may completely change its appearance due to manipulation of the organs.

We propose a visual laparoscope-tracking method which is simple and robust (Arbter & Wei, 1996), (Arbter & Wei, 1998). The laparoscope may be a mono-laparoscope or stereo-laparoscope. A mono-laparoscope enables the robot to track the instrument in the lateral directions left/right and up/down, while a stereo-laparoscope provides depth information and can be used to control the distance between the tip of the laparoscope and the instrument. Due to the multiplicity of problems with shape analysis, we do not check for the presence of any particular shape or structure. Instead, we use colour information alone for instrument segmentation. The non-uniqueness of the instrument colour inspires us to use an artificial colour-marker to distinguish the instrument (Fig. 12a). To mark the instrument, the colour distribution of typical laparoscopic images is analysed and a colour is chosen which does not appear in the operational field (the abdomen here). With colour image segmentation, the marker can be correctly located in the image and used to control the robot motion. Thus, even if only a very small part of the marker is visible, reliable data can still be obtained for robot control.

To build up an experimental system, only commercially available hardware was used, with the instruments from Bausch Inc., Munich, Germany, the stereo-laparoscope system from Laser Optic Systems Inc., Mainz, Germany, the AESOP 1000 robot from Computer Motion, Goleta, USA, the MaxVideo 200 image processing system from Datacube Inc., USA, and a M68040/25MHz host-CPU from Motorola Inc., USA. The coloured markers have been placed on the instruments by the manufacturer. The electronic components are integrated into an electronic radiation protecting cabinet being mobile and used as transportation car for the robot arm, too.

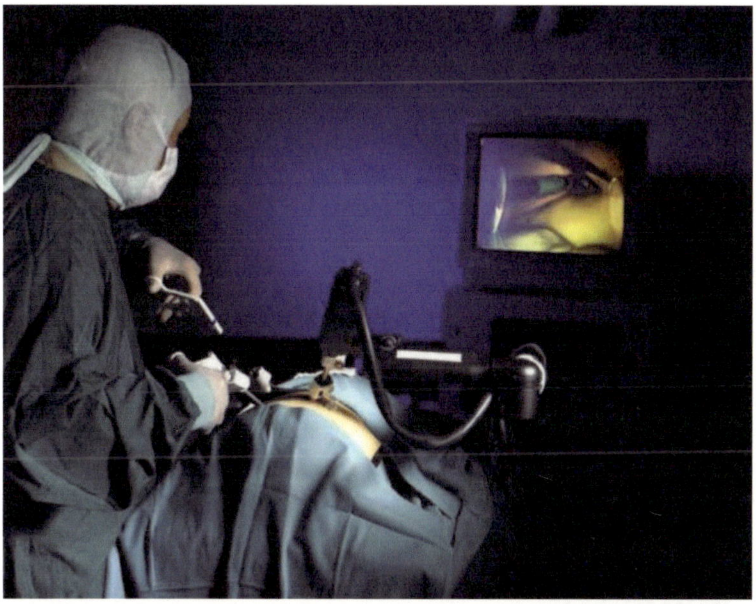

Figure 8. DLR automated camera guidance scenario with AESOP robot

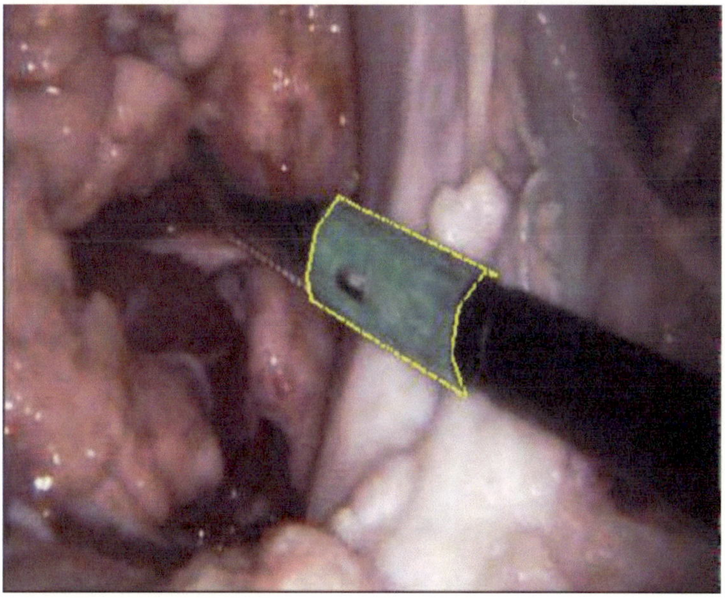

Figure 9. Laparoscopic instrument with colour marker (DLR)

For the initial period of clinical tests the system was evaluated in 20 laparoscopic cholecystectomies and compared with those using human camera control.

In the following, the image processing module, the robot controller module, and the experimental results are presented.

4.2 Image Processing

Figure 10 shows a block diagram of the image processing module. The inputs are the analog video *RGB-signals,* either from the CCD-camera pair of the stereo-laparoscope, or from only one CCD-camera of a mono-laparoscope. The inputs are **time multiplexed** at the video frame rate of 25 Hz (CCIR) in order to spend only one image processing hardware to process the stereo-images. Then the analog signals are converted into digital *RGB-signals* of 8 bits each. The *RGB* data stream is **converted** to the *HSV* format (Hue, Saturation, Value) for reasons explained below. The **classifier** separates two classes of pixels, those having the colour of the marker and those not. The result is a binary image containing the object separated from the background. The classifier is the kernel of the image processing module and will be explained in detail below. The **localiser** computes the bounding box and the centre of gravity of the object pixels as well as their number (size of region). The bounding box is then used to define the region of interest (ROI) for segmentation of the next frame. The use of an ROI speeds up the segmentation procedure and improves the robustness against misclassification. Figure 11 shows a stereo-laparoscopic image (of an experimental environment) superimposed by the centres of gravity and bounding boxes of the segmented marker.

4.2.1 Colour representation

A colour can be represented by its red, green, and blue components *(RGB).* In digital 8bit-images, the *RGB* values are between 0 and 255. Thus colours can be represented by the points within the *RGB* cube of size 256 x 256 x 256. The *RGB* colour space can be transformed to another colour space, the *HSV* colour space (Hue, Saturation, Value) where only two components *H* and *S* are directly related to the intrinsic colour and the remaining component *V* to the intensity. Different *RGB-to-HSV* transformations are known in video technology and computer graphics. We have used the following one (Foley et al., 1990):

$$r = R/R_{\max}, \qquad g = G/G_{\max}, \qquad b = B/B_{\max} \tag{1}$$

$$\min = \text{Minimum}\{r, g, b\} \tag{2}$$

$$\max = \text{Maximum}\{r, g, b\} \tag{3}$$

$$\Delta = \max - \min \tag{4}$$

$$H = \begin{cases} 60^o\ (g-b)/\Delta & : \max = r \\ 60^o\ (b-r)/\Delta + 120^o & : \max = g \\ 60^o\ (r-g)/\Delta + 240^o & : \max = b \end{cases} \tag{5}$$

$$S = (\max - \min)/\Delta \tag{6}$$

$$V = \max \tag{7}$$

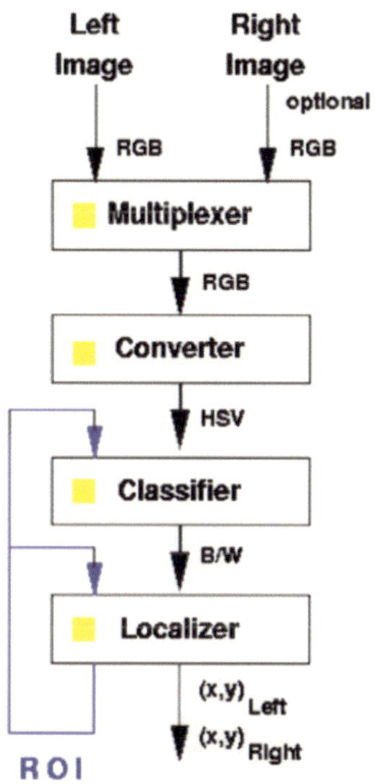

Figure 10. Structure of the image processing module

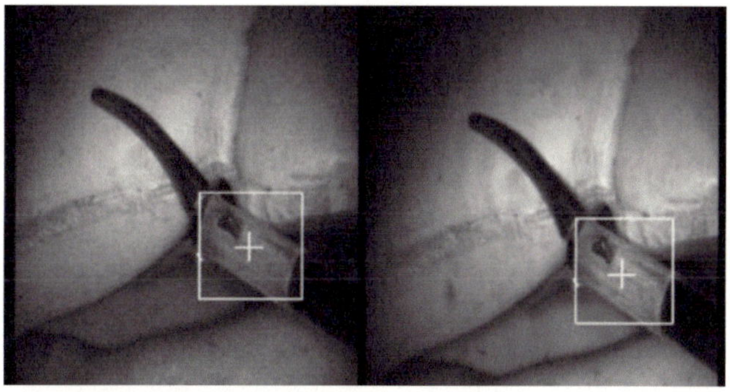

Figure 11. A stereo laparoscopic image superimposed by the centres of gravity and bounding boxes of the segmented marker

In laparoscopic surgery, we would like the image segmentation results to be insensitive to the strength of illumination. The *H* and *S* are insensitive to the strength of illumination, if only one light source, having a certain colour temperature, is used, as is the case in laparoscopy. One advantage of the *H S* colour space is its 2-dimensionality in contrast to the 3-dimensionality of the *RGB* colour space, so that the colour signature of a colour image can be directly analyzed in the *H S* plane. Figure 12d shows a colour space of the *H S* representation, filled with the corresponding colour, where the brightness is set to 255. In this coordinate system, the *H* value is defined as the angle from the axis of red colour, and the *S* value (normalised to the range of zero to one) is the length from the origin at the centre.

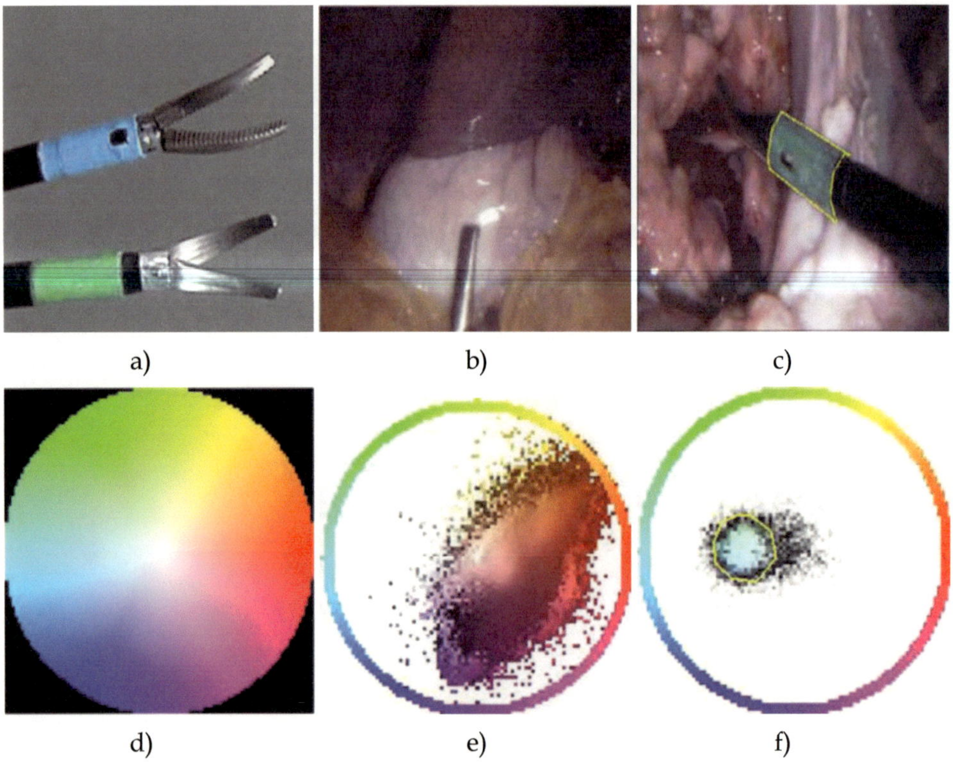

Figure 12. (a) Distal ends of colour coded minimally invasive surgical instruments (b) A typical laparoscopic image (c) Marker image with polygonal boundary (d) HS colour space (e) Colour Histogram of the abdominal scene (f) Colour histogram of the marker superimposed by the polygonal classifier boundary (cluster-polygon)

4.2.2 Marker colour selection

To choose the colour to be brought onto the instrument, we analyzed the colour components of real laparoscopic images recorded on a video tape. Typical abdominal images containing variations of colours are manually selected. Figure 12b shows one of the 17 images used in our colour analysis. An array of counters in a quantised *HS* domain is set to zero at the start. Then, for each pixel in the images, we compute its *HS* values and increment the counter by 1 at the corresponding *HS* position. The result is a 3-D histogram, which indicates the frequency of occurrence of all the colours in the analyzed images. To give an intuitive perception of the histogram, we display it in a colour image format, with the brightness (V) set proportional to the frequency of occurrence and the *HS* values equal to the *HS* coordinates in the *HS* plane. Figure 12e shows such a histogram, where the ring near the image boundary is used to help perceive the overall colour distribution. The crescent bright region within the ring represents the colours that do not appear in the images and can thus be used as the colour to be marked on the instrument. For the marked colour to be optimally distinguishable from those present in the image, the colours near the cyan are preferred, as can be seen in Fig. 12e. After the admissible colours have been determined, we have to consider the material which carries the desired colour, its commercial availability, and its biocompatibility. On account of these factors, we have used a near-cyan plastic ring, as shown in Fig. 12c.

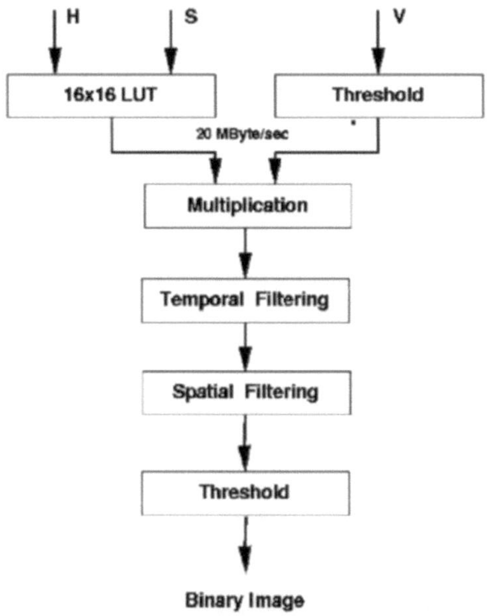

Figure 13. Classifier structure

4.2.3 Colour training selection

Due to the colour distortion through laparoscopes, we have to locate the actual position of the chosen colour in the *H S* plane. We select a set of typical images showing the marker in different situations, e.g., near, far, slanted, or orthogonal to the view direction, and calculate the colour histograms from the marker regions only. We first manually outline the marked instrument in the image with a polygonal boundary as shown in Fig. 12c. Then, the pixels within the polygon are used to compute the colour distribution in the *H S* plane. Figure 12f shows the colour cluster of the marker.

To represent the corresponding individual marker colour space, we again use a polygonal approximation of the cluster boundary Fig. 12f. By backprojection of the enclosed colours to the original training set and by modifying the boundary, we iteratively minimise the number of misclassified background pixels by simultaneously maximizing the number of correctly classified marker pixels. We repeat this procedure for all the images out of the training set, resulting in a set of colour regions. The union of the individual regions represent the marker colour space, and we call its border cluster-polygon. The above process is called colour training, and is of the type of supervised learning.

4.2.4 Colour classifier

The kernel of the colour classifier (Fig. 13) is a 16-bit look-up table (LUT). This LUT is the implementation of the region beeing bounded by the cluster-polygon. Its input is a data stream of 16-bit *HS* values, which are formed by concatenating the 8-bit *H* and 8-bit *S* values. Its output is binary and indicates whether the input value falls within the cluster-polygon or not. Low intensity pixels do not provide reliable *H S* values and are themselves of no interest. Thus, pixels beeing classified as marker pixels, but having an intensity below a certain threshold are reset to zero (background) by multiplication of the LUT output with the thresholded intensity *V*. This step of postprocessing would not be necessary, if *RGB* values would be used as input. But the use of a 16-bit LUT requires to reduce the resolution to 5 bits for each *RGB* component. This is an other reason, why we preferred the *HSV* colour space. Fig. 14 shows the initial segmentation of Fig. 12c using the cluster-polygon of Fig. 12f. It can be seen from Fig. 14 that most of the marker pixels are correctly classified, yet some of them and a few background pixels are misclassified. Misclassification of marker pixels is much less critical than of background pixels and can be accepted up to a considerable amount since no shape analysis is used. Although we could avoid false segmentations of background pixels by choosing a smaller cluster-polygon, but this would also eliminate too many pixels belonging to the marker. The classification errors tend to be scattered, as well in the space as in the time domain. Furthermore, the space-frequency bandwidth of the marker region is much lower than the bandwidth of the scattered errors. Therefore the inital segmentation can efficiently be improved by spatio-temporal lowpass postprocessing. We add successive binary frames (time-domain lowpass) and convolve the result with a 7 x 7 box operator (space-domain lowpass, local 7 x 7average). By thresholding the low-pass filtered image, not only misclassified background pixels are removed, but also misclassified marker pixels are recovered, thus the marker region becomes more compact, as shown in Fig. 15. A special colour classifier design tool (CCDT) has been developed, which allows for an easy design of a colour classifier (Arbter & Kish, 2004).

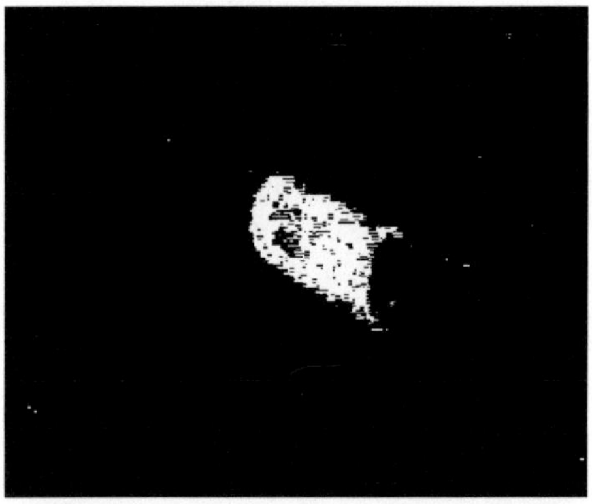

Figure 14. Colour segmented marker

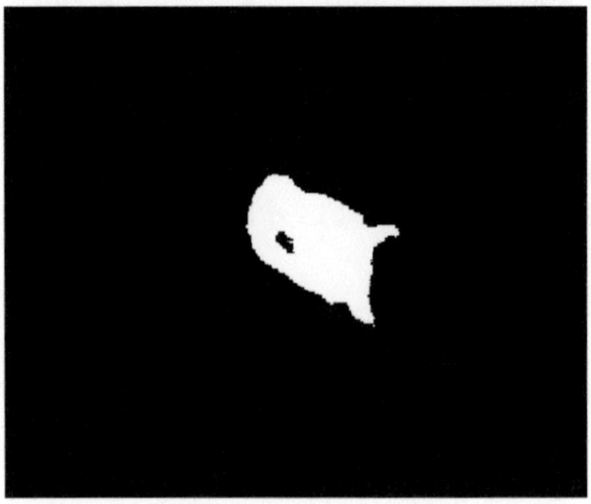

Figure 15. Postfiltered segmentation result

4.3 Robot Controller

The task of the controller is to bring the actual image of the instrument to a desired location at the monitor screen by smoothly moving the robot according to the incoming signals from the image processing system. The desired location is either prestored, or it can be redefined on-line by moving the instrument to the desired monitor position, while the tracking mode is switched off. In the second case the image processing module extracts the actual location values and stores them as reference coordinate values for the future.

As input to the robot controller, we have used the centers of gravity as well as the corners of the bounding boxes. We made the experience that corners are much more reliable in most cases than centres of gravity, especially in the case where the marker is partially occluded.

Since the AESOP 1000 robot system (Computer Motion Inc., 1994) provides direct motion control in the image plane, no user-involvement in the robotic kinematics is necessary. The commands **MoveLeft ()** and **MoveRight ()** specify robot motions such that the laparoscopic image moves to the left and right of the human eyes looking at the monitor image; that is, they specify the *x*-direction motion in the image coordinate system. Similarly, **MoveUp ()** and **MoveDown ()** control the motion in the *y*-direction in the image plane. Motions orthogonal to the image plane (longitudinal *z*-direction motions) are specified by the **Zoomln ()** and **ZoomOut ()** commands.

Suppose (x_L^0, y_L^0) and (x_R^0, y_R^0) are the reference coordinate values in the left and right images, respectively. Suppose (x_L, y_L) and (x_R, y_R) are the current coordinate values of the colour marker location in the left and right camera images, respectively. Then, we determine the 3D-speed command of the robot motion as follows:

$$\begin{aligned} v_x &= \alpha[(x_L - x_L^0) + (x_R - x_R^0)] \\ v_y &= \alpha[(y_L - y_L^0) + (y_R - y_R^0)] \\ v_z &= \beta[\sqrt{(x_L - x_R)^2 + (y_L - y_R)^2} - \\ &\quad \sqrt{(x_L^0 - x_R^0)^2 + (y_L^0 - y_R^0)^2}]. \end{aligned}$$

The equations reduce in the case of mono-laparoscope to:

$$v_x = \alpha(x - x^0), \qquad v_y = \alpha(y - y^0).$$

This intermediate commands are then converted to the specific **Move . . . (speed)** commands by separating magnitudes and signs for speed and direction.

With this control law the closed loop system has approximately a first order low-pass transfer function. The bandwidth (dynamics) depends on the values *a* for lateral motions and *0* for longitudinal motions, respectively, and may easily be adapted to the surgeon's needs. The system follows asymptotically slow instrument motions, as they occur if the surgeon changes the operational field, but damps fast motions, as they occur if the surgeon treats the tissue. This behavior provides the surgeon with smoothly moving images in the first case and with quasi-stable images in the second case, as is desired.

4.4 Robustness

Safety is of the highest priority in surgery. The correct segmentation of instruments is crucial for correct visual guidance. A problem particular to laparoscope images is that the received light by the narrow lens system is usually very weak, so that the CCD signal (including noise) has to be highly amplified. For this reason, the signal-to-noise ratio is considerably lower than that of a standard CCD-camera. In our system, the high rate of correct colour segmentation in the presence of noise is attributed to the use of spatio-temporal low-pass filtering.

Occlusion of instruments occurs very often during surgical operations. It can be caused either by another instrument or by organs. As far as the lateral motion control is concerned, partial occlusion is by no means a hindrance, since no precise motion control is necessary. Besides, partial occlusion does not affect image-tracking either, because no shape analysis is used in the tracking. In the case of complete occlusion, the colour code can be re-allocated, when it re-appears, at almost the same speed as it is tracked. It may happen that in few critical situations, e.g., when the colour code is too far away from the laparoscope, either the left or the right colour code is not fully segmented due to uneven illuminations. In such a case, the computed disparity provides wrong information about depth. In our sytem the bounding boxes are permanently checked with respect to their difference in size. If this difference is greater than a threshold, e.g., 40 pixels, the z -direction motion control is blocked.
Another characteristic of laparoscope images is that saturation may occur caused by too intensive illumination, or by specular reflections at moist organ surfaces. The highly saturated part in the image is white in colour. When saturation occurs on the instrument, e.g., when the instrument is placed too near to the laparoscope, the saturated part loses its original colour of the colour-code. But since the instrument is cylindric in shape, i.e., the surface normals vary in a wide range, the probability of complete saturation of the colour-marker is extremely low. Particulary those regions where the normals are oriented towards the light source tend to be saturated. In this sense, saturation is similar to partial occlusion.
Furthermore, due to the use of the region of interest (ROI) in the classifier, the segmentation result will not be disturbed by any events outside ROI. For instance, the visual attention of the robot will not be redirected toward the image boundary when a second instrument appears there. Also, the reaction time of the robot assures image stability. Any quick movement of the instrument, e.g., due to instrument change, will not cause the robot to follow. Still, as the statistics processor provides the number of colour-marker pixels, we use it as another security check. If the pixel number is less than a threshold, e.g., 50, then a decision is made that no object is reliably segmentable, and the robot remains stationary.

4.5 Performance characteristics

The image processing system MaxVideo is a pipeline processor working at 20 MHz. Its image processing components such as colour transformation, colour classification (LUT), temporal filtering, spatial filtering,
localisation, and bounding box extraction are working in parallel. The result is transferred via VME-Bus to the host CPU where the robot controller, safety check, and the interface to the AESOP robot are implemented. The system works asynchronously at a maximum rate of 34 Hz for mono-images and of 17 Hz for stereo-images when the region of interest has been found, and at a minimum rate of 15 Hz for stereo-images, when the region of interest is the whole image of 512x512 pixels for each of the two images. The rate might be doubled by using double buffering technique, in which image acquisition and image processing work in parallel, too. But this is not necessary for our task.
A recent implementation of the system runs on a standard PC (Intel Pentium 4,2.6 GHz Xeon) in realtime for stereo-laparoscopic images delivered at a framerate of 25 Hz.

4.6 Experiments and evaluation

The system has first been tested in a dummy abdomen used for surgical training. Artificial (plastic) organs as well as as real organs (of pigs) have been used. During this phase the surgeons learned to use the system. Furthermore system parameters, as dynamic behavior, have been tuned to the surgeons needs, and the classifier could have been refined (LUT, thresholds).

The system was then tested on pigs at the Klinikum rechts der Isar, Technical University of Munich. Of particular importance where the tests of the system performance under the following typical disturbances:

- partial occlusion by organs or another instrument,
- staining by blood or gall juice,
- rinsing fluid,
- smoke caused by electro-dissection and coagulation.

The visual guidance in the cavity of the pigs was very successful and there were no cases in which the robot was wrongly guided.

During the initial period of clinical evaluation, that followed, 20 laparoscopic cholecystectomies on humans have been performed and compared to 58 laparascopic cholecystectomies under human assistance. The evaluation included the parameters set up time, operation time, frequency of lens cleaning, frequency of camera correction, and incidence of intraoperative complications. Student's test was used for the statistical analysis and values of $p < 0.05$ were considered to be significant. After laparoscopic surgery using the robotic system, the surgeon completed a questionnaire to asses subjectively the performance of the robotic system compares to a human assistant.

The set up time for the robot system was defined as the interval from the point at which the robot arm was attached to the side of the operation table until laparoscopy started. This time period was compared to that needed without the robot, namely the interval between connection of the sterilised tubes to the equipment and the initial insertion of the laparoscope into the abdominal cavity. The surgical time was defined as the interval from the beginning of the cholecystectomy and the moment when the laparoscope was finally extracted. Contamination of the optical lens caused by contact with internal organs or intraperitoneal fluid is very bothersome because in this case the laparoscope has to be extracted and to be cleaned. The frequency [events/hour] of lens cleaning is therefore an important assessment parameter in laparoscopic procedures as well as the frequency of camera corrections by the surgeon. With the robotic system those corrections are necessary if the reaches the border of his working space. If the human assistant misguides the laparoscope then the surgeon intervents sometimes manually but mostly by a verbal instruction to the assistant.

The mean set up time for the robot system (21 minutes) was considerably longer than that without the robot (9 minutes). But, before the system was integrated into the mobile cabinet, the setup time was up to 55 minutes. With the integrated system the setup time was reduced to around 15 minutes.

The surgical time using the robot was between 35 and 70 minutes. The mean value of 54 minutes was 6 minutes shorter than with human assistance, although the difference between the two was not statistically significant (p>0.05).

The mean frequency of interruptions for lens cleaning was only I/hour compared to 6.8/hour with the human assistance (p<0.0001). This improvement is a consequence of the utilization of a stereo laparoscope within an automatic control loop which maintains the distance between the lens and the marker, and which stops longitudinal motion if the marker becomes inivisibile in at least one image of the stereo image pair.

Similarly the mean frequency of interventions of the surgeon for correcting the position/orientation of the camera decreased from 15.3/hour with human assistance to 2.2/hour with the robotic system. This improvement is basically the consequence of the automatic guidance concept.

	Units	Robot Assistance n=20	Human Assistance n=58	Statistical Significance P
Setup time	minutes	21 [10-55]	9	<0.0001
Operation time	minutes	54 [35-70]	60	>0.05
Lens cleaning	events/h	1.0	6.8	< 0.0001
Camera	events/h	2.2	15.3	< 0.0001
Complications	technical anatomical	2 1		

Table 1. Clinical evaluation results

The procedures were successfully completed in 17 cases with the robot camera assistant, but were interrupted in the 3 remaining cases. In two of the latter cases robot camera control had to be changed to human camera control, and the remaining one case was converted to open surgery because of anatomical reasons. In the first case that was transferred to human camera control the reason was insufficient white balancing of the laparoscope. In the second case, there was a problem in positioning of the robotic arm, which disturbed the free movement of the surgeon. The troubles that arose in these two cases were avoided in future operations.

Subjective assessment by the surgeon revealed that the robot camera control performed worse in 12.5% , equal in 12.5%, and better in 71% of the cases. This statistical result is dominated by the two cases mentioned above, where the procedure was interrupted due to technical reasons, which are not relevant in the future. Furthermore the smoothness of motion was emphasised as an important improvement, supporting the surgeons concentration. For more details see (Ungeheuer et al., 1997) and (Omote et al., 1999).

4.7 Conclusion

We have described an autonomous, real-time visual guidance system for laparoscopic surgery. The system is based on commercially available hardware components. We proposed to use colour marking on the instrument for simple and reliable segmentation. The cost of manufacturing the extra colour-marker on the instrument is expected to be negligible in comparison to the price of the instrument itself. No special sterilization is needed. The system is very robust, both in the case of partial occlusion, and when the camera is very near to the instrument. Clinical experiments have demonstrated that the system can be reliably used for laparoscopic surgery. Automated laparoscope guidance promises to give back the surgeon his autonomy, particularly at standardised routine laparoscopic procedures as cholecystectomy fundoplication, hernia repair, or diagnostic laparoscopy.

5. Motion compensation of the beating heart

This section deals with motion compensation of the beating heart. The scenario and clinical background is introduced first, describing why beating heart surgery is beneficial for the patient and why robotic systems are required to advance surgery in this field. Next, a region-based motion tracking scheme for the beating heart is described, with special focus on robustness of the approach. Finally, motion compensation is dealt with, before concluding with a summary and perspectives for future research.

5.1 Introduction

Tracking the motion of organs poses particular demands to the imaging system, since the target objects are deformable, as discussed above in section 2.3. This section starts with the stabilisation of organs and introduces the field of robotically assisted heart surgery thereafter.

5.1.1 Stabilisation of organs

While e.g. bone surgery allows for stereotactic fixation of the operating field, a complete stabilisation of the organ of interest is, in general, not possible in soft tissue sugery. The occurring motions are mainly due to respiration and heart beat, which is continued by the pulsating flow of blood in the vessels. Furthermore, organs are exposed to external forces during surgery, as e.g. when insufflating the abdomen with CC>2 during laparoscopic surgery or when tissue is drawn during surgery. These forces can cause the organs to change their position and to deform.

To perform surgery on the beating heart, a mechanical stabiliser is used to restrict motion in the operating field on the heart surface (Jansen, 1998). Since the heart tissue is elastic and deformable, this does not enable a complete fixation of the surface of the beating heart, however (Jacobs et al., 2003). The remaining motion is significant, especially for minimally invasive surgery at the beating heart, and a limiting factor to perform beating heart TECAB (totally endoscopic coronary artery bypass grafting, see below). The goal of the project described in the following is to compensate for this remaining motion of the beating heart.

5.1.2 Robot-assisted cardiac surgery

About three quarters of all annual heart surgeries in Germany (about 100 000) are bypass surgeries due to coronary heart diseases (800 000 cases worldwide) (Borst, 2001). During this kind of surgery the narrow part of a coronary vessel is bypassed with an healthy vessel, which is usually a vene from the leg or from the thoracic wall.

The conventional surgical technique brings along high strain for the patient, because the the thoracs is widely opened at the sternum to provide access the heart. To arrest the heart during the intervention the use of the heart-lung machine is necessary, in order to maintain the blood circulation. This brings along the danger of complications such as neurological disturbances by microembolies. Furthermore, the contact of blood with artificial surfaces can lead to general inflammation reactions. Also there are risks because of blood heparinisation to avoid thromboses. The overall high degree of traumatisation of the patient can lead to serious complications and accounts for a relatively high convalescence time of 2-3 months (Borst, 2001).

The high strain for the patient is approached to be reduced by two strategies:

On the one hand, surgery at the beating heart avoids the use of the heart-lung machine and thus also the risks that come with it. For beating heart surgery, the operating field is stabilised by a mechanical stabiliser, e.g. the Octopus™ system by Medtronic, which is fixed to the heart surface with small sucking mechanisms. (Jansen, 1998).

On the other hand, minimally invasive surgery avoids the highly traumatic sternotomy by using small incisions between the rips to access the heart. The surgical instruments and an endoscopic camera are inserted through these so-called "ports". This surgical technique is known as TECAB (Totally Endoscopic Coronary Artery Bypass), and endoscopic robot systems are applied, with which the surgon controls the instruments inside the patient at an input console (cf. Fig. 6). The daVinci™system is an endoscopic surgerical robotic system which has been available for a few years (Guthart & Salisbury, 2000). The newly designed DLR surgical KineMedic robot (Ortmaier et al., 2006) will be able to to perform these tasks as well and adds a number of improvements (cf. section 3.4.

Minimally invasive surgery at the beating heart has been investigated at a few heart centres, such as Leipzig (heart centre, Prof. Dr. F. Mohr, PD Dr. V. Falk) (Mohr et al., 1999; Falk et al., 1999), Hamburg (University, Prof. Dr. H. Reichenspurner, PD Dr. D.H. Bohm, formerly in Munich-Grosshadern) (Reichenspurner et al., 1999b; Boehm et al., 1999), or in Canada (University of Western Ontario, Dr. W. Douglas Boyd) (Boyd et al., 2000).

Beating heart TECAB brings along considerable benefits for the patient, such that the convalescence time is reduced to a few days only. The surgical technique, however, poses strongly increased demands: In contrast to open surgery at the arrested heart, the contact to the operating field has to be established by a surgical robot system, the working space at the heart itself is very limited, and also the mechanically stabilised areas on the heart surface shows significant residual motions, which impede fast and safe interventions (Reichenspurner et al., 1999a; Jacobs et al., 2003).

5.1.3 Related work on motion compensation of the beating heart

The importance of motion compensation of the beating heart has been recognised and investigated in international research groups. Research has especially been performed by (Nakamura et al., 2001) and (Ginhoux et al., 2004). Both approaches, however, use artificial markers for motion estimation, which have to be fixed to the surface of the heart and the insertion and usage in the operating field of which brings along further difficulties. Therefore, using natural landmarks to estimate the motion of the beating heart ((Groger et al., 2002), section 5.3) is especially attractive. Moreover, region-based tracking of natural landmarks yields a particular texture unique for each landmark. This easily allows to track several landmarks concurrently, whereas using identical artifical landmarks bears the danger of ambiguities.

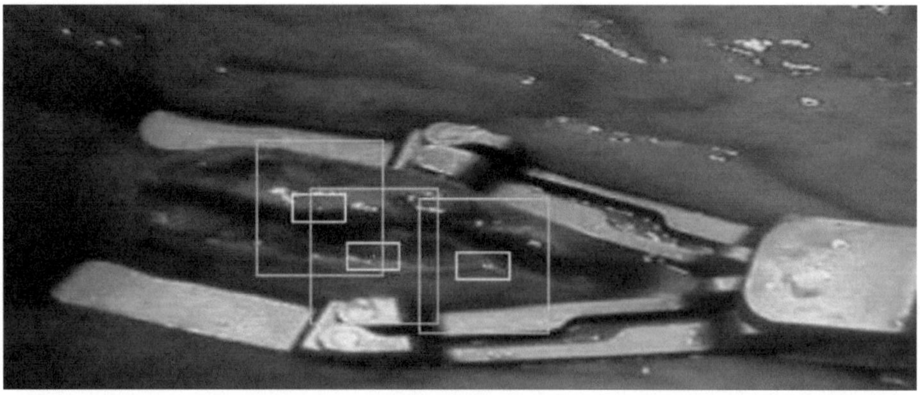

Figure 16. Mechnically stabilised heart with landmarks and tracking areas (from left to right LM2, LM8, and LM1)

Related work on motion compensation of the beating heart only allows for global correction of the image motion by moving the viewing camera according to motion captured (Nakamura et al., 2001; Ginhoux et al., 2004). However, as shown in (Groger & Hirzinger, 2006b), the motion of the beating heart cannot be fully reduced by compensating the occurring motion with a constant image correction factor.

5.2 Overview of the motion compensation scheme

Figure 17 gives a schematic overview of a possible solution for motion compensation in minimally invasive robotic surgery: The robot compensates the heart motion, such that the relative pose between the heart surface and the tool centre point of the surgical instrument remains constant (grey part of Fig. 17). The surgeon can then work on a virtually stabilised heart as he was used to in on-pump surgery, in which the heart does not move and the heart-lung machine is used to sustain the circulation. The following paragraphs describe this scheme in more detail.

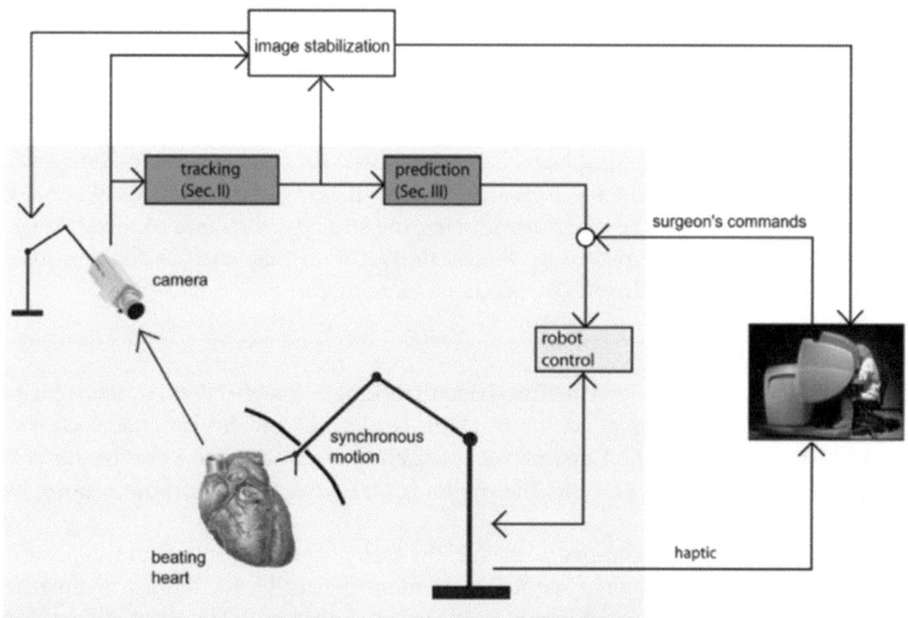

Figure 17. Schematic overview of motion compensation scheme

The surgeon's commands are superimposed on the motion of the instrument robot, which are calculated as shown in the inner part of Fig. 17. To perform the surgery it is not only necessary to move the surgical instruments according to the heart motion, but also to provide the surgeon with a stabilised image (see right part of Fig. 17 and (Falk et al., 1999)). Image stabilisation itself can be achieved either electronically by appropriate image warping algorithms or by moving the laparoscope robot in a way similar to the instrument robot, as indicated in the upper part of Fig. 17. Additionally, the surgeon can be provided with haptic (tactile or kinesthetic) feedback if appropriate surgical instruments at the slave side and displays at the master side are available (Kubler et al., 2005), (Preusche et al., 2001).

Before motion compensation in beating heart surgery can be performed, organ motion arising from the patient's respiration or heart beat has to be coped with. Therefore, the reliable measurement of this motion is an essential part of an advanced minimally invasive robotic surgery system (tracking block in the inner part of Fig. 17). Algorithms are presented which are able to track the motion of the 2-D projection of the beating heart surface by exploiting natural landmarks (see section 5.3). Motion tracking is made more robust by the prediction algorithms (inner part of Fig. 17) introduced in section 5.3.4, which are able to compensate for short failures of the motion estimation scheme. Furthermore, prediction is necessary to overcome the delays (data acquisition and processing, communication, etc.) which deteriorate the performance of the visual servoing control loop closed in the inner part of Fig. 17. Robust motion compensation (i.e. synchronous movement of heart surface and instrument, such that the relative distance /orientation between the instrument pose and selected frames lying on the heart surface remains almost constant) can be achieved only if these delays are eliminated. The robot control block is necessary for Cartesian control of the surgery robot as well as for taking the kinematic constraint at the entry point of the instrument into the human body into account. This is described in detail in (Ortmaier & Hirzinger, 2000) and will not be repeated here.

5.3 Motion tracking of the heart

Tracking the motion of the beating heart is the basic step for an approach to compensate the motion. This section introduces a region-based tracking strategy based on natural landmarks (Groger et al., 2002). After introducing the strategy, the issue of robust tracking is described and a few algorithms are presented to deal with this, such as the elimination of specular reflections and a multisensory prediction strategy.

5.3.1 Tracking model

As introduced in 2.1, region- and feature based tracking strategies can be distinguished. A region-based approach seems good for tracking landmarks on the heart surface, since all information should be used and geometric constraints on the tracking environment would be hard to establish. In the following, the model for tracking motion on the beating heart is introduced.

Parametric Model Given a reference pattern r, the task of tracking is to find the position of r in subsequent frames of an image sequence, or more generally, to find a transformation T mapping a pattern p in the current image to the original pattern r. The dissimilarity between two image patterns is expressed by the sum of squared differences (SSD) and is applied to determine suitable parameters of the transformation T:

$$J_{\mathrm{SSD}}(r,p) = \sum_{i \in \mathrm{dom}(r)} \left(r(i) - p(i)\right)^2 , \tag{8}$$

where r and p are two image patterns and dom(r) denotes the domain of pattern r.

Searching for the best match of a reference pattern r in subsequent images, an image region p is allowed to be transformed according to the parameters of the model. The optimum motion parameter vector μ_{opt} minimising the dissimilarity between the reference and transformed patterns is given by

$$\mu_{\text{opt}} = \underset{\mu \in M}{\operatorname{argmin}} J_{\text{SSD}}(r, T_\mu(p)), \tag{9}$$

where M is the set of all parameter vectors to the transformation T_μ, i.e. the search space to find μ_{opt}.

Affine Motion Model Although heart tissue is distorted nonlinearly, an affine motion model as in (Hager & Belhumeur, 1998) can be applied if the pattern is small enough to allow linear approximation. With the motion parameter vector μ, written as $\mu = (t_x, t_y, s, \phi, \tau, \alpha)^T$, the affine transformation i' of an image position vector $i = (i_x, i_y)^T$ is given by

$$i' = A \cdot i + t, \tag{10}$$

where $t = (t_x, t_y)^T$ is the translation vector, and the warping matrix A can be decomposed as

$$A = s \cdot \begin{pmatrix} \cos\phi & -\sin\phi \\ \sin\phi & \cos\phi \end{pmatrix} \cdot \begin{pmatrix} \cos\alpha & \sin\alpha \\ -\sin\alpha & \cos\alpha \end{pmatrix} \cdot \begin{pmatrix} 1 & 0 \\ 0 & \tau \end{pmatrix} \cdot \begin{pmatrix} \cos\alpha & -\sin\alpha \\ \sin\alpha & \cos\alpha \end{pmatrix}, \tag{11}$$

where s is the scaling parameter, ϕ the rotation angle, and τ and α are the shear parameter value and direction.

Illumination Model A linear compensation model is used to cope with illumination changes. It is applied to each pattern before the SSD measure is calculated to compare the reference and tracked patterns. Only mean compensation is demanded

$$\text{mean}(p) \overset{\text{def}}{=} \sum_{i \in \text{dom}(p)} p(i) = 0, \tag{12}$$

which is achieved by shifting the intensities of a given pattern p such that their mean value is zero. Further compensation such as the normalisation of the standard deviation relating to the local contrast does not significantly improve tracking in the given heart images.

5.3.2 Elimination of specular reflections

The wet and glossy surface of the beating heart gives rise to frequent specular reflections of the light source, which disturb the tracking scheme considerably: These highlights are not bound to a particular surface structure and move according to the change in orientation between the light source and the heart surface. Strategies to detect the specular reflections and to reconstruct the underlying structure are developed and evaluated in (Groger et al., 2001, 2005): Structure inside specular areas is reconstructed using local structure information determined by the structure tensor, which provides a reliable measure of the orientation of structures. The reconstruction scheme uses intensity information mainly from boundary pixels along the current local orientation and interpolates linearly between these intensities. Thus, surface structure in the image is continued and smooth transitions at the boundaries are ensured. Preprocessing endoscopic heart images by this scheme makes the subsequent tracking considerably more robust toward specular reflections (Groger et al., 2001). The results given below are based on video sequences processed in this way.

5.3.3 Motion trajectories

Investigations show that the affine motion model described by Eq. 10 can be simplified from six to two degrees of freedom (i.e. a two-dimensional translation vector) to capture the heart motion

in the stabilised area (Groger et al., 2002). To determine the significance of the parameters of the motion model, the parameter space is searched exhaustively to find the best match.
The quality of tracking and the appropriateness of the suggested tracking model is shown by an analysis of the trajectories of the parameters associated with the tracked pattern. This analysis assesses the occurrence of outliers from the expected trajectory and the strength of the signal indicated by the appearance of dominant frequency components in the amplitude spectrum of the trajectory. Outlier measures developed in (Groger et al., 2002) calculate the total number of outliers and the distance of a given trajectory from its smooth version.

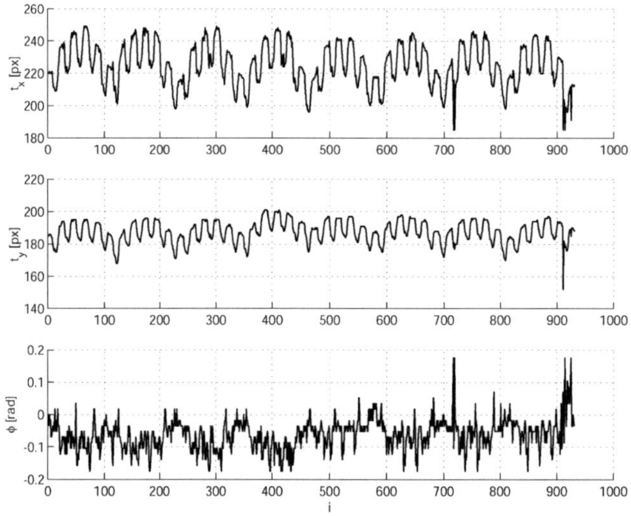

Figure 18. Selected trajectories of the affine parameters of landmark LM2. The temporal resolution is 40 ms (25 Hz frame rate). Translation in x and y are given in pixel [px], rotation ϕ in radians [rad]

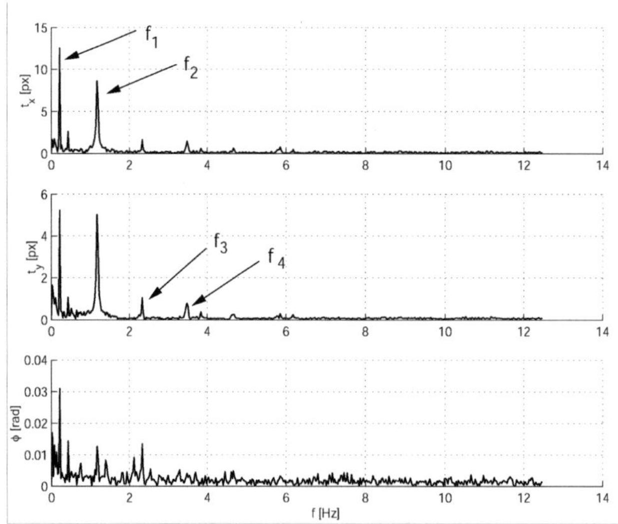

Figure 19. Amplitude spectrum of selected affine parameters at landmark LM2

The quasi-periodic progression of the translational parameters is presented in Fig. 18. The other parameters are strongly disturbed and thus hardly contain any useful information (see Fig. 18 for the rotational parameter ϕ. Reduction of dimensions of the parameter search space to only two translational degrees of freedom allows to efficiently obtain the optimum $\mu_{opt} \in M$ (section 5.3.1, Eq. 9. Moreover, this enables realtime implementation on a standard computer with simultaneous tracking of several landmarks as in section 5.3.4. The small search space allows for exhaustive search for μ_{opt} in realtime, thus avoiding errors by local minima.
The results presented here are confirmed by details given in (Groger et al., 2002). Tracking of e.g. 332 equally distant landmarks over 931 frames in the stabilised area of Fig. 16 with the proposed translational tracking model shows that more than 97% of all positions and frames are tracked without outliers.
The amplitude spectrum of the translation parameters shows two dominant peaks at f_1 = 0.24 Hz and f_2 = 1.18 Hz (see Fig. 19). The frequency f_1 corresponds to the respiration rate of the patient, f_2 to the heart rate. The influence of respiration on the measured heart motion becomes clear if the patient anatomy is considered. The respiration effect causes the diaphragm moving up and down, which yields an additional motion superimposed to the motion caused by the heart beat itself. The distribution of the dominant peaks depends on the current setup, e.g. the image coordinate system or the placement of the mechanical stabiliser. In addition to f_1 and f_2, the first and second harmonics of the (non-sinusoidal) heart beat can be extracted from the amplitude spectrum: f_3 = 2.36 Hz and f_4 = 3.54 Hz. The amplitude spectrum of the rotational parameter shows similar behaviour, but the dominant frequencies are much less pronounced.
The spectrum analysis shows that the trajectories of tracked positions are strongly correlated with heart beat and respiration. Since the amplitude spectrum only provides a global view of the trajectory, natural changes of the physiological parameters are not taken into account. Therefore, the spectrum is only used to show the correctness of the applied tracking model but not considered in the proposed motion tracking scheme.

5.3.4 Motion prediction

The motion parameters of a mechanically stabilised beating heart can be captured by exploiting natural landmarks as shown before. Nevertheless, landmarks may be occluded for a short time (e.g., by surgical instruments) and cause tracking to fail. To guarantee robust motion parameter estimation under these circumstances, algorithms were developed which are able to predict these parameters if no tracking information is available. This will not only bridge missing tracking information, but also allow dynamic positioning of the tracking search area. Additionally, prediction is useful for motion compensation: it helps to overcome the delay time of the closed controller loop (including video capturing, data processing, and data transmission) and, thus, increases the bandwidth of the robotic system and, therefore, improves the quality of motion compensation.
As illustrated in Fig. 20, if tracking information is not available, the prediction scheme estimates the expected position of a given landmark from its past trajectory. Therefore, the best matching "embedding" vector is calculated (for more detail see (Ortmaier et al., 2002), (Ortmaier et al., 2005)).
This enables to predict the motion of a landmarks with high accuracy over a number of frames. The extension of the prediction approach to multiple landmarks (Ortmaier et al., 2005) also takes the trajectories of the remaining landmarks into account. Thus, motion can

be predicted for a longer period, as is the case with short-time occlusion by an instrument. To increase robustness of motion estimation even more, and to account for larger occlusions as well, which several landmarks can be concerned of, additional sensor signals such as the respiration pressure signal and the ECG of the patient contribute to a multisensory prediction strategy (Ortmaier et al., 2005).

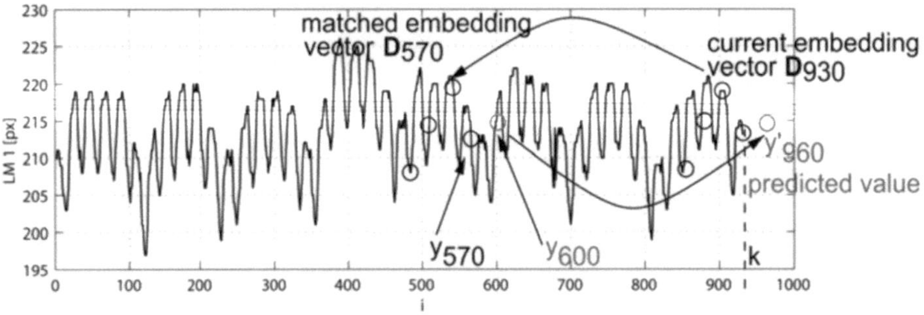

Figure 20. Illustration of the local prediction scheme

5.4 Motion compensation of the heart

As introduced in section 5.2, the motion compensation of the beating heart requires a robotic system, capable of both sufficient accuracy and dynamics to follow the motion of the beating heart. As one possible strategy the robot can move the endoscope to stabilise the motion of the beating heart in a global stabilisation approach. However, since the motion of the heart surface varies locally, this method is not sufficient to fully stabilise the motion of the heart surface as shown in (Groger & Hirzinger, 2006b). Another strategy is to compensate heart motion digitally, i.e. by stabilising the image presented to the surgeon. A special approach to achieve this is presented in (Groger & Hirzinger, 2006a). It is based on robust motion estimation of natural landmarks on the heart surface and uses an efficient interpolation strategy to build dense field of motion correction for the image. Results show that the image motion can be significantly reduced by this approach (Groger & Hirzinger, 2006a). The degree of image motion correction has to be performed in accordance to motion compensation of the surgical instrument, which requires the system to maintain a high degree of consistency in the motion compensation strategy.

Further investigations will involve the the new KineMedic robot (Ortmaier et al., 2006), which provides a considerably higher degree of accuracy and dynamics than existing medical robotic systems, which is required for the task of motion compensation of the beating heart.

6. Conclusion

Motion tracking in minimally invasive surgery is a fundamental issue to adapt medical robotic systems to the changing environment of the operating field. The two example scenarios show that the intelligent and adaptive robotic systems can contribute considerably to make surgery more gentle to the patient by reducing traum and to assist the surgeon with the increased demands and difficulaties of minimally invasive surgery, in which direct contact is lost to the operating field.

Automated laparoscope guidance fulfills the assistant surgeon's task of camera guidance in a reliable and non-exhausting manner, and represents an important step towards minimally invasive solo surgery. Motion compensation of the beating heart is a key step towards beating heart TECAB, a cardiac surgical technique, which is most beneficial to the patient. Further investigations of the described projects involve the newly developed DLR KineMedic robotic system.

7. Acknowledgements

In particular, the authors would like to thank the clinical projects partners: Prof. Dr. H. Feussner from the Department of Surgery at the Klinikum rechts der Isar (MRIC) of the Technical University of Munich contributed the medical part to the automated laparoscopic guidance project. PD Dr. D.H. Bohm from the Department of Cardiovascular Surgery at the University Hospital of Hamburg-Eppendorf (UKE), Germany, is the clinical partner for the project on motion compensation of the beating heart.

8. References

Arbter, K. & Kish, D. (2004). Bin Entwurfswerkzeug fur Farbklassifikatoren in Echtzeitanwendungen, in: *10. Workshop Farbbildverarbeitung,* Koblenz, Germany

Arbter, K. & Wei, G.Q. (1996). Verfahren zum Nachfuhren eines Stereo-laparoskopes in der minimal invasiven Chirurgie, German patent no. 19529950

Arbter, K. & Wei, G.Q. (1998). Method of tracking a surgical instrument with a mono or stereo laparoscope, US patent no. 5820545

Bardinet, E.; Cohen, L. & Ayache, N. (1996). Tracking medical 3D data with a deformable parametric model, in: *Proc. European* Con/. *Computer Vision,* vol. 1, pp. 317-328

Bargar, W.; Bauer, A. & Borner, M. (1998). Primary and revision - total hip replacement using the robodoc system, *Clinical Orthopaedics and Related Research,* vol. 354:pp. 82-91

Black, M. & Yacoob, Y. (1995). Tracking and recognizing rigid and non-rigid facial motions using local parametric models of image motion, in: *International Conference on Computer Vision (ICCV),* pp. 374-381

Boehm, D.H.; Reichenspurner, R.; Gulbins, H.; Detter, C.; Meiser, B.; Brenner, P.; Habazettl, H. & Reichart, B. (1999). Early experience with robotic technology for coronary artery surgery, *Annals of Thoracic Surgery,* vol. 68:pp. 1542-1546

Borst, C. (2001). Operieren am schlagenden Herz, *Spektrum der Wissenschaft,* pp. 50-55

Boyd, W.; Rayman, R. & Desai et al., N. (2000). Closed-chest coronary artery bypass grafting on the beating heart with the use of a computer-enhanced surgical robotic system, *J Thorac Cardiovasc Surg,* vol. 120:pp. 807-809

Casals, A.; Amat, J.; Prats, D. & Laporte, E. (1995). Vision guided robotic system for laparoscopic surgery, in: *Proc. 7th Int.* Con/, *in Advanced Robotics, ICAR'95,* pp. 33-36, Sant Feliu de Guixols-Spain

Computer Motion Inc., 130-B Cremona Drive, G.C..U. (1994). AesoplOOO users guide

Corke, P. (1993). Visual control of robot manipulators - a review, in: K. Hashimoto (Ed.), *Visual Servoing,* pp. 1-31, World Scientific

Doignon, C.; Nageotte, F. & de Mathelin, M. (2004). Detection of grey regions in color images: application to the segmentation of a surgical instrument in robotized laparoscopy, in: *Proceedings of the IEEE/RSJ International Conference on Intelligent Robots and Systems,* pp. 3394-3399, Sendai, Japan

Doignon, C.; Nageotte, F. & de Mathelin, M. (2006). Segmentation and guidance of multiple rigid objects for intra-operative endoscopic vision, in: *International Workshop on Dynamical Vision, in conjunction with ECCV 2006,* Springer, Graz, Austria

Falk, V; Diegeler, A.; Walther, T.; Loscher, N.; Vogel, B.; Ulmann, C.; Rauch, T. & Mohr, F.W. (1999). Endoscopic coronary artery bypass grafting on the beating heart using a computer enhanced telemanipulation system, *Heart Surg Forum,* vol. 2:pp. 199-205

Foley, J.; van Dam, A.; Feiner, S. & Hughes, J. (1990). *Computer Graphics: Principles and Practice,* 2nd ed., Addison-Wesley, Reading, Massachusetts

Ginhoux, R.; Gangloff, J.; de Mathelin, M.; Soler, L.; Sanchez, M.A. & Marescaux, J. (2004). Beating heart tracking in robotic surgery using 500 Hz visual servoing, model predictive control and an adaptive observer, in: IEEE *International Conference on Robotics and Automation (ICRA),* pp. 274-279, New Orleans, USA

Groger, M. & Hirzinger, G. (2006a). Image stabilisation of the beating heart by local linear interpolation, in: K. Cleary & R. Galloway (Eds.), *Medical Imaging 2006: Visualization, Image-Guided Procedures, and Display,* vol. 6141 of *Proceedings ofSPIE,* San Diego, USA

Groger, M. & Hirzinger, G. (2006b). Optical flow to analyse stabilised images of the beating heart, in: A. Ran-chordas; H. Araujo & B. Encarnacao (Eds.), *International Conference on Computer Vision Theory and Applications (VISAPP),* pp. 237-244, INSTICC Press, Setubal, Portugal

Groger, M.; Sepp, W; Ortmaier, T. & Hirzinger, G. (2001). Reconstruction of image structure in presence of specular reflections, in: B. Radig & S. Florczyk (Eds.), *Pattern Recognition, Proc. 23rd DAGM Symposium,* vol. 2191 of *LNCS,* pp. 53-60, Springer, Munich, Germany

Groger, M.; Ortmaier, T.; Sepp, W. & Hirzinger, G. (2002). Tracking local motion on the beating heart, in: S.K. Mun (Ed.), *Medical Imaging 2002: Visualization, Image-Guided Procedures, and Display,* vol. 4681 of *Proceedings ofSPIE,* pp. 233-241, San Diego, USA

Groger, M.; Sepp, W. & Hirzinger, G. (2005). Structure driven substitution of specular reflections for realtime heart surface tracking, in: IEEE *International Conference on Image Processing (ICIP),* vol. 2, pp. 1066-1069, Geneva, Italy

Guthart, G. & Salisbury, J. (2000). The Intuitive telesurgery system: Overview and application, in: IEEE *International Conference on Robotics and Automation (ICRA),* pp. 618-621, San Francisco, USA

Hager, G. (1997). A modular system for robust hand-eye coordination using feedback from stereo vision, IEEE *Transactions on Robotics and Automation,* vol. 13(4):pp. 582-595

Hager, G. & Belhumeur, P. (1998). Efficient region tracking with parametric models of geometry and illumination, IEEE *Transactions on Pattern Analysis and Machine Intelligence,* vol. 20(10)

Hirzinger, G.; Albu-Schaffer, A.; Hahnle, M.; Schafer, I. & Sporer, N. (2001). A new generation of torque controlled light-weight robots, in: IEEE *International conference on Robotics and Automation (ICRA),* pp. 3356-3363, Seoul, Korea

Hurteau, R.; DeSantios, S.; Begin, E. & Gagner, M. (1994). Laparoscopic surgery assisted by a robotic cameraman: Concept and experimental results, in: *Proc. IEEE Int.* Con/. *Robotics and Automation (ICRA),* pp. 2286-2289, San Diego

Hutchinson, S.; Hager, G. & Corke, P. (1996). A tutorial introduction to visual servo control, IEEE *Transactions on Robotics and Automation,* vol. 12(5):pp. 651-670

Jacobs, S.; Holzhey, D.; Kiaii, B.; Onnasch, J.; Walther, T.; Mohr, F. & Falk, V (2003). Limitations for manual and telemanipulator-assisted motion tracking - implications for endoscopic beating-heart surgery, *Ann Thome Surg,* vol. 76:pp. 2029-2035

Jansen, E. (1998). *Towards minimally invasive coronary arterry bypass grafting,* Brouwer Uithof, Utrecht Kazanzides, P.; Mittelstadt, B.; Musits, B.L.; Bargar, W.L.; Zuhars, J. & et al. (1995). An integrated system for cementless hip replacement, IEEE *Eng. Med. Biol. Mag.,* vol. 14:pp. 307-313

Kiibler, B.; Seibold, U. & Hirzinger, G. (2005). Development of acutated and sensor integrated forceps for minimally invasive robotic surgery, *International Journal of Medical Robotics and Computer Assisted Surgery,* vol. 1(3):pp. 96-107

Lee, C; Wang, Y.; Uecker, D. & Wang, Y. (1994). Image analysis for automated tracking in robot-assisted endoscopic surgery, in: *Proc. Int.* Con/. *Pattern Recognition,* pp. A:88-92

Mclnerney, T. & Terzopoulos, D. (1995). A dynamic finite element surface model for segmentation and tracking in multidimensional medical images with application to cardiac 4d image analysis, *Computerized Medical Imaging and Graphics,* vol. 19(l):pp. 69-83

Mclnerney, T. & Terzopoulos, D. (1996). Deformable models in medical image analysis: A survey, *Medical Image Analysis,* vol. 1(2):pp. 91-108

Mittelstadt, B.; Kazanzides, P.; Zuhars, J.; Williamson, B.; Cain, P.; Smith, F. & Bargar, W. (1996). *Computer-Integrated Surgery,* chap. The evolution of a surgical robot from prototype to human clinical use, pp. 397-407, MIT Press, Cambridge, MA

Mohr, F.W.; Falk, V.; Diegeler, A. & Autschbach, R. (1999). Computer enhanced coronary artery bypass surgery, / *Thorac Cardiovasc Surg,* vol. 117:pp. 1212-1213

Moran, M. (1993). Stationary and automated laparoscopically assisted technologies, *Journal of Laparoendoscopic Surgery,* vol. 3(3):pp. 221-227

Nakamura, Y; Kishi, K. & Kawakami, H. (2001). Heartbeat synchronization for robotic cardiac surgery, in: IEEE *International Conference on Robotics and Automation (ICRA),* pp. 2014-2019, Seoul, Korea

Omote, K.; Feussner, H.; Ungeheuer, A.; Arbter, K.; Wei, G.Q.; Siewert, J.R. & Hirzinger, G. (1999). Self-guided robotic camera control for laparoscopic surgery compared with human camera control, *The American Journal of Surgery,* vol. 117:pp. 321-324 Ortmaier, T. &

Hirzinger, G. (2000). Cartesian control issues for minimally invasive robot surgery, in: IEEE *Int. Conference on Intelligent Robots and Systems (IROS),* Takamatsu, Japan

Ortmaier, T.; Reintsema, D.; Seibold, U.; Hagn, U. & Hirzinger, G. (2001). The DLR minimally invasive robotics surgery scenario, in: G. Fa'rber & J. Hoogen (Eds.), *Workshop on Advances in Interactive Multimodal Telepresence Systems,* pp. 135-147, Munich, Germany

Ortmaier, T.; Groger, M. & Hirzinger, G. (2002). Robust motion estimation in robotic surgery on the beating heart, in: *Computer Assisted Radiology and Surgery (CARS),* pp. 206-211, Paris, France

Ortmaier, T.; Groger, M.; Boehm, D.; Falk, V. & Hirzinger, G. (2005). Motion estimation in beating heart surgery, IEEE *Transactions on Biomedical Engineering (TBME),* vol. 52(10):pp. 1729-1740

Ortmaier, T.; Weiss, H.; Hagn, U.; Grebenstein, M.; Nickl, M.; A. Albu-Schaffer, C. Ott, S.J.; Konietschke, R.; Le-Tien, L. & Hirzinger, G. (2006). A hands-on-robot for accurate placement of pedicle screws, in: IEEE *International Conference on Robotics and Automation (ICRA),* pp. 4179-4186, Orlando, USA

Preusche, C.; Ortmaier, T. & Hirzinger, G. (2001). Teleoperation Concepts in Minimal Invasive Surgery, in: *Proceedings of 1st IFAC Conference on Telematics Application in Automation and Robotics,* VDI/VDE - GMA, Weingarten, Germany

Reichenspurner, H.; Boehm, D.H.; Welz, A.; Schulze, C.; Gulbins, H. & Wildhirt, S. (1999a). 3D-Video- and robot-assisted port access mitralvalve surgery, *Annals of Thoracic Surgery*

Reichenspurner, H.; Damiano, R.; Mack, M.; Boehm, D.H.; Gulbins, H.; Meiser, B.; Elgafi, R. & Reichhart, B. (1999b). Experimental and first clinical use of the voice-controlled and computer-assisted surgical system ZEUS for endoscopic coronary artery bypass grafting, *Journal of Thoracic and Cardiovascular Surgery,* vol. 118:pp. 11-16

Sackier, J. & Wang, Y. (1996). *Computer-Integrated Surgery,* chap. Robotically Assisted Laparoscopic Surgery: From Concept to Development, pp. 577-580, MIT Press, Cambridge, MA, USA

Shi, J. & Tomasi, C. (1994). Good features to track, IEEE *Conference on Computer Vision and Pattern Recognition,* pp.593-600

Taylor, R.; Paul, H.; Mittelstadt, B. & et al. (1989). A robotic system for cementless total hip replacement surgery in dogs, in: *Proc. 2nd Workshop Medical and Healthcare Robotics,* Newcastle-on-Tyne, U. K.

Taylor, R.; Funda, J.; Eldridge, B.; Gomory, S.; Gruben, K. & et. al (1995). A telerobotic assistant for laparoscopic surgery, IEEE *Engineering in Medicine and Biology,* vol. 14:pp. 279-288

Taylor, R.H.; Paul, H.; Kazandzides, P.; Mittelstadt, B.; Hanson, W; Zuhars, J.; B.Williamson; Musits, B.; Glassman, E. & Bargar, W. (1994). An image-directed robotic system for precise orthopaedic surgery, IEEE *Trans. Robot. Automat.,* vol. 10:pp. 261-275

Taylor, R. & Stoianovici, D. (2003). Medical robotics in compter-integrated surgery, IEEE *Transactions on Robotics and Automation,* vol. 19(5):pp. 765-781

Tonet, O.; Thoranaghatte, R.; Megali, G. & Dario, P. (2007). Tracking endoscopic instruments without a localizer: A shape-analysis-based approach, *Computer Aided Surgery,* vol. 12(l):pp. 35-42

Troccaz, J. (1994). Robots in surgery, in: *Proc. Int. Symposium on Robotics Research,* Herrsching, Germany Turner, D. (1995). Solo surgery with aid of a robotic assistant, in: *Proc. Int.* Con/. *Telemedicine and Telecare,* pp. 83-86, London, U.K.

Ungeheuer, A.; Arbter, K.; Omote, K.; Feussner, H.; Wei, G.Q.; Siewert, J.R. & Hirzinger, G. (1997). Selbststeuernde farbcodierte Kamerafiihrung bei laparoskopischen Eingriffen, *Minimal invasive Chirurgie,* vol. 6.3:pp. 41-47

Voros, S.; Orvain, E.; Cinquin, P. & Long, J.A. (2006). Automatic detection of instruments in laparoscopic images: a first step towards high level command of robotized endoscopic holders, in: *First IEEE/RAS- EMBS International Conference on Biomedical Robotics and Biomechatronics (BioRob)*

Wei, G.Q.; Arbter, K. & Hirzinger, G. (1997). Real-time visual servoing for laparoscopic surgery, IEEE *Engineering in Medicine and Biology,* vol. 16(l):pp. 40-45

Wintermantel, E. & Ha, S.W (Eds.) (2001). *Biokompatible Werkstoffe fur die therapeutische Medizintechnik,* Springer Verlag

Y. S. Kwoh, J.H. & et al., E.A.J. (1988). A robot with improved absolute positioning accuracy for ct-guided stereotactic brain surgery, IEEE *Trans. Biomed. Eng.,* vol. 35:pp. 153-161

11

Surgical Skills Training For Robotic Assisted Surgery

Juan D. Hernandez R.[1], Fernando Bello[2] and Ara Darzi[2]
[1]Universidad de los Andes School of Medicine,
[2]Imperial College London Faculty of Medicine
[1]Colombia, [2]United Kingdom

1. Introduction

The enormous impact of technology in medicine has a remarkable example in the introduction of robotic systems in minimally invasive surgery approximately a decade ago. With relatively small modifications to the commercial systems originally introduced, the field of robotic surgery is now established and growing. Several thousand procedures have been practiced successfully in areas like general surgery, thoracic and cardiovascular surgery, urology, gynaecology, and others. Research in robotic surgery is growing exponentially, and its future is promising. The systems employed by the specialties mentioned above are known as telemanipulator systems due to their technical configuration and interaction with the surgeon. Although there are other robotic systems employed in, for example, orthopaedic and urologic surgery, this chapter will focus on the use of telemanipulator systems for laparoscopic or minimally invasive surgery, and that is what will be meant when using the expression robotic surgery

Possible limitations to massive use of surgical telemanipulator systems could be the cost, technical capabilities of hospitals around the world and surgical expertise and training. The aim of this chapter is to explore this last issue, which, in the end, will determine if these systems are widely accepted by the surgical community and its use is extended beyond hospitals and academic centres in the developed world. It will set up to find if surgeons require new abilities to practice surgical procedures using telemanipulator systems; if there is an advantage for already trained laparoscopic surgeons or if surgical trainees can easily learn the use of this equipment. It will also discuss if this technology has an impact on the learning curve of advanced laparoscopic procedures, and how scientists and surgeons are working to improve its performance.

2. Ergonomic limitations of laparoscopic surgery (LS)

Since the massive expansion and use of minimally invasive surgery (MIS) in the early 1990's shortly after its introduction, extensive evidence has demonstrated its advantages over open surgery in different procedures (McMahon et al, 1994; Williams et al, 1993; Z'graggen et al, 1998): Faster recovery and short hospital stay with less pain and fewer complications. These factors, together with good surgical results, have resulted in procedures such as laparoscopic cholecystectomy, Nissen's fundoplication and adrenalectomy becoming gold

standard techniques for those surgeries (National Institutes of Health 1993, Heemskerk et al, 2007).
However, the swift developments of MIS after the first laparoscopic cholecystectomies were presented to the world (Ostrosky & Jacobs, 2003; Muhe, 1992), led to the introduction of instruments and equipment by the industry, but little thought was spent in making them user friendly from an ergonomic point of view. They have been basically the long-shaft versions of the traditional instruments used in open surgery, many of them unchanged since the 19th century. As a result, surgeons may experience nerve compression with an area of paresthesia in the thumb (Kano et al, 1995), produced by the position of the finger in the instrument and the force or pressure applied to it.
MIS has some other ergonomic implications for the surgeon that make it very challenging, and for some surgeons difficult enough as to discourage them from learning advanced laparoscopic skills. In spite of that, authors consider laparoscopic surgery the best approach to a large number of procedures, at least until robotic surgery proves otherwise. However, there are characteristics of LS that could be improved through RS.
The drawbacks of MIS are several. First, long instruments placed through fixed entry points create a fulcrum effect, with the tip of the instrument moving in the opposite direction of the hands. This situation is made worse in obese patients (Yu et al, 2006). In these cases, the reverse movement is summed to the high resistance of a very thick abdominal wall. Second, the surgical field is viewed on a 2-D screen often positioned on either side of the patient, not where the actual surgical field really is. Additionally, the camera acting as the surgeon's eyes is held by an assistant, who may not have full knowledge of the procedure, or may get distracted or tired. All these elements create an unnatural environment where the surgeon has lost orientation, the eye-hand-target axis and visual depth perception (Falk et al, 1999; Smith et al, 2001). Finally, the surgeon is no longer in direct contact with tissues, but through an instrument that drastically reduces its tactile perception. This is due to its length and the fact that the instrument's shaft goes trough a port that creates friction.
Other problems appear by uncomfortable and sometimes awkward positions assumed during long procedures, producing pain and muscular fatigue of the back, shoulders, elbows and wrists (Galleano et al, 2006). Other appliances often cause discomfort, for example, foot pedals for instruments that use energy. There is not only physical but mental fatigue and strain, attributed to the effort of adapting to 2-D vision (Byrn et al, 2007). These working conditions may not only have long term effects on surgeon's health, but also affect performance in terms of time and outcomes.
As none of the abovementioned conditions are present in open surgery, or for that matter, in any usual daily activity humans have learned to do, they reduce the surgeon's normal dexterity and limit his ability to deal with difficult situations (Cadière et al, 2001). MIS procedures in confined spaces such as pelvis and retroperitoneum, but particularly in the thoracic cavity, are extremely difficult, and in some cases, simply impossible to complete. This is especially true if they include manoeuvres like suturing, which requires movements in different angles, including a 180 degrees action, which would be parallel to the shaft of the instrument (Bann et al, 2003).
A long learning curve has been the only existing path to overcome these difficulties (Smith et al, 2001), and many surgeons have failed to make the transition from open to MIS even in their area of expertise, since laparoscopic surgery requires a whole new set of skills many are not willing to learn.

3. MIS Skills acquisition and learning curve development

The term "learning curve" is now an obliged element in medical publications, especially in the surgical field. It is used in reference to the process of gaining knowledge and improving skills in performing a specific procedure (Ramsay et al, 2000). It could be concluded that at some point a surgeon should reach a plateau. If the surgeon practices the same procedure frequently, he should keep a flat line, with occasional peaks and valleys which are normal to human performance.

Several authors have published learning curves of different surgical procedures based on their results through time. Outcomes like surgical time, mortality, morbidity, in-hospital stay, etc. have been used to establish the improvement of a group or an independent surgeon in performing a specific operation or technique (Watson et al, 1996). Advanced MIS has not been embraced by all surgeons as would be expected considering its advantages. This could be attributed to the important effort that needs to be invested in order to overcome long learning curves for most procedures (Yu et al, 2006).

In a systematic review, Ramsay et al comment that using outcomes like patients survival or complications, and quality assurance aspects like time to complete the surgical procedure and hospital stay as "proxies of learning" is inappropriate, since they are too general and do not provide accurate or objective definition of learning (Ramsay et al, 2000; Watson et al, 1996; Darzi et al, 1999).

The learning curve assessment should be based on factors more closely related to the surgeon's skills rather than in variables that are either too general, too difficult to control or not a direct reflection of learning. These measurements should be both quantitative and qualitative to capture a wide array of human learning manifestations, and ideally should have numerical representation to actually depict them as a curve. Examples of more appropriate parameters to objectively measure learning and improvement in surgical skills are number of movements, path length, time, number of errors. Such variables are reproducible and easily compared in different studies or when comparing LS and RS.

The reason these parameters have been considered useful to measure surgeons' learning curves is because an experienced surgeon practicing either a specific task or a whole surgical procedure performs a smaller number of movements and he is more precise, therefore having a shorter path length for the instruments and spending less time than a novice. As the surgeon or student in training practices, these variables resemble more and more those of the expert, and a learning curve can be defined.

At the authors institution (St Mary's Hospital), the parameters number of movements, path length and time spent, have been calculated in open and laparoscopic surgery on bench models. This is known as motion tracking analysis, and for the purpose of these measurements, the ICSAD (Imperial College Surgical Assessment Device) was developed. ICSAD uses an electromagnetic field to track the hand coordinates and to analyse objective measures for the assessment of surgical skills (Datta et al, 2001). The same concept has been applied to the assessment of robotic surgical skills using the Da Vinci telemanipulator system and ROVIMAS (Robotic Video & Motion Analysis Software) (Dosis et al, 2003), bespoke software offering advanced motion and video analysis capabilities for open, laparoscopic and robotic surgical skills assessment. ROVIMAS can calculate and display the hand kinematics, the time, the total path length of hands, the number of movements made, the hand directions, velocities etc. It also synchronises these hand kinematics with simultaneously recorded procedural video.

4. RS Skills acquisition and learning curve development

Contrary to the general perception of robots, surgical robots are not independent in their actions; they cannot move on their own and only respond to human direct commands. Current existing robotic systems used in general surgery (MIS) are known as master-slave telemanipulator systems. Commercially available FDA-approved systems are the Zeus System (Computer Motion, Inc., Goleta, CA) and the da Vinci™ Surgical System (Intuitive Surgical, Sunnyvale, California). Since Computer Motion was taken over by Intuitive Surgical, the only widespread commercial master-slave telemanipulator currently being sold and updated is the da Vinci system, and therefore will be the focus of this paper.

The da Vinci system is composed of a console where the surgeon sits (master), rests his arms and grabs the instruments controls; a computer interface where surgeon movements are transmitted to the instruments; a patient-side cart holding up to 4 robotic arms (slave) and a video cart consisting of the standard laparoscopic monitor, Xenon lights, insufflation equipment and video processing system. The robotic arms hold the camera and up to three instruments, two for surgeon's left and right hands, and the other to assist the surgeon. The workstation allows the surgeon to setup the system at the beginning of the surgery, to change the camera position and focus, and adjust the distance and position of the controls. It also has diathermy function pedals. To activate the controls, the surgeons forehead must remain at the headrest allowing him to comfortable see through the vision device, a binocular viewer that projects the images from a dual-lens scope with independent light sources and cameras for each eye. The images obtained are therefore in real time and three-dimensional. The computerized interface is able to filter and scale surgeon movements, avoiding natural tremor and allowing the intuitive, natural hand movements to be reproduced in the small surgical field at an appropriate scale.

During the rapid introduction of MIS, higher incidence of common bile duct injuries in laparoscopic as compared to open cholecystectomy were recorded (Deziel et al, 1993, Shea et al, 1996; Z'graggen et al, 1998). These lesions are found more frequently in the initial cases of a number of surgeons. It is possible that these surgeons did not appreciate the unique skills required to practice laparoscopic surgery competently, leading to this situation. As mentioned before, some technically demanding tasks cannot be done safely or accurately enough using conventional laparoscopic instruments (Damiano et al, 2000; Loulmet et al, 1999), for example coronary artery bypass grafting in the confined spaces of the thorax. It is with this background that telemanipulators appear in laparoscopic surgery.

The feasibility of carrying out different surgical procedures with robotic systems has been demonstrated in different fields (Cadière et al, 1999; Chitwood et al, 2001; Falcone et al, 2000), with special emphasis in cardiac surgery (Falk et al, 1999) using both the Zeus and the da Vinci, with more than 2000 procedures performed just two years after their introduction (Ruurda et al, 2002), and a calculated 20,000 by the end of 2004 (Mehrabi et al, 2006). Both Zeus (no longer in production) and da Vinci have similar characteristics in their final forms: a set of robotic arms holding the camera and instruments, 3D visualization of the surgical field and instruments with "wrists" in their tips that allow complex movements in confined spaces, giving surgeons seven degrees of freedom instead of the four available in MIS (Bann et al, 2003; Falk et al, 1999).

Several authors have tested the advantages of the da Vinci™ Surgical System in clinical practice in a large number of surgical procedures (Cichon et al, 2000; Loulmet et al, 1999; Munz et al, 2003a; Heemskerk et al, 2007), and it has been reported that it allows surgeons to perform more complex tasks restoring surgical dexterity, hand-eye alignment and depth perception (Falk et al, 2001; Byrn et al 2007). When the surgeon sits at the workstation, it recreates the eye-hand motor axis that is lost in MIS (Ban et al, 2003), giving the surgeon the impression that when he moves his hands, the instruments move right in front of his eyes with similar degrees of freedom, mimicking his movements on the handles. Due to the position of the head in the viewing device, he feels immersed in the surgical field. It is in delicate and complex procedures, like cardiac surgery, where the virtues of the system are more evident. Tremor is eliminated through bandwidth filtering and there is improved visualization with the availability of three-dimensional viewing directly controlled by the surgeon. All these, combined with improved ergonomics for the operating surgeon in the seated position at the console, make clear advantages over the laparoscopic surgery setting (Bann et al, 2003). However, it remains to be proven if these advantages have an impact on patients outcomes.

There are important setbacks in telemanipulators that also need evaluation and the establishment of strategies to deal with these obstacles. Very importantly, the surgeon has no direct tissue tactile feedback whatsoever, and therefore he has to trust only what he sees (Munz et al, 2004) and in visual cues that experience give when dealing with tissues and suture materials. Having no sense of tension, pressure or grasp on tissues and sutures increases the probability of a wide array of lesions or errors during tasks and surgical procedures for which a learning process is needed. It is therefore an important consideration when comparing LS and RS to keep in mind that there is a learning curve to a safe and accurate use of the robotic telemanipulator. An additional point to bear in mind is that, no matter how intuitive and user-friendly a telemanipulator system might be, it is still a tool, and therefore the operator needs to know the task or procedure beforehand if the system's usefulness is to be evaluated.

In order to avoid the problems that occurred with the introduction of laparoscopic surgery, (Scott et al, 2001; Shea et al, 1996; Watson et al, 1996) appropriate training and assessment need to be established for this new technology to ensure good outcomes. It is important therefore, that both the impact on the learning curve and any possible advantages over the standard laparoscopic technique be recognized, tested and objectively measured. Only using this approach its widespread use by the surgical community would be justified and supported.

4.1 Learning robotic surgery skills

Learning the basic use of the da Vinci system is very intuitive. Once a surgeon sits on the console, holds the controls and looks through the vision device, is perfectly able to move the instruments and practice simple tasks from the onset. They could reproduce the movements they typically do in open surgery. On the other hand, the main disadvantage is the total lack of tactile feedback. It forces the surgeon to trust only in his vision (3-D). It should be pointed out that in papers where subjects with no surgical experience are tested doing surgical tasks, they may not only be learning to use the robot, but learning the surgical task itself. Therefore, comparisons need to control for these variables in order to be valid. Such studies show advantages and disadvantages of the use of robots in surgery, better defining the systems current and future role. We now review some of the published studies. These were chosen from different specialties for their relevance in skill acquisition, attention to learning curves, number of cases and design.

Obek (Obek et al, 2005), published a study where twenty students with no knowledge of laparoscopic surgery where divided in two groups to determine if there was transfer of skills between robotic and laparoscopic surgery. After observing knot tying on the da Vinci with and without previous training in LS, they concluded that there is reciprocal transfer of skills between LS ad RS, although it is incomplete. They considered that training with LS previously is better than training with RS alone. Interesting findings were that novices learning intracorporeal suturing with the robot were faster and more precise than those learning with conventional laparoscopic instruments. As their attention was focused on skills transfer, they found that those who learned with LS did better in their last tasks on the da Vinci.

Heemskerk, in a study with medical students (Heemskerk et al, 2007), compared the skill acquisition in robotic and traditional laparoscopy. Subjects were randomized to start with RS or LS on three rather simple tasks and on knot tying as the fourth task. Researchers found that a steeper learning curve was achieved with LS, but RS allowed a faster and more accurate performance. Comparing with other studies, they suggested that the tendency to a flat learning curve in RS would be explained by a better performance from the start with RS, leaving little room for improvement. They also comment that RS may be more beneficial to surgeons with little or no experience in LS, and that benefit of robotic assistance would be more evident in complex surgical procedures.

Mehrabi et al designed a set of four training tasks for subjects with different surgical experience (Mehrabi et al, 2006). They were asked to practice four procedures in a pig, and then practice each of them in rats. After the training, they had to repeat all four procedures in a pig. They were able to demonstrate a learning curve and a significant improvement in quantitative and qualitative scores similar to all participants. They mention that learning process was independent of the subject's confidence on the surgical technique, and considered the learning process closer to open rather than to laparoscopic surgery. They recommend that every surgeon should go through an animal model training course before clinically using the da Vinci system.

Ruurda published the initial experience of the Utrecht group with 208 different procedures (Ruurda et al, 2005). They practiced a variety of procedures with a small number of complications and results at least as good as with laparoscopic surgery. Setup time and positioning of the robot were improved as they practiced different surgical interventions, of different degrees of complexity. They conclude that the application of the current generation of telemanipulators should be reserved to procedures with complex dissection and suturing, and that future systems will need to reduce their size, complexity and cost.

An exceptional example of a complex MIS procedure is the Roux-en-Y gastric bypass for morbid obesity. Multiple bowel anastomoses and a major rearrangement of the gastrointestinal tract make it a great challenge. Mechanical sutures help reduce the burden of intracorporeal suturing, but even so, the learning curve is long and steep. Describing a teaching environment for RS, Ali (Ali et al, 2007) trained an MIS fellow in RS, making the experience progressive in complexity. He found that the fellow's performance exceeded the senior members of the team during their own learning curve. In this study, the team opted for a hand-sewn anastomosis, which greatly raises the difficulty. During his clinical practice, the fellow had no complications originated on technical errors. This group considered possible to reduce the learning curve of a complex surgical procedure using the telemanipulator system within an organized training program. Yu et al reported the learning curve for 100 cases (Yu et al, 2006). They found that every twenty patients operating time was reduced, and on the last twenty patients was less than average. Another significant finding was that they had no leaks and no deaths and a smaller rate of strictures than other series. The 0% leak rate is important since other series have reported 7%. They suggested the use of the da Vinci to train surgeons and help them overcome the learning curve.

This evidence shows that learning to use the robot requires a short exposure to the system as compared to laparoscopic surgery, and may have its main impact on complex procedures and in the performance of surgeons with no experience in LS.

4.2 Learning curve and differences in RS performance according to LS surgical expertise

An issue that has become of great importance in RS is that of the performance of subjects with different degrees of knowledge and experience in LS. A number of authors have explored this issue with different approaches. Zorn followed the learning curve of an experienced laparoscopic surgeon starting his practice of robotic radical prostatectomy (Zorn et al, 2007). He found that the results and learning curve were similar to a group of urologists who switched to RS, and whose previous experience was only in open surgery and not in LS. In other words, Zorn's study suggest that laparoscopic experience is not a requirement to practice RS proficiently, and that surgeons with expertise in an open surgical technique will perform as good as laparoscopic surgeons practicing RS, both during the learning curve and when reaching the plateau.

Munz et al presented a bench model experiment of cardiac surgery, in which a left internal mammary artery was anastomosed to the left anterior descending artery of the heart (Munz et al 2003b). The procedure was repeated five times by expert cardiac surgeons, and then compared to the open approach by the same subjects. Qualitative analysis of video recordings and quantitative motion tracking analysis with ROVIMAS (da Vinci) and ICSAD (open surgery) showed an important improvement in performance represented by time taken, number of movements, path length, circumference to area ratio and overall performance for robotic surgery. Although it is not mentioned in the paper, the cardiac surgeons taking part in this study were not experienced in minimal access cardiac surgery. In a related paper, another British team established a progressive programme to introduce robotic cardiac surgery (Trimlett et al, 2003). They started with pig hearts, then live animals and finally went into clinical practice. In the process, they found that the learning curve is short and can be reproduced when comparing different subjects and that moving to clinical practice is rapidly achievable.

On another St. Mary's group experiment (Hernandez et al, 2004), 13 surgeons naïve to the telemanipulator system were divided in two groups and their learning curves on a bench model experiment were followed. One group was formed by experienced laparoscopic surgeons and the other by surgeons and surgical registrars without laparoscopic experience. The model was composed of two segments of synthetic small bowel assembled in a jig and fixed in a standardized position in a closed box. Surgeons had to complete an anastomosis with interrupted stitches in a single layer. The bowel anastomosis model was chosen because it simulates a complex procedure that requires forward planning and the use of a significant range of skills, and entails a longer learning process. It should resemble the practice of a complex surgical procedure, which is the real purpose of the robot. Results showed clearly an improvement for every subject in all variables measured (time and motion tracking analysis and quality of performance), which clearly depicted a learning curve in just five repetitions of the task (Fig. 1). A surprising finding was that between the two groups there was not a significant difference at the final task in any of the measurements. In other words, by the end of the experiment an after only five procedures completed using the da Vinci system, novice surgeons performed as well as the experienced laparoscopic surgeons. It is worth underlining that some of the trainees had to be taught how to do intracorporeal knot-tying from scratch.

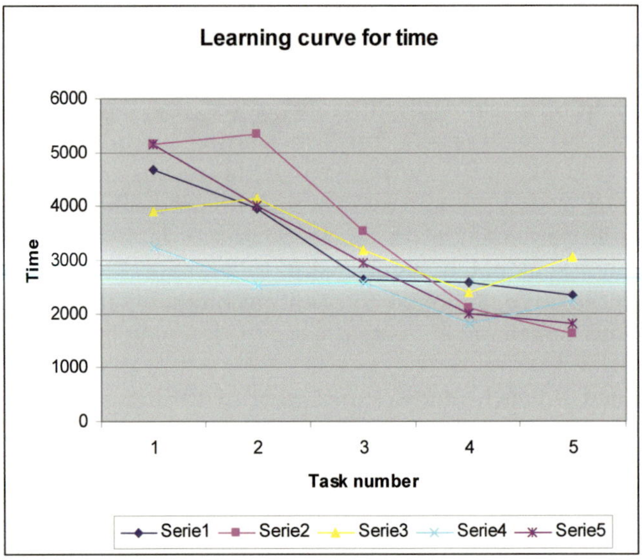

a)

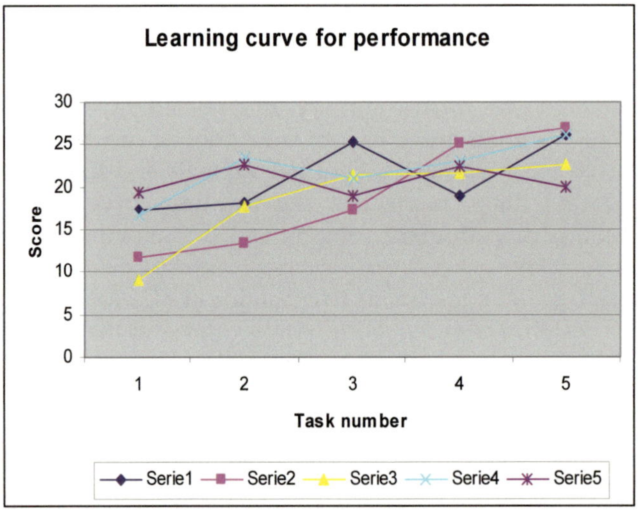

b)

Figure 1. Graphics representing the learning curves for five subjects from both groups for time (a) and for quality of performance (b). Same color lines in a) and b) represent one surgeon

Closer examination of the curves shown in Fig. 1 reveals that there are differences in learning from one surgeon to another. For example, surgeon represented as series 2 (pink line/squares) showed a rapid and clear progress in the learning curve with the most important reduction in time of the study and a marked improvement in the score achieved. Series 1 (blue line/diamond) had an important improvement in time taken to complete the five tasks, but in terms of quality had a very uneven performance, with the third task scored as good as the fifth, but with a poor score for the fourth. Series 5 (Purple line, stars) had a steep reduction in time but an almost flat line for score. In spite of the differences, every single surgeon had a better time and score when comparing first and last task, and it was possible to draw a learning curve for each of them. This is an important achievement for a complex task in just five repetitions. It is the authors' opinion that this performance was possible due to the special characteristics of the da Vinci system.

In a clinical study of robot-assisted laparoscopic aorto-iliac bypasses (Diks et al, 2007), the authors showed a clear improvement after the eighth of seventeen patients. The learning curve was shorter when compared with other studies, since the aortic clamp time and aortic anastomosis time were significantly reduced. It remained a long and very complex procedure even with robotic assistance.

Based on these studies, it is then possible to say that the learning curve for complex tasks on the da Vinci system is shorter than expected as compared to LS, and that there may not be a difference between experienced and non-experienced surgeons. This seems to be truth only after the non-experienced surgeons have learned the procedure itself, a fact that constitutes a variable in the first tasks. These studies also seem to show that results are more favorable to robotic use when the task or surgical procedure complexity is higher.

4.3 Comparison in clinical practice of LS and RS

Several studies have compared laparoscopic and robotic surgery in specific procedures, especially in urologic surgery.

In an interesting study, Link et al compared robotic and laparoscopic pyeloplasty (Link et al, 2006). Laparoscopic pyeloplasty is a complex procedure because extensive, precise suturing is necessary, and therefore advanced skills are a requirement. The authors compared 10 procedures practiced with the da Vinci system by an urologist expert in laparoscopic surgery and ten laparoscopic pyeloplasties by the same surgeon. They found that time, complications and quality of the procedure were comparable, rendering the robotic assistance unnecessary for experienced laparoscopic surgeons. Additionally, cost was clearly higher in RS. In their conclusion they consider the system would be useful to surgeons without training in laparoscopic intracorporeal suturing.

Following the same line, El Nakadi et al compared robotic and laparoscopic Nissen's fundoplication in a randomized controlled trial (El Nakadi et al, 2006). They followed 20 patients randomized in two groups, evaluating complications during a one-year period. Operative time was longer with the robot, and there was no difference in complications and postoperative symptoms. Costs were several times higher with RS. The authors consider there is no advantage in using the robot for Nissen's, and numbered as disadvantages of the system the lack of appropriate instruments, high costs and longer setup times.

In another Nissen's study, Draaisma (Draaisma et al, 2006) found no differences in operating time, quality of life, oesophageal manometry and pH monitoring and symptoms. They found that surgeons comfort and visualization had an important improvement, but they conclude that the use of the da Vinci for the Nissen fundoplication is not justified.

The use of telemanipulators by expert surgeons in less demanding procedures does not seem to bring any particular advantage. The explanation could be that expert surgeons use visual cues and references that allow them to practice even complex procedures accurately, safely and in short times. Therefore, they seem to have successfully overcome the limitations of LS addressed by RS and, consequently, robot assistance does not appear to be useful for them.

5. Technological developments that enhance RS performance and safety

When using a telemanipulator system, the surgeon has to relay only in what he is seeing, since he is not having any physical contact with the patient when sitting at the console, and therefore he cannot count on the partial feedback that exists in MIS. It has been proved that 3-D vision enhances surgical performance and reduces errors (Munz et al, 2004). Additionally, motion scaling, tremor abolition and instruments with "wrists" improve performance by 50%, and when 3-D vision is added, time spent is reduced by 20% and dexterity is enhanced by 15% (Moorthy et al, 2004). However, there are additional technical features that could improve the performance of robotic surgery even more, making the experience more realistic and immersive.

There is ongoing investigation to improve the surgeon's performance in robotic surgery and to bring additional technical capabilities in order to perform surgical procedures more safely and accurately.

5.1 Motion tracking

Following the successful application of motion analysis using the ICSAD, the same concept has been applied to the assessment of robotic surgical skills using the Da Vinci telemanipulator system. The ROVIMAS software (Dosis et al, 2003) can calculate and display all the variables of motion tracking analysis and is able to provide facilities such as a video player synchronized with the hand kinematics. The latter enables the comprehensive assessment of surgical skills, since every task can be watched through the video with simultaneous real-time displays of dexterity measures (Dosis et al, 2004).

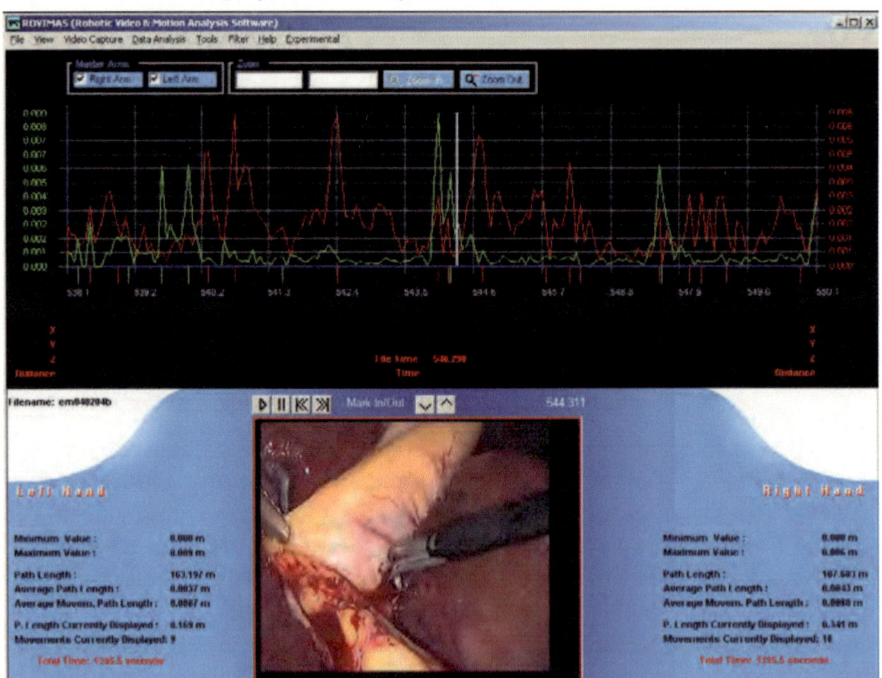

Figure 2. Sample screen image of surgical video synchronized with motion analysis graphics and data. Published with authorization of the Revista Colombiana de Cirugía

The analysis of real-time kinematic data coming from the master arms holding the instruments and streamed from the computer interface of the da Vinci system displays distance and velocity graphics calculated from the robotic positional data. It can also analyse and produce graphics on trajectory, give statistical results and allows zooming-in to observe specific movement patterns. The use of ROVIMAS on the da Vinci and the ICSAD on laparoscopic and open surgery make an accurate comparison between the three surgical approaches possible, reducing methodological bias. Some of the studies carried out at the Imperial College London and included in this chapter have used this technology.

Figure 2 represents the layout of a computer screen showing the ROVIMAS data. This data may be specific for left and right hand, can show time taken, path travelled by instrument tips and number of movements. In the example, the observer could zoom-in at a graphic's segment and review specific movements, and compare those movements with the synchronized image to check for errors or very small movements. In that sense, the assessors will instantly know when, why and in which part of the procedure the surgeon manipulated with higher hand velocity (for example, when dealing with a bleeding situation).

The purpose of this project has been to research and enhance the motion analysis system with stochastic models to discriminate levels of expertise in real and complex procedures. Hidden Markov Models are widely used for this purpose in speech, hand and other pattern recognition research areas and it is currently used in this project to recognize different steps in a procedure, different levels of expertise and to model surgical movements.

Dosis published a clinical experience of the use of ROVIMAS (Dosis et al, 2005). They recorded ten laparoscopic cholecystectomies practiced by five surgeons with different levels of training, in gallbladders with different degrees of difficulty. ROVIMAS allowed authors to discriminate expert from novice surgeons and also to demonstrate that the system can be used in an operating theatre without interfering with the procedure.

Apart from obtaining individual learning curves, these data could be used in the assessment of surgical performance of trainees or for surgeon's certification; to create simulations based in experts' performances or to compare novices to experts and this way setting minimum standards in robotic training, both in simulated or clinical settings. These aspects will have great impact in skill assessment and RS training.

5.2 Augmented reality provision for robotic minimally invasive surgery.

Augmented reality combines synthetic objects with the real world, in real-time. The presence of augmented reality will enable the surgeon to perceive, in real-time, supplementary information intra-operatively without turning away from the operating scene. In one of the possible scenarios, 3D models will be reconstructed from a patient's pre-operative CT/MRI scans and integrated with the intra-operative endoscopic video stream (Wang et al, 2004).

Several issues need to be addressed when producing augmented reality facilities: calibration, registration and tracking. Calibration determines the properties of the camera being used to view the operating field. These properties are required when creating the simulated scene. The next stage of the process is to accurately align the virtual objects with their counterparts within the video sequences. This matching of real and virtual is known as registration. Once this blending has occurred, the dynamics of the surgical scene must be taken into account. Any deformation of structures, especially those due to tissue-tool interactions, need to be tracked. The virtual objects can then be updated accordingly and re-rendered onto the display (Wang et al, 2006).

It is hoped that by providing augmented reality facilities to the da Vinci surgical system, the enhanced visualization will allow for robotic image guided surgery. It will also advance the education of trainee surgeons by allowing them to carry out simulated robotic procedures with the aid of these extra capabilities.

A form of augmented reality would actually give surgeons back part of the sensory information lost partially in LS and completely in RS. Force and tactile feedback would require adapting sensors to the tips of the instruments. This would let the surgeon know if he is applying to much pressure or traction to a tissue or suture material. For example, to introduce the needle in a coronary artery during cardiac surgery requires feeling the tissue being pierced by the needle, then carefully passing the suture trough it and delicately tying a knot with the application of the right amount of pressure (Okamura AM, 2004).

An elegant experiment by a team from Johns Hopkins (Akinbiyi et al, 2006.) has combined a tracking system attached to the instruments of the da Vinci system with an augmented reality array based on haptic feedback. The variation is that instead of sending haptic feedback directly to the surgeon's hands, they used what is called sensory substitution. The force surgeon is applying to tissue is graphically represented and overlaid on the streaming video from the camera that the surgeon is viewing on the visor device of the console. They were able to demonstrate that using the force feedback with sensory substitution, forces were applied consistently, there were fewer errors and not one suture was broken due to excessive traction, and knots were tied accurately.

In a series of experiments, Reiley was able to prove that the use of visual force feedback produced lower suture breakage rates, in expert and novice robotic surgeons and in subjects with no surgical training (Reiley CE, 2007). She suggested that the use of these aides would reduce novice surgeons' learning curves.

Finally, a method called active constraint or haptic visual fixtures creates limits for the movement of the instruments within or outside certain boundaries. Dedicated to minimally invasive surgery in the heart, two types of active constraint were developed by Borelli et al at Imperial College London: the inner and the outer regions. The aim of "active constraints" in the inner-regions is to constrain the cutting tool inside the boundary of a desired area, while in the outer-regions the entry of the cutting tool is prevented within the central delimited area. In both cases there is an intermediary third region, modelled by a spring and damper, which allows the cutting tool to transition from the allowed to the forbidden region, without causing instability [Borelli et al, 2003].

All these future supporting tools should improve surgeons' performance on the system, especially for those who are in training, but will also make procedures safer reducing the chance for human error.

6. Telerobotics, telementoring and telesurgery

Tele-surgical procedures have been practiced using satellite links between Europe and the US and Asia and the US (Chitwood et al, 2001; Smith et al, 2001), and some of them via terrestrial fiberoptic networks (Marescaux et al, 2002). In a master-slave telemanipulator system setup, the surgeon does not need to be by the patient; furthermore, the system allows the surgeon not only to be remote from the slave, but also from the operating room (Cadiere et al, 1999). This has important implications for training surgeons in new procedures (Bann et al, 2003) and for space program or military use, but will require high-speed linkups via telephone or satellite (Lee et al, 1998; Fabrizio et al, 2000; Marescaux et al, 2002). Fabrizio (Fabrizio et al, 2000) have examined the effect of time delay that occurs with telemonitoring: programmed incremental time delays were made in audiovisual acquisition and robotic controls. They concluded a time delay of less than 700 ms was acceptable. Above this time the number of errors increased; although the general consensus suggests shorter times—300 ms (Marescaux et al, 2001; Marescaux et al, 2002).

To study the effect of time delay as it would present in telesurgery, Thompson designed a laboratory-based experiment using laparoscopic tasks (Thompson et al, 1999). They were able to show that video time delays significantly affected performance, and that this effect was magnified when haptic devices were also affected by the time delay.

Interest in telesurgery remains, but it is dampened by the lack of appropriate, widely available technology that will reduce the time delay of video and audio signals transmission. The potential for use in remote areas including the battlefield and space are enormous. It has to be kept in mind however, that for the currently available systems, there must be a laparoscopic trained surgeon by the side of the robotic arms cart, and therefore, at the patient side. The reason is that the port placement selection and introduction are done by him, not by the system alone. This is an obstacle to remote surgery that would have to be addressed with future systems or through specialized personnel training.

7. Conclusions

Robotic surgery using telemanipulator systems has been proved to be feasible and safe in several tens of thousands of procedures carried out around the world. It has demonstrated its utility in complex procedures in vascular, urological and bariatric surgery, amongst other specialties. As a matter of fact, a totally laparoscopic coronary artery bypass is not feasible without the robot. However, current evidence does not favour the widespread use of telemanipulators in general surgery, since the time and outcomes do not differ from laparoscopic surgery, and costs are excessively high. Another factor against is the current size and design of the system. Da Vinci's robotic arms are large and cumbersome, making setup times prolong surgeries.

It can be suggested that comparative studies between LS and RS have been conducted with expert laparoscopic surgeons, which would have two effects. First, laparoscopic performance for these subjects is excellent, since they have overcame the difficulties LS places to novice surgeons, therefore, the experts do not feel a great difference between both environments. Second, as they are experts, the learning curve in RS will tend to be flat, making any difference non-significant.

In spite of these difficulties, it is good to keep in mind that we are seeing just the first generation of commercial surgical telemanipulators, and is possible to think that they could follow a similar path in development as personal computers and cellular telephones, of course in a different proportion.

Several authors support the theory that robotic surgery's greatest impact in performance will be found in trainees or in surgeons with no laparoscopic experience. These surgeons will go through learning curves that are shorter than the ones they would have learning the same procedure laparoscopically. As most surgeons in the world only perform cholecystectomy through a laparoscopic approach, the potential population is very numerous. The challenge of this technology is to attract them by improving the aforementioned problems.

The future success of robotic surgery largely depends on new generation of telemanipulator systems that should be cheaper, smaller in size, easy to use and with a wide range of instruments and functions.

8. References

Akinbiyi T, Reiley CE, Saha S, Burschka D, Hasser CJ, Yuh DD, Okamura A (2006). Dynamic augmented reality for sensory substitution in robot-assisted surgical systems. *28th IEEE EMBS Annual International Conference, Conference Proceedings* pp. 567-570.

Ali MR, Rasmussen J, BhaskerRao B (2006). Teaching robotic surgery: a stepwise approach. *Surg Endosc,* 21: 912-915.

Bann S, Khan M, Hernández JD, Munz Y, Moorthy K, Datta V, Rockall T, Darzi A(2003). Robotics in surgery. *J Am Coll Surg,* 196(5): 784-795.

Borelli J, Bello F, Rodriguez y Bena F, Davies B (2003). An active constraint environment for minimally invasive Heart Surgery: early experience of a cutting operation. *Procs. Medicine Meets Virtual Reality* 12, IOS Press, ISSN: 0926-9630

Byrn JC, Schluender S, Divino CM, Conrad J, Gurland B, Shlasko E, Szold A (2007). Three-dimensional imaging improves surgical performance for both novice and experienced operators using the da Vinci robotic system. *Am J Surg,* 193: 519-522.

Cadiere GB, Himpens J, Vertruyen M, Favretti F (1999) The world's first obesity surgery performed by a surgeon at a distance. *Obes Surg* 9: 206-209

Cadiere GB, Himpens J, Germay O, Izizaw R, Degueldre M, Vandromme J, Capelluto E, Bruyns J (2001) Feasibility of robotic laparoscopic surgery: 146 cases. *World J Surg* 25: 1467-1477.

Chitwood RW, Nifong LW, Chapman WHH, Felger JE, Bailey BM, Ballint T, Mendleson KG, Kim VB, Young JA, Albrecht RA (2001) Robotic surgical training in an academic institution. *Ann Surg* 234: 475-486.

Cichon R, Kappert U, Schneider J, Schramm I, Gulielmos V, Tugtekin SM, Schuler S (2000) Robotic-enhanced arterial revascularization for multivessel coronary artery disease. *Ann Thorac Surg* 70: 1060-1062

Damiano RJ, Ehrman WJ, Ducko CT, Tabaie HA, Stephenson ER, Kingsley CP, Chambers CE (2000) Initial United States clinical trial of robotically assisted endoscopic coronary artery bypass grafting. *J Thorac Cardiovasc Surg* 119: 77-827,

Darzi A, Smith S, Taffinder N (1999) Assessing operative skills. *BMJ* 318: 887-888.

Datta VK, Mackay SM, Mandalia M, Darzi AW (2001). The use of electromagnetic motion tracking analysis to objectively measure open surgical skill in the laboratory-based model. *J Am Coll Surg,* 193: 479-485.

Deziel DJ, Millikan KW, Economou SG, Doolas A, Ko ST, Airan M (1993). Complications of laparoscopic cholecystectomy: a national survey of 4,292 hospitals and an analysis of 77,604 cases. *Am J Surg*, 165: 9-14.

Diks J, Nio J, Jongkind V, Cuesta MA, Rauwerda JA, Wisselink W (2007). Robot-assisted laparoscopic surgery of the infrarenal aorta, the early learning curve. Surg Endosc, March 1. Epub ahead of print. PMID: 17332959.

Dosis A, Bello F, Rockall T, Munz Y, Moorthy K, Martin S, Darzi A (2003). ROVIMAS: A software package for assessing surgical skills using the da Vinci telemanipulator system. *ITAB 2003: 4Th International IEEE Embs Special Topic Conference on Information Technology Applications in Biomedicine, Conference Proceedings - New Solutions for New Challenges*, pp. 326-329.

Dosis A, Bello F, Moorthy K, Munz Y, Gillies D, Darzi A (2004). Real-time synchronization of kinematic and video data for the comprehensive assessment of surgical skills. Newport Beach, Los Angeles, California, *Stud Health tech Inform. Medicine Meets Virtual Reality 12 (MMVR). Conference Proceedings*, 98: 82-88.

Dosis A, Aggarwal R, Bello F, Moorthy K, Munz Y, Gillies D, Darzi A (2005). Sinchronized video and motion analysis for the assessment of procedures in the operating theater. *Arch Surg*, 140: 293-299.

Draaisma WA, Ruurda JP, Scheffer RCH, Simmermacher RKJ, Gooszen HG, Rijnhart-de Jong HG, Buskens E, Broeders IAMJ (2006). Randomized clinical trial of standard laparoscopic versus robot-assisted Nissen fundoplicationfor gastro-oesophageal reflux disease. *British J Surg*, 93: 1351-1359.

El Nakadi I, Mélot C, Clsset J, DeMoor V, Bétrune K, Feron P, Lingier P, Gelin M (2006). Evaluation of da Vinci Nissen fundoplication clinical results and cost minimization. *World J Surg*, 30: 1050-1054.

Fabrizio MD, Lee BR, Chan DY, Soianovici D, Jarrett TW, Yang C, Kavoussi LR (2000). Effect of time delay on surgical performance during telesurgical manipulation. *J Endourol*, 14: 133-138.

Falcone T, Goldberg J, Margossian H, Stevens L (2000) Robotic-assisted laparoscopic microsurgical tubal anastomosis: a human pilot study. *Fertil Steril* 73: 1040-1042

Falk V, McLoughlin J, Guthart G, Salisbury JK, Walther T, Gummert J, Mohr FW, (1999) Dexterity enhancement in endoscopic surgery by a computer-controlled mechanical wrist. *Minim Invasive Therap & Allied Technol* 8: 235-242.

Falk V, Mintz D, Grünenfelder J, Fann JI, Burdon TA (2001) Influence of three-dimensional vision on surgical telemanipulator performance. *Surg Endosc* 15: 1282-1288

Galleano R, Carter F, Brown S, Frank T, Cuschieri A(2006). Can armrests improve comfort and task performance in laparoscopic surgery? *Ann Surg*, 243: 329-333.

Heemskerk J, van Gemert WG, de Vries J, Greve JW, Bouvy ND (2007). Learning curves of robot-assisted laparoscopic surgery compared with conventional laparoscopic surgery an experimental study evaluating skill acquisition of robot-assisted laparoscopic tasks compared with conventional laparoscopic tasks in inexperienced users. *Surg Laparosc Endosc Percutan Tech*, 17: 171-174.

Hernández J, Bann SD, Munz Y, Moorthy K, Martin S, Dosis A, Bello F, Datta V,

Rockall T, Darzi A (2004). Qualitative and quantitative analysis of the learning curve of a simulated surgical task on the da Vinci system. Surgical Endoscopy; 18: 372-378.

Kano N, Yamakawa T, Ishikawa Y, Miyajima N, Ohtaki S, Kasugai H(1995). Prevention of laparoscopic surgeon's thumb. *Surg Endosc*, 9: 738-739.

Lee BR, Bishoff JT, Janetschek G, Bunyaratevej P, KamolPronwijit W, Cadeddu JA, Ratchanon S, O'Kelley S, Kavoussi LR (1998). A novel method of surgical instruction international telementoring. *World J Urol*, 16: 367-370.

Link RE, Bhayani SB, Kavoussi LR (2006). A prospective comparison of robotic and laparoscopic pyeloplasty. Ann Surg, 243: 486-491.

Loulmet D, Carpentier A, d'Attellis N, Berrebi A, Cardon C, Ponzio O, Aupecle B, Relland JYM (1999) Endoscopic coronary artery bypass grafting with the aid of robotic assisted instruments. *J Thorac Cardiovasc Surg* 118: 4-10.

Marescaux J, Leroy J, Gagner M (2001). Transatlantic robot-assisted telesurgery. Nature; 413: 379-380.

Marescaux J, Leroy J, Rubino F, Smith M, Vix M, Simone M, Mutter D (2002) Transcontinental robot-assisted remote telesurgery: feasibility and potential applications. *Ann Surg* 235: 487-492

McMahon AJ, Russell AT, Baxter JN, Ross S, Anderson JR, Morran CG, Sunderland G, Galloway D, Ramsey G, O'Dwyer PJ (1994). Laparoscopic versus minilaparotomy cholecystectomy: a randomized trial. *Lancet*, 343: 135-138.

Mehrabi A, Yetimoglu CL, Nickkholgh A, Kashfi A, Kienle P, Konstantinides L, Ahmadi MR, Fonouni H, Schemmer P, Friess H, Gebhard MM, Buchler MW, Schmidt J, Gutt CN (2006). Development and evaluation of a training module for the clinical introduction of the da Vinci robotic system in visceral and vascular surgery. *Surg Endosc*, 20: 1376-1382.

Moorthy K, Munz Y, Dosis A, Hernández JD, Martin S, Bello F, Rockall T, Darzi A(2004). Dexterity enhancement with robotic surgery. *Surgical Endoscopy*, 18: 790-795.

Muhe E (1992). Long-term follow-up after laparoscopic cholecystectomy. *Endoscopy*, 24: 739-808.

Munz Y, Moorthy K, Kundchadkar R, Hernandez JD, Martin S, Darzi A, Rockall T. Robotic assisted rectopexy. *Am J Surg* 2003; 187: 88-92.

Munz Y, Dosis A, Lo B, Wang DA, Moorthy K, Pandey V, Stanbridge R, Casula R, Martin S, Bello F, Yang GZ, Darzi A, Rockall T (2003b). Objective assessment of performance of robotic assisted LIMA to LAD anastomosis in a bench-model. *Heart Surg Forum* 6: S24

Munz Y, Moorthy K, Dosis A, Hernández JD, Bann S, Bello F, Martin S, Darzi A, Rockall T (2004). The benefits of stereoscopic vision in robotic-assisted performance on bench models. *Surgical Endoscopy*; 18: 611-616.

National Institutes of Health (1993). National Institutes of Health consensus development conference on gallstones and laparoscopic cholecystectomy. *Am J Surg*, 165: 390-396.

Obek C, Hubka M, Porter M, Chang L, Porter JR (2005). Robotic versus conventional laparoscopic skills acquisition: implications for training. *J Endourol*, 19: 1098 - 1103.

Okamura AM (2004). Methods for haptic feedback in tele-operated robot assisted surgery. *Ind Rob*, 31: 499-508.

Ostrosky J, Jacobs M (2003). History of laparoscopy. In: *Laparoscopic surgery*, Cueto-Garcia J, Jacobs M, Gagner M (Ed.), pg 3-4., McGraW-Hill Publishing, ISBN 0-07-136481-1, New York.

Ramsay CR, Grant A, Wallace SA, Garthwaite PH, Monk AF, Russell IT (2000) Assessment of the learning curve in health technologies. *Intl J of Technol Assess Health Care* 16: 1095-1108.

Reiley CE (2007). Evaluation of augmented reality alternatives to direct force feedback in robot-assisted surgery: visual force feedback and virtual fixtures. *Thesis to the Johns Hopkins University*, April 2007. Pp. 134-138.

Ruurda JP, Vroonhoven ThJ, Broeders IA (2002) Robot-assisted surgical systems: a new era in laparoscopic surgery. *Ann R Coll Surg Engl* 84: 223-226.

Ruurda JP, Draaisma WA, van Hillensberg R, Borel Rinkes IH, Gooszen HG, Janssen LW, Simmermacher RK, Broeders IA (2005). Robot-assisted endoscopic surgery: a four-year single-center experience. *Dig Surg*, 22: 313-320.

Scott DJ, Young Wn, Tesfay ST, Frawley WH, Rege RV, Jones DB (2001) Laparoscopic skills training. *Am J Surg* 182: 137-142

Shea JA, Healey MJ, Berlin JA, Clarke JR, Malet PF, Staroscik RN, Schwartz JS, Williams SV (1996) Mortality and complications associated with laparoscopic cholecystectomy. A meta-analysis. *Ann Surg* 224: 609-620

Smith CD, Farrell TM, McNatt SS, Metrevel RM (2001) Assessing laparoscopic manipulative skills. *Am J Surg* 181:547-550.

Thompson JM, Ottensmeyer MP, Sheridan TB (1999). Human factors in telesurgery: effects of time delay and asynchrony in video and control feedback with local manipulative assistance. *Telemed J*, 5: 129-137.

Wang D, Faraci A, Bello F, Darzi A (2006). Simulating tele-manipulator controlled tool-tissue interactions using a nonlinear FEM deformable model. *Stud Health Technol Inform*. 119: 565-567.

Wang D, Bello F, Darzi A (2004). Augmented reality provision in robotically assisted minimally invasive surgery. *Proc. of the 18th computer assisted radiology and surgery (CARS)*. Pp. 527-532.

Wang D, Faraci A, Bello F, Darzi A (2006). Simulating tele-manipulator controlled tool-tissue interactions using a nonlinear FEM deformable model. Stud Health Technol Inform. 119: 565-567.

Watson DI, Baigrie RJ, Jamieson GG (1996) A learning curve for laparoscopic fundoplication: Definable, avoidable, or a waste of time? *Ann Surg* 224: 198-203

Williams LF, Chapman WC, Bonau RA, McGee EC, Boyd RW, Jacobs JK (1993) Comparison of laparoscopic cholecystectomy with open cholecystectomy in a single center. *Am J Surg* 165: 459-465.

Yu SC, Clapp BL, Lee MJ, Albrecht WC, Scarborough TK, Wilson EB (2006). Robotic assistance provides excellent outcomes during the learning curve for laparoscopic Roux-en-Y gastric bypass: results from 100 robotic-assisted gastric bypass. *Am J Surg*, 192: 746-749.

Z'graggen K, Wehrli H, Metzger A, Buehler M, Frei E, Klaiber C (1998) Complications of laparoscopic surgery in Switzerland. *Surg Endosc* 12: 1303-1310.

Zorn KC, Orvieto MA, Gong Em, Mikhail AA, Gofrit ON, Zagaja GP, Shalhav AL (2007). Robotic radical prostatectomy learning curve of a fellowship-trained laparoscopic surgeon. *J Endourol*, 21: 441-447.

12

Medical Robotics in Cardiac Surgery

Stephan Jacobs and Volkmar Falk
Department of Cardiac Surgery, Heartcenter, University of Leipzig
Germany

1. Introduction

Surgical telemanipulators are obviously used in cardiac surgery to provide the surgeon in a confined space the same stereoscopic vision, full dexterity, unimpaired hand-eye-alignment and tactile feedback, as in open surgery. This is the basic concept that enables the controlled fine soft tissue manipulation that is needed in bypass grafting, valve surgery, ASD Closure and Cardiac Tissue Ablation for Atrial Fibrillation.
When computer-enhanced telemanipulation systems were introduced into the field of cardiac surgery some 8 years ago there was obviously a lot of enthusiasm and expectations were high. As with any new technology early adopters strived for scientific recognition and the use of robotics in the cardiac surgical suite received a great deal of media attention. With more experimental and clinical experience, the potential benefits but also the limitations of the currently available technology became visible [1,2]. Initially two systems were available but the Computer Motion Zeus system soon proved to be of limited clinical use due to the fact that the system offered only limited dexterity making endoscopic reconstructive microsurgery (such as performing a coronary anastomosis) difficult. Intuitive's da Vinci system is therefore the only Surgical Telemanipulator that is currently being used. A total of 2984 endoscopic cardiac procedures world wide (reported in a company based registry) have been performed in 2005 and increase steadily. This includes Totally Endoscopic Coronary Artery Bypass Grafting (TECAB) procedures or small access single- or multivessel coronary artery bypass procedures with endoscopic uni- or bilateral ITA harvest (1784 procedures).

2. Development of Robotic Cardiac Surgery

Computer enhanced Telemanipulation systems have enabled total endoscopic coronary artery bypass grafting both on the arrested and more recently also on the beating heart, a procedure that was unthinkable only few years ago. Every new technique in the medical sector runs through an evolutionary process. Thoracoscopic ITA-take down was followed by a Minimally Invasive Direct Coronary Artery Bypass Grafting (MIDCAB) procedure. After an initial learning curve that was demonstrated in all centers using the telemanipulator, the totally endoscopic coronary bypass grafting procedure on pump was achieved. The conversion rate to MIDCAB was in the range of 30%. At the same time computer assisted mitral valve repair (MVR) was established. Successful MVR has been performed with all critical steps of the repair procedure being performed intracorporeally

[3]. Because of the necessity of a small right thoracotomy, the advantages of this procedures compared to a conventional minimal invasive access are small. The number of MVR increased within 450 cases in 2004 over 600 in 2005 to approximately 950 in 2006 (reported in a company based registry).
After the development of endoscopic stabilizers which allow free articulation of the pads and thus provide easier placement, coronary artery bypass grafting on the beating heart was feasible. The conversion rate (elective conversion to a MIDCAB procedure) with this approach was high (>50%) in the beginning and LAD occlusion times exceed those reported for MIDCAB procedures [4]. Among the difficulties determination of optimal anastomotic site, excessive target vessel calcification and incomplete vessel occlusion limitations have been overcome with a new generation of stabilizer and with a sufficient irrigation system for back-bleeding from septal branches. The conversion rate in overall patients was about 30% but decreased over the time to nearly 10%. The efficacy of TECAB tested by angiography was similar to conventional bypass procedures. Confirming data of a European multicenter registry including 220 TECAB procedures will be published soon. From these data, it can be concluded that the use of the daVinci telemanipulation systems is safe, provided the user has a low threshold for conversion.

3. System Setup and Operative Details of TECAB Procedure

The patient is placed in a supine position with a small positioning roll placed caudal of the left scapula to lift the thorax and drop the left shoulder. The patient is draped in a way to allow for standard sternotomy and saphenous vein harvesting or a left lateral minithoracotomy if required. The lower axillary line needs to be accessible for port placement. A holding arm for the endostabilizer is mounted to the OR table rail on the patient's right side and the operating table is rotated 10° to 15° to raise the patient's left side.
The camera port is placed in the 5th intercostals space 2cm medial of anterior axillary line. A 30° scope angled up is inserted and the thoracic cavity is scanned for anatomical landmarks and to exclude the presence of adhesions. The surgical cart is then brought to the table and the camera attached to the central arm (Figure 1). Under direct vision, the right instrument port is placed in the third intercostal space medial to anterior axillary line and thus in the center of a triangle which is created by the manubrium, acromion and the camera port. Insertion of the trocar is monitored by endoscopic vision.
The left instrument port is placed in the seventh intercostal space medial to the anterior axillary line (Figure 2). The instrument arms are centred for optimal range of motion, by adjusting the respective set-up joints, and the instruments are inserted. The instruments are moved along the entire length of ITA to evaluate for external collisions between patient's body and instrument arms; instrument arms and camera arm. The ideal position for the setup joints of the instrument arms is 90° between the primary and secondary axis ("shoulder") and 45° between the secondary and tertiary axis ("elbow"). For the camera arm the net-sum of angles should be 0° resulting in straight alignment of the scope and the central column. With this setup there should be only little if no necessity to move the setup joints during the procedure. The remote centers should be placed correctly within the ports to provide the highest precision and lowest friction.
In order to maximize space in a closed chest environment single lung ventilation of the right lung is required. CO_2-insufflation is necessary to increase the available space between the sternum and the heart and enhance exposure. After single right-lung ventilation is initiated

CO_2-insufflation is begun for adequate visualization. Insufflation pressures in the range of 10-12mmHg are usually well tolerated, despite an increase in right ventricular filling pressures, a decrease of intrathoracic blood volume index and right ventricular ejection fraction. Cardiac output and blood pressure may decrease despite a compensatory increase in heart rate.
After the set-up of the system the surgical procedure starts with dissection of the left internal thoracic artery (LITA). The anatomic structures (anatomic landmarks) such as the phrenic nerve and the subclavian artery are easily identified. LITA take down starts by retracting and incising the facia immediately covering the LITA with low power monopolar cautery. The LITA is always in view during blunt dissection moving from the lateral to medial edge keeping a pedicle including the lateral veins without the facia. Dissection is performed from the first intercostal space down to the level of the bifurcation. Side branches are cut using low energy cautery.
The pedicle is not detached from the chest wall until the anastomosis is finally performed to avoid torsion of the graft and any interference during pericardiotomy. The mediastinal and diaphragmatic attachments of the pericardium are bluntly dissected to allow the pericardial sac to drop and to facilitate insertion of the endostabilizer later during the procedure. The epicardial fat is removed beginning medially. Care must be taken to avoid injury of the phrenic nerve. The pericardiotomy is performed with a longitudinal incision in pericardium over the suspected course of the left anterior descending artery (LAD). The pericardiotomy should not be extended to far lateral and over the apex as the heart may drop out of the pericardial sac. Identification of the LAD is facilitated by identifying anatomical landmarks such as the apex of the heart, the grove between the medial aspect of the left atrial appendage and pulmonary artery and the ventricular septum that can be identified by differences in the contractile pattern of the right and left ventricles. The ideal site for the anastomosis is then determined by absence of visible atheromatous plaques and avoiding proximity to bifurcations. The range of motion for the left and right instrumente is verified in the anastomotic region to ensure freedom from collisions or singularities and to allow for set up changes at this point if required. It maybe necessary to flip the endoscope from 30°, angled up to 30°, angled down to enhance visualization. At this time the ideal length of the graft can be assessed. The distal end is then prepared for the anastomosis. This is done leaving the concomitant veins intact to provide counter traction during LITA preparation and to keep the orientation of the graft. The distal end of the LITA is skeletonized. It is advantageous to free the distal end (up to 2cm) of all adventitial tissue to facilitate suturing.
After heparinization (an Activated Clotting Time (ACT) of 300 seconds is recommended) a vascular clamp is placed approximately 2cm proximal to the transection site of the LITA. The clamp maybe attached to the chest wall in order to provide additional counter traction and to facilitate exposure of the graft during the initial stitches for the anastomosis. The LITA is clipped distally and cut and spatulated in preparation for the anastomosis. Markers on the scissors allow for assessment of the correct length of the cut. Graft patency is confirmed by briefly releasing the vascular clamp. In case of insufficient flow, the procedure should be converted to open. Further endoscopic manipulation of a graft with insufficient flow is strongly discouraged. A 12mm subxyphoid cannula is inserted under endoscopic vision. Before introduction of the Endostabilizer, temporary silastic occlusion tapes and a 7cm 7-0 double-armed Prolene suture are inserted and stored in the mediastinum. The Endostabilizer is then introduced under endoscopic vision by the patient side surgeon and positioned above the LAD target site. Vacuum lines and irrigating saline line are connected

and the Multilink Irrigator is advanced into the field of view. The console surgeon then positions the stabilizer feet parallel to the LAD target site. After suction is applied, the feet are locked into position externally. After blunt dissection of the anastomotic target site, the silastic tapes are placed proximal and distal to the anastomotic site. It is helpful to cut the epicardium with the blunt knife before the dull needle is placed through the underlying muscle. Care must be taken to leave enough space (2 cm) between the two occlusion tapes. The LAD is occluded by lowering the self-locking plate onto the vessel and anchoring the silastic tape. Using a 15° sharp blade the arteriotomy is performed and enlarged with Potts Scissors. The initial incision should be very limited to allow control of residual bleeding from septal branches or incomplete vascular occlusion. Spots of visible atheroma should be avoided. Transection of the LITA is completed at this time and the graft is brought in close proximity of the target site. If graft length is critical a stay suture to the epicardium may prevent excess tension at the anastomotic site. The anastomosis is best performed by beginning at the middle of the medial wall distant to the surgeon suturing inside-out on the LITA and outside-in on the LAD towards and around the heel. This way, there is less resistance for needle penetration through the less fixed graft tissue. The anastomosis is completed using the second needle going inside-out on the LAD and outside-in on the LITA around the toe. During suturing it is important to tense the suture after each stitch in order to avoid anastomotic leakage. After the needles are broken off, an instrument knot is tied. Since there is only limited tactile feedback, visual control is of utmost importance. The occlusion tapes and the vascular clamp are released and evacuated through an instrument port. After pleural effusion is drained under vision, the stabilizer and instruments are withdrawn and the left lung is ventilated.

4. Results

TECAB was performed initially on the arrested heart using the Port-Access technique with femoro-femoral bypass, endoaortic balloon clamping and applying cardioplegic arrest. CPB time and cross-clamp time were in the range of 80-120 and 40-60 minutes respectively. The reported patency rate for the TECAB procedure on the arrested heart ranged from 95 to 100% prior to discharge and 96% at 3 months follow-up angiography and thus equalled the patency rates of conventional bypass surgery. However, operating times were in the range from 4 to 6 hours for a single bypass graft. In a more recent analysis angiographic patency rate in selected patients was 98,2% (61/62) and the conversion rate was 23% (27/111), mostly related to problems with the Port-Access system or peripheral cannulation [5].
Endoscopic coronary artery bypass grafting on the beating heart is technically more challenging [6,7]. In a recent multicenter registry the data of five centers were accumulated. Based on an intention-to-treat, the conversion rate (elective conversion to a MIDCAB procedure) was 33% (37/117). Conversions were mostly due to the inability to locate or dissect the LAD, the presence of heavy target vessel calcification and rarely other conditions such as arrhythmia or hemodynamic instability [5]. Take-down of the LITA is now a routine procedure that can be performed in 30 to 40 minutes. Time is lost for setting up the stabilizer and preparing the anastomotic area. LAD occlusion times are usually in the range of 25-40 minutes and thus exceed those reported for MIDCAB procedures. Total operating times for a beating heart TECAB procedure range from 2.5 to 3.5 hours. The patency rates for completed beating heart TECAB procedures are in the range of 92 to 94% [5].

The use of a telemanipulation system is currently restricted to few indications (single vessel bypass grafting of the LAD, occasionally double vessel grafting) but it is conceivable that it may be used for endoscopic multi-vessel procedures in the near future [8]. A number of steps that occur between ITA take-down and performing the anastomosis are still challenging due to the lack of assistance, limited space, the lack of fine tactile feedback and a limited number of instruments. Among the difficulties are the handling of excessive epicardial fat, determination of the optimal site for an anastomosis, target vessel calcification, and back-bleeding from septal branches. In addition, difficulties with positioning of the stabilizer or incomplete immobilization, render beating heart closed chest bypass grafting difficult. A low threshold for conversion is mandatory to avoid any risk to the patient. Elective conversion is safe and should not be considered a failure.

5. Current potential Solutions

It is the ultimate wish of the patient for less invasive therapy that has driven the development for endoscopic cardiac surgery.
There is room for improvement and the fact that technical developments usually occur in incremental steps and may take time to become clinically available, limits acceptance. Over the years a number of iterations both in soft- and hardware components have been implemented in the system based on critique and input from surgeons around the world. With the second generation of the telemanipulation system, the daVinci S, some difficulties, that arise from design constraints inherent to the architecture, are solved with the development of a stabilization device, placed on the 4th robotic cart arm.The application of multi-modal 3D imaging, surface registration and computational modeling of the range of motion of the robotic arms in an individual patient data-set optimizes preoperative planning of the procedure and allow for intraoperative navigation [9].
Beside good results, one reasons for conversion to MIDCAB was inability to perform the anastomosis due to lack of orientation. Identifying coronary pathology and to define the ideal location for an anastomosis in the absence of tactile feedback was observed and procedures failed. To solve these problems a distal endoscopic Coupling Device, a simple yet effective and time saving technique for anastomotic coupling was introduced to facilitate beating heart TECAB. The endoscopic "Ventrica system" was evaluated at the Heartcenter Leipzig in the animal lab and clinically used by the Frankfurt group [10].

6. Perspectives

The use of intraoperative imaging is growing due to the need of updated information in order to perform finer, more challenging interventions. Current uses of intraoperative imaging require the surgeon to interpret the images and decide what the next action should be. It has been shown to be advantageous to assist the surgeon by performing semi-automatic image-guided instrument control in certain interventional steps and allow the surgeon to concentrate on more important aspects. The surgeon is released from some simple and repetitive tasks which in turn increases his situational awareness and produces an improvement of the human factors, as well as of the patient safety. Therefore integrations of "automated or semi-automated components" for soft tissue manipulation might be the solution. Involving automation in a highly variable, deformable moving environment is still

technically challenging and automation will clearly not be the answer in cardiac surgery. But shared anatomy, dividing the control of the robotic
system into the user and the system itself, provides the benefit of each component. These are the cognitive abilities of the human and the high precision and less inertia of the machine. Based on intraoperative imaging and feedback control, a soft tissue manipulation is semi-automatically possible and may prove beneficial in selected applications.

7. Conclusion

The DaVinci Telemanipulation system has been introduced to provide the human operator with dexterity in confined space. After successfully beginning with IMA-takedown and achieving some TECAB cases on pump, the technique was underestimated by surgeons. The lack of rapid improvement and the time consuming procedure led to frustration and many centers did not proceed. Minimally invasive cardiac surgery is challenging and it takes a lot of experience to get used to the system to complete a TECAB procedure. With a step by step program and the sensibility to overcome some limitations, forcing developments of new technology, the computer enhanced surgery can be successfully performed. With refinements in telemanipulator technology and the development of adjunct devices to enhance exposure the technique of computer enhanced endoscopic cardiac surgery will further evolve and may prove beneficial for selected patients.

8. Figures

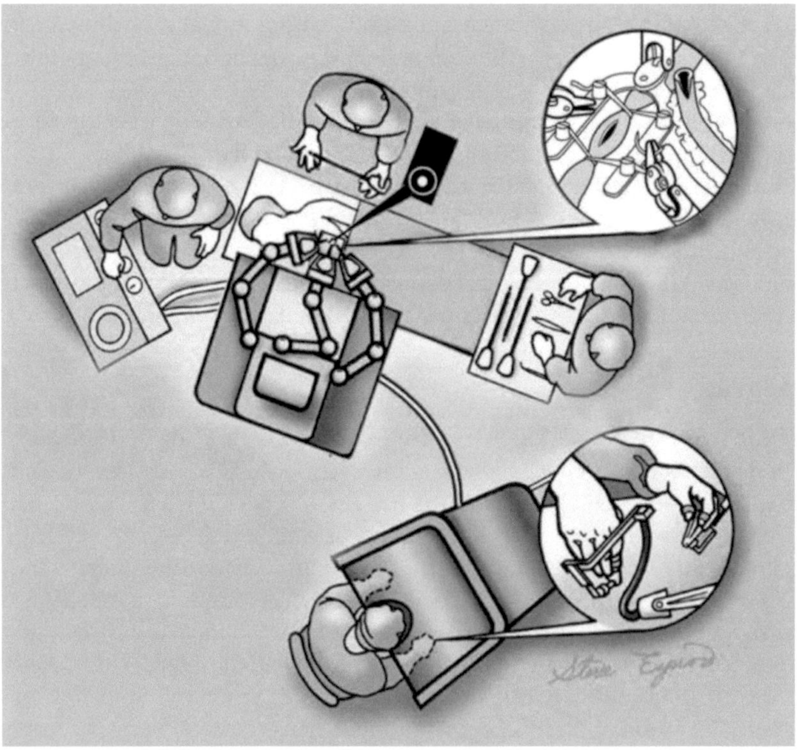

Figure 1. Schematic illustration of operating room setup

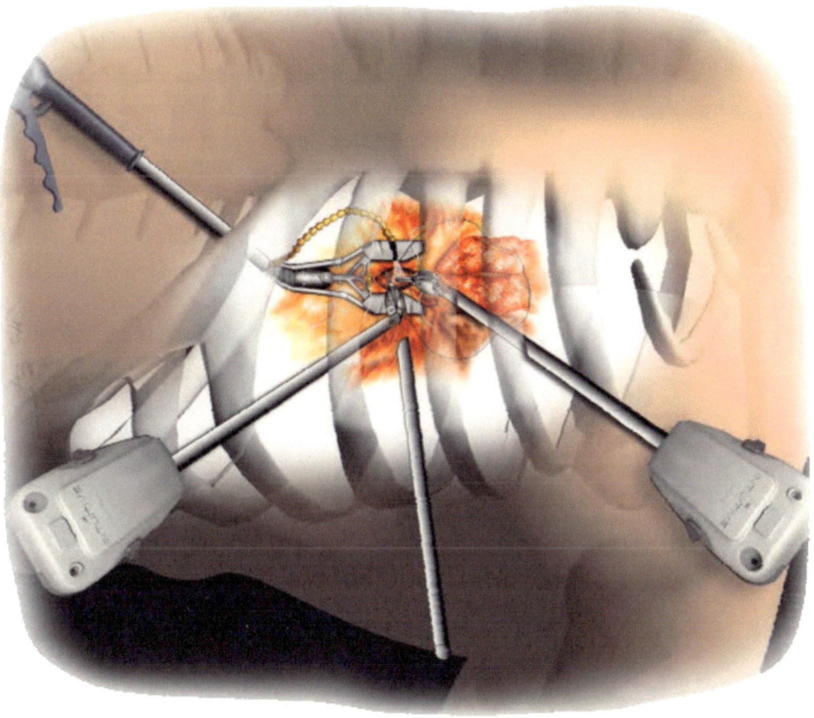

Figure 2. Schematic semitransparent illustration of port set-up in relation to the target site

9. References

Falk V, Diegeler A, Walther T, Bannusch J, Bucerius J, Raumans J, Autschbach R, Mohr FW: Total endoscopic coronary artery bypass grafting. *Eur J Cardiothorac Surg* 2000;17:38-45 [1]

Falk V, Fann JI, Grünenfelder J, Daunt D, Burdon TA,: Total endoscopic computer enhanced beating heart coronary artery bypass grafting. Ann Thorac Surg 2000;70:2029-2033 [2]

Rodríguez E, Kypson AP, Moten SC, Nifong LW, Chitwood WR. Robotic mitral surgery at East Carolina University: a 6 year experience *Int J Med Robot.* 2006 Sep;2(3):211-5 [3]

Jacobs S, Falk V, Holzhey D, Mohr FW: Perspectives in endoscopic cardiac surgery. *Comput Biol Med.* 2006 Dec 19 [4]

De Cannière D, Wimmer-Greinecker G, Cichon R, Gulielmos V, Van Praet F, Seshadri-Kreaden U, Falk V. Feasibility, Safety and Efficacy of Closed Chest CABG:Early European Experience. *.J Thorac Cardiovasc Surg* submitted [5]

Kappert U, Cichon R, Schneider J, Gulielmos V, Tugtekin SM, Matschke K, Schramm I, Schüler S: Closed chest coronary artery bypass surgery on the beating heart with the use of a robotic system. *J Thorac Cardiovasc Surg* 2000;120:809-811[6]

Falk V, Diegeler A, Walther T, Jacobs S, Raumans J, Mohr FW: Total endoscopic off-pump coronary artery bypass grafting. *Heart Surgical Forum* 2000;3:29-31 [7]

Stein H, Cichon R, Wimmer-Greinecker G, Ikeda M, Hutchinson D, Falk V: Totally endoscopic coronary artery bypass surgery using the da vinci surgical system: a feasibility study on cadaveric models. *Heart Surg Forum* 2003;6:E183-190 [8]

Falk V, Mourgues F, Adhami L, Jacobs S, Thiele H, Nitzsche S, Mohr FW, Coste-Manière E. Cardio Navigation - Planning, Simulation and Augmented Reality in Robotic assisted endoscopic bypass grafting. *Ann Thorac Surg* 2005;79:2040-7 [9]

Falk V, Walther T, Stein H, Jacobs S, Walther C, Rastan A, Wimmer-Greinecker G, Mohr FW: Facilitated Endoscopic Beating Heart Coronary Bypass Grafting using a Magnetic Coupling Device. *J Thorac Cardiovasc Surg* 2003 Nov;126(5):1575-9 [10]

13

Robotic Neurosurgery

Karas, CS, M.D. and Baig, MN, M.D., Ph.D.
Department of Neurological Surgery, Ohio State University
USA

1. Introduction

The field of neurosurgery has made a concerted effort in adapting and incorporating advancing technologies into the operative field, adapting new techniques and devices successfully in an effort to increase the safety and efficacy of brain and spine surgery. Diligent efforts are made to minimize normal tissue trauma during surgical intervention while maximizing clinical outcomes. Among these adaptations are the emphasis on surgical robotics. That surgical robots have not found widespread clinical utilization in neurosurgical procedures is debatable, because the term "robot" itself has several definitions. For our purpose, we will focus our discussion to mechanical devices used in the operating field of neurosurgery that ultimately give the operator, i.e. surgeon, ability to control the device through automation or remote control.

Name	Type	Function	Advantages	Disadvantage
Automated Positioning System	Supervisory controlled	Radiosurgery	Precision	Limited function
NeuroMate	Supervisory controlled	Biopsy, MDS	Precision	Limited function, cost
Minerva	Supervisory controlled	Biopsy	Precision	Limited function, safety issues
Evolution 1	Shared control	Pedicle screws, ETV, transsphenoidal	Dexterity enhancement	Lack of sensory feedback, cost
da Vinci	Telesurgical	Urologic, gynecologic, and general surgery	Dexterity enhancement	Lack of sensory feedback, not equipped for bone/disc work
NeuRobot	Telesurgical	Tumor resection	Dexterity enhancement	Lack of sensory feedback, cost
Cyberknife, RoboCouch	Supervisory controlled	Radiosurgery	Precision	Limited function
SpineAssist	Supervisory controlled	Pedicle screws	Precision	Limited function, cost

Table 1. Robotic surgical devices with FDA-approved and experimental neurosurgical applications

Technological advances in the field of robotics had clearly been incorporating into the operating room through the use of microscopy, navigation, instrumentation, optics, and imaging (Nathoo et al., 2005). However, the use of a mechanical device, whether through automation or remote control, to ultimately manipulate the instruments directly in contact with a patient is relatively new to brain and spine surgery. Since Kwoh et al. attempted a robotic brain biopsy in the late 1980s, growing interest in this field and its potential clinical benefits has encouraged the development of multiple systems (Kwoh et al., 1988). As with all novel instrumentation, the role of these systems must be clearly defined.
Among neurosurgeons this is particularly challenging, because the concepts of manual microsurgical techniques are already embedded effectively and successfully in standard practice. Approaching central nervous system pathology within millimeters through small working channels surrounded by vital tissue almost defines the subspecialty. Manual dexterity and minimization of coarse movement are an essential part of neurosurgery. Integration of surgical robotics is, therefore, an interesting dilemma and great promise. Although its theoretical advantages seem most suited to neurosurgical disease, the state of the art and technology has not yet matched the theory and expectations. Despite these practical hindrances, advances coupling clinical, and scientific discovery, continue to expand the notion of what is possible. This paper reviews some of the more promising systems in neurosurgical robotics, including brain and spine applications, in use and in development (Table 1).

2. Brain Surgery

There has been multiple robotic approaches to address the specific challenges associated with interventions on the brain (Benabid et al., 1987; Benabid et al., 1992; Drake et al., 1991; Karas and Chiocca, 2007; Kwoh et al., 1998; Nathoo et al., 2005). Deep intracranial pathology requiring manipulation of or direct trauma to the parenchyma has inspired devices that may minimize damage to normal tissue (Drake et al., 1991; Kwoh et al., 1988). While this is not meant to serve as a review of surgical robotics in general, an understanding of the subtypes of system available may be helpful. Nathoo et al. eloquently propose a classification based on the robot–surgeon interaction (Nathoo et al., 2005). Three systems are described. The first is a supervisory-controlled robotic system in which the robotic intervention is preplanned and programmed and then supervised by the surgeon as it carries out its programmed movements autonomously. The second is a robotic telesurgical system in which the robot is manipulated by the surgeon in real time through remote control, with limited feedback to the operator. The third is a shared control system in which the surgeon directly controls the movements of the robot as the robot enhances the surgeon's skills through dexterity enhancement, a term that generally describes mechanical solutions to human limitations, including physiologic tremor reduction.
As previously stated, development efforts have been focused on gaining access to deep pathology or structures (such as the third ventricle) with limited trauma to the normal brain. Coupling these devices, therefore, with image-based navigation systems and developing controlled, precise target-acquisition capabilities have been crucial advances in attempting intracranial procedures. In general, with these resources, existing models focus their technology on specific tasks.
The most widely used and simplest example of robotic assisted neurosurgery for the brain pathology is the latest model of the Leksell Gamma Knife Radiosurgical system. This is as supervisory-controlled robot that uses a Automated Positioning System (APS) (Elekta, Stockholm, Sweden) to adjust the patient's head within a collimator automatically, based on a

predetermined stereotactic radiosurgical plan. Thus this latest model of Leksell Gamma Knife eliminates multiple manual steps that were required by the Neurosurgeon and the Radiation Oncologist of confirmation and reconfirmation of the head position prior to delivery of the therapy. Most patients requiring Gamma Knife therapy need multiple doses of different intensity and position for proper therapeutic effect, thus confounding the manual manipulation dilemma. Several studies have confirmed the benefits of such automation, confirming shorter treatment times, reduced exposure of patients and personnel to radiation, and greater ability to deliver radiation to an increased number of smaller isocenters, thereby reducing the maximum dose to the target (Regis et al., 2002; Tlachacova et al, 2005).

For the purpose of lesion biopsy within the brain, navigation with image-guidance systems is common practice. To take this a step further, attempts to automate the brain biopsy procedure with robotic arms have been performed. The NeuroMate (Integrated Surgical Systems, Sacramento, CA, USA) robotic surgical system was the first FDA-approved robotic device for neurosurgery (Benabid et al., 1987). This system involved a passive robotic arm which moves in a pre-programmed direction to a specific site defined by integrated neuronavigation systems for stereotactic biopsy or functional neurosurgical applications. The Minerva (University of Lausanne, Lausanne, Switzerland) which followed, attempted to account for brain shift by placing the robotic arm within a CT scanner to provide real-time image guidance (Glauser et al., 1995). Safety issues forced the discontinuation of this device (Nathoo et al., 2005). Indications for the NeuroMate continue to expand as image-guidance technology advances. Recent studies have proven its localization and targeting capabilities are comparable with those of standard localizing systems (Li et al., 2002). Varma et al. achieved good accuracy with a frameless application of this system in microelectode placement for treatment of Parkinson's disease (Verma et al., 2003).

Another system, the Evolution 1 robotic system (Universal Robot Systems, Schwerin, Germany) has been tested for several neurosurgical applications. Its been used successfully for endoscope-assisted transphenoidal pituitary ademona resections. However it has been deemed too cumbersome and time-consuming to justify their use (Nimsky et al., 2004). More recently this system has been used for endoscopic third ventriculostomy (ETV) in six patients with hydrocephalus secondary to aqueductal stenosis (Zimmerman et al., 2004). Specifically, the robotic arm was used to precisely and reliably guide an endoscope to visualize the floor of the third ventricle. The ventriculostomy was performed manually by the surgeon through working channels in the endoscope, which was held rigidly by the robot. Theoretical advantages of this system over surgeon-alone ETV are precision targeting through image-guidance coupling and dexterity enhancement, which eliminates micro movements of a hand-held scope. Thus far there is no evidence supporting a clinical or outcome benefit of robotic over manual ETV, despite the measured differences.

Asides from the interventions requiring a single instrument or endoscope-stabilization solutions, telesurgical systems with multiple arms for both variable instrumentation and endoscopy are currently available in other surgical specialties (Nathoo et al., 2005; Stoianovici, 2000). The Neurobot telerobotic surgical system has been used successfully in complex procedures requiring simultaneous retraction and dissection (Hongo et al., 2002). Goto et al. describe a robot-assisted craniotomy in which the NeuRobot is used to resect superficial portions of an intraaxial tumor on a live human subject, citing dexterity enhancement as one of the potential advantages (Goto et al., 2003). At our institution several da Vinci surgical systems are available for both clinical use and research purposes. It has become standard instrumentation for prostatectomy and other urological procedures, and is

FDA-approved for general and gynecologic surgery also. Given its tremor reduction, motion scaling capabilities, multiple working arms, and patented Endowrist (Intuitive Surgical, Sunnyvale, CA, USA) technology which enables for full range of motion at the instrument head comparable with that of the human wrist, this device was tested at our institution for several neurosurgical procedures also. In our experience with cadaveric trials of end-to-end ulnar nerve reanastomosis, lumbar discectomy, intradural spinal dissection, and complex intraventricular surgery, significant obstacles to brain and spine applications still remain (Oral Presentation, AANS/CNS Section on Pediatrics, Denver, USA, 2006).

These obstacles, however, do provide insight into some of the necessities of robotic neurosurgery, which require both software and hardware changes. Specifically, the traditional endoscope with working channels allows for one tract through normal tissue to the ventricles rather than multiple tracts to accommodate instrumentation. This traditional model coupled with Endowrist technology may provide the added benefit of a greater range of motion within the ventricular system, which is otherwise impossible to achieve manually. Robotic devices focused on accurate localization may also move, or be manipulated, in such a way as to precisely acquire a target at a deep location at the expense of normal tissue at a more superficial level. For example, an endoscope positioned robotically to view the floor of the third ventricle may pivot dangerously at the cortex or foramen of Monroe and fornix. Docking after target acquisition, therefore, with continued mobility only distally is ideal. Finally, a clear disadvantage within all categories of surgical-robotic models is the lack of feedback to the operator. Although visual feedback has improved significantly with advances in optics and image-guidance, other sensory feedback is lagging. Position, velocity, or acceleration of the instruments may be recognized through a combination of visual cues and, for telesurgical or shared-surgical models, proprioceptive cues. Without complete sensory feedback, however, other significant sensations are lost, including force on adjacent structures or characteristics of manipulated tissues, for example compliance, texture, pulsatility, or elastisticy. Active research in this aspect of robotics continues and will be crucial in the integration of these systems into neurosurgery given the arguably absolute necessity of such feedback when operating within the central nervous system (Gray & Fearing, 1996).

3. Spine Surgery

There is a growing interest in the field of spine surgery to incorporate a robotic arm to image-guidance in order to assist with surgical interventions on bony landmarks. Several robotic systems have been developed to address the challenges encountered in spinal surgery. As with brain applications, these devices are enhanced significantly by advances in intraoperative image-guidance. In general, research in this area has focused on accurate placement of spinal instrumentation, citing the theoretically increased accuracy that robotics offers (Garcia-Ruiz et al., 1998; Goto et al., 2003; Taylor et al., 1999). In radiosurgery, robotic solutions to spine motion with respiration have also been extremely useful (Adler et al., 1999).

As with intracranial radiosurgical applications, the most common robotic subtype in spinal stereotactic radiosurgery is a supervisory-controlled system. Cyberknife (Accuracy, Sunnyvale, CA, USA) relies on a predetermined plan which targets spinal pathology for focused beam radiotherapy. By use of feedback mechanisms this system can adjust its trajectory to correct for patient movement, most of which result from respiration. This novel use of robotics has been expanded to intracranial use also, given the possibility of brain shift. A recent addition to the Cyberknife system is the RoboCouch Patient Positioning System (Accuracy), which uses similar technology to reposition the patient during the course of treatment.

Other supervisory-controlled systems have been developed for conventional spinal surgery as well (Chop et al., 2000; Lieberman et al., 2006). Specifically, devices coupled with image-guided navigation systems have been tested for accurate pedicle screw placement. Most recently, Lieberman et al. tested the SpineAssist (MAZOR Surgical Technologies, Caesarea, Israel) miniature robot for both pedicle and translaminar facet screw placement (Lieberman et al., 2006). Again, this device consists of a passive arm, which mounted on a fixed part of the axial skeleton. Motion of the robotic arm is defined by preoperatively planned screw trajectories, and is supervised by the surgeon. This and other robots with similar functionality have been tested successfully on human subjects, and the SpineAssist device is currently FDA-approved for spinal instrumentation.
As stated previously, we have tested several procedures with the da Vinci Surgical System at our institution, including lumbar discectomy, and intradural dissection. Because of the focused function of most robotic devices, it is clear that operations requiring both bony and soft tissue manipulation at different stages would also require human intervention at some point or multiple limited-function robots. Even the multifaceted design of the da Vinci telesurgical robot with multiple arms is limited in spinal surgery. The range of forces provided by this device, while adequate for abdominal or gynecologic surgery, does not enable use of a drill for bone remodeling, nor does it facilitate extraction of disc material. Without this capability, discectomy is nearly impossible, and intradural intervention requires conventional manual laminectomy. In a cadaveric study, after laminectomy, the da Vinci robot was used to open and close the dura and to separate nerve roots in the cauda equina from the filum (Karas & Chiocca, 2007). These maneuvers were performed with relatively little trauma despite only visual feedback.

4. Conclusion

Surgical robots have clearly affected the current practice of neurosurgery through several FDA-approved devices, most notably in the realm of radiosurgery. It is clear, however, that while the field of surgical robotics advances, attention must be given to the details of brain and spine surgery and surgical anatomy. Integrations of new focused technologies then can be adapted more easily into the neurosurgeon's already highly specialized operating environment. Creating the future of dexterity enhancement, automation, and sensory feedback, is of most value to surgical robotics if it can be studied in the context of each specialty. The robots most widely used in neurosurgery have been products of this contextual research, which concentrated on central nervous system-specific solutions. Attempts to adapt other instrumentation for neurosurgical use have proven to be less effective.

5. References

Adler JR, Murphy MJ, Chang SD et al (1999) Image-guided robotic radiosurgery. Neurosurgery 44:1299–1307

Benabid AL, Cinquin P, Lavelle S et al (1987) Computer driven robot for stereotactic surgery connected to CT scan, and magnetic resonance imaging: technological design and preliminary results. *Appl Neurophysiol* 50:153–154

Benabid AL, Hoffman D, Munari C et al (1992) Potential use of robots in endoscopic neurosurgery. *Acta Neurochir Suppl* 54:93–97

Chop WW, Green B, Levi A (2000) Fluoroscopic guided targeting system with a robotic arm for pedicle screw insertion. *Neurosurgery* 47:872–878

Drake JM, Joy M, Goldberg A et al (1991) Computer and robot-assisted resection of thalamic astrocytomas in children. *Neurosurgery* 29:27–31

Garcia-Ruiz A, Gagner M, Miller JH (1998) Manual versus robotically assisted laparoscopic surgery in the performance of basic manipulation and suturing tasks. *Arch Surg* 133:957–961

Glauser D, Frankhauser H, Epitaux M et al (1995) Neurosurgical robot Minerva: first results and current developments. *J Image Guid Surg* 1:266–272

Goto T, Hongo K, Kakizawa Y et al (2003) Clinical application of robotic telemanipulator system in neurosurgery. *J Neurosurg* 99:1082–1084

Gray BL, Fearing RS (1996) A surface micromachined microtactile sensor array. Presented at the *IEEE international conference on robotics and automation*, Minneapolis, USA

Hongo K, Kobayashi S, Kakizawa Y et al (2002) Neurobot: telecontrolled micromanipulator system for minimally invasive microneurosurgery-preliminary results. *Neurosurgery* 51:985–988

Kwoh YS, Hou J, Jonckheere EA, Hayati S (1988) A robot with improved absolute positioning accuracy for CT guided stereotactic brain surgery. *IEEE Trans Biomed Eng* 35(2):153–160

Li QH, Zamorano L, Pandya A et al (2002) The application accuracy of the neuromate robot—a quantitative comparison with frameless and frame-based surgical localization systems. *Comput Aided Surg* 7(2):90–98

Lieberman IH, Togawa D, Kayanja MM et al (2006) Bone-mounted miniature robotic guidance for pedicle screw and translaminar facet screw placement: part 1-technical development and a test case result. *Neurosurgery* 59:641–648

Moy G, Wagner C, Fearing RS (2000) A compliant tactile display for teletaction. Presented at the *IEEE international conference on robotics and automation*, San Francisco, USA

Nathoo N, Cavusoglu MC, Vogelbaum MA et al (2005) In touch with robotics: neurosurgery for the future. *Neurosurgery*, 56:421–433

Nimsky J, Rachinger H, Iro R, Fahlbusch (2004) Adaptation of a hexapod-based robotic system for extended endoscope-assisted transsphenoidal skull base surgery. *Minim Invasive Neurosurg* 47:41–46

Regis J, Hayashi M, Porcheron D et al (2002) Impact of the model C and automatic positioning system on gamma knife radiosurgery: an evaluation in vestibular schwannomas. *J Neurosurg* 97(Suppl 5):588–591

Stoianovici D (2000) Robotic surgery. *World J Urol* 18:289–295

Taylor RH, Jensen P, Whitcomb LL et al (1999) A steady-hand robotic system for microsurgical augmentation. *Int J Robot Res* 18:1201–1210

Tlachacova D, Schmitt M, Novotny J et al (2005) A comparison of the gamma knife model C and the automatic positioning system with leksell model B. *J Neurosurg* 102(Suppl):25–28

Varma TR, Eldridge PR, Forster A et al (2003) Use of the neuromate robot in a frameless mode for movement disorder surgery. *Stereotact Funct Neurosurg* 80(1–4):132–135

Zimmerman M, Krishnan R, Raabe A (2004) Robot-assisted navigated endoscopic ventriculostomy: implementation of a new technology and first clinical results. *Acta Neurochir* 146:697–704

14

The Use of Software Systems for Visualized Treatment Objectives in Orthognatic Surgery

Zafer Ozgur Pektas, Beyza Hancioglu Kircelli and Ulkem Cilasun
Baskent University
Turkiye

1. Introduction

Maxillomandibular harmony constitutes a major component of the ideal facial aesthetics. Improvement of facial aesthetics is one of the main reasons that patients request surgical correction of dentofacial deformities. Orthognathic surgery enables the correction of dentofacial skeletal or occlusal discrepancies. The need for this type of surgery has increased recently, as more adult patients are seeking orthodontic treatment (Nattrass & Sandy, 1995). Orthognathic surgery differs from other procedures of maxillofacial surgery procedures in a way that, the esthetic and psychosocial impact plays an important role in the patient perception of a successful treatment outcome. Therefore, a satisfying outcome of orthognathic surgery includes not only the decisive surgical technique and intermaxillary correction but also the accomplishment of the aesthetic goals that are successful to both patients and professionals (Sarver et al., 1988; Sarver & Johnston, 1990; Proffit & White, 1991). However, the concept of the ideal result is rather subjective and mainly determined by the consequency between the patient expectations and the actual result.

Without a visual reference, it is hard for the patients to visualize the outcomes of the surgical procedures and to contribute to the treatment plan in the preoperative planning session (Turpin, 1995; Cunningham et al.1995). In this manner, visualized treatment objectives (VTO) are important predictive tools to interpret the patients' perspectives of esthetics and to give an acceptable preview of the result. Furthermore, these VTOs facilitate the communication between the treatment team and the patient as well as provide guidance to the desired result. They also determine the need for bimaxillary versus single-jaw procedures and whether adjunctive treatments including rhinoplasty, genioplasty, liposuction or augmentation are necessary.

Lateral cephalometric radiographs are commonly used to predict the surgical treatment outcomes. Visualized treatment prediction began with manual profile predictions. Tracing overlay approach or using templates are the two methods for profile prediction by pencil drawing. Tracing overlay approach involves manual repositoning of the overlaid tracings and is limited to simulate the effects of mandibular surgeries. In this method, cephalometric film is traced including all teeth with their occlusal surfaces on an acetate paper. Subsequently, the structures that will not be moved by mandibular surgery are traced over the original tracing with a new sheet of acetate paper. After sliding the overlay tracing so that the mandibular teeth can be seen in their desired postsurgical position, lower teeth and jaw is traced. By superimposing the overlay tracing back on the cranial base, it can be measured how far the lower incisor and chin is moved. The lower lip will move 2:3 as far. Also, soft tissue chin will move 1:1 with bone. Finally, soft tissue outline can be traced regarding to these reference ratios (Profitt & Sarver, 2003). Besides, manual prediction method by using templates consists of cutting different parts of the acetate tracings and repositioning them over the original cephalometric tracing to simulate the surgical treatment. This method is compulsory when the maxilla will be positioned vertically and useful when major movements of the teeth must be simulated. Although templates can be used for any type of prediction, preparing them is more time-consuming rather than proceeding directly to a finished prediction tracing, as is done with the overlay method in uncomplicated mandibular surgery. With these two aforementioned methods, the predicted posttreatment soft tissue outline is drafted based on the reported changes of soft tissue/hard tissue ratios. Whatever the prediction method is, producing the predicted soft tissue outline is more of an art form than a scientific exercise (Profitt & Sarver, 2003). Although, manual prediction methods are relatively informative to the professionals, as they presented only the "line drawing" profile of the surgical simulation and they can not provide a realistic image of the treatment results to the patients (Sinclair et al., 1995) (Fig. 1).

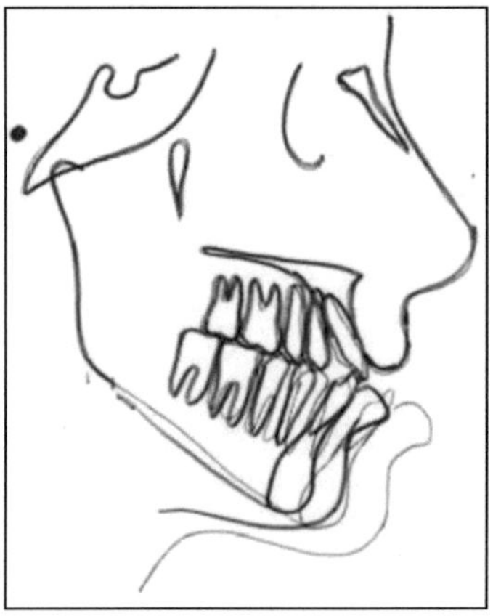

Figure 1. A manual prediction with overlay tracing method

Later on, computer-based analysis were introduced in the 1980s, where cephalometric landmarks could be digitized and the repositioning could be monitorized. This has facilitated the prediction, shortened the time and was more practical and accurate than the manual techniques (Harradine & Birnie, 1985; Walters & Walters, 1986). With these programs, measurements, calculations and analyses were performed by the computer. These cephalometric radiographic digitizing programs use the data from the published studies of the soft tissue reaction to the hard tissue movements. They incorporate these data into prediction algorithms that can provide excellent single-line profile drawings predicting the final treatment goal. As mentioned for the manual techniques, also this method is relatively more acceptable to professionals, but again, it can only present the line drawing profile of the surgical simulation, which is of minor concern to the patient. Patient is often essentially interested in determining what he or she will look like after treatment (Proffit & White, 1991; Sarver et al., 1988; Sarver & Johnston, 1990; Turpin, 1995; Cunningham et al., 1991).

The initial uses of computerized technology involved basic image modifications (Sarver et al., 1988) of both profile and frontal images obtained with a video camera, a digital camera, a scanner or a 35-mm slide scanner. Computer assisted cut-and-paste image modifications are useful to show significant facial changes expected after orthognatic surgery, however they do not provide the clinician the ability to determine the underlying hard tissue and intermaxillary dental relationship.
By the rapid improvement in computer technology and software systems, the integration of photographic images with cephalograms is enabled (Sarver & Johnston, 1990; Turpin, 1990). Digital tracing can be accomplished either by direct digitization of the cephalogram or a previously traced image, or by indirect digitization of the image which is monitorized. The softwares superimpose the patients' profile photographs on the digitized cephalometric tracings and the computer-based estimation displays both line drawing tracings and the corresponding facial images (Fig.2). The main purposes of calibrating the cephalometric radiographs to the patient's digital photographs are relating the underlying hard tissue to the overlying soft tissue; allowing quantification of both hard and soft tissue movements and applying the algorithmic response ratios between them.

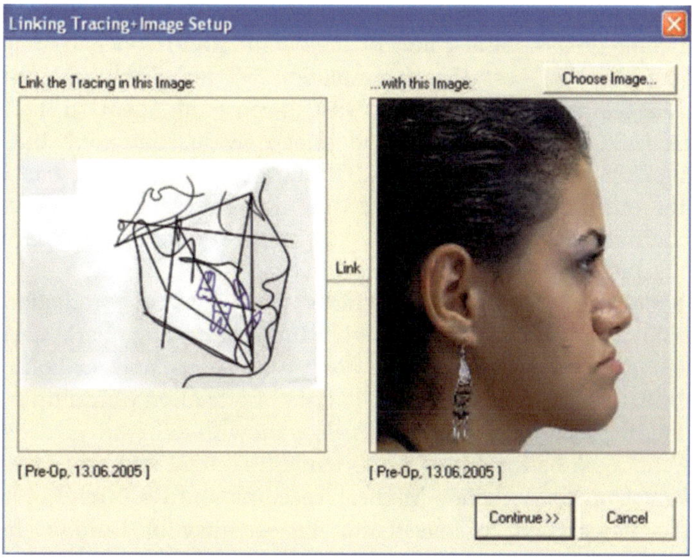

Figure 2. Screen view of linking the cephalogram with digital photograph of a patient

The Quick Ceph (Quick Ceph Systems, San Diego, CA) (Schendel et al.,1976), Dentofacial Planner (Dentofacial Software, Toronto, Canada) (Loh et al.,2001), Orthognathic Treatment Planner (Pacific Coast Software, Pacific Palisades, CA) (Jacobson & Sarver, 2001), Prescription Portrait (Rx Data Inc) (Jacobson & Sarver, 2001), Vistadent AT (GAC International) (Syliangco et al.,1997), Portrait Planner (Rx Data Inc., Ooltwah, Tenn), TIOPS™ (Total Interactive Orthodontics Planning System) and OPAL™ (Orthognatic Prediction Analysis) are some of these softwares which were developed to allow the clinicians to manipulate the digital representations of hard and soft tissue profile tracings and subsequently process the preoperative image to simulate the treatment.
Studies on the accuracy of these computer-assisted predictions were started with Hing in 1989. In this study, the accuracy of Quick Ceph (Hing 1989) is evaluated on 16 mandibular

advancement patients. The prediction tracings were produced from the preoperative cephalograms and then compared with the 1 year postoperative tracings. The results indicated that the horizontal landmark positions were overestimated and the vertical landmark positions were underestimated for the anterior mandible.

Kazandjian and colleagues compared the accuracy of two video imaging systems (Quick Ceph Image and Portrait Planner). Again, both programmes were noted to underestimate the amount of lower lip retraction and prediction was more superior than the actual result. Also the prediction errors in the vertical plane were grater than those in the sagittal plane (Smith et al., 2004; Kazandjian et al., 1999).

Smith and colleagues investigated perceived differences in the ability of current softwares to simulate the actual outcome of orthognathic surgery. They chose 10 difficult test cases with vertical discrepancies and "retreated" them using the actual surgical changes. Five programs—Dentofacial Planner Plus, Dolphin Imaging, Orthoplan, Quick Ceph Image, and Vistadent—were evaluated, by using both the default result and a refined result created with each program's enhancement tools. Three groups (orthodontists, oral-maxillofacial surgeons, and laypersons) judged the default images and the retouched simulations by ranking the simulations in side-by-side comparisons and by rating each simulation relative to the actual outcome on a 6-point scale. For the default and retouched images, Dentofacial Planner Plus was judged the best default simulation 79% and 59% of the time, respectively, and its default images received the best (lowest) mean score (2.46) on the 6-point scale. It also scored best (2.26) when the retouched images were compared, but the scores for Dolphin Imaging (2.83) and Quick Ceph (3.03) improved. Retouching had little impact on the scores for the other programs. However, the authors emphasize other considerations including the performance, ease of use, cost, compatibility, and image and practice management tools (Smith et al., 2004).

At present, a wide variety of computer-assisted cephalometric prediction softwares are available and Dolphin Imaging System (Dolphin Imaging, Canoga Park, CA) is one of these programs which is gaining popularity amongst surgeons and orthodontists. Dolphin Imaging Version 10.0 software, enables the indirect digitization of multiple dental, skeletal and soft-tissue landmarks of the scanned cephalogram with a cursor.

A group of patients who had received orthodontic treatment and underwent orthognathic surgery at Baskent University Adana Medical Teaching and Research Center during April 2003–April 2006, are studied to investigate the accuracy of Dolphin Imaging System software in predicting the soft tissue response subsequent to skeletal changes in a variety of orthognathic surgery cases. 11 patients (four males, seven females) with a mean age of 23.5 years (range 18–35 years) were included in the study and those who had adjunctive corrective procedures, such as genioplasty, rhinoplasty or liposuction, were excluded.

Case selection was made on the basis of the following inclusion criteria:

1. Availability of complete records, including lateral cephalometric radiographs and profile photographs, taken preoperatively, after orthodontic preparation, immediately before surgery and postoperatively at least 1 year after surgery.
2. Availability of lateral cephalograms allowing identification of selected hard and soft tissue cephalometric landmarks.
3. No history of cleft lip and/or palate.
4. No history of temporomandibular joint surgery.

The preoperative and postoperative lateral cephalograms were obtained using a Planmeca PM 2002 EC Proline X-ray machine (Helsinki, Finland), with a dosing period of 0.4 s, 66 KV and 12 mA, using Kodak MXG General Purpose Green films (Colorado, USA). Only cephalograms displaying distinctive and clear anatomical landmarks were included for each patient. The registration and standardization of the preoperative and postoperative scans were accomplished with the patients registered to the cephalostat in the natural head position, looking at their own eyes in a mirror placed in front, at a certain distance, during the cephalometric imaging, providing a repeatable head position (Usumez & Orhan 2001). Also, patients were asked to close their jaws in the centric occlusion, which also provided a repeatable registration regarding the mandibular position. A treatment plan was constituted for each patient, based on clinical and cephalometric evaluation and preoperative study models. All patients underwent one or a combination of the following surgical procedures:

1. Le Fort I maxillary impaction (three patients) or downfracture (three patients).
2. Le Fort I maxillary advancement (six patients).
3. Bilateral sagittal split osteotomy for mandibular advancement (three patients) or set-back (six patients).

Again, all of them had been treated with pre- and postsurgical fixed orthodontic appliances, and the same method of fixation (plate and screw fixation) was used to stabilize the osteotomized segments, in either maxillary or mandibulary osteotomies. The surgical procedures with the demographic data of the patients are given in Table 1.

	Patient	Age / Sex	Surgical procedure
1	S.B.	26 / F	Maxillary advancement with downfracture; mandibular setback
2	D.Y.	19 / F	Mandibular setback
3	H.V.	20 / M	Mandibular advancement
4	S.I.	35 / F	Maxillary advancement with impaction; mandibular setback
5	H.Y.	26 / M	Mandibular advancement
6	H.E.	25 / F	Maxillary advancement with impaction
7	S.O.	18 / M	Maxillary advancement with impaction; mandibular setback
8	S.T.	21 / F	Maxillary advancement with downfracture; mandibular setback
9	Z.S.	25 / F	Mandibular advancement
10	C.H.U.	19 / F	Maxillary advancement with downfracture
11	M.N.	26 / M	Mandibular setback

Table 1. Demographic data and type of surgical procedure

2. Digital tracing

The diagnostic records included the lateral cephalometric radiographs which were obtained immediately before surgery and at least 1 year after surgery, in order to eliminate the effect of soft tissue oedema (range 12–22 months). The preoperative and postoperative cephalometric radiographs were scanned using an Epson Expression 1680 Color Graphics Scanner (Epson, Long Beach, CA) into a digital format at 400 dpi, with a 100 mm calibration ruler, and displayed on a high-resolution monitor (Philips 107E61, NVIDIA Geforce4 MX4000, 1024 × 768 pixels). All the scanned images of the radiographs were then digitized, entered to a Pentium-based computer (Intel Pentium IV, 3.00 GHz, Windows XP Professional version 2002; Microsoft Corporation, Redmond, WA) and processed by one investigator (B.H.K.), using Dolphin Imaging Software version 10.0. To enable optimal landmark identification digitally, all tracings and digitations were performed in a darkened room. On the software, the digitization was started following the selection of the Ricketts and Steiner Analyses from the analysis toolbar. The landmarks were digitized as prompted by the Dolphin system directly on-screen, using a mouse-controlled cross-hair locator after locating two fiducial points placed 100 mm apart on the calibration ruler (Fig. 3).

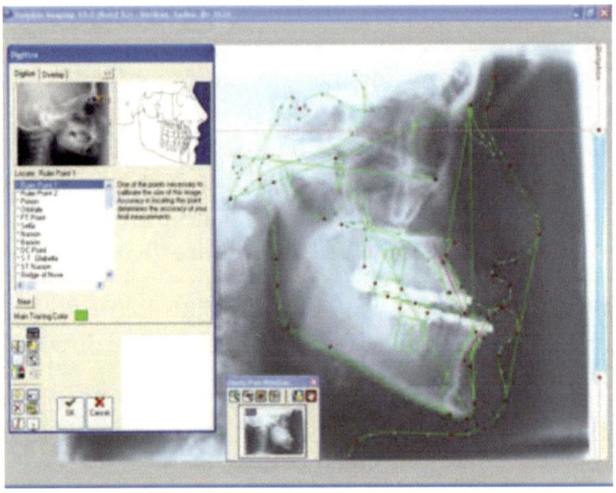

Figure 3. Screen view of the digitized cephalogram

Image enhancement tool functions involving blur/sharpen brightness and contrast options were used to assist in point identification when difficulty was encountered. Both preoperative and postoperative cephalograms were digitized and traced according to the selected analyses. In order to achieve the comparison of the actual postoperative outcome and the treatment simulation outcome from the software, preoperative and postoperative cephalogram tracings were first superimposed on the sella-nasion plane registered at sella. In order to enhance the superimposition accuracy, any structures and landmarks that have not moved during the surgical treatment, such as sella, nasion, basion, orbitale and porion, were simply transferred directly from the preoperative tracing to the postoperative cephalogram during the tracing session. Although the patients were registered according to the natural head position, any different positioning was corrected with a rotation option incorporated in the software. Hence, before transferring the stable points to the postoperative cephalogram, tracing of the preoperative cephalogram was overlaid, aligned and superimposed according to those anatomical points that had not moved during the surgery, such as sella, nasion, basion and orbitale, by using the rotation, enlarge or shrink options of the software. Preoperative and postoperative superimpositions were used to obtain a landmark movement spreadsheet indicating the exact amount of movement of each point after the surgical treatment. The location of any cephalometric landmark is expressed in terms of *x,y* coordinates, according to a selected centre point which can be determined by the user. In this study, the point sella was determined as the centre.

Secondly, a treatment simulation was generated according to the data on this spreadsheet and prediction tracings were obtained using the postoperative actual displacement amounts. Finally, actual posttreatment tracings and prediction tracings were superimposed on the sella–nasion plane registered at sella. The differences between the actual postoperative tracings and the prediction tracings were measured on these superimpositions and the measurements in the horizontal and vertical planes were again obtained as a spreadsheet according to an *x,y* coordinate system.

The facility of transferring the unchanged cranial structures during the surgical treatment to the posttreatment cephalogram, by overlaying the pretreatment tracing to the posttreatment cephalogram and displaying a millimetric landmark movement spreadsheet with respect to a *x,y* coordinate system, which is operated by the 'Tracing differences analysis dialog' toolbar, are two newly-added features of Dolphin Imaging Software version 10.0 that provide further enhancement for the analysis in this latest version.

Comparisons between the predicted tracing and the actual profile for the soft tissue analysis were performed on seven cephalometric landmarks, including the tip of the nose, subnasale, soft tissue point A, upper lip, lower lip, soft tissue point B and soft tissue pogonion; the definitions for both cranial and soft tissue landmarks are shown in Figure 4. The preoperative profile view, computer assisted prediction and final postoperative profile view, with cephalometric tracings of four representative patients, are shown in Figures 5–8.

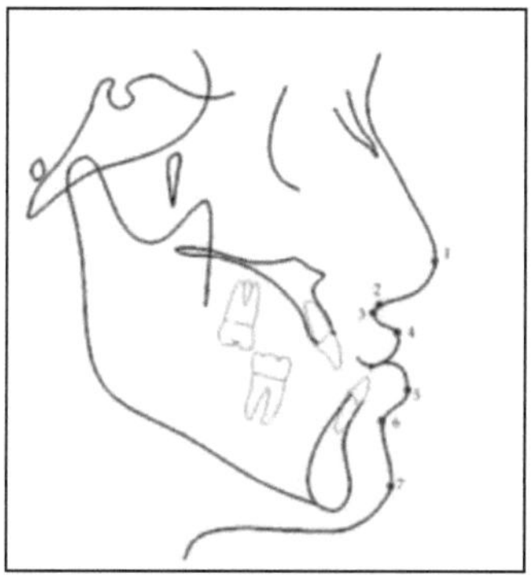

Figure 4. Cephalometric soft tissue landmarks and definitions used for analysis: 1. Tip of nose, point of the anterior curve of the nose; 2. Subnasale, point where the nose connects to the center of upper lip; 3. Soft tissue A-point, most concave point between subnasale and the anterior point of the upper lip; 4. Upper lip, most anterior point on the curve of the upper lip; 5. Lower lip, most anterior point on the curve of the lower lip; 6. Soft tissue B-point, most concave point between the lower lip and the soft tissue chin; 7. Soft tissue pogonion, point on the anterior curve of soft tissue chin

The differences in soft tissue outline between the predicted tracing and the actual profile achieved by surgery were evaluated mainly in the sagittal (*x* axis) and vertical (*y* axis) planes individually. The first analysis comprised the total group of patients and heterogeneous types of surgery, whereas the remaining analysis was performed with homogeneous groups, which were established based on the same type of surgery (maxillary advancement, mandibular setback or mandibular advancement).

The results for the total study group and heterogeneous types of surgery are given in Table 2. Although the magnitude of mean differences are presented in the first analysis, the pattern and direction of the prediction errors with respect to the sagittal and vertical planes (overestimations or underestimations) are not included, as this would result in a methodological error in a heterogeneous group. According to Table 2, the mean differences between the prediction and actual final result were < 1 mm in four of seven soft tissue measurements, including the tip of nose, subnasale, soft tissue point A and soft tissue pogonion in the sagittal plane. In general, predictions were found to be more accurate for the sagittal plane than for the vertical plane.

Cephalometric landmark	Sagittal Plane (mm)	Vertical Plane (mm)
Tip of nose	0.5 ± 0.4	1.4 ± 1.3
Subnasale	0.9 ± 0.7	0.9 ± 1.4
Soft tissue A	1.0 ± 0.8	1.3 ± 1.1
Upper lip	1.5 ± 1.4	1.4 ± 1.1
Lower lip	1.0 ± 0.7	2.5 ± 1.7
Soft tissue B	0.6 ± 0.5	1.6 ± 1.2
Soft tissue pogonion	0.7 ± 0.5	1.6 ± 0.9

Table 2. Comparisons concerning total treatment group, regardless of the type of surgery. Values are given as mean (average of differences between the prediction and actual final result) ± SD (standard deviation of differences between prediction and actual final result)

Cephalometric landmark	Sagittal Plane (mm)	Vertical Plane (mm)
Tip of nose	-0.7 ± 0.5	-2.2 ± 1.2
Subnasale	-1.4 ± 0.4	-1.6 ± 1.7
Soft tissue A	-1.5 ± 0.6	-1.9 ± 1.2
Upper lip	+2.0 ± 1.5	+1.8 ± 1.2

Table 3. Differences for maxillary advancement in 6 patients

Cephalometric landmark	Sagittal Plane (mm)	Vertical Plane (mm)
Lower lip	+1.1± 0.8	-2.0 ± 2.1
Soft tissue B	-0.6 ± 0.5	-1.9 ± 1.3
Soft tissue pogonion	-0.7 ± 0.5	-2.0 ± 1.1

Table 4. Differences for mandibular setback in 6 patients

Cephalometric landmark	Sagittal Plane (mm)	Vertical Plane (mm)
Lower lip	+0.6 ± 0.3	-3.1 ± 1.3
Soft tissue B	-0.7 ± 0.4	+0.6 ± 0.4
Soft tissue pogonion	+0.7 ± 0.7	-1.2 ± 0.3

Table 5. Differences for mandibular advancement in 3 patients

Tables 3, 4 and 5 present the evaluations for unique types of surgeries, including maxillary advancement, mandibular setback and mandibular advancement, respectively. These comparisons also include the pattern and direction of the prediction errors with respect to the sagittal and vertical planes (overestimations or underestimations). The (+) values present the overestimations (predicted landmarks were anterior or inferior with respect to actual result), whereas the (−) values present the underestimations (predicted landmarks were posterior or superior with respect to actual result) of the predictions.
The analysis of Table 3 provides data for the maxillary advancements. In general, the computer generated predictions tended to underestimate the differences for the tip of nose, subnasale and soft tissue point A, whereas the upper lip was predicted to be more protrusive and inferiorly positioned with respect to the actual outcome in both sagittal and vertical planes.

	Sagittal plane; x-axis (%)			Vertical plane; y-axis (%)		
	<1 mm	**1-2 mm**	**>2 mm**	**<1 mm**	**1-2 mm**	**>2 mm**
Tip of nose	82	18	-	46	27	27
Subnasale	45	55	-	82	-	18
Soft tissue A	46	36	18	55	27	18
Upper lip	55	18	27	36	36	28
Lower lip	55	27	18	18	27	55
Soft tissue B	73	27	-	36	18	46
Soft tissue pogonion	73	27	-	9	64	27
Overall	**61**	**30**	**9**	**40**	**28**	**32**

Table 6. Frequency of predicted errors. Predicted errors are shown as 3 groups; error <1 mm, error between 1-2 mm, and error >2 mm. Overall value is the average of all predicted errors

Comparisons regarding the mandibular setback surgeries are given in Table 4; the computer-generated predictions in the sagittal plane were closer to the actual surgical results than those in the vertical plane. Table 5 shows comparisons between the computer based predictions and the actual results in the mandibular advancement group. The predictions in the vertical plane were found to be less accurate than those in the sagittal plane. The distribution of frequencies of computer-based prediction errors are given in Table 6 and the results are quantified in three groups as errors <1 mm, 1-2 mm and >2 mm. In general, the prediction errors in the sagittal plane were smaller than those reported for the vertical plane. None of the prediction errors was greater than 2 mm for the tip of the nose, subnasale, soft tissue point B point and soft tissue pogonion in the sagittal plane. The majority of errors for the tip of the nose was <1 mm in the sagittal plane. The distribution of prediction errors present a wider range in the vertical plane; the analysis of all landmarks exhibits prediction errors >2 mm, whereas subnasale has a relatively high accuracy, with 82% of the errors <1 mm.
In general, the results of this study reveal that the computer-based predictions were more accurate in the sagittal plane than those observed in the vertical plane for all predetermined soft tissue landmarks. The frequency of prediction errors <2 mm is 91% for the sagittal plane, whereas 68% of the prediction errors were <2 mm for the vertical plane. These results

were proved to be satisfactory, as errors of 1–2 mm were previously reported to be clinically acceptable by orthodontists, surgeons and lay people (Kazandjian et al., 1999). The literature review also reveals a number of studies using former versions of Dolphin Imaging software. A recent study by Gossett *et al.* (Gossett et al., 2005), in which the prediction accuracy of computer assisted surgical VTOs is compared with conventional VTOs, revealed a statistical significant difference of only 1 in angular and 2 in linear measurements, including the interincisal angle, upper incisor to nasion-A line and lower incisor to nasion-B line, respectively. They used Dolphin Imaging System version 8.0 for image analysis, but this study differs by their method of excluding soft tissue predictions, as the early postoperative radiographs were thought to be prone to errors due to postoperative soft tissue oedema. They concluded that this system was comparable to conventional VTO in its prediction accuracy. However, conventional VTO was found to be relatively more reliable for predictions of the mandibular arch when compared with the Dolphin Imaging System.

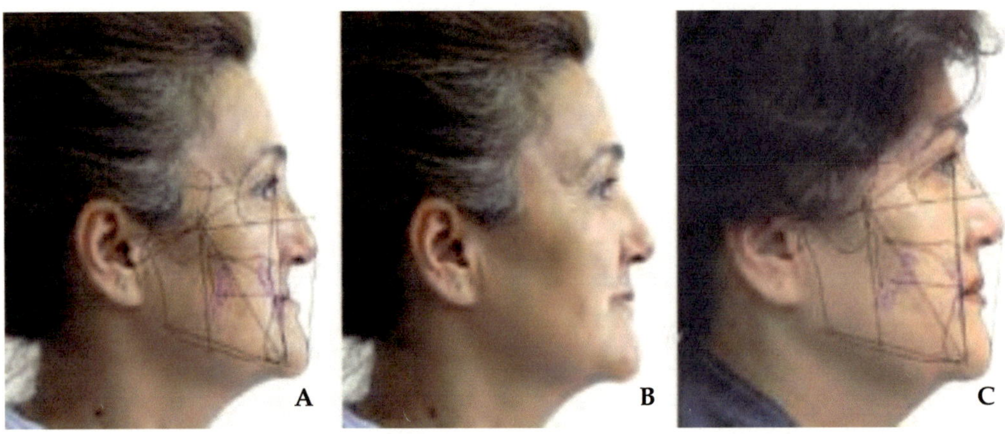

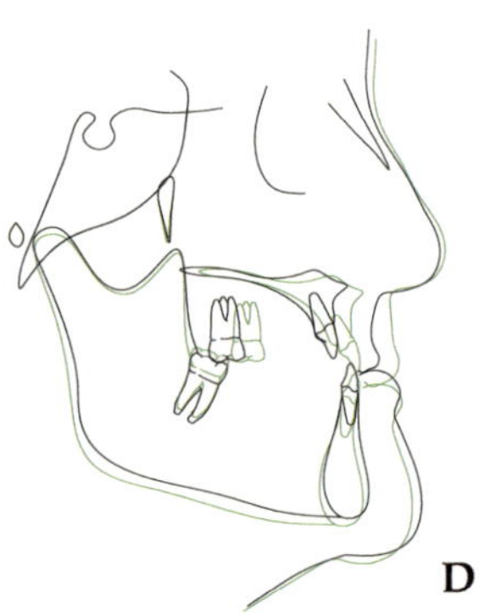

- **A.A; 50 years, 3 months**
- **Treatment planning (VTO);**
  - LeFort Ost: (H:+5.4 mm V:+1.7 mm)
  - Auto-rotate Md: -1.5 Deg

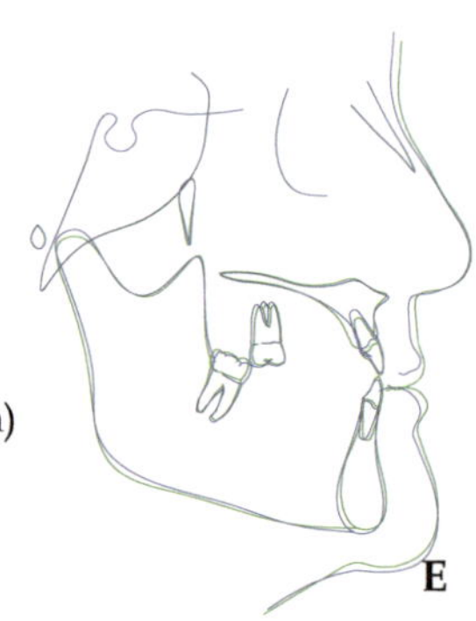

H: Horizontal movement; V: Vertical movement; Md: Mandible.

Figure 5. The preoperative profile view (A), computer assisted prediction (B) and final postoperative profile view (C), initial (black) and final (green) cephalometric tracings superimposition (D), predicted (blue) and final (green) cephalometric tracings superimposition (E)

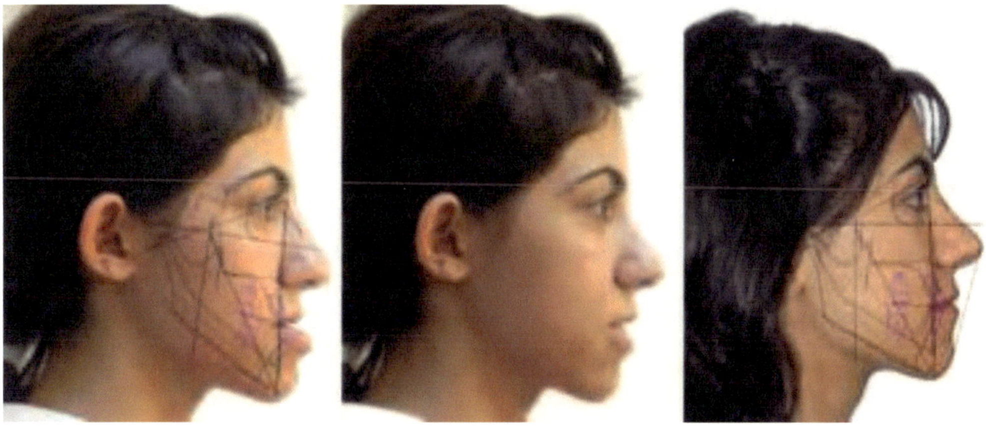

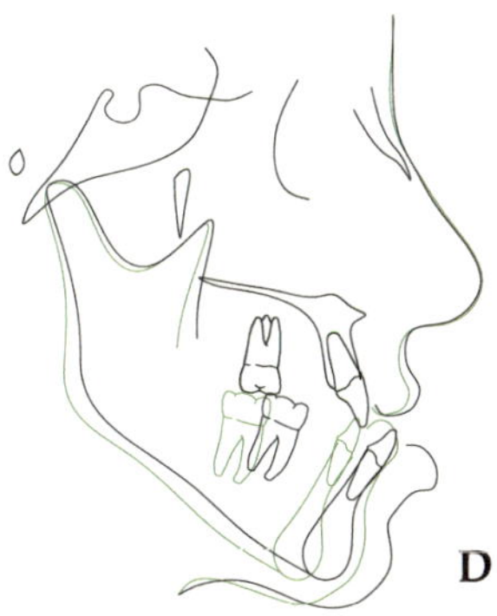

- **D.Y; 19 years, 11 months**
- **Treatment planning (VTO);**
  - BSSO: (H:-9.4 mm V:-0.9 mm)

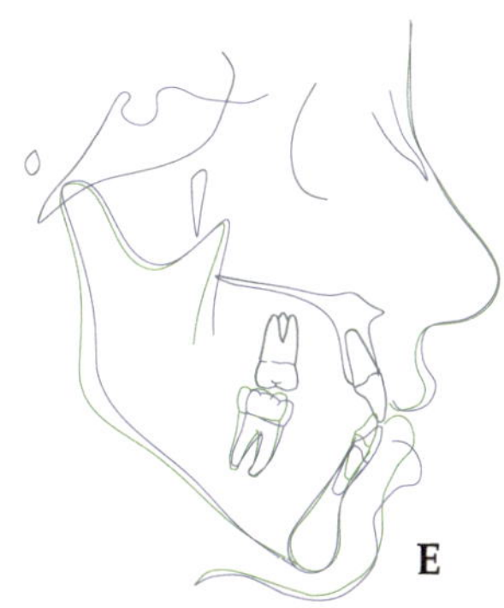

H: Horizontal movement; V: Vertical movement; BSSO: Bilateral sagittal split osteotomy.

Figure 6. The preoperative profile view (A), computer assisted prediction (B) and final postoperative profile view (C), initial (black) and final (green) cephalometric tracings superimposition (D), predicted (blue) and final (green) cephalometric tracings superimposition (E)

In another study, Lu *et al.* (Lu et al., 2003) also used the Dolphin Imaging System version 8.0 to predict soft tissue outcomes after orthognathic surgery on patients who underwent simultaneous maxillary and mandibular setback operations. The results showed a disagreement with our study, in that the software predictions of surgical profile changes were more accurate in the vertical plane than in the sagittal plane. Predictions directed to tip of the nose and subnasale revealed these sites as the most reliable ones that the software could predict, whereas the least accurate predicted landmark was the lower lip, measured in the sagittal plane. These results display an agreement with our results for the tip of the nose; however, unlike Lu *et al.* (Lu et al., 2003), the prediction for the upper lip in the sagittal plane and for the lower lip in the vertical plane were reported as the least accurate landmarks in the presented study.

A considerable number of studies carried out with various prediction imaging programs reveals a consensus towards the variability in lower lip predictions (Sinclair et al., 1995; Eales et al., 1994; Konstiantos et al., 1994; Kolokitha et al. 1996; Schultes et al., 1998; Csaszar et al., 1999). The influence of incisor position and angulation, soft tissue thickness and tonicity, perioral musculature and muscle attachments were considered as possible explanations for the low accuracy rates for lower lip predictions (Syliangco et al., 1997; Stella et al. 1989). When compared with previous studies (Syliangco et al., 1997; Hing, 1989), we observed that the accuracy of lower lip prediction was high in the sagittal plane, whereas the vertical plane measurements revealed greater prediction errors for mandibular advancement surgeries. In this context, Dolphin Imaging offers the 'auto lip adjustment feature', which enables the user to adjust both lips simultaneously in the vertical and horizontal planes (Fig.9).

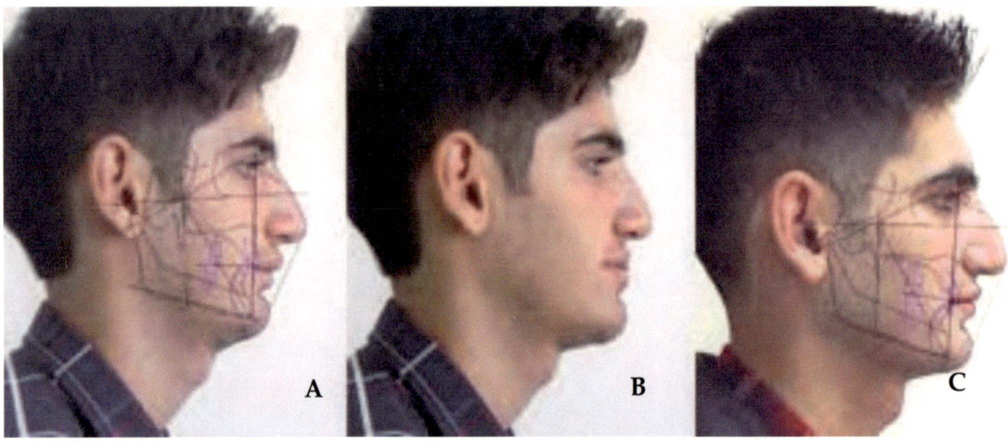

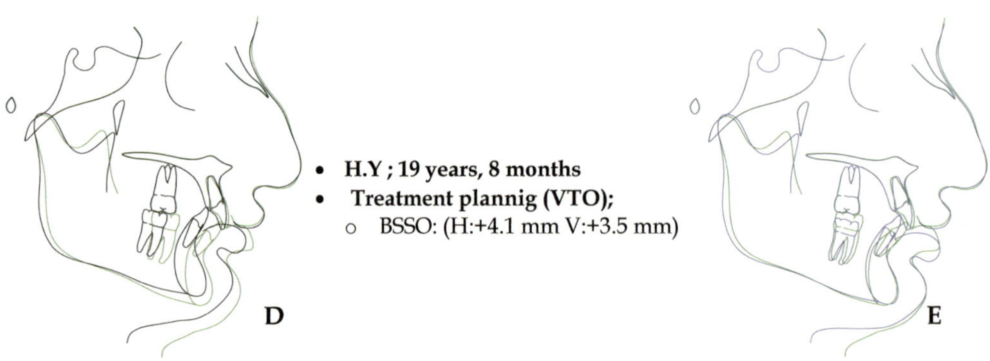

H: Horizontal movement; V: Vertical movement; BSSO: Bilateral sagittal split osteotomy.

Figure 7. The preoperative profile view (A), computer assisted prediction (B) and final postoperative profile view (C), initial (black) and final (green) cephalometric tracings superimposition (D), predicted (blue) and final (green) cephalometric tracings superimposition (E)

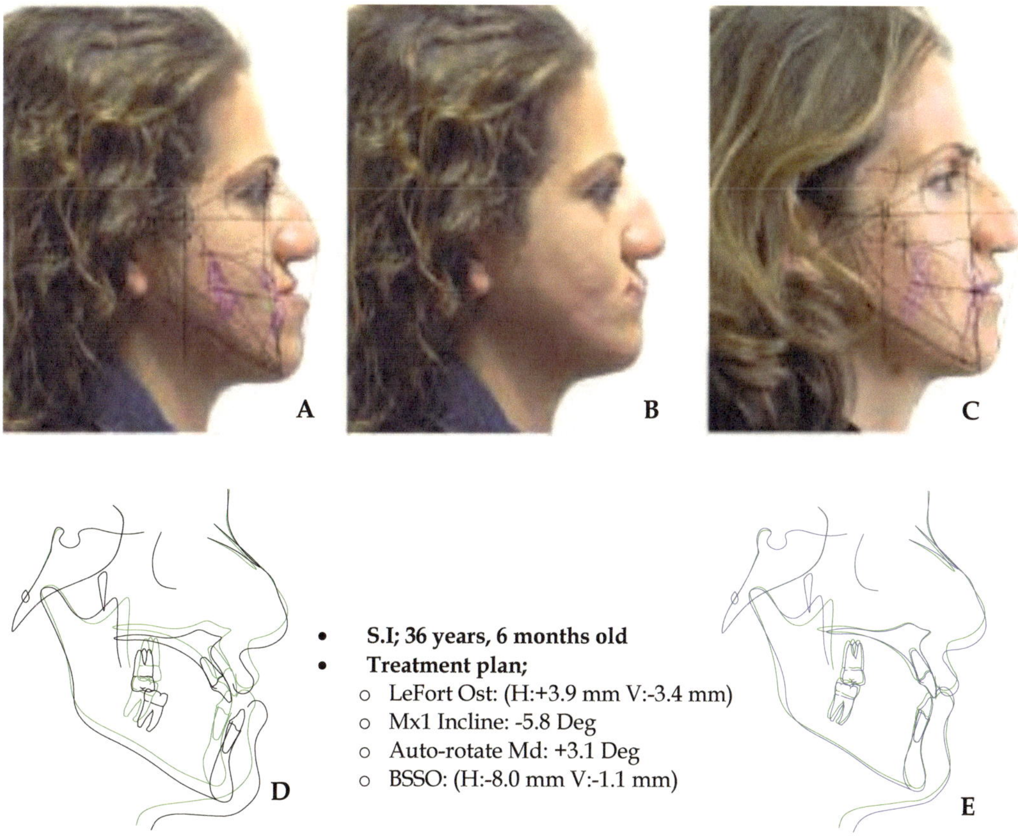

H: Horizontal movement; V: Vertical movement; Mx1:Maxillary incisor; Md:Mandible; BSSO: Bilateral sagittal split osteotomy.

Figure 8. The preoperative profile view (A), computer assisted prediction (B) and final postoperative profile view (C), initial (black) and final (green) cephalometric tracings superimposition (D), predicted (blue) and final (green) cephalometric tracings superimposition (E)

The favourable effects of visualized treatment objectives on patients' perception have led to computer-assisted cephalometric predictions being an integral part of orthognathic surgery treatment planning. However, besides many advantages of these systems, it should be kept in mind that the presentation of these predictions to patients should be done carefully, to avoid unrealistic expectations of the surgical outcome, as some authors have some concerns about predictions might imply a guaranteed outcome (Pospisil, 1987). Philips *et al.* (Philips et al., 1995) reported higher self-image expectation for patients for whom the video-image case presentation was performed when compared with a standard case presentation group. However, Sarver *et al.* (Sarver et al.1988) have found that 89% of a sample of patients judged video images to be realistic and 83% of the patients benefited from image analysis in determining whether to undergo the operation.

Although we have attempted to provide standardized material for this current study, with the precautions described and with the facilities of a newer version of the software, it may still be prone to some errors due to individual intersubject variations; differences in the exact time period from preoperative to postoperative imaging for each case, or soft tissue profile changes due to effects other than surgery (weight gain or weight loss), variations in the image quality or prediction algorithms may be considered as the possible sources of errors.

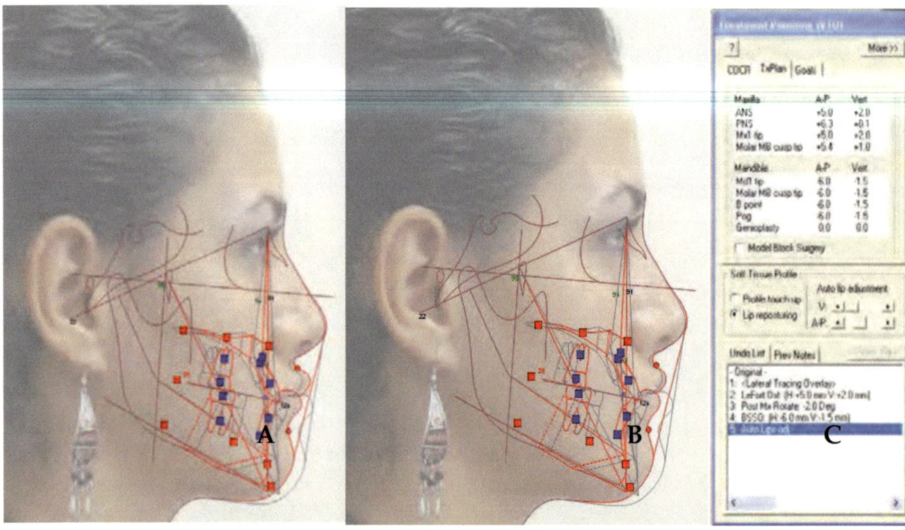

Figure 9. A computer assisted visual treatment planning (VTO). Unrealistic upper lip projection (A) , the computer assisted visual treatment planning with lip adjustment. Note the upper lip correction (B), and treatment planning window of the software (C)

The progression in computer science is a rapid and ongoing process. Novel techniques use three-dimensional colour photographs, algorithms and reconstructed 3D CT scans to enhance the prediction accuracies of these systems (Xia et al., 2000). Holberg *et al.* compared 3D prediction based on finite element method with a two-dimensional prediction programe (Dentofacial Planner Plus™) and found the prediction accuracy to be satisfactory. In addition to profile prediction, they reported that the procedure allowed a differentiated 3D assessment of esthetically important regions such as cheeks, nasolabial folds and the nasal wings without an additional x-ray radiation (Holberg et al., 2005).
Further investigations are also required to incorporate individual patient variability in order to integrate these systems to our current use.

3. References

Burstone C, James RB, Legan H, Murphy GA, Norton LA. (1978). Cephalometrics for orthognathic surgery. *J Oral Surg* , 36, 4, 269–277, 0022-3255.

Csaszar GR, Bruker-Csaszar B, Niederdellmann H. (1999). Prediction of soft tissue profiles in orthodontic surgery with the Dentofacial Planner. *Int J Adult Orthod Orthognath Surg*, 14, 4, 285–290, 0742-1931.

Cunningham SJ, Hunt NP, Feinmann C. (1995). Psychological aspects of orthognathic surgery: a review of literature. *Int JAdult Orthod Orthognath Surg*, 10, 3, 159-177, 0742-1931.

Eales EA, Newton C, Jones ML, Sugar A. (1994). The accuracy of computerized prediction of the soft tissue profile: a study of 25 patients treated by means of the Le Fort I osteotomy. *Int J Adult Orthod Orthognath Surg*, 9, 2, 141–152, 0742-1931.

Gossett CB,Preston CB, Dunford R, Lampasso J. (2005). Prediction accuracy of computer-assisted surgical visual treatment objectives as compared with conventional visual treatment objectives. *J Oral Maxillofac Surg*, 63, 5, 609–617, 0301-0503.

Harradine NW, Birnie DJ. (1985). Computerized prediction of the results of orthognathic surgery. *J Maxillofac Surg*, 13, 6, 245-249, 0301-0503.

Hing NR. (1989). The accuracy of computer generated prediction tracings. *Int J Oral Maxillofac Surg*, 18, 3, 148-51, 0901-5027.

Holberg C, Heine AK, Geis P, Schwenzer K, Rudzki-Janson I. (2005). Three-dimensional soft tissue prediction using finite elements. Part II: Clinical application. *J Orofac Orthop*, 66, 2, 122-134, 1434-5293.

Jacobson R, Sarver DM. (2001). The predictability of maxillary repositioning in Le Fort I orthognathic surgery. *Am J Orthod Dentofacial Orthop*, 122, 2, 142-154, 0889-5406.

Kazandjian S, Sameshima GT, Champlin T, Sinclair PM. (1999). Accuracy of video imaging for predicting the soft tissue profile after mandibular set-back surgery. *Am J Orthod Dentofacial Orthop*, 115, 4, 382–389, 0889-5406.

Kolokitha OE, Athanasiou AE, Tuncay OC. (1996). Validity of computerized predictions of dentoskeletal and soft tissue profile changes after mandibular setback and maxillary impaction osteotomies. *Int J Adult Orthod Orthognath Surg*, 11, 2, 137–154, 0742-1931.

Konstiantos KA, O'Reilly MT, Close J. (1994). The validity of the prediction of soft tissue profile changes after Le Fort I osteotomy using the Dentofacial Planner. *Am J Orthod Dentofacial Orthop*, 105, 3, 241–249, 0889-5406.

Loh S, Heng JK, Ward-Booth P, Winchester L, McDonald F. (2001).A radiographic analysis of computer prediction in conjunction with orthognathic surgery. *Int J Oral Maxillofac Surg*, 30, 4, 259–263, 0901-5027.

Lu CH, Ko EWC, Huang CS. (2003). The accuracy of video imaging prediction in soft tissue outcome after bimaxillary orthognathic surgery. *J Oral Maxillofac Surg*, 61, 3, 333–342, 0301-0503.

Nattrass C, Sandy JR. (1995). Adult orthodontics. *Br J Orthod*, 22, 4, 331–337, 0301-228X.

Phillips C, Hill BJ, Cannac C. The influence of video imaging on patients' perceptions and expectations. (1995). *Angle Orthod*, 65, 4, 263-270, 0003-3219.

Pospisil OA. (1987). Reliability and feasibility of prediction tracing in orthognathic surgery. *J Craniomaxillofac Surg*, 15, 2, 79–83, 1010-5182.

Proffit WR, White RP. (1991). The need for surgical orthodontic treatment, In: *Surgical Orthodontic Treatment,* Proffit WR, White RP Jr, 2-24, Mosby–Year Book, St Louis, MO, USA.

Proffit WR, Sarver DM. (2003). Treatment Planning: Optimizing Benefit to the Patient, In: *Contemporary Treatment of Dentofacial Deformity,* Proffit WR, White RP Jr, Sarver DM, 172-244, Mosby–Year Book, 0-323-01697-9, St Louis, MO, USA.

Sarver DM, Johnston MW, Maturas VJ. (1988). Video imaging for planning and counseling in ortho surgery. *J Oral Maxfac Surg*, 46, 1, 939–945, 0301-0503.

Sarver DM, Johnston MW. (1990).Video-imaging: techniques for superimposition of cephalometric radiography and profile images. *Int J Adult Orthod Orthognath Surg*, 5, 4, 241-248, 0742-1931.

Sarver DM (2000). The Application of Video Imaging Technology to Orthognatic Surgery, In: *Oral and Maxillofacial Surgery,* Fonseca JR, 57-81, W.B. Saunders Comp., 0-7216-9633-3, Philadelphia, USA.

Schendel SA, Eisenfeld J, Bell WH, Epker BN. (1976). Superior repositioning of the maxilla. Stability and soft tissue osseous relations. *Am J Orthod,* 70, 6, 663–674, 0889-5406.

Schultes G, Gaggl A, Karcher H. (1998). Accuracy of cephalometric and video-imaging program Dentofacial Planner Plus in orthognathic surgical planning. *Comput Aided Surg*, 3, 3, 108–114, 1092-9088.

Sinclair PM, Kilpelainen P, White R, Rogers L, Sarver D. (1995). The accuracy of video-imaging in orthognathic surgery. *Am J Orthod Dentofacial Orthop*, 107, 2, 177–185, 0889-5406.

Smith JD, Thomas PM, Proffit WR. (2004). A comparison of current prediction imaging programs. *Am J Orthod Dentofacial Orthop*, 125, 5, 527–536, 0889-5406.

Stella JP, Streater MR, Epker BN, Sinn DP. (1989). Predictability of upper soft tissue changes with maxillary advancement. *J Oral Maxillofac Surg*, 47, 7, 697–703, 0301-0503.

Syliangco ST, Sameshima GT, Kaminishi RM, Sinclair PM. (1997). Predicting soft tissue changes in mandibular advancement surgery: a comparison of two video-imaging systems. *Angle Orthodont*, 67, 5, 337–346, 0003-3219.

Turpin DL. (1990). Computers coming on line for diagnosis and treatment planning. *Angle Orthod*, 60, 3, 163-164, 0003-3219.

Turpin DL. (1995). The need for video imaging. *Angle Orthod*, 65, 4, 243–244, 0003-3219.

Usumez S, Orhan M. (2001). Inclinometer method for recording and transferring natural head position in cephalometrics. *Am J Orthod Dentofacial Orthop*, 120, 6, 664-670, 0889-5406.

Walters H, Walters DH. (1986). Computerized planning of maxillofacial osteotomies: The program and its clinical application. *Br J Oral Maxillofac Surg*, 24, 3, 178-189, 0266-4356.

Xia J, SammanN, UeungRW, *et al.* (2000). Computer-assisted threedimensional surgical planning and simulation. 3D soft tissue planning and prediction. *Int J Oral Maxillofac Surg*, 29, 4, 250–258, 0901-5027.

15

Intelligent Laparoscopic Assistant Robot through Surgery Task Model: How to Give Intelligence to Medical Robots

Dong-Soo Kwon, Seong-Young Ko and Jonathan Kim
Korea Advanced Institute of Science and Technology
Republic of Korea

1. Introduction

Laparoscopy has become one of the most popular surgical techniques since the 1990s due to its surgical effectiveness, fast recovery and good cosmetic outcome. From simple to more complex surgeries, the proportion of laparoscopic to open procedures is continuously increasing. Due to small incision, patients can regain health without much trauma and hospitalization; however, the operating surgeons suffer from limited range of motion, reduced flexibility, loss of tactile sensation and limited depth perception compared to open surgery. One of the important issues for successful surgery is the cooperation between the operating surgeon and the assistant as it is directly related to how the surgeon can perform surgical tasks. Manipulating vessels and organs using long tools without direct visual feedback requires utmost attention and the assistant should maneuver the laparoscope without disrupting the operating surgeon. Novice assistants often suffer from: (a) the difficulty in properly positioning the laparoscope in three-dimensional space based on the projected images on a monitor, (b) the presence of the fulcrum effect at the trocar insertion point, and (c) the hand tremor caused by fatigue. To alleviate the effect of these difficulties, some surgical robotic systems (Franzino, 2003; Ghodoussi et al., 2002; Guthart & Salisbury, 2000; Mitsuishi et al., 2003) and laparoscopic assistant robot systems such as AESOP(Wang et al., 1996), Endo*Assist*(Finlay, 1996) and so forth(Berkelman et al., 2002; Kobayashi et al., 1999; Taylor et al., 1995) were developed.
Despite the applicability in real surgeries, these systems exhibit some common limitations or constraints that should be resolved. These systems are known to occupy a voluminous space in the operating room and the external motion of links tends to interfere or come in close contact with the surgeon and surgical staff. In order to develop a compact robot and to reduce possible interference with surgical staff, we adopted an internally bending mechanism. This internally bending mechanism confines the majority of motions inside the patient's abdomen and also reduces the size of the robotic system. The proposed laparoscopic assistant robot system, KaLAR (KAIST Laparoscopic Assistant Robot), will be explained in detail later.
Although most of the robotic assistants can substitute for the role of human assistant, clinical studies revealed that a considerable number of voice commands are needed to control the robot, while only a handful of voice commands is sufficient with a human

assistant. Another modality of control such as the use of surgeon's head motion can be used, but this does not completely eliminate the need for voice commands and may introduce additional physical stress (Nishikawa et al., 2001). Surgery requires delicate handling of tissues at the surgical site and the burden of controlling the robot should be kept minimal. Since lesser control burden is imposed on the operating surgeon when aided by a human assistant, a skillful human assistant is a good example of how a robotic assistant should behave. A key difference between a human assistant and a robotic assistant lies in the degree of preliminary knowledge of the surgery. Therefore, in order for the robot to become an intelligent assistant rather than a motorized surgical tool, it should have preliminary surgical knowledge similar to a well-trained human assistant. The ideal method may be to develop a complete human-like robot with both human-level artificial intelligence and interaction capability; however, considering the state-of-the-art in current robotic technology, this remains a distant goal. Although achieving a general surgical intelligence may be difficult, it is possible to achieve *task-specific* intelligence for laparoscopic assistant robot through a surgery task model, considering its specific task domain and restrictive behavior patterns.

The remains of this chapter will present the laparoscopic assistant robot system and the interaction method based on a surgery task model. In section 2, the details of the robot system will be explained. Section 3 will describe the concept and implementation of the interaction method based on a surgery task model. Section 4 will demonstrate the preliminary result of the proposed robotic system and the interaction scheme based on a surgery task model. Finally, conclusions and discussions for future work are presented in section 5.

2. Compact Assistant Robot for Adjusting Laparoscope View

2.1 Basic Concepts and Workspace Requirements

In this section, our compact laparoscopic assistant robot, KaLAR, will be explained(Kim et al., 2004; Lee, 2004). KaLAR makes the use of a bending mechanism that is composed of several articulated joints. The robotic system can generate 3-DOF motion, including 2-DOF internal bending motion and 1-DOF external linear motion. Until now, various bending mechanisms have been developed for application in laparoscopic surgery(Ikuta et al., 2003; Simaan et al., 2004; Yamashita et al., 2003). These mechanisms were mainly focused on improving the mechanical characteristics of the bending mechanism for performing surgical manipulation rather than controlling a laparoscope. Although our system does not require high accuracy in position control, it requires relatively wide area of open space for electronic wires for CCD module, mechanical wires for articulated joints and optical fiber bundle for light source and therefore, a much simpler bending mechanism consisting of many thin, hollow cylindrical links (Tanaka, 1978) was adopted.

To determine the range of viewing angle in conventional laparoscopy, we made observations during human cholecystectomies. Cholecystectomy is the surgical removal of the inflamed or stoned gallbladder and is the most common procedure for laparoscopy. In general, 4-DOF motion is available in conventional laparoscopic surgery (Çavuşoğlu et al., 2001). There are mainly two rotations (up/down and left/right) about two axes on the incision surface, a translation (in/out) along the axis perpendicular to the incision surface, and an axial rotation. Since the axial rotation is not fully utilized, we have not implemented this feature in our system.

Our observation shows that the ranges of up/down and left/right movements are within 30 degrees while the range of in/out movement is approximately 100mm during normal operation, as shown in figure 1. The range of this in/out motion is in accordance with the result reported by Riener et al. using an electromagnetic position sensor (Riener et al., 2003). Based on this observation of the necessary workspace, we have developed a laparoscopic assistant robot that can cover the full range of view required for human cholecystectomy.

2.2 Design of Compact Laparoscopic Assistant Robot

The overall design of the developed robot is as shown in figure 2. The direction of views can be altered by changing the alignment of the articulated joints while magnification/ reduction of view can be altered by moving closer or away from the surgical site using a linear actuator. Since KaLAR itself functions as a laparoscope, a CCD camera module and a bundle of optical fibers are installed at the tip of the bending section as shown in figure 2 and they are directly connected to the image capturing unit and a xenon light source.

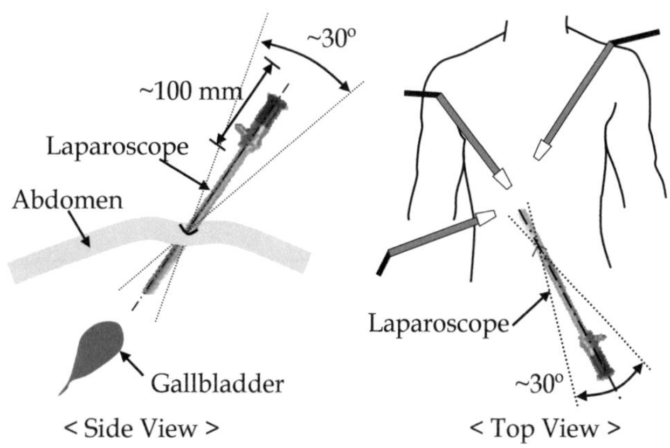

Figure 1. Range of motions in human cholecystectomy

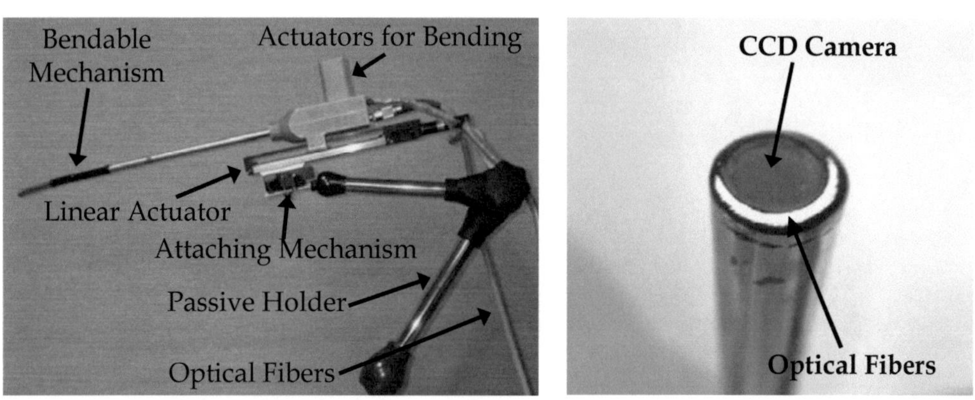

Figure 2. The developed compact laparoscopic assistant robot

2.2.1 Bending Motion

The bending mechanism consists of a series of thin, hollow cylindrical links connected by small joints and each link has two or four guiding holes inside as shown in figure 3. For internal bending motion, the most distal link is connected to two wheels through two pairs of steel wires, which are guided by guiding holes in the joints. There are 2 guiding holes inside each link except two links on both ends of the bending mechanism. The two links on both ends have 4 guiding holes and the wires passing through the guiding holes are distally connected to the CCD module and proximally to two wheels. The two wheels of different sizes are directly attached to corresponding motors as shown in figure 4. For controlling the bending mechanism, rotation of the motor changes the tension in the wires and thus, changes the orientation of each joint as shown in figure 5. For safety and initialization, two stoppers and photo sensors are placed to fix the bending range as shown in figure 4.

We have determined the range of motions of a rigid laparoscope in section 2.1 and comparable range of motion must be possible with the bending mechanism. To determine how much of bending is required for comparable viewing range, we have simulated the motion using approximated parameters in laparoscopy and design constraints. For installation of a CCD module and a bundle of optical fibers at the tip, approximately 70 mm of length is required. From the observation, the distance between the navel and the gallbladder is approximately 200 mm and in some cases, laparoscope may be placed 30~50 mm apart from the gallbladder during surgery. The bending section is 23 mm long and it is composed of 7 circular links connected by 6 joints. In conjunction with an assumption that bending of links will form a circular shape with a constant radius, we can compute the

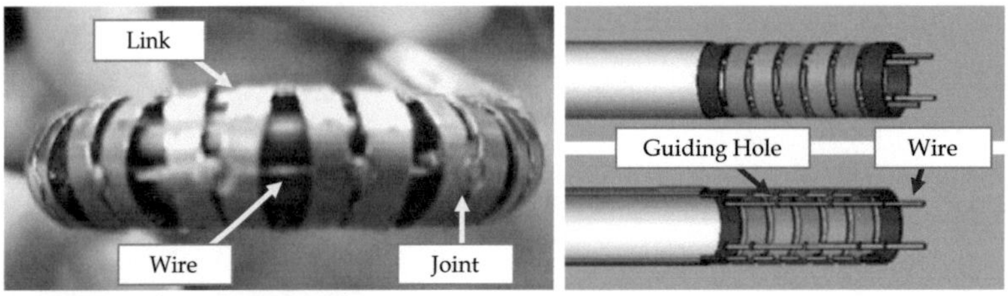

Figure 3. Wire-driven bending mechanism

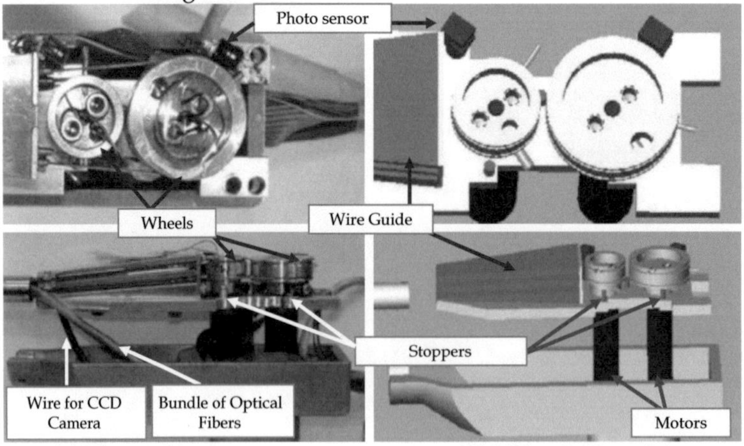

(a) The real image (b) The designed image

Figure 4. Configuration of wheels and motors for bending motion

required bending angle for comparable viewing range. As shown in figure 6, about 30 degrees of bending angle will have the equivalent viewing angle as a rigid laparoscope rotates 15 degrees about the insertion point. If the robot is positioned farther than 30 mm from the region of interest, the viewable range will be greater than that of a rigid laparoscope. For making the installation procedure more flexible, we've configured two limit sensors so that bending can take place from -60 to +60 degrees in each direction.

2.2.2. In/Out Motion and Sterilization

For moving closer and away from the surgical site, a linear actuator consisting of a linear motion guide, a ball screw, and a brushed DC motor was installed. In order to cover the necessary workspace, we chose the linear actuator with 130mm stroke length. This linear actuator is connected to a passive laparoscope holder by a connector similar to the one used to join a camera and a tripod as shown in figure 7. The use of this passive holder allows the surgeon to readily install the robot to the bedside.

To sterilize the KaLAR system, moving portion of the robot, which includes the upper part and the linear actuator, is made separable from the passive holder unit and thus, both the robot and the passive holder can be easily sterilized with ethylene oxide gas.

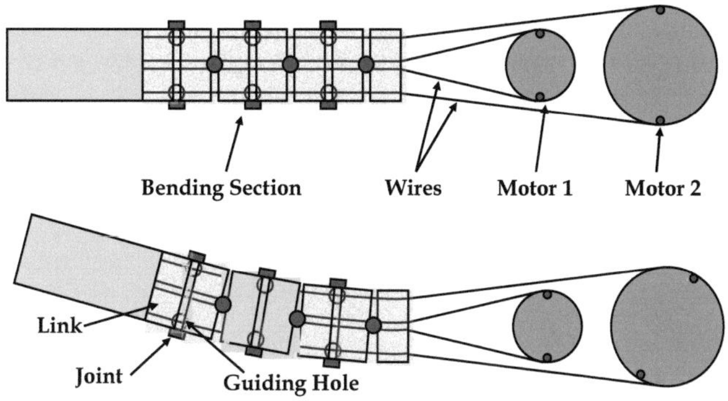

Figure 5. Wire-driven bending mechanism with motors

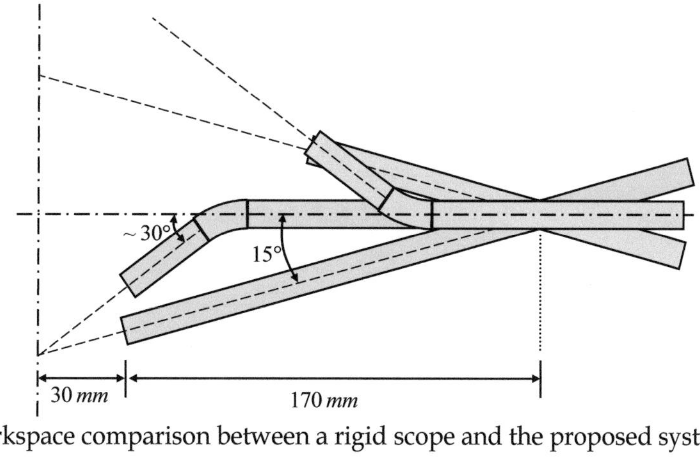

Figure 6. Workspace comparison between a rigid scope and the proposed system

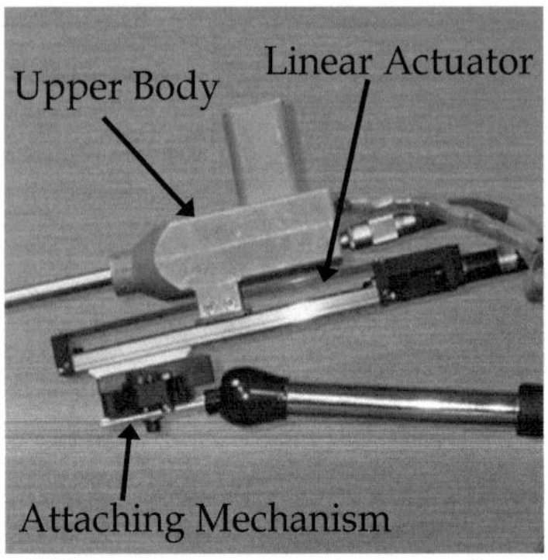

Figure 7. 2-DOF upper body and linear actuator connected to a passive laparoscope holder using attaching mechanism

2.3 Hysteresis Compensation in Bending Mechanism

Interesting characteristics of the bending mechanism are the linearity and hysteresis. Ideal mathematical modeling of the bending mechanism shows that its bending angle ($\theta_{up/down}$, $\theta_{left/right}$) moves highly linear relative to wire length variation ($\Delta lw_{up/down}$, $\Delta lw_{left/right}$) (Ko et al., 2007a). However, since the real bending mechanism has a play in joints and guiding holes, the behavior of the bending mechanism has considerable hysteresis. Figure 8 shows the block diagram of a low-level control structure including the hysteresis compensation. The compensation is conducted by adding the measured average offset value to the desired input only if the input is increasing. This compensation scheme can be expressed by (1). In case of the linear (zoom-in/-out) motion, no compensation is made due to no observed hysteresis effect.

$$\Theta_{comp,i} = \Theta_{hys,i} \times \frac{sign(\dot{\theta}_{des}) + 1}{2} \tag{1}$$

where $\Theta_{comp,i}$ indicates the value of hysteresis compensation of each motor, $\Theta_{hys,i}$ indicates the value of measured hysteresis and $\dot{\theta}_{des}$ indicates the velocity of the desired input.

This simple hysteresis compensation scheme may produce a discontinuity in the desired value. Since the discontinuity causes an abrupt and unstable transition between views,

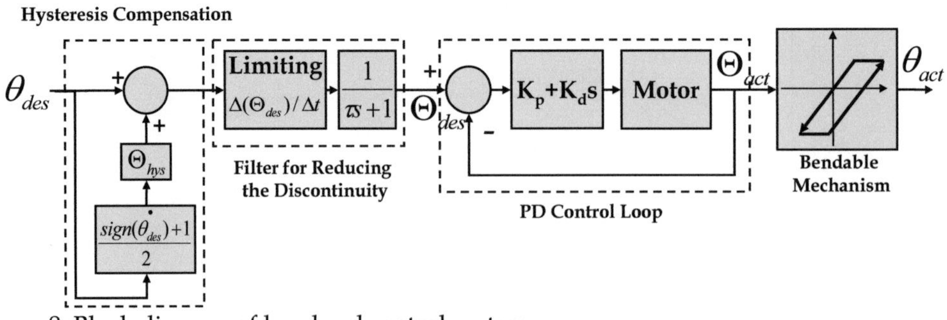

Figure 8. Block diagram of low-level control system

maximum deviation of the desired value is limited to a predefined maximum speed ($\dot{\theta}_{\max}$). We've determined these values to be roughly 11.2°/sec for bending motion and 8mm/sec for linear motion. This method can be expressed by (2) to (4).

$$\Delta_d(k) = \theta_{des}(k) + \Theta_{comp}(k) - \Theta_{beforeLPF}(k-1) \tag{2}$$

$$if(|\Delta_d(k)| > \dot{\theta}_{\max} \times \Delta T)$$

$$\Theta_{beforeLPF}(k) = \Theta_{beforeLPF}(k-1) + \dot{\theta}_{\max} \times \Delta T \times sign(\Delta_d(k)) \tag{3}$$

$$else$$

$$\Theta_{beforeLPF}(k) = \theta_{des}(k) + \Theta_{comp}(k) \tag{4}$$

where $\Theta_{beforeLPF}$ indicates the desired position value, Θ_{comp} indicates the value calculated by (1), θ_{des} indicates the desired input and ΔT is the sampling time.

The $\Theta_{beforeLPF}$ obtained by equation (3) or (4) goes through a first order low pass filer with τ= 0.03sec for eliminating the discontinuity in velocity and the result value is regarded as the final desired input Θ_{des} for a PD controller. As shown in figure 8, the low-level controller does not form a perfect closed loop but it is sufficiently controllable under the assumptions that there is no external force acting on the moving tip and that the surgeon can see the laparoscopic view on the monitor. Figures 9(a) and 9(b) show the tracking performance during the left/right swing motion before and after the hysteresis compensation.

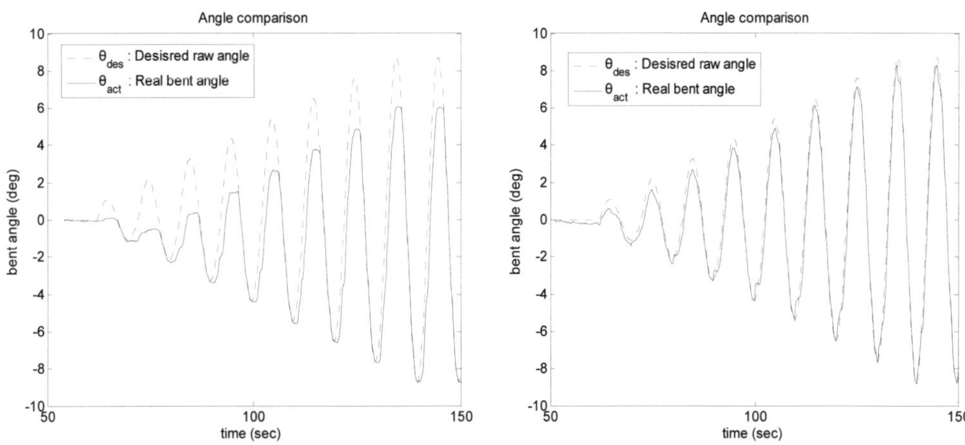

(a) Without hysteresis compensation
($error_{max}$ = 3.86 °, $error_{min}$ = -0.38 °, $error_{std}$ = 1.36 °)

(b) With hysteresis compensation
($error_{max}$ = 1.76 °, $error_{min}$ = 0.0 °, $error_{std}$ = 0.51 °)

Figure 9. Tracking performance without and with hysteresis compensation

2.4 High Level Control Method : A User Interface

This section explains a higher-level control method of the KaLAR system, which is related to the generation of the desired position (θ_{des}) from the surgeon's command. We adopted both a voice interface and a visual-servoing method to control the system. Voice recognition is implemented based on a speaker-independent software module and thus, requires no training. Since voice interface is one of the most intuitive control methods, it is used in many laparoscopic assistant systems (Allaf et al., 1998), but it has a limitation of requiring many voice inputs in case continuous view changes are required. To overcome this shortcoming, a visual-servoing method (Casals et al., 1996; Nishikawa et al., 2003; Wang et al., 1996; Wei et al., 1997) was developed. But the sole use of visual-servoing is not sufficient for the complete control of the robotic system. Therefore, we've combined the voice interface and the visual-servoing. The operating surgeon can choose between the voice interface and visual-servoing using a voice command. It can be also determined automatically based on the surgery task model, which will be explained in section 3 in detail.

2.4.1 Voice Interface

As shown in figure 10, voice commands are used to determine the robot's state and the control mode. After an initialization process, the system is in the *pausing state* and waits for the surgeon's command. Upon "start" command by the surgeon, the robot system is placed in the *controlling state* where the robot can be physically activated for specific movement and image processing. To pull the robot out of the *controlling state,* "pause" command is required. In the *controlling state,* the surgeon can choose the control mode using voice commands "tracking mode" or "voice mode." In the *voice command mode,* the surgeon manipulates the surgical view using the commands "go up," "go down," "go left," "go right," "zoom in," and "zoom out." These commands move the robot toward the corresponding direction by predetermined amounts, about 4 degrees per command for bending and 20 mm per command for a linear motion. The *auto-tracking mode* is for tracking the primary surgical instrument marked with color markers. In this mode, 2-DOF bending motion is controlled by visual-servoing while the in and out motion with respect to the abdomen is still controlled by the voice commands "zoom in" and "zoom out." For additional convenience, 2-position memory function is also implemented using the commands "remember position 1," and "remember position 2," and the stored positions can be retrieved by the commands "go to position 1" and "go to position 2."

2.4.2 Visual-Servoing

Visual-servoing is expected to alleviate the surgeon from issuing a great number of voice commands in times of frequent change of camera views. The visual-servoing algorithm is based on the result of other researchers (Casals et al., 1996; Nishikawa et al., 2003; Wang et al., 1996; Wei et al., 1997). Unlike the previous works, a color marker composed of two-color band is placed at the tip to locate the tip of the instrument in the captured image and to identify the tool's type as shown in figure 11 (Ko et al., 2007a). The two-color band is composed of three parts: *near*(P_1), *middle*(P_2) and *far*(P_3) part, named by the distance from the tip. The near and the far parts from the tip are marked with bright cyan for it is rarely found in the internal organs (Wei et al., 1997). These parts have different thickness and are used to locate the direction and position of the tool tip. Since the real distances (D_{1t} and D_{12}) between markers and the tip in figure 11(b) are known, we can obtain the tip position with a simple equation (5), in which the effect of a perspective view is neglected for the sake of simplification. The color of the middle part is used for identifying the type of the tool that is inserted and thus, is utilized to verify the marker detection and to upload the geometric information of the tool.

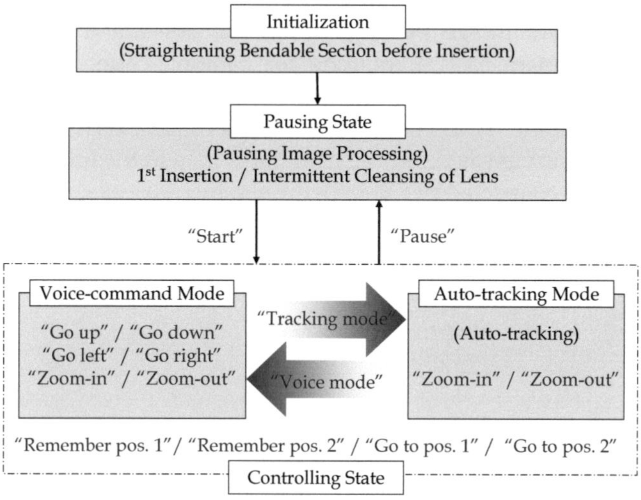

Figure 10. Robot's states and available voice commands

$$P_t = P_1 + |P_2 - P_1| \frac{D_{1t}}{D_{12}} \frac{P_1 - P_3}{|P_1 - P_3|} \tag{5}$$

To avoid the surgeon's motion sickness, visual-servoing is activated only when the tip is moved out of the small portion at the center of a monitor screen. The size of the portion and the maximum bending speed during *in vivo* porcine cholecystectomies were determined by the operating surgeons' preference before the surgery began and were approximately 11.2deg/sec and 30% of the monitor screen, respectively.

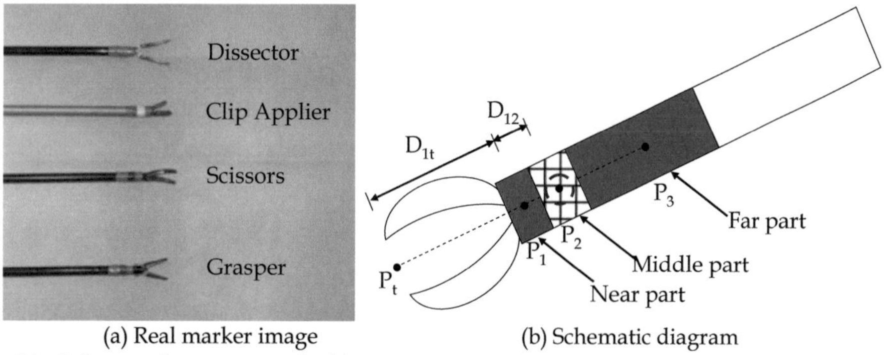

(a) Real marker image (b) Schematic diagram

Figure 11. Color markers on surgical instruments

2.5 Overall System Configuration

The main controller is based on a Pentium 4 2.8GHz PC running under Windows 2000. Model 626 board from Sensoray Co. Inc. is utilized for performing low-level position control and for generating hardware interrupts. VoiceEZ software from Voiceware Co. Ltd. is utilized for recognizing the surgeon's voice commands and for synthesizing voice instructions. For convenience, a wireless headset from Inter-M Co. Ltd. is used. Matrox Meteor-II frame grabber board from Matrox Co. and a small CCD camera (IK-M43S) from

Toshiba Co. are used for image processing. In the developed software module, three threads were implemented, each accounting for position control, voice recognition and image process. Sampling in the PD controller is conducted at 1000Hz and image processing is done at the minimum rate of 25 Hz. Since the CCD camera module can support multiple outputs, the laparoscopic view is delivered simultaneously to the image grabber and a super VHS recorder, which is connected to a high definition monitor, as shown in figure 12.

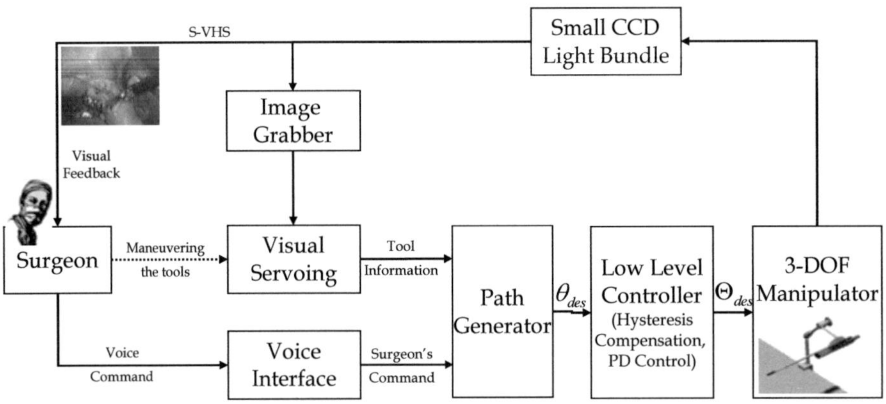

Figure 12. Overall system configuration

3. Surgery Task Model based Interaction

3.1 A Basic Concepts and Backgrounds

As mentioned in Introduction, we believe that an intelligent assistant robot should have the preliminary surgical knowledge similar to that of a well-trained human assistant. A structured preliminary surgical knowledge is defined as a *surgery task model*. Based on this premise, figure 13 illustrates the basic concept of our interaction scheme based on a surgery task model. Unlike other previous assistant robot systems that only follow a surgeon's direct commands, the robot system having the surgery task model responds to surgeon's behavior and performs predefined tasks. This concept can be considered as a specific form of a general human-robot interaction (HRI) structure proposed for an ultimate service robot system with relatively high cognition (Lee et al., 2005; Yoon, 2005). The proposed structure insisted that the HRI should include a task model, a user model, a mental model, a needs model and an interaction model. In case of surgical assistant robot, whose work domain is relatively specific and has restrictive behavior, the interaction scheme with only a task model is sufficient to be applied to a laparoscopic assistant robot. This assistant robot with a surgery task model can acquire information of the surgical environment, estimate current surgical task based on the task model, and finally can suggest appropriate actions, such as maneuvering of a laparoscope.

Some methods for task analysis and task modeling have been developed. In efforts to analyze tasks efficiently, Goals, Operators, Methods and Selection (GOMS), Task Action Grammar (TAG), and so forth have been studied by human-computer interaction research groups (Johnson, 1992). In order to describe a discrete event system, modeling methods based on state-transition models such as automata, Petri-net, and etc. have been studied (Cassandras & Lafortune, 1999). Recently, these task analysis methodologies have been applied

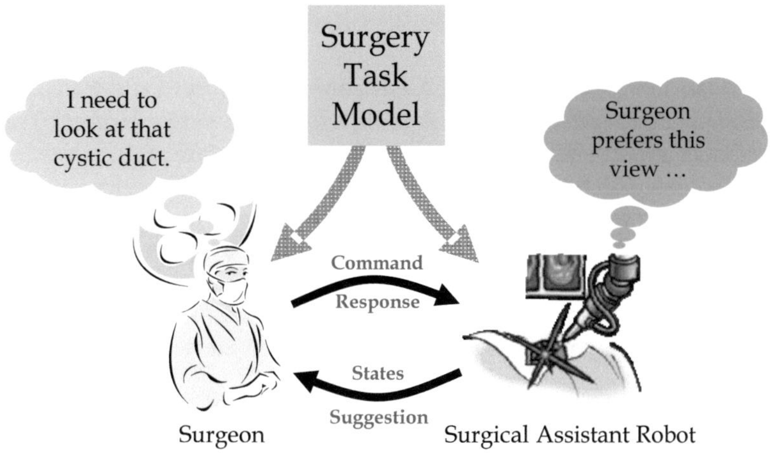

Figure 13. Basic concept of the interaction between a surgeon and a surgical assistant robot

to medical and medical robotics fields. MacKenzie and his colleagues constructed a hierarchical decomposition of Nissen fundoplication, a type of laparoscopic surgery for stopping the reflux of stomach acid, based on a hierarchical task analysis (HTA) (MacKenzie et al., 2001). The procedure was broken down into a sequence of surgical steps and these steps were further broken down into surgical sub-steps, tasks, sub-tasks, and finally primitive motions. Their work showed that a surgical procedure can be expressed with a sequence of decomposed surgical steps, and this decomposition provides a method to evaluate the effectiveness of a surgical procedure, including the procedure with new surgical techniques or new tools. However, this model did not consider the variance in surgery and the role of the surgical robot. Ohnuma and his colleagues suggested a model for an operating scenario based on timed automata including a surgical task, a surgeon, a scrub nurse or a scrub nurse robot, a patient, and their interaction(Ohnuma et al., 2005). This model was integrated into a scrub nurse robot for control. However, it deals with a simplified surgical procedure and the associated analysis is not applicable for controlling a laparoscope. Rosen et al. proposed a modeling method for minimally invasive surgery using a discrete Markov model for assessing surgical performance(Rosen et al., 2006). Their modeling method is a bottom-up approach; they constructed a discrete Markov model from a sequence of tool motions, which are defined by the position and orientation of the tool and the exerted force and torque. Their modeling approach provides a generalized method for decomposing a surgical task. However, it can only assess surgical performance and thus, cannot be applied to surgeon-robot interaction.

In this section, a surgery task model, which can cope with variance in the surgical procedures, is proposed for a laparoscopic assistant robot.

3.2 Definition of Surgery Task Model

A *surgery task model* is defined as a structured form of surgical knowledge that is necessary for a surgeon to perform a specific surgery, including *surgical procedures, input information* for identifying the current surgical states, and *action strategies* at each surgical state(Ko et al., 2007b). While it would be an onerous task to standardize or quantify each step of surgery, simple surgical procedures such as a cholecystectomy can be decomposed into discrete steps.

To allow the task model to include the variance in surgery, state-transition modeling method is utilized. States are defined as sub-procedures, i.e. *surgical stages*. Transitions are defined as changes among surgical stages. The transitions are triggered when the *input information* of the external environment satisfies the predefined conditions. Each surgical stage has a specific *action strategy*. Considering that the model will be applied to a laparoscopic assistant robot, the surgical view captured by a laparoscope and the surgeon's commands were determined as the input information. The type of tool is identified from the surgical view and utilized to trigger transitions between the surgical stages, and the tool position and the surgeon's voice commands are utilized to determine the surgical view based on predefined action strategies.

3.3 Surgical Procedure

As a first step, 8 cases of human-assisted human cholecystectomy were recorded and analyzed in terms of laparoscopic view and operating room view. Using both views, each surgical procedure was decomposed into meaningful surgical stages based on their goal and primary surgical tools in use as shown in Table 1.

No. of Surgical Stages	The Primary Goal	The Primary Surgical Tools/Devices
0	Start	Forceps & Trocar for Lap.
1	Preparing Laparoscope	Positioning a Laparoscope
2	Inserting Trocar for Right Hand and Examining Briefly	Forceps & Scalpels & Trocar
3	Inserting Trocars for Left Hand	Forceps & Scalpels & Trocar
4	Lifting Liver	Ratchet Grasper / Dissector
5	Exposing Artery/Duct	Dissector
6	Clipping Artery/Duct	Clip Applier
7	Cutting Artery/Duct	Scissors
8	Separating Gallbladder(GB) with Dissector	Dissector
9	Separating GB with Cautery	Cautery
10	Inserting Pouch	Extracting Laparoscope & Inserting Plastic Pouch
11	Collecting GB	Dissector
12	Extracting Trocars	Trocars
13	Extracting Laparoscope	Laparoscope
14	Extracting GB	Scissors & Suction
15	Suturing Ports	Needles & Forceps
16	Applying a Hemostatic	Hemostatic
17	Irrigating	Irrigator
18	Stanching by Cautery	Cautery
19	Extracting Lap. for Cleaning	Extracting Laparoscope & Cleaning it with clean Gauze
20	Doing Unrelated Works	-
21	End	-

Table 1. Definitions of surgical stages in human cholecystectomy

Sequential flow of surgical stages was analyzed and a complete surgical procedure was determined and represented by a state-transition diagram as shown in figure 14. Since the surgical procedure is not deterministic procedure and has a little variance, the diagram includes the probability and the occurrence of traversing from one stage to another as shown in figures 14 and 15. In figure 15(a), white and black boxes indicate 0% and 100% probability, respectively. Figure 15(b) shows the occurrence of the transitions, and white and black boxes indicate 0 and 2.63 times/case, respectively. However, since the variance of the surgical procedure is not extreme, you can see that the probabilistic map is very sparse. In order to find out the dominant surgical stages and the dominant sequence, one or two transitions with the highest probability at each stage are chosen as shown in figure 16. The chosen transitions and the stages can be considered as the *normal surgical procedure* of human cholecystectomy.

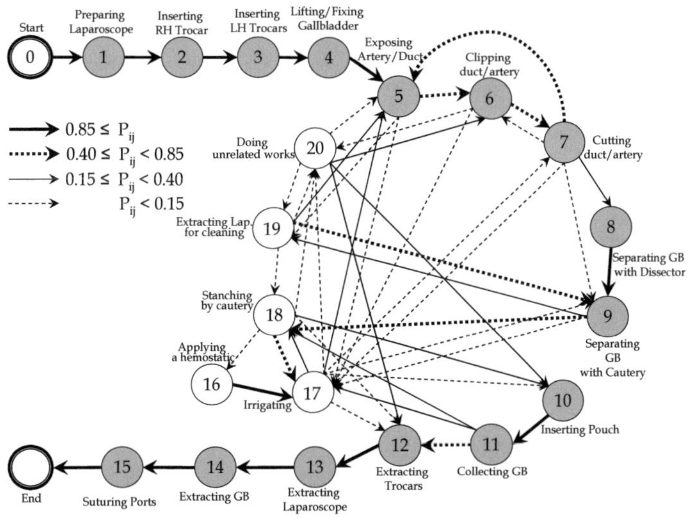

Figure 14. Surgical procedure represented in state-transition diagram with classified robability value of each transition

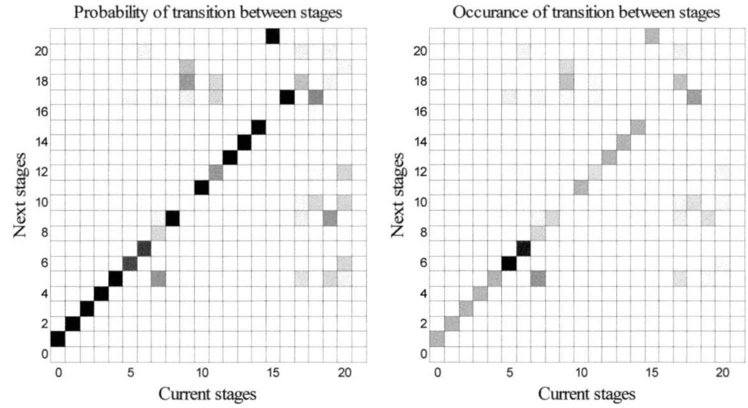

(a) Probability : White 0 %, Black 100% (b) Occurrence : White 0 times, Black 2.63 times

Figure 15. Probability and occurrence of transition between stages

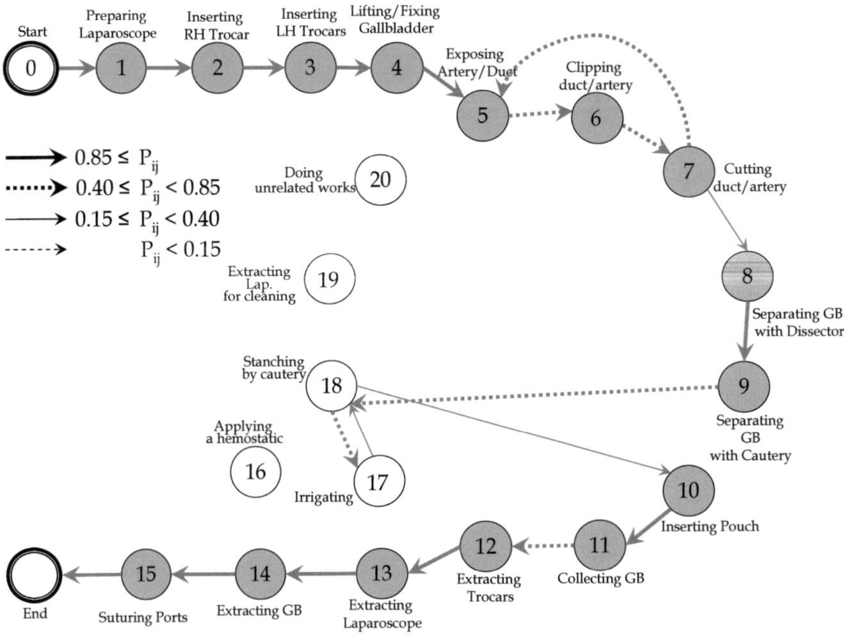

Figure 16. Normal procedure (frequent stages) in human cholecystectomy

3.4 Action Strategies: Desired Camera Viewpoint and Viewing Method

Considering that our surgery task model will be applied to a laparoscopic assistant robot, the action strategy should be related to the optimal camera view. Among the characteristics related to the camera view, the viewing method and the desired camera viewpoint at each stage were considered. To find the preferred view of the surgeon at each stage, the normal procedures of a cholecystectomy was observed through video analysis and consultation with a surgeon. These observations revealed that there are distinctive relations among the tools being utilized, tasks being performed, and the preferred camera view. At some stages, the surgeon wants the laparoscope to follow the tool tip and an assistant positions the laparoscope so that the tool tip is positioned at the center of the monitor. In some stages, the surgeon prefers the laparoscope to remain steady so as to maintain a steady view of the surgical site. The relationship among surgical stages, tools, and camera viewpoints is summarized in figure 17. This information allows us to estimate the current stage by looking at the inserted tool and the information of the previous stage.

As shown in figure 17, current stage is highly related to the tool in use. This allows us to utilize the surgical tool as a major transition condition to estimate the current surgical stage. In addition to the tool change, insertion and extraction of the laparoscope or tools are also considered as transition conditions. The only transition conditions for the normal surgical procedure are listed in table 2.

3.5 Input Information: Laparoscopic View and Surgeon's Commands

Since the type of surgical tool is a key feature for the transition condition and the tip position of the tool is important for the tool tracking capability, the laparoscopic view is determined as one of the input modalities. The method to extract the information from the laparoscopic

view is identical with the one described in section 2.4.2. The color of the middle part of the marker is also utilized to identify the inserted tool's type.
Surgical information from the laparoscopic view may not be sufficient to completely control the laparoscope throughout the surgery. Some kind of manual intervention to regulate the motion of the robot is sometimes needed. Therefore, the surgeon's voice commands are utilized to modify the view whenever the view is not satisfactory. Although the preferred camera views may have many parameters that are not explicitly represented in figure 17, i.e. tracking speed, exact location of the surgical target, the views can be generally classified as two modes: *site-keeping* mode and *tool-tracking* mode. In case of the site-keeping mode, it is

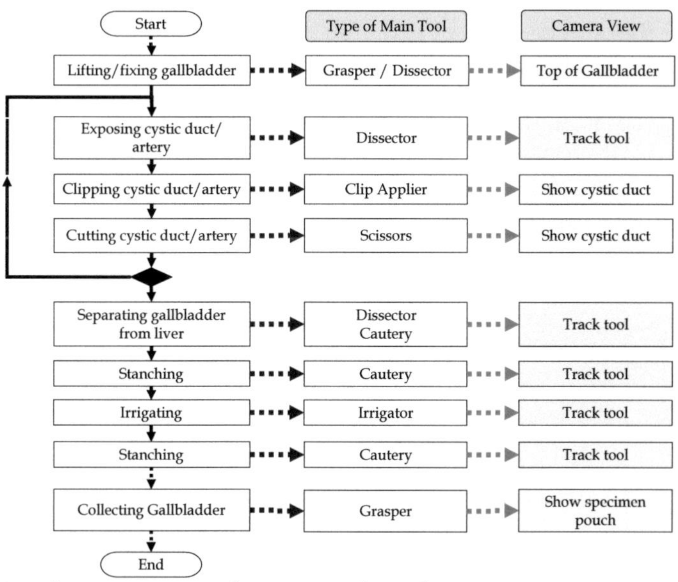

Figure 17. Relations between surgical stages, tools and camera viewpoints

Current stage	Next stage	Transition condition	Current stage	Next stage	Transition condition
0	1	Starting insertion of Lap. trocar	9	18	Finishing the separating procedure
1	2	Starting insertion of RH trocar	10	11	Inserting lap. after plastic pouch
2	3	Starting insertion of LH trocar	11	12	Starting extracting trocar
3	4	Detecting LH ratchet grasper or dissector	12	13	Starting extracting laparoscope
4	5	Detecting LH grasper	13	14	Starting extracting gallbladder
5	6	Detecting clip applier	14	15	Starting suturing ports
6	7	Detecting scissors	15	21	Finishing suturing ports
7	5	Detecting dissector	17	18	Detecting cautery
7	8	Detecting dissector	18	10	Starting extracting laparoscope
8	9	Detecting cautery	18	17	Detecting irrigator

Table 2. Transition conditions between surgical stages of the normal surgical procedure

necessary to accurately recognize the surgical site for showing the desired view. Recognition of the surgical site is left for the future works. For the time being, the desired view is determined by surgeon's voice commands. On this account, the robot's control diagram is very similar to one described in figure 10 except the viewing method is determined automatically based on the surgery task model.

3.6 Implementation and Simulation of the Surgery Task Model

To implement the surgery task model outlined in sections 3.3 to 3.5, we've composed the data in figures 15 and 16 and table 2 into a set of structured data, as shown in figure 18. The surgery task model has the total number of stages, task being performed at each stage, viewing characteristics at each stage, and a possible transition route at a given stage. The surgical tools are used as a dominant factor for estimating the transition to next stage. In this simulation, we used a normal surgical procedure shown in figure 16, rather than all procedures in general laparoscopic surgery represented by figure 14.

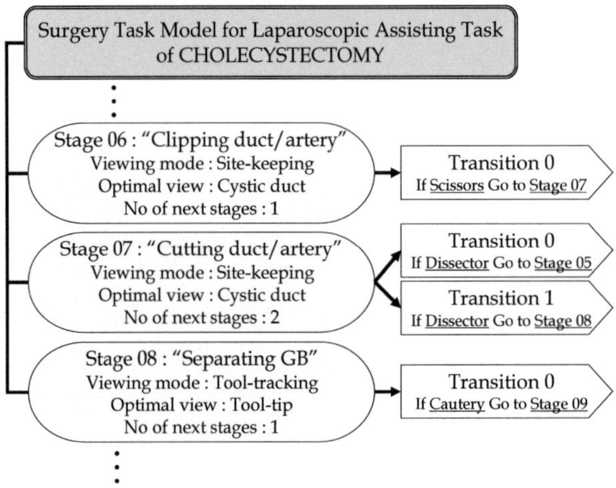

Figure 18. Data structure of surgery task model

It is possible that two or more possible next stages exist. In such case, we consider all possibilities at the given stage. In the normal cholecystectomy procedure shown in figure 16, it occurs at a "Cutting duct/artery" stage (stage 7). The next stage may be either "Separating GB with Dissector" (stage 8) or "Exposing duct/artery" (stage 5), because both the transition conditions for stages 5 and 8 are a dissector. Fortunately, the action strategies for these cases are the same, i.e. the preferred view is to "track tool," as shown in figure 17. However, since the preferred views of all possible routes at other surgeries can be different from each other, this issue should be resolved in the future work.

To verify the possibility of estimating the present stage when the state of the last stage and the type of currently inserted tool are given, a simplified simulation was performed. Since the checking mechanism related to insertion/extraction of the laparoscope and the left-hand tool is not implemented yet, this information was provided by a keystroke. The result of this simulation is shown in figure 19. Similar to the normal surgical procedure, the surgical tools are inserted into the simulated environment of the abdomen in the following order:

Dissector, Clip applier, Scissors, Dissector, Clip applier, Scissors, Dissector, Cautery, Irrigator, Cautery, and Dissector.

Each tool is given a unique ID (1 - Dissector, 2 - Clip applier, 3 - Scissors, 4 - Cautery and 5 - Irrigator), as shown on the right side of figure 19(b). The identified tool type is plotted with respect to time in figure 19(b) and the estimated surgical stages during that period are plotted in figure 19(a). For example, when the clip applier is inserted during a 36~43 sec. period (marked by ①), the estimated surgical stage can be found by tracking the symbols in figure 19(a) ("clipping duct/artery"). This prediction process uses only the information about the previous stage and the tool type, and two different stages for a given period may be expected. For example, during a 48~53 sec. period (marked by ②), the proposed interaction scheme defines the present stage as either "separating GB with Dissector" or "exposing duct/artery." However, since the next instrument is identified as the clip applier, the next stage can be estimated as the "clipping duct/artery" stage (stage 6).

The prediction process is conducted only when the tools are identifiable. When the tool is not detected or identified, the scheme does not change the current stage. At the beginning and end of the surgery, where no tool-stage relationship is defined, a time sequence is used to represent the preparation (stages 0~3) and wrap-up procedures (stages 12~15 and 21).

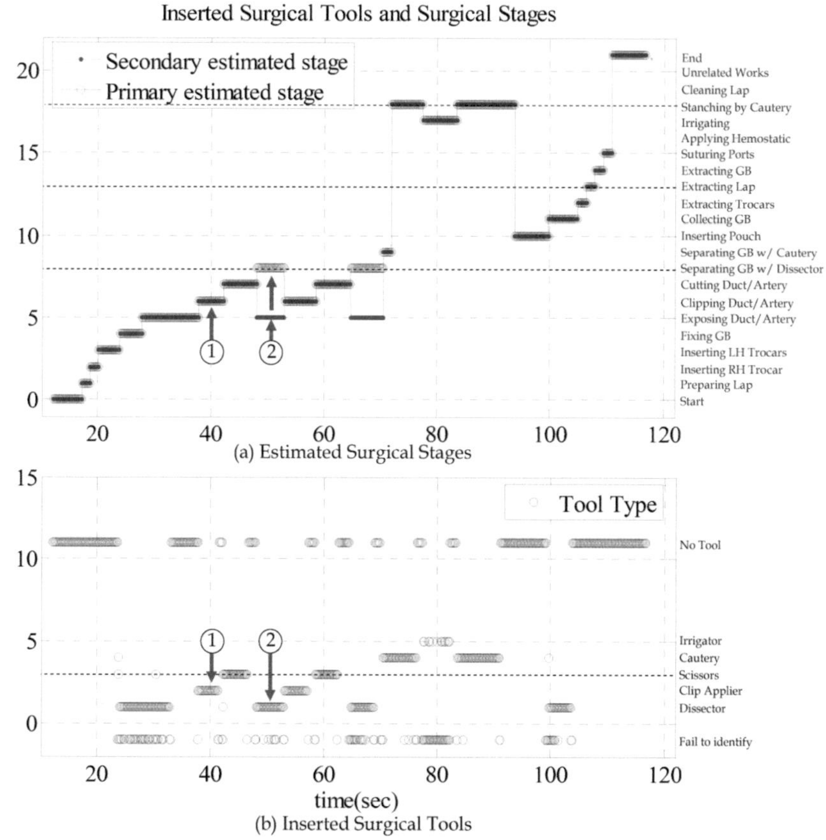

Figure 19. Implemented interaction based on the proposed surgery task model

4. *In Vivo* Experiments

4.1 Verification of Mechanical Properties

Three cases of porcine cholecystectomy were performed to evaluate the performance of KaLAR. The objective of these trials are: (a) to determined if the workspace covered by the robot is sufficient for cholecystectomy, (b) to see if solo-surgery is possible with the proposed control scheme, and (c) the time required to complete the surgery is comparable to other robot-assisted and human-assisted cholecystectomy. The materials used were three female pigs of 3~4 months old and weigh approximately 30 kg. The size of their abdominal cavity was smaller than that of an adult person and thus, the trocar for laparoscope had to be placed below the navel. Since the KaLAR's initial position influences the motion range, it is necessary to place it carefully during the initialization procedure. The cholecystectomy mainly deals with the gallbladder located beneath the liver. Thus, KaLAR's position was adjusted with a passive holder so that it shows the lower part of the liver. All three surgeries were performed by one surgeon as shown in figure 20 and all the surgical procedures were in accordance with the guidelines enforced by the local ethics committees.

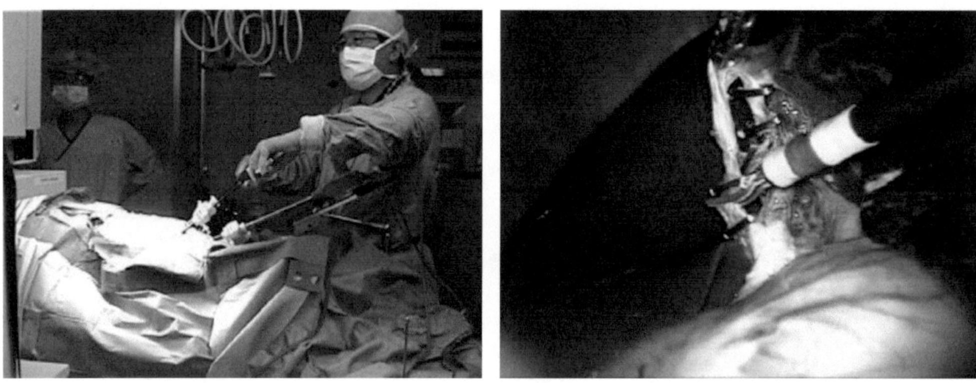

(a) Solo-surgery (b) Internal View

Figure 20. Porcine cholecystectomy with KaLAR

Through animal tests, we were able to confirm that the workspace covered by KaLAR is sufficient for porcine cholecystectomy and the control of the robot using voice commands and visual-servoing is effective enough for solo-surgery. The surgical time comparison with other robot-assisted and human-assisted porcine cholecystectomies is summarized in Table 3, where the surgical time was defined as the time between initial insertion and final extraction of KALAR. The surgical times described in the work by Kobayashi et al. were recalculated in terms of our definition, that is, we have subtracted the trocar insertion time from the total operating time(Kobayashi et al., 1999). Although we only have a limited number of surgeries and the time measurement can only be used for a rough estimate of the robot's performance, the time spent for porcine cholecystectomy can be said to be comparable to other robot-assisted and human-assisted porcine cholecystectomy. Note that the time difference for between experiments with KaLAR and the other system seems to be mainly caused by the surgeon's expertise level, considering our surgeon's operating time (23.3±9.9 minutes for four cases) for the human cholecystectomy with a conventional rigid scope is slightly shorter than for these experiments using KaLAR.

Target and material	Time (min)
On a pig with Kobayashi's system (Kobayashi et al., 1999)	38 (one case)
On a pig with a human assistant (Kobayashi et al., 1999)	41.6 (ten cases)
On a pig with the KaLAR system	26.7±8.3 (three cases)

Table 3. Surgical time for porcine cholecystectomy

4.2 Preliminary Experiment with Surgery Task Model

This section will describe the results of the *in vivo* tests from the perspective of the proposed interaction scheme. For this purpose, the second and third experiments of were analyzed and compared because they were performed with different interaction schemes. In the third experiment (Exp. A), the surgeon arbitrarily determined the control mode at different stages of surgery by issuing "tracking mode" or "voice mode" command. In the second experiment (Exp. B), simplified version of the proposed interaction method was implemented and the surgeon had no control over the control mode. In this test, only the normal surgical procedure was considered and the camera view was selected mainly based on the tool-viewpoint relation shown in figure 17. We measured the surgical time and the number of voice commands issued during each surgery. Table 4 indicates that the surgical time was increased but the number of voice commands was reduced with the proposed scheme. In Table 4, the number of issued voice commands is counted excluding the commands during preparation stages. While the results do not provide conclusive evidence of the efficacy of the proposed scheme, it may be worthwhile to conduct more experiments to see if the proposed scheme can reduce the number of commands and thus, less control burden.

	Operating Time (min.)	No. of Voice Commands
In vivo experiment with surgeon's ability to decide viewing mode (Exp. A)	20	71
In vivo experiment with the proposed interaction scheme (Exp. B)	24	50

* The operating time and the number of voice commands are measured excluding the results during the preparation procedure.

Table 4. Results of *in vivo* porcine cholecystectomy

5. Conclusion and Discussion

To develop an intelligent laparoscopic assistant robot, the mechanism should be designed so that the robotic system can be easily handled in real operation environment, and to give *task-specific* intelligence to medical robot, the robotic system should have well-structured task model of the surgery. On these grounds, this chapter describes the intelligent laparoscopic assistant robot, KaLAR, focusing on (a) its compactness and convenience, and (b) its novel interaction scheme through a surgery task model. Unlike previous robotic systems, the robot uses an internally bending mechanism and constrains the motions within the abdomen. This approach is expected to reduce the potential risk of interfering with surgical staff. The inherent hysteresis characteristics of the mechanism were compensated for more accurate control. In order to facilitate easy operation, a voice interface and a visual-servoing method were introduced and implemented. To verify the applicability of KaLAR, three solo-surgeries on porcine cholecystectomy were performed. These *in vivo* animal tests show that the mechanical structure of the KaLAR system is acceptable in the surgical environment and has sufficient workspace to provide necessary views during cholecystectomy.

In order to implement a task-specific intelligence for assistant robot, we proposed a surgery task model, which includes the surgical procedure (sequence of surgical stages), input information on the surgical environment, and actions strategies composed of proper viewing mode and viewpoint at each stage. We believe that the surgery task model makes it possible to realize ideal surgeon-robot interaction. In this model, the surgical procedure is extracted through a video analysis and represented as a state-transition diagram. For input information, the laparoscopic view and the operating surgeon's voice commands are utilized. To verify the possibility to realize the interaction scheme based on the surgery task model and to assess the effectiveness of the scheme, the model was integrated to the KaLAR system. Although the issued voice commands were not remarkably reduced, the surgery task model's applicability in real surgery is demonstrated through an *in vivo* porcine cholecystectomy. Although statistically insufficient, the results of our preliminary experiments show that the proposed interaction has the potential to reduce the surgeon's control burden and allow the surgeon to control the robot naturally.

Despite KaLAR's applicability, several issues should be solved. In case of the mechanical issues, the length of the bending tip should be shortened because its lengthiness can restrict the reachable area. There is the potential harmfulness caused by the robot's malfunction, especially during the zooming motion. To reduce the possibility of the malfunction, we will introduce the additional sensor to confirm the actuators' position measured in the zooming motion. Next, for the issues related to the interaction scheme, the optimal view in the site-keeping mode needs to be determined in a more systematic manner and an identification method for insertion/extraction of the laparoscope and the left-hand tools are required to make the proposed scheme more effective. In dealing with the variance in surgery, a method to utilize the whole model described in figure 14 should be considered. Also, the possibility of misidentification of the transition condition and the robustness of the surgical procedure should be investigated. Finally, more *in vivo* tests are required for more quantitative evaluation and for its extensibility to other minimally invasive surgeries

6. References

Allaf, M. E.; Jackman, S. V.; Schulam, P. G.; Cadeddu, J. A.; Lee, B. R.; Moore, R. G. & Kavoussi, L. R. (1998). Laparoscopic visual field : Voice vs foot pedal interfaces for control of the AESOP robot, *Surgical Endoscopy*, Vol.12, (pp. 1415-1418), 0930-2794

Berkelman, P.; Cinquin, P.; Troccaz, J.; Ayoubi, J.; Letoublon, C. & Bouchard, F. (2002). A Compact, Compliant Laparoscopic Endoscope Manipulator, *Proceedings of IEEE International Conference on Robotics & Automation*, pp. 1870-1875, 0-7803-7272-7, Washington, DC, May, 2002

Casals, A.; Amat, J. & Laporte, E. (1996). Automatic Guidance of an Assistant Robot in Laparoscopic Surgery, *Proceedings of the IEEE International Conference on Robotics and Automation*, pp. 895-900, 0-7803-2988-4, Minneapolis, Minnesota, April, 1996

Cassandras, C. G. & Lafortune, S. (1999). *Introduction to Discrete Event Systems*, Kluwer Academic Publishers, 0-7923-8609-4, Norwell, MAÇavuşoğlu, M. C.; Villanueva, I. & Tendick, F. (2001). Workspace Analysis of Robotic Manipulators for a Teleoperated Suturing Task, *Proceedings of the IEEE/RSJ International Conference on Intelligent Robots and Systems*, pp. 2234-2239, 0-7803-6612-3, Maui, HI, October - November, 2001

Finlay, P. A. (1996). Clinical experience with a goniometric head-controlled laparoscope manipulator, *Proceedings of IARP Workshop on Medical Robotics*, Vienna, Austria

Franzino, R. J. (2003). The Laprotek surgical system and the next generation of robotics, *Surgical Clinics of North America*, Vol.83, (pp. 1317-1320), 0039-6109

Ghodoussi, M.; Butner, S. E. & Wang, Y. (2002). Robotic Surgery - The Transatlantic Case, *Proceedings of IEEE International Conference on Robotics & Automation*, pp. 1882-1888, 0-7803-7272-7, Washington, DC, May, 2002

Guthart, G. S. & Salisbury, J. K. (2000). The Intuitive™ Telesurgery System: Overview and Application, *Proceedings of IEEE International Conference on Robotics & Automation*, pp. 618-621, 0-7803-5886-4, San Francisco, CA, April, 2000

Ikuta, K.; Hasegawa, T. & Daifu, S. (2003). Hyper Redundant Miniature Manipulator "Hyper Finger" for Remote Minimally Invasive Surgery in Deep Area, *Proceedings of IEEE International Conference on Robotics &Automation*, pp. 1098-1102, 0-7803-7736-2, Taipei, Taiwan, September, 2003

Johnson, P. (1992). Human-Computer Interaction: Psychology, Task Analysis and Software Engineering, McGRAW-HILL Book Company Europe, 0077072359, UK

Kim, J.; Lee, Y.-J.; Ko, S.-Y.; Kwon, D.-S. & Lee, W.-J. (2004). Compact Camera Assistant Robot for Minimally Invasive Surgery: KaLAR, *Proceedings of IEEE/RSJ International Conference on Intelligent Robots and Systems*, pp. 2587-2592, 0-7803-8463-6, Sendai, Japan, Sept.-Oct., 2004

Ko, S.-Y.; Kim, J.; Lee, W.-J. & Kwon, D.-S. (2007a). Compact laparoscopic assistant robot using a bending mechanism, *Advanced Robotics*, Vol.21, No.5-6, (pp. 689–709), 0169-1864

Ko, S.-Y.; Kim, J.; Lee, W.-J. & Kwon, D.-S. (2007b). Surgery Task Model for Intelligent Interaction between Surgeon and Laparoscopic Assistant Robot, *International Journal of Assistive Robotics and Mechatronics* Vol.8, No.1, (pp. 38-46), 1975-0153

Kobayashi, E.; Masamune, K.; Sakuma, I.; Dohi, T. & Hashimoto, D. (1999). A New Safe Laparoscopic Manipulator System with a Five-Bar Linkage Mechanism and an Optical Zoom, *Computer Aided Surgery*, Vol.4, No.4, (pp. 182-192), 1092-9088

Lee, K.; Kim, H.-R.; Yoon, W. C.; Yoon, Y.-S. & Kwon, D.-S. (2005). Designing a human-robot interaction framework for home service robot, *Proceedings of IEEE International Workshop on Robot and Human Interactive Communication*, pp. 286-293, 0-7803-9275-2, Nashville, TN, August, 2005

Lee, Y.-J. (2004). Development of a Compact Laparoscopic Assistant Robot: KaLAR, *Master's thesis*, Korea Advanced Institute of Science and Technology, Daejeon Korea

MacKenzie, C. L.; Ibbotson, J. A.; Cao, C. G. L. & Lomax, A. J. (2001). Hierarchical decomposition of laparoscopic surgery : a human factors approach to investigating the operating room environment, *Minimally Invasive Therapy and Allied Technologies*, Vol.10, No.3, (pp. 121-127), 1364-5706

Mitsuishi, M.; Arata, J.; Tanaka, K.; Miyamoto, M.; Yoshidome, T.; Iwata, S.; Warisawa, S. & Hashizume, M. (2003). Development of a Remote Minimally-Invasive Surgical System with Operational Environment Transmission Capability, *Proceedings of IEEE International Conference on Robotics & Automation*, pp. 2663-2670, 0-7803-7736-2, Taipei, Taiwan, September, 2003

Nishikawa, A.; Asano, S.; Fujita, R.; Yohda, T.; Miyazaki, F.; Sekimoto, M.; Yasui, M.; Takiguchi, S. & Monden, M. (2003). Robust Visual Tracking of Multiple Surgical Instruments for Laparoscopic Surgery, *Proceedings of Computer Assisted Radiology and Surgery*, London, UK

Nishikawa, A.; Hosoi, T.; Koara, K.; Negoro, D.; Hikita, A.; Asano, S.; Miyazaki, F.; Sekimoto, M.; Miyake, Y.; Yasui, M. & Monden, M. (2001). Real-Time Visual Tracking of the Surgeon's Face for Laparoscopic Surgery, *Lecture Notes in Computer Science*, Vol.2208, (pp. 9-16), 0302-9743

Ohnuma, K.; Masamune, K.; Yoshimitsu, K.; Shinohara, K.; Vain, J.; Fukui, Y. & Miyawaki, F. (2005). Surgical Scenario for Lapsaroscopic Surgery with Timed Automata and Development of Scrub Nurse Robot - Application of Human Adaptive Mechatronics to surgical support system, *Proceedings of the 2nd COE workshop on Human Adaptive Mechatronics(HAM)*, pp. 163-166, Japan, March, 2005

Riener, R.; Reiter, S.; Rasmus, M.; Wetzel, D. & Feussner, H. (2003). Acquisition of arm and instrument movements during laparoscopic interventions, *Minimally Invasive Therapy & Allied Technologies*, Vol.12, No.5, (pp. 235-240), 1364-5706

Rosen, J.; Brown, J. D.; Chang, L.; Sinanan, M. N. & Hannaford, B. (2006). Generalized Approach for Modeling Minimally Invasive Surgery as a Stochastic Process Using a Discrete Markov Model, *IEEE Transactions on Biomedical Engineering*, Vol.53, No.3, (pp. 399-413), 0018-9294

Simaan, N.; Taylor, R. & Flint, P. (2004). High Dexterity Snake-Like Robotic Slaves for Minimally Invasive Telesurgery of the Upper Airway, *Lecture Notes in Computer Science*, Vol.3217, (pp. 17-24), 0302-9743

Tanaka, H. (1978). Articulated, Four-way Bendable Tube Structure, US Patent 4108211

Taylor, R. H.; Funda, J.; Eldridge, B.; Gomory, S.; Gruben, K.; LaRose, D.; Talamini, M.; Kavoussi, L. & Anderson, J. (1995). A Telerobotic Assistant for Laparoscopic Surgery, *IEEE Engineering in Medicine and Biology*, Vol.14, No.3, (pp. 279-288), 0739-5175

Wang, Y.-F.; Uecker, D. R. & Wang, Y. (1996). Choreographed Scope Maneuvering in Robotically-Assisted Laparoscopy with Active Vision Guidance, *Proceedings of IEEE Workshop on Applications of Computer Vision*, pp. 187-192, 0-8186-7620-5, Sarasota, FL, December, 1996

Wei, G.-Q.; Arbter, K. & Hirzinger, G. (1997). Real-Time Visual Servoing for Laparoscopic Surgery : Controlling Robot Motion with Color Image Segmentation, *IEEE Engineering in Medicine and Biology*, Vol.16, No.1, (pp. 40-45), 0739-5175

Yamashita, H.; Kim, D.; Hata, N. & Dohi, T. (2003). Multi-Slider Linkage Mechanism for Endoscopic Forceps Manipulator, *Proceedings of the IEEE/RSJ International Conference on Intelligent Robots and Systems*, pp. 2577-2582, 0-7803-7860-1, Las Vegas, Nevada, October, 2003

Yoon, W. C. (2005). Cognitive Human-Robot Interaction: Groping for Dialogue Intelligence, *Robot and Human : Korea Robotics Society Review*, Vol.2, No.3, (pp. 29-43), 1738-4796, *(Written in Korean)*

16

Miniature robotic guidance for spine surgery

Y. Barzilay, L. Kaplan and M. Liebergall
Spine Unit, Department of Orthopaedic Surgery,
Hadassah-Hebrew University Medical Center, Jerusalem
Israel

1. Introduction

Instrumented spinal fusion surgery is increasingly performed in the treatment of degenerative disorders, Spondylolisthesis, deformity, trauma and tumors affecting the spine (Davis, 1994; Katz, 1995). In-vitro and In-vivo studies using the free hand or fluoroscopically assisted techniques documented breaching of the pedicle in 3-55% (Amiot et al., 2000; Belmont et al., 2001; Belmont et al., 2002; Boachie-Adjei et al., 2000; Carbone et al., 2003; Castro et al., 1996; Esses et al., 1993; Farber et al., 1995; Gertzbein & Robbins, 1990; Laine et al., 1997a; Laine et al., 1997b; Laine et al., 2000; Liljenqvist et al., 1997; Lonstein et al., 1999; Odgers et al., 1996; Schulze et al., 1998; Suk et al., 1995; Vaccaro et al., 1995a; Vaccaro et al. 1995b; Weinstein et al., 1998; Xu et al., 1998)

Clinically significant screw misplacements however occur in 0-7% (Amiot et al. 2000; Belmont et al.2002; Belmont et al. 2001; Boachie-Adjei et al. 2000; Carbone et al. 2003; Castro et al. 1996; Esses et al. 1993; Farber et al. 1995; Gertzbein & Robbins, 1990; Laine et al. 2000; Laine et al. 1997a; Liljenqvist et al. 1997; Lonstein et al. 1999; Odgers et al. 1996; Schulze et al. 1998). Neuro-monitoring, neuro-stimulation, and computed assisted navigation systems reduce the incidence of screw misplacement, however none of them has gained significant popularity in spine surgery, mainly due to logistical and cost-effectiveness issues such as the need for dynamic referencing and a line-of sight, extra staff, expensive tools and cumbersome procedures, longer operation time and the high cost of the capital equipment (Berlermann et al. 1997; Bolger & Wigfield, 2000; Carl et al. 1997; Choi et al. 2000; Digioia et al. 1998; Ebmeier et al. 2003; Foley & Smith, 1996; Girardi et al. 1999; Glossop et al. 1996; Kalfas et al. 1995; Kim et al. 2001; Laine et al. 1997b; Merloz et al. 1998; Mirza et al. 2003; Rampersaud et al. 2001; Rampersaud and Foley, 2000; Raynor et al. 2002; Reidy et al. 2001; Schlenzka et al. 2000; Schwarzenbach et al. 1997; Simon and Lavallee, 1998; Welch et al. 1997).

Surgical robots have emerged during the 1990's and offer distinct added value in terms of accuracy and minimally-invasiveness of the surgical procedure. However, current systems are extremely expensive and large in size, and typically require immobilization of the patient (Taylor & Stoianovici, 2003). The SpineAssist® (Shoham et al. 2003) (Mazor Surgical Technologies, Caesarea, Israel) is a bone-mounted miniature robotic guidance system, clinically and experimentally validated for spinal surgery (Barzilay et al. 2006, Lieberamn et al 2006; Togawa et al. 2007). It facilitates image-based semi-active guidance for providing high accuracy in the positioning of surgical tools and implantable devices such as Pedicle screws, Kyphoplasty needles, tumor evacuators and more. To the best knowledge of the authors, no other clinically validated robotic system is available today for spine surgery. In a recent publication (Barzilay et al. 2006) technical issues as well as patient-related and surgeon-related issues encountered during the clinical development phase were analyzed and lead to improvements in software and in robotic tools. Ways were offered to reduce errors and shorten the learning curve when new users are introduced to this system. In this chapter, a short summary of the clinical development phase and an overview of the early routine clinical use of the SpineAssist in procedures involving pedicle screws insertion, kyphoplasty, vertebroplasty and biopsy of the spine are presented. Also describes is the very early usage of the system in deformity surgery.

The SpineAssist® (SA) (Fig. 1) is a miniature bone-mounted robot - 2.5 inch diameter, 250 gram - featuring a six-degree-of-freedom parallel design.

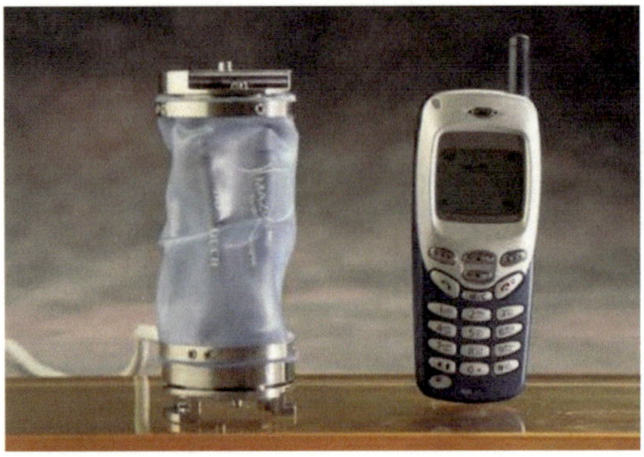

Figure 1. The SpineAssist miniature robot

The miniature robot is connected to the SA workstation (Fig. 2), which controls its motion and runs specially designed graphic user-interface software.

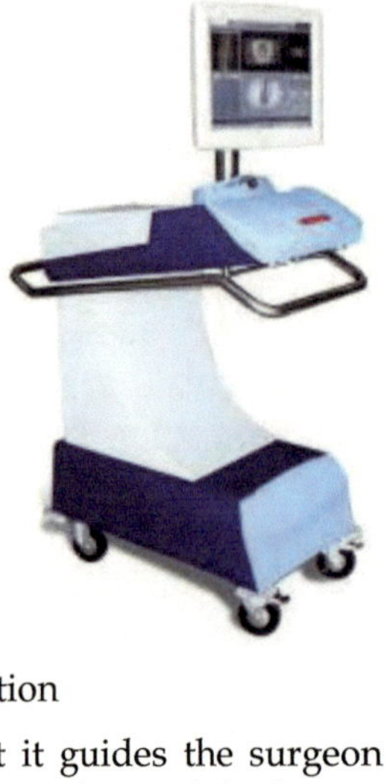

Figure 2. The SpineAssist Workstation

The system is semi-active, in that it guides the surgeon to the desired implant positions according to his/her preoperative plan, while leaving the actual surgical act in the physician's hands. The concept is of pre-operative planning and intra-operative execution. The planning is done on a 3-D model of the patient's spine generated by the system based on a CT scan (Fig. 3). The plan includes implant sizing and placements for all the levels of the spine to be operated on, and can be done on the workstation itself or on the physician's laptop or desktop computer.

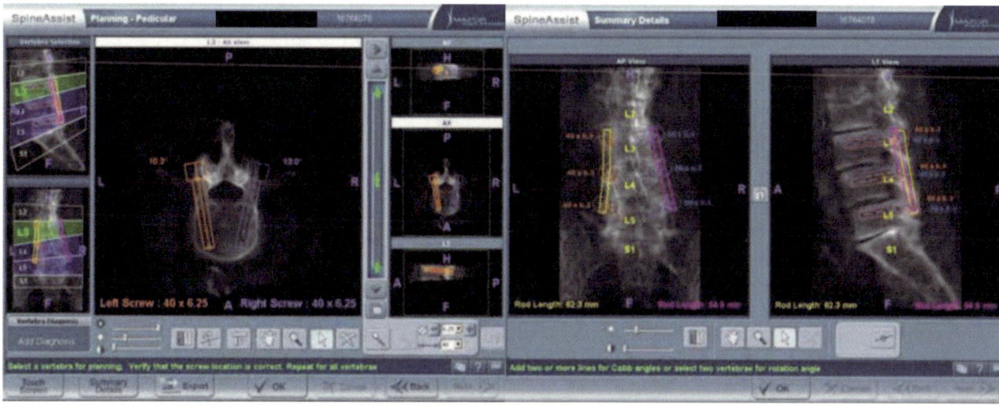

Figure 3. 3D planning of pedicle screws to be introduced into L3 vertebra and a summary of a plan for L3-4-5 fusion

In preparation for the intraoperative execution of the plan, the SA workstation is connected by means of a BNC video cable to a C-Arm fluoroscopy imaging machine and two blank images - anterior-posterior (AP) and 60° Oblique - are taken with a special Image Calibrator attached to the image intensifier of the C-Arm. These two "blank" images are used by the system to automatically compensate for distortions due to ambient magnetic fields and other sources of distortion to the intraoperative fluoroscopy images. The miniature robotic device is also verified for calibration prior to every case by using a specially designed jig with 3 marker holes at positions that are known to the software. The entire process of image and robot calibration takes about 10 minutes and is performed by the radiology technician during the setup of the OR for surgery - parallel to other preparations and prior to bringing the patient in. As the operation begins, a minimally-invasive Hover-T® frame or a less-invasive spinous-process clamp (Fig. 4) is attached to the patient's bony anatomy.

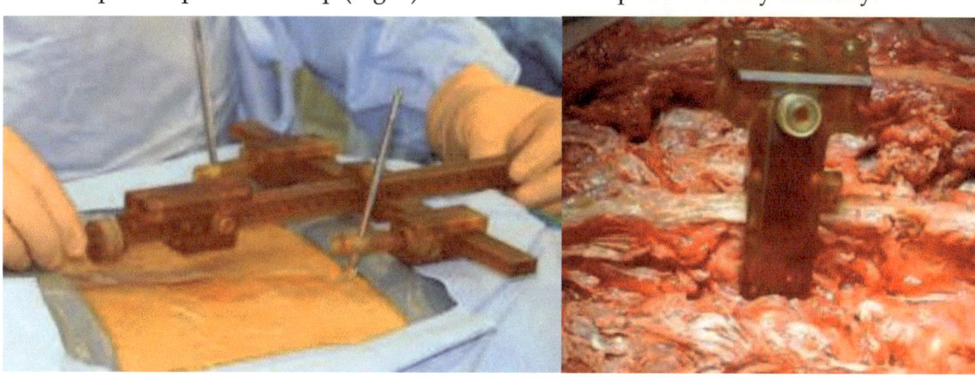

Figure 4. The clamp (right) and the Hover-T frame (left) firmly connect the robot to the patient's body

Two fluoroscopic images are taken - AP and 60° oblique - with a targeting device attached to the Hover-T / Clamp. The system performs automatic, per-vertebra, matching of these intra-operative fluoroscopic images with the pre-operative CT. The accuracy of this process, also referred to as the image registration process, is visually verified by the surgeon; the first level to be operated on is then selected. The target is removed, the SA device is mounted onto the clamp/frame and the system controls its motion so that it points to the exact entry point and trajectory according to the surgeon's pre-operative plan. Based on the known kinematical properties of the system and the desired entry point relative to the robot base the system instructs the surgeon to attach one of three guiding arms (short-1 medium-2 or long-3) to the top plate of the robotic platform, through which surgical tools are inserted by the surgeon to facilitate introduction of the implant. The three arms cover the entire workspace necessary for a variety of spinal procedures. An open approach may be used (Fig. 5), as well as MIS (minimally invasive) and percutaneous approaches (Fig. 6).

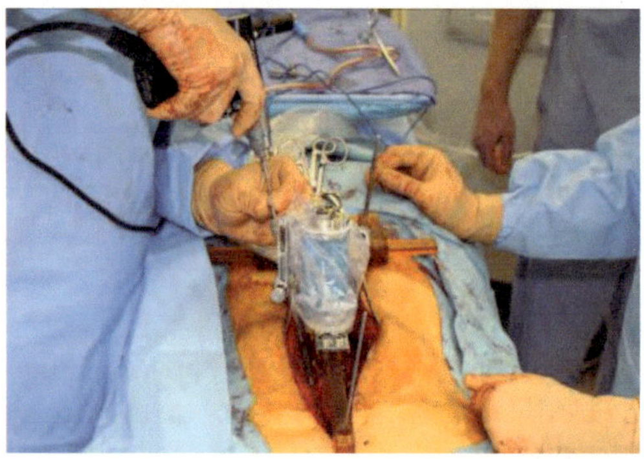

Figure 5. Intraoperative open approach, notice the tool guide through which the surgical tools are inserted

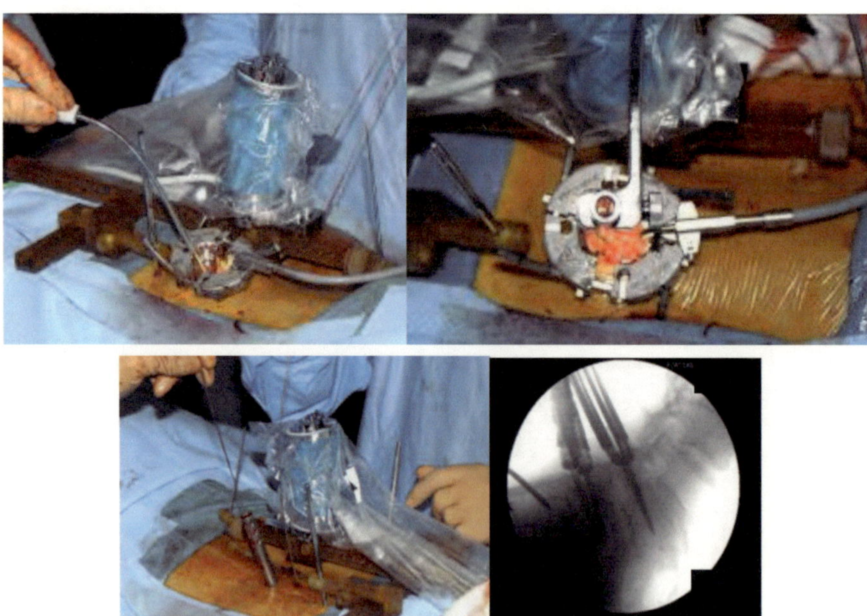

Figure 6. Intraoperative minimally invasive surgery (MIS, upper left and right) and percutaneous (lower left and right) approaches

Fifteen patients were operated on during the clinical development phase of the Spine Assist in two spine centers (March to November 2005) with obstacles occurring in 9 cases (Barzilay et al. 2006). These obstacles were defined as related to surgeon, technique, software or equipment. Conclusions drawn during this period led to improvements in all aspects mentioned. The software was improved, making it more robust, easier to use and better in terms of pre-operative planning. Improvement in the robot's tools made them more user friendly and less prone to skiving by soft tissues. As for surgeon related errors - The clamp must be secured tightly to the spinous process in order to avoid unwanted mobility leading to errors in entry point and trajectory. Minimal force should be used when using the SA and no foreign bodies (i.e. surgical gauze) should be left in the surgical field during acquisition of fluoroscopy images or during operation of the robot. Routine clinical usage of the SA in the authors institution commenced in September 2006. The SA guidance was used by the authors in 24 procedures including 19 spinal fusions, 4 kyphoplasy/vertebroplasty and 1 biopsy. The demographic data and indications for surgery of the study group are summarized in table 1.

Number of patients	24	18 F 6 M
Age (Years)	61 (24-75)	
Indications	Related to degenerative disorders	19
	Vertebral compression fractures	Osteoporotic 3 Metastatic 1
	Infection	Spondylodiscitis 1

Table 1. Demographic data and indications for surgery

Total	**Primary**	**Revisions**		
24	21	3		
Procedure	**1-Level**	**2-Level**	**3-Level**	**4-Level**
TLIF + Posterior fixation	8	7		1
PDPLF	2			
Vertebroplasty	2			
Kyphoplasty	2			
Craig needle biopsy	1			

Table 2. SpineAssist guided surgical procedures

A detailed account of each surgery was taken during the procedure, with attention being paid to system and team performance during all preoperative and intraoperative stages. The ability of the system to successfully accomplish each stage of the procedure was recorded, including importing patient's CT, planning, C-Arm and robot calibration, fluoro acquisition, CT-to-fluoro registration, finding the appropriate kinematical solution for guidance, utility of the surgical accessories and overall accuracy of placements. Surgical data included time measurements of total procedure, time from attachment of clamp/hover-t to detachment, time of fluoro utilization, number of planned screw/needles and the number of executed screws/needles. Parallel to the routine use of the SA in "simple" fusion cases, Kyphoplasty and biopsy, the system was used in three deformity cases, one Scheuermann's kyphosis (80 degrees Cobb T3-T12), one Juvenile idiopathic scoliosis of 78 degrees with pedicle diameter ranging from 3 to 4.5 mm and one case of congenital scoliosis with a hemi vertebra of L2-3 partially segmented from L2. Data from these cases were excluded from results as they were not considered routine. These cases will be further discussed later in this chapter. Table 2 summarizes the surgical procedure performed with SA guidance.

Three cases are presented in figures 10 to 12; these cases demonstrate the abilities of the SA to accurately guide implants or needles. In the first case (Fig. 10) the vertebroplasty needle was aimed at a void in the lower end plate of L3 caused by an osteoporotic fracture.

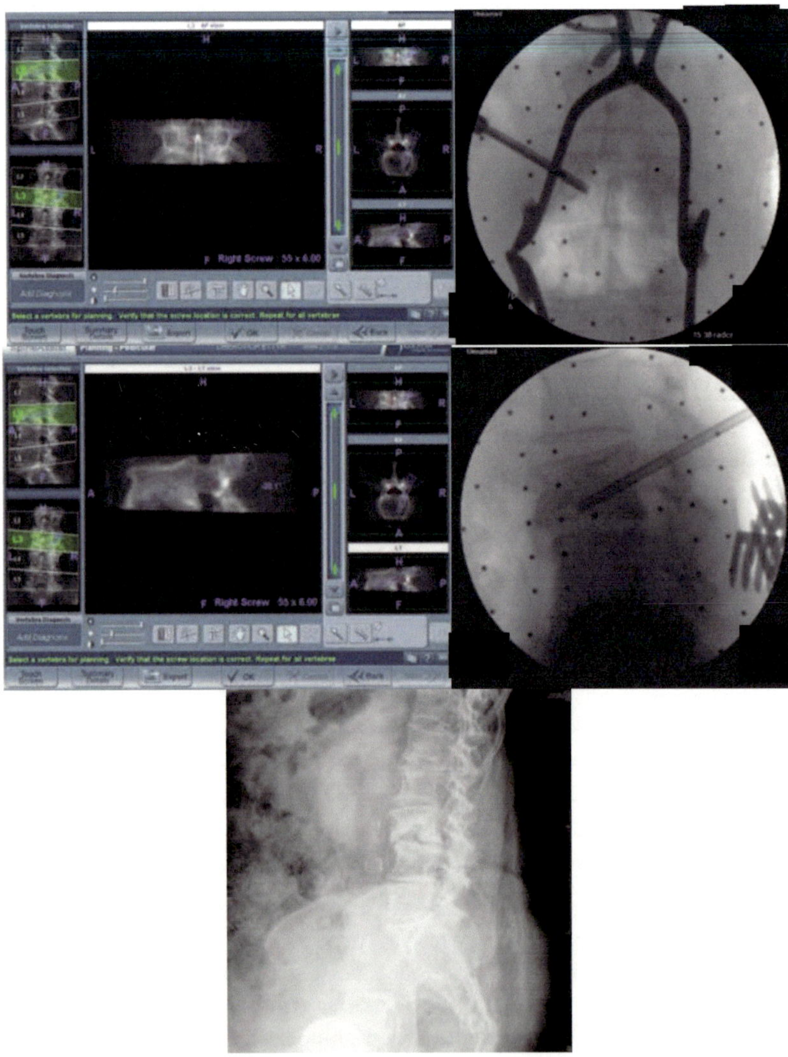

Figure 10 a-f. A 60 years old lady with corticosteroid induced osteoporotic fracture of the inferior endplate of L3 and recess stenosis of L4 presented with intractable low back pain and rt L4 radicular pain unresponsive to non operative treatment. She underwent SA guided L3 Vertebroplasty followed by bilateral L3-4 decompression. The vertebroplasty needle was aimed at a void in the inferior endplate of L3. Axial planning and AP fluoro are reversed in directions, but represent same anatomical sides

In the second case (Fig. 11), 4 cannulated pedicular screws were implanted with SA guidance, again according to the preoperative plan.

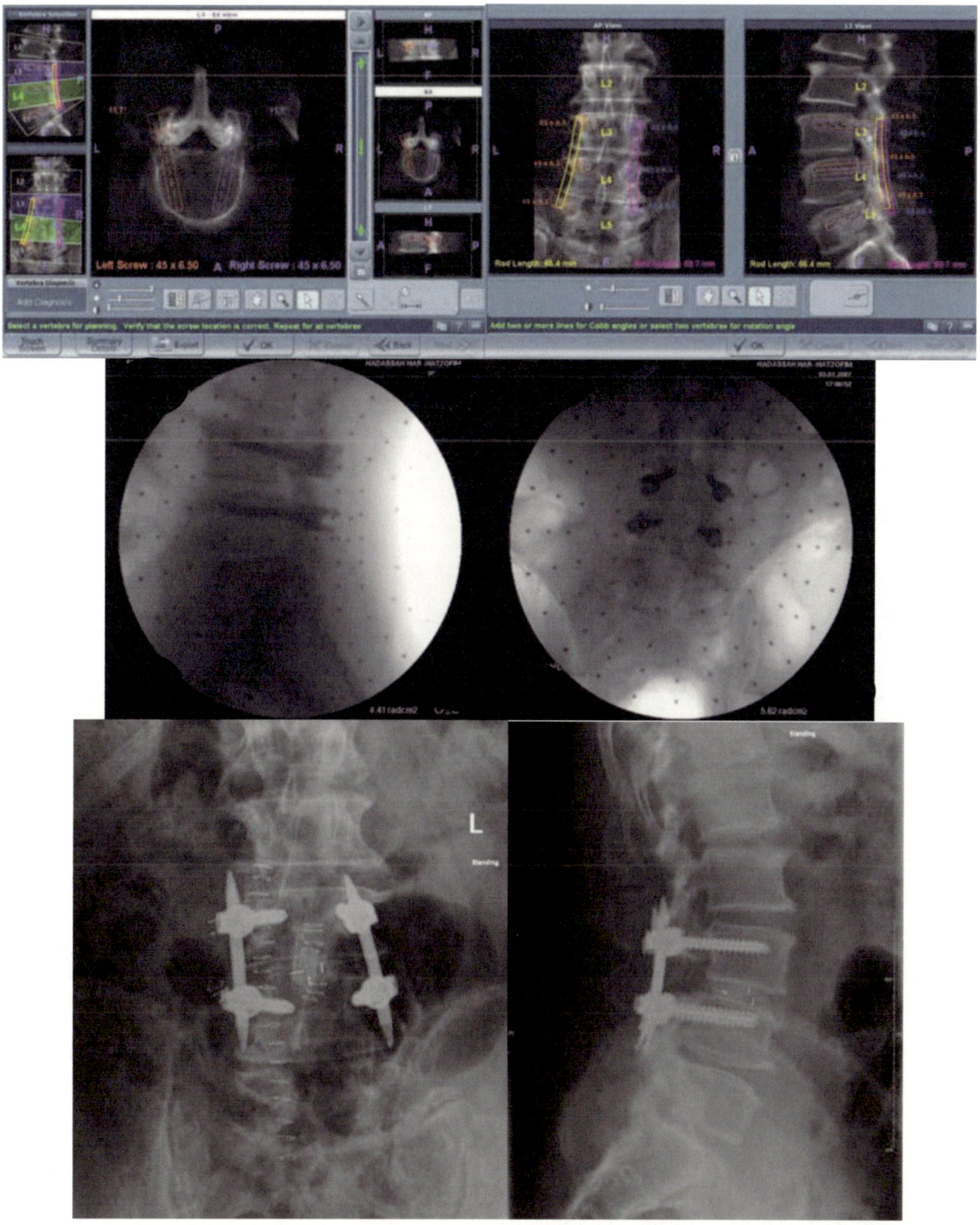

Figure 11 a-f. Preplanning and execution of L3-4 fusion, using cannulated screws. The L5 screws were planned in order to improve the segmentation process of the SA work station

In the third case (figure 12), pedicular screws were used in a lady with lumbar scoliosis de-novo. The intra-operative fluoroscopy images document how close the execution is to the plan.

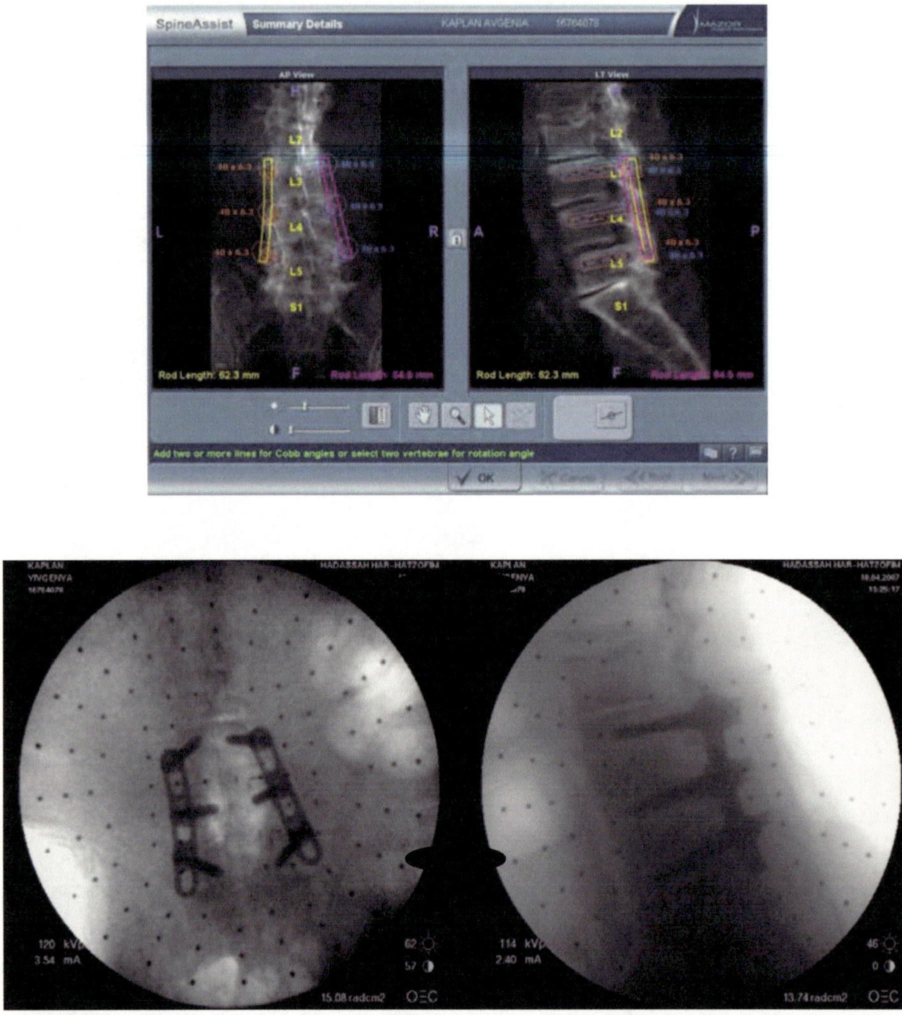

Figure 12 a-c. Planning summary and execution on a 70 years old lady with back pain and spinal intermittent claudication with lumbar scoliosis de-novo and spinal stenosis of L3-5. The surgical procedure included TLIF of L3-4 L4-5, bilateral decompression and SA guided posterior fixation of L3-4-5. The fluoroscopy images represent true AP and Lateral views of the operated levels

Data summarizing the SA usage is shown in tables 3 and 4. Table 3 contains data regarding time measurement in the use of the SA, including time from clamp attachment to detachment (instrumentation time without plates) and total procedure. Table 4 details clinical success (defines as screw in acceptable clinical position and according to plan).

	Average	Range
Screws per case	3.7	1-6
Total case time (Min)	186	47-298
SpineAssist time per case = instrumentation time without plates (Min)	39	17-95
SpineAssist Time per screw (Min)	10.2	4.25-38

Table 3. SA usage compared to whole procedure, instrumentation time in total and per-screw

	Total	Range
Entry points	89	1-6 (3.7 average per-case)
Success rate	85%	0-100%**
Success rate excluding technical failures*	95%	66-100%***

* Technical failures leading to abandonment of SA procedure
** 0% and 25 success rates in 2 cases where technical failures prevented robot usage
***66% in a case where gauze was left in the field, blocking the robot's arm from attaching to the bone, deviating two entry points

Table 4. Clinical success rates

The SA was first used in one level, "simple" fusion cases. Each step was carried out with great care, paying attention to every technical detail, which led to prolonged procedures. A strategic decision was taken to drill the entry point under fluoro guidance (AP and Lateral) in a similar manner to needle insertion in vertebroplasty, and then to verify the drill hole using probes and finders. In the first few cases entry point were found to be higher and lateral relative to the accessory process. Comparing the planning screen to the entry point position, it was found that the robot executed the plan accurately. These early planning errors led to further software improvements - the planning screen now enables a "film" in axial, coronal and sagittal planes, improving surgeon's 3-D understanding of planned implant position. Implementation of the lessons learned in the first few cases led to higher success rates, quicker procedures and minimized fluoroscopy usage (range of SA procedure time and success rates - tables 3 and 4). Later on in the series the SA was used in more levels and in cases with degenerative deformities such as Spondylolisthesis and lumbar scoliosis de-novo. After gaining enough confidence and experience, percutaneous cannulated pedicular screws were inserted, leading to a smaller surgical exposure, easier recovery and a better cosmetic result. Of the 24 procedures in the series, technical failures were encountered in two, and surgeon related errors occurred in two. These failures and possible solutions for future users are summarized in table 5.

Case #	Failure	Solution
1	Technical failure of robot arm	Production process modified
16	Gauze left in field	Check before mounting clamp Gauze seen on fluoroscopy
17	Faulty cable	Have extra set of equipment
24	Clamp moved	Check clamp stability If wrong entry point reassess Re-position and repeat fluoro acquisition

Table 5. Failure analysis and solutions for future users

As mentioned above, the system was used in 3 cases of spinal deformity. In the first case of a teenaged male with painful Scheuermann's kyphosis measuring 80 degrees the Hover-T frame was used, the system passed all stages successfully but, being attached to a rigid frame, relatively far away from the patient's body, the robot was unable to reach the desired angles and the procedure was aborted. In the second case- a teenaged boy with progressive lumbar congenital scoliosis (Hemi vertebra L2-3 RT) the clamp was used. The system guided excellent entry points into the pedicles above the hemi vertebra, but failed to recognize entry points distal to the hemi vertebra. This case is being studied at the R&D department. In the 3rd case of a teenage patient with idiopathic scoliosis measuring 80 degrees and with tiny pedicles (3-4.5mm) registration failed using the Hover-T frame. However, when the clamp replaced the Hover-T the system performed well leading to perfect entry points and trajectories. At this stage the authors consider the usage of the SA in cases with deformity as early learning curve. A new Hover-T frame with more flexibility in positioning and an improved range of motion may enable percutaneous screw insertion in deformity cases and will upgrade these difficult procedures substantially. Another technical difficulty encountered during this series was the acquisition of high quality AP fluoroscopy images in the transition area between the chest support of the Jackson frame and air surrounding the abdomen, especially in patients with osteoporosis. In short procedures such as vertebroplasty, involving T7-10, the authors prefer to use the OSI plate, having a uniform "background", leading to easier fluoroscopy acquisition.

In conclusion, the SpineAssist is a highly accurate surgical guidance system, incorporating a bone-mounted miniature robot and unique image registration software. The system has been validated, is routinely used in the author's institution and is undergoing further evolution, expanding its work volume and the indication for its use. At the same time, it is a delicate system, especially sensitive to mechanical overload. While excess forces exerted to different parts of the robot and its attachments will generally not damage it, they may well affect the system's accuracy in guiding the surgeon to the desired position. Special care should be taken to follow the recommended, gentle, surgical technique and to utilizing the appropriate tools and surgical accessories. Careful attention should also be given to the pre-operative plan - which becomes an integral part of the surgery - and to intra-operatively acquiring high-quality fluoroscopic images. When these simple rules are followed, and simple errors mentioned earlier are avoided, excellent results should be expected. Looking forward into the future we recommend that the working volume of the robot be increased, for example by means of modified designs of the guiding arms and robot attachments to the body; this will facilitate the utilization of the system for patients with extreme deformities or with tiny tumors (i.e. osteoid osteoma) in "unreachable" locations, in which we believe it will have a significant added value.

2. References

Amiot, L.P. et al. (2000). Comparative results between conventional and computer-assisted pedicle screw installation in the thoracic, lumbar, and sacral spine. *Spine*, Vol. 25, No. 5, (March 2000) 606-614, ISSN: 0362-2436

Barzilay, Y. et al. (2006). Miniature robotic guidance for spine surgery - introduction of a novel system and analysis of challenges encountered during the clinical development phase at two spine centres. *Int J Med Robot*, Vol. 2, No. 2, (June 2006) 146-53, ISSN: 1478-5951

Belmont, P.J. et al. (2001). In vivo accuracy of thoracic pedicle screws. *Spine*, Vol. 26, No. 21, (November 2001) 2340-2346, ISSN: 0362-2436

Belmont, P.J. et al. (2002). Accuracy of thoracic pedicle screws in patients with and without coronal plane spinal deformities. *Spine*, Vol. 27, No. 14, (July 2002) 1558-1566, ISSN: 0362-2436

Berlermann, U. et al. (1997) Planning and insertion of pedicle screws with computer assistance. *J Spinal Disord.*, Vol. 10, No. 2, (April 1997) 117-124, ISSN: 0895-0385

Boachie-Adjei, O. et al. (2000). Safety and efficacy of pedicle screw placement for adult spinal deformity with a pedicle-probing conventional anatomic technique. *J Spinal Disord.*, Vol. 13, No. 6, (December 2000) 496-500, ISSN: 0895-0385

Bolger, C. & Wigfield, C. (2000). Image-guided surgery: Applications to the cervical and thoracic spine and a review of the first 120 procedures. *J Neurosurg*, Vol. 92, No. 2, (April 2000) 175-180, ISSN: 0268-8697

Carbone, J.J., Tortolani, P.J., & Quartararo, L.G. (2003). Fluoroscopically assisted pedicle screw fixation for thoracic and thoracolumbar injuries: Technique and short-term complications. *Spine*, Vol. 28, No. 1, (January 2003) 91-97, ISSN: 0362-2436

Carl, A.L. et al. (1997). In-vitro simulation: Early results of stereotaxy for pedicle screw placement. *Spine*, Vol. 15, No. 22, (May 1997) 1160-1164, ISSN: 0362-2436

Castro, W.H. et al. (1996). Accuracy of pedicle screw placement in lumbar vertebrae. *Spine*, Vol. 21, No. 11, (June 1996) 1320-1324, ISSN: 0362-2436

Choi, W.W., Green, B.A., & Levi, A.D.O. (2000). Computer-assisted fluoroscopic targeting system for pedicle screw insertion. *Neurosurgery*, Vol. 47, No. 4, (October 2000) 872-878, ISSN: 0148-396X

Davis, H. (1994). Increasing rates of cervical and lumbar spine surgery in the United States 1979-1990. *Spine*, Vol. 19, No. 10, (May 1994) 1117-1124, ISSN: 0362-2436

DiGioia, A., Jaramaz, B., & Colgan, B. (1998). Computer Assisted Orthopaedic Surgery: Image Guided and Robotic Assistive Technologies. *Clin Orthop Relat Res,* Vol. 354, (September 1998) 8-16, ISSN: 0009-921X

Ebmeier, K., Giest, K., & Kalff, R. (2003). Intraoperative computerized tomography for improved accuracy of spinal navigation in pedicle screw placement of the thoracic spine. *Acta Neurochir Suppl.,* Vol. 85, (2003) 105-113, ISSN: 0065-1419

Esses, S.I., Barton, L.S., & Vadim, D. (1993). Complications associated with the technique of pedicle screw fixation: A selected survey of ABS members. *Spine,* Vol. 18, No. 15, (November 1993) 2231-2239, ISSN: 0362-2436

Farber, G.L. et al. Accuracy of pedicle screw placement in lumbar fusions by plain radiographs and computed tomography. *Spine,* Vol. 20, No. 13, (July 1995) 1494-1499, ISSN: 0362-2436

Foley, K.T., & Smith, M.M. (1996). Image-guided spine surgery. *Neurosurg Clin N Am,* Vol. 7, No. 2, (April 1996) 171-186, ISSN: 1042-3680

Gertzbein, S.D., & Robbins, S.E. (1990). Accuracy of pedicular screw placement in vivo. *Spine,* Vol. 15, No. 1, (January 1990) 11-14, ISSN: 0362-2436

Girardi, F.P. et al. (1999). The placement of lumbar pedicle screws using computerised stereotactic guidance. *J Bone Joint Surg Br.,* Vol. 81, No. 5, (September 1999) 825-9, ISSN: 0301-620X

Glossop, N.D., Hu, R.W., & Randle, J.A. (1996). Computer-aided pedicle screw placement using frameless stereotaxis. *Spine,* Vol. 21, No. 17, (September 1996) 2026-2034, ISSN: 0362-2436

Kalfas, I.H. et al. (1995). Application of frameless stereotaxy to pedicle screw fixation of the spine. *J Neurosurg.,* Vol. 83, No. 4, (October 1995) 641-7, ISSN: 0022-3085

Katz, J.N. (1995). Lumbar spine fusion. Surgical rates, costs and complications. *Spine,* Vol. 20, No. 24, (December 1995) 78S-83S, ISSN: 0362-2436

Kim, K.D. et al. (2001). Computer-assisted thoracic pedicle screw placement: An *in vitro* feasibility study. *Spine,* Vol. 26, No. 4, (February 2001) 360-364, ISSN: 0362-2436

Laine, T. et al. (1997a). Accuracy of pedicle screw insertion: a prospective CT study in 30 low back patients. *Eur Spine J,* Vol. 6, No. 6, (1997) 402-405, ISSN: 0940-6719

Laine, T. et al. (1997b). Improved accuracy of pedicle screw insertion with computer-assisted surgery: A prospective clinical trial of 30 patients. *Spine,* Vol. 22, No. 11, (June 1997) 1254-1258, ISSN: 0362-2436

Laine, T. et al. (2000). Accuracy of pedicle screw insertion with and without computer assistance: A randomized controlled clinical study in 100 consecutive patients. *Eur Spine J,* Vol. 9, No. 3, (June 2000) 235-240, ISSN: 0940-6719

Lieberman, I.H. et al. (2006). Bone-mounted miniature robotic guidance for pedicle screw and translaminar facet screw placement: Part I--Technical development and a test case result. *Neurosurgery.* Vol. 59, No. 3, (September 2006) 641-650, ISSN: 0148-396X

Liljenqvist, U.R., Halm, H.F., & Link, T.M. (1997). Pedicle screw instrumentation of the thoracic spine in idiopathic scoliosis. *Spine,* Vol. 22, No. 19, (October 1997) 2239-2245, ISSN: 0362-2436

Lonstein, J.E. et al. (1999). Complications associated with pedicle screws. *J Bone Joint Surg Am,* Vol. 81, No. 11, (November 1999) 1519-1528, ISSN: 0021-9355

Merloz, P. et al. (1998). Pedicle screw placement using image-guided techniques. *Clin Orthop Relat Res,* Vol. 354, (September 1998) 39-48, ISSN: 0009-921X

Mirza, S.K. et al. (2003). Accuracy of thoracic vertebral body screw placement using standard fluoroscopy, fluoroscopic image guidance, and computed tomographic image guidance: A cadaver study. *Spine*, Vol. 28, No. 4, (February 2003) 402-413, ISSN: 0362-2436

Odgers, C.J. et al. (1996). Accuracy of pedicle screw placement with the assistance of lateral plain radiography. *J Spinal Disord.*, Vol. 9, No. 4, (Aug. 1996) 334-8, ISSN: 0895-0385

Rampersaud Y.R., Foley K.F. (2000). Image-guided spinal surgery. *Op Tech Orthoped*, Vol. 10, (2000) 64-8

Rampersaud, Y.R., Simon, D.A., & Foley, K.T. (2001), Accuracy requirements for image-guided spinal pedicle screw placement. *Spine*, Vol. 26, No. 4, (February 2001) 352-359, ISSN: 0362-2436

Raynor ,B.L. et al. (2002). Can triggered electromyograph thresholds predict safe thoracic pedicle screw placement? *Spine*, Vol. 27, No. 18, (September 2002) 2030-2035, ISSN: 0362-2436

Reidy, D.P. et al. (2001). Evaluation of electromyographic monitoring during insertion of thoracic pedicle screws. *J Bone Joint Surg Br*, Vol. 83, No. 7, (September 2001) 1009-1014, ISSN: 0301-620X

Schlenzka, D., Laine, T., & Lund, T. (2000). Computer-assisted spine surgery. *Eur Spine J*, Vol. 9, No. 1, (February 2000) S57-S64, ISSN: 0940-6719

Schulze, C.J., Munzinger, E., & Weber, U. (1998). Clinical relevance of accuracy of pedicle screw placement. A computed tomographic-supported analysis. *Spine*, Vol. 23, No. 20, (October 1998) 2215-2221, ISSN: 0362-2436

Schwarzenbach, O. et al. (1997). Accuracy of computer-assisted pedicle screw placement: An in-vivo computed tomography analysis. *Spine*, Vol. 22, No. 4, (February 1997) 452-8, ISSN: 0362-2436

Simon, D.A., & Lavallee, S. (1998). Medical Imaging and Registration in Computer Assisted Surgery. *Clin Orthop Relat Res*, Vol. 354, (September 1998) 8-16, ISSN: 0009-921X

Shoham, M. et al. (2003). Bone-Mounted Miniature Robot for Surgical Procedures: Concept and Clinical Applications *IEEE Transactions on Robotics and Automation*, Vol. 19, No. 5, (October 2003) 893-901, ISSN: 1042-296X

Suk, S. et al. (1995). Segmental pedicle screw fixation in the treatment of thoracic idiopathic scoliosis. *Spine*, Vol. 20, No. 12, (June 1995) 1399-1405, ISSN: 0362-2436

Taylor, R. H., & Stoianovici, D. (2003). Medical Robotics in Computer-Integrated Surgery, *IEEE Transactions on Robotics and Automation*, Vol. 19, No. 5, (October 2003) 765-781, ISSN: 1042-296X

Togawa, D. et al. (2007). Bone-mounted miniature robotic guidance for pedicle screw and translaminar facet screw placement: part 2--Evaluation of system accuracy. *Neurosurgery*, Vol. 60, No. 2, (February 2007) ONS129-139, ISSN: 0148-396X

Vaccaro, A.R. et al. (1995a). Placement of pedicle screws in the thoracic spine: Part I. Morphometric analysis of the thoracic vertebrae. *J Bone Joint Surg Am*, Vol. 77, No. 8, (August 1995) 1193-1199, ISSN: 0021-9355

Vaccaro, A.R. et al. (1995b). Placement of pedicle screws in the thoracic spine: Part II. An anatomical and radiographic assessment. *J Bone Joint Surg Am*, Vol. 77, No. 8, (August 1995) 1200-1206, ISSN: 0021-9355

Weinstein, J.N. et al. (1988). Spinal pedicle fixation: Reliability and validity of roentgenogram-based assessment and surgical factors on successful screw placement. *Spine*, Vol. 13, No. 9, (September 1988) 1012-1018, ISSN: 0021-9355

Welch, W.C. et al. (1997). Evaluation with evoked and spontaneous electromyography during lumbar instrumentation: A prospective study. *J Neurosurg,* Vol. 87, No. 3, (September 1997) 397-402, ISSN: 0022-3085

Xu, R. et al. (1998). Anatomic considerations of pedicle screw placement in the thoracic spine: Roy-Camille technique versus open lamina technique. *Spine,* Vol. 23, No. 9, (1998) 1065-1068, ISSN: 0021-9355

17

Nerve Sparing Axillary Dissection using the da Vinci Surgical System

Susan M L Lim, Cheng-Kiong Kum and Foong-Lian Lam
Centre for Breast Screening and Surgery, Centre for Robotic Surgery
Singapore

1. Abstract

We would like to describe a new minimally invasive method of axillary dissection via a periareolar incision and an 8mm incision in the axilla using the da Vinci Surgical System. The ten times (10X) magnification and three dimension (3D) image, together with the versatility and precision of the robotic telemanipulators has enabled us to perform nerve-sparing axillary dissection in 14 patients with carcinoma of the breast with lymph node metastases undergoing segmental mastectomy or total mastectomy and requiring level I and II axillary dissection. The time for the robotic axillary dissection ranged from 25 to 110 minutes with an average of 53 minutes. The average number of lymph nodes retrieved was 18 (range from 8 to 28). Postoperatively all patients recovered well. The robotic system can enhance the surgeon's ability by providing a high-definition, magnified, three-dimensional view of the operative field, intuitively controlled articulating instruments, and elimination of tremors, and has potential benefits for the patient.

2. Introduction

For women with breast cancer, the status of axillary node involvement is the single best predictor of survival, and important treatment decisions are based on this information. (Bland et al., & Maibenc et al., 1999) While much progress and innovation has been made in the surgical approach to the breast (Veronesi et al., 1994), there has been less progress made in the surgical approach to the axilla. For women with breast cancer, the presence of metastatic disease in the regional basin significantly decreases five-year survival. (Schottenfeid et al., 1976) A level I and II axillary dissection is recommended for staging purposes as well as for local control. (Recht et al., & Houlihan, 1995) However, axillary dissection has been associated with significant morbidity which includes pain, paresthesia, swelling, shoulder dysfunction, and lymphoedema. Multiple reports have shown that axillary dissection was associated with paresthesia (60%), pain (45%), weakness (40%), swelling (26%), stiffness (12%) and lymphoedema in up to 43% of patients. (Taylor & Armer, 2004) The logical step in the advancement of breast cancer surgery would be to decrease the morbidity of the axillary dissection without necessarily sacrificing on lymph node retrieval for accurate staging. Less invasive treatment modalities have been evaluated in order to lower the morbidity of axillary lymph node dissection. These have included the sentinel node biopsy (Veronesi et al., 2003) (SLNB) and endoscopic axillary lymph node dissection. (Tsangaris et al., 1999; Paepke et al., 2003; Kuehn et al., 2001; Brunt et al., 1998; Avrahami et al., 1998) SLNB in particular is rapidly being accepted by many centres as a low morbidity method of identifying possible spread to the axilla. Since March 2003, we performed minimal access axillary dissection in patients with breast cancer, and noted significant patient benefits in terms of less pain and paresthesia, and improved shoulder mobility (unpublished results). However, the procedure itself was cumbersome and non-ergonomic, given the reduced range of motion and instrument dexterity of the standard laparoscopic instrument, and 2-dimensional view of the operative field. In recent years, there has been a rapid growth of surgical procedures performed using the da Vinci Surgical System (Intuitive Surgical, Sunnyvale, CA, USA). (Hazey & Meivin., 2004; Bodner et al., 2004; Undre et al., 2004; Menon et al., 2003) The system uses a master-slave robot concept where the surgeon controls telemanipulators to perform the operation, hence the commonly used term 'robotic surgery'. The advantages of robotic surgery using this system include 10X magnification , three-dimensional vision, elimination of tremor, use of instruments with seven degrees of freedom (d.o.f.) of movement, and the ability of the surgeon to perform the procedure comfortably seated with armrests for support. Procedures demanding superior visualization or requiring complex reconstruction obtain the greatest benefit from robotics over conventional laparoscopy. This is our report of 14 patients with carcinoma of the breast and lymph node metastases who underwent a level I and II axillary dissection using the da Vinci Surgical System. The objective was to develop a technique of axillary dissection which could visualize the cutaneous nerves and lymphatics in the axilla, and aid in fine dissection with preservation of the nerves.

3. Patients and Methods

Between 19 November 2004 and 15 November 2006,14 robotic axillary dissections using the da Vinci Surgical System (Intuitive Surgical, Sunnyvale, CA, USA) were successfully performed on 14 patients with carcinoma of the breast and lymph node metastases who underwent segmental mastectomy or total mastectomy. All patients were comprehensively informed about the technique, and signed informed consent. The age range was 32-74 years. The tumour size ranged from 1.5 cm to 8.0 cm. The tumour location was in the upper, outer quadrant (6 patients), upper inner quadrant (2 patients), lower outer quadrant (1 patient), upper half of breast (3 patients) and lateral half of breast (1 patient). One patient only had axillary dissection as her mastectomy had been performed at another medical facility. General anaesthesia with endotracheal intubation was employed and the patient was positioned supine with the arm abducted to 120 degrees. A large soft roll was positioned under the side of the patient to elevate that side from the table 30 degrees. Segmental excision of the tumour was first performed through a periareolar incision. Following the excision of the tumour with clear margins, the breast cavity was washed with saline, and hemostasis achieved prior to commencement of the axillary dissection. The axillary space was created as follows: the clavipectoral-axillary fascia was gently opened by blunt dissection and a "closed-open" scissors introduced gently into the axillary space through the opening. This opening provided the working space and access to the axilla for the endoscope and instrument arm of the surgical system. The surgical cart of the da Vinci Surgical System containing the camera arm and the left and right instrument arms, was positioned over the shoulder. A zero degree 3D endoscope (InSite™ Vision System, Intuitive Surgical, Sunnyvale, USA) was placed through the periareolar incision and targeted toward the axillary vein. A bi-polar coagulating forceps, placed in the left arm of the robot, was also positioned through the same incision. A cautery hook or cautery spade, connected to unipolar diathermy was placed in the contralateral arm of the robot and inserted through an 8mm incision in the axilla. A self-retaining retractor was placed in the incision to maintain the axillary space. In the 7 cases of total mastectomy procedures, the access of the robotic instruments and camera was through the mastectomy incision (circumareolar, skin sparing). Once the axillary space was achieved with good visuals, axillary dissection was performed. Once all three nerves (intercostobrachio-cutaneous, long thoracic, thoracodorsal) had been identified and dissected free from the axillary contents, the axillary fat pad was dissected in a lateral and inferior direction to the anterior border of the latissimus dorsi muscle, and divided. Hemostasis was achieved with uni- or bi-polar coagulation. The specimen and lymph nodes contained within were extracted through the breast incision and submitted to pathology. The breast incision was closed with 4/0 vicryl and steristrips. No surgical drainage was required for the axilla. The stab incision in the axilla was closed with steristrips. All patients were admitted following surgery. For patients with tumour in the lateral quadrants of the breast, oncoplastic reconstruction of the lumpectomy defect was performed using a flap of fatty tissue overlying the serratus anterior muscle, supplied by a branch of the thoracodorsal artery which was identified and preserved. (Denewer & Farouk ,2007) This is a very useful thin fascial flap for distant coverage. The thoracodorsal artery is identified proximally, and branches coursing medially toward the serratus are identified and preserved. The fascial flap to be elevated is then outlined and incised. This is a very thin flap that is dissected off the underlying serratus anterior muscle. Dissection continues from distal to proximal and includes the branches of the thoracodorsal artery. Branches extending into the serratus muscle are cauterized with the bipolar electrocoagulation unit. Care should be taken to preserve the long thoracic nerve. The fascia is dissected away, leaving the nerve intact (see figure 1).

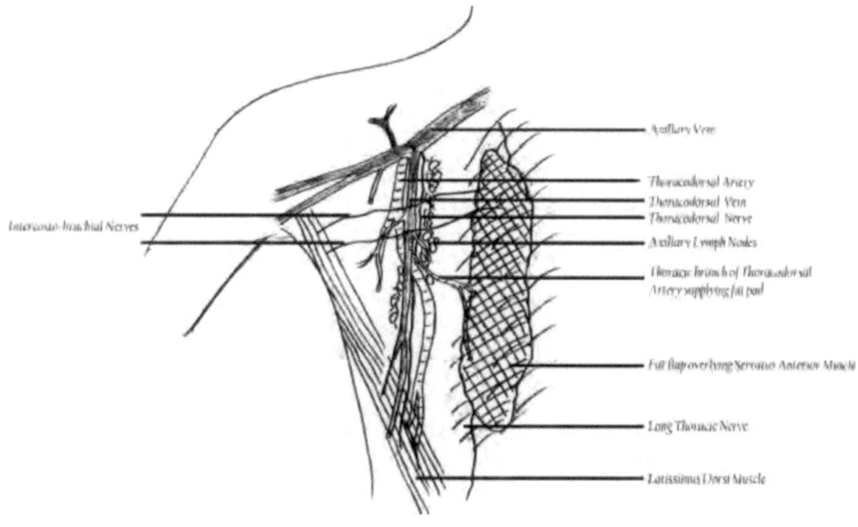

Figure 1. Contents of Axilla

4. Results

14 patients underwent robotic axillary dissection following segmental mastectomy or total mastectomy for carcinoma of the breast. The set up times for the da Vinci system ranged from 3 to 20 minutes, mean operative duration for the robotic axillary dissection was 53

minutes (range from 20 to 110 minutes); and the mean total operative time for both the breast and axillary surgery (measured from the time of the initial skin incision to the last subcutaneous stitch was completed) was 149 minutes (range 105-240 minutes). There were no intraoperative technical failures of the da Vinci telemanipulator system. Blood loss was negligible in all cases. In patients who had segmental mastectomy performed (6 patients), the margins of resection of the breast tissue were free of tumour in all patients. The average number of lymph nodes removed was 18 (range from 8 to 28). In those patients who underwent oncoplastic reconstruction using the flap of fatty tissue overlying the serratus anterior muscle, the branch of the thoracodorsal artery was easily identified in all cases and preserved. All patients were hospitalized following surgery. There were no intra- or post-operative complications such as hematoma, wound infection, or injury to nerves and vessels. Out of the 14 patients operated upon, 2 had no seroma formation post-operatively. 8 patients had seroma formation for 2 weeks and 4 patients for one month documented on ultrasound. In all these patients, the seroma resolved over time. Axillary pain and paresthesia of upper arm were also noted to be minimal, with the major advantage, often realized by the patient and surgeon immediately after surgery, being the improved mobility of the operated arm. The patients reported full range of movement of the upper limb without any stiffness or pain. The patients who had the oncoplastic reconstruction performed using the flap of fatty tissue overlying the serratus anterior muscle supplied by the branch of the thoracodorsal artery had excellent cosmesis post-operatively.

5. Discussion

Improved surgical techniques in breast cancer surgery have evolved over the years, which include skin and areolar-sparing mastectomy, segmental mastectomy, oncoplastic breast procedures, and reconstructive options. (Simmons et al., 2003; Gerber et al., 2003) This increased use of breast-conserving therapy for treatment of breast cancer has nearly eliminated the major morbidity of loss of the breast. The present focus of postoperative morbidity has shifted to the axillary dissection, a procedure which for many women has become the major cause of long-term morbidity after local therapy for breast cancer. (Harris et al., 1999) In the surgical approach to the axilla however, apart from the sentinel node biopsy, there have been few innovations in techniques to spare the common complications of an axillary dissection, which range from seroma or hematoma formation to injury to the nerves that course through the axilla. Injury to the long thoracic nerve may result in a winged scapula or palsy of the serratus anterior muscle and occurs in approximately 10% of cases, (Bennion & Love, 1997) while injury to the thoracodorsal nerve will lead to weakness of the latissimus dorsi muscle. Injury to the intercostobrachial nerve may cause permanent numbness in the lateral axilla and medial portion of the upper arm. These injuries, while distressing to patients, are probably underestimated, as they are not life-threatening and do not require hospitalization. (Ivens et al., 1992) In this report, we have shown that axillary lymph node dissection with the da Vinci Surgical System is a precise, gentle, and safe alternative to lymphadenectomy performed via a standard axillary incision. The authors embarked on this technique after finding that the robotic approach yielded better precision and visualisation that could result in less morbidity following axillary dissection. This ergonomic master-slave system offered three-dimensional visualization, wristed instrumentation, intuitive finger-controlled movements and a comfortable seated position for the surgeon. While the increase in operating time reflects the initial small learning curve, the advantages of dissection using telemanipulators were striking to the surgeon and appeared to have significant positive impact on patient outcome. Surgeon advantages included a 3D view of the axilla, 10X magnification, and an ergonomical operating position with seven d.o.f. of movement of the instruments with elimination of tremor. A potential disadvantage of this technology is the added cost, and the lack of tactile sensation, but three-dimensional visualization compensated for this handicap. Patient outcome may be improved as the enhanced view facilitates identification and preservation of the nerves in the axilla; the long thoracic nerve on the medial wall, thoracodorsal nerve on the posterior wall, and especially the intercostobrachial nerves which course through the axilla. In addition, lymph nodes and lymphatic channels are better visualized, adding to the completeness of the lymphatic dissection. The reason for minimal seroma is probably due to the better visualisation and more meticulous and precise dissection using a 'no-touch' technique i.e. the tissues were only handled with the robotic instruments. The aesthetic result was also better as a separate axilla incision was avoided. The 10X magnification also enabled the fat overlying the serratus anterior muscle to be harvested as a flap with its own blood supply from the thoracic branch of the thoracodorsal artery. The harvested fat flap allows for immediate reconstruction of the segmental mastectomy defect in patients with tumours located in the lateral quadrants of the breast. Sentinel lymph node biopsy remains a good management option for patients with early breast cancer, with low morbidity. We believe that robotic axillary dissection is a useful complement to this technique when there is an oncoplastic requirement for a complete axillary dissection. There are distinct advantages with robotic axillary dissection and this could be added to the repertoire of procedures in a hospital that has purchased the robot for use in other types of surgery.

6. Conclusion

Nerve-sparing axillary dissection with the da Vinci Surgical System is feasible and can be performed within the current oncological standards. Access to the axillary space is obtained through the initial incision for breast tumour removal and eliminates the necessity for a second main axillary incision. The three dimensional view, magnified 10X, and the robotic telemanipulators can enhance the surgeon's ability with better vision, intuitive instrument control and depth perception, and elimination of tremors, and can possibly reduce postoperative complications for the patient. We conclude that robotic axillary lymph node dissection can be safely and selectively introduced into a breast cancer surgery program.

7. References

Armer J, Fu MR, Wainstock JM, Zagar E, Jacobs LK (2004): Lymphedema following breast cancer treatment, including sentinel lymph node biopsy. *Lymphology. Jun;* 37(2): 73-91.

Avrahami R, Nudelman I, Watenberg S, Lando O, Hiss Y, Lelchuk S (1998): Minimally invasive surgery for axillary dissection. Cadaveric feasibility study. *Surg Endosc May;* 12(5):466-8.

Bennion RS, Love SM (1997): Treatment of breast disease. In Diagnosis of diseases of the breast. *WB Saunders Company;* 521-45.

Bland KI et al (1999): Axillary dissection in breast-conserving surgery for stage I and II breast cancer: a National Cancer Data Base study of patterns of omission and implications for survival. *JAm Coll Surg Jun;* 188(6):586 - 95.

Bodner J, Wykypiel H, Wetscher G, Schmid T (2004): First experiences with the da Vinci operating robot in thoracic surgery. *Eur J Cardiothorac Surg. May;* 25(5): 844-51

Brunt LM, Jones DB, Wu JS, Brunt EM, Radford DM (1998): Endoscopic axillary lymph node dissection: an experimental study in human cadavers. *J Am Coll Surg. Aug;* 187(2):158-63.

Denewer A, Farouk O (2007): Can Nipple-sparing Mastectomy and Immediate Breast Reconstruction with Modified Extended Latissimus Dorsi Muscular Flap Improve the Cosmetic and Functional Outcome among Patients with Breast Carcinoma? *World J Surg; Jun;* 31(6):1169-1177

Gerber B, Krause A, Reimer T, et al (2003): Skin-sparing mastectomy with conservation of the nipple-areola complex and autologous reconstruction is an oncologically safe procedure. *Ann Surg Jul;* 238(1):120-7.

Giuliano AE, Jones RC, Brennan M, et al (1997): Sentinel lymphadenectomy in breast cancer. */ Clin Oncol Jun;* 15(6):2345-2350.

Harris JR, Lippman ME, Morrow M, et al (1999): Diseases of the breast. 2nd ed., *Baltimore, Lipponcott Williams & Wilkens,* p 403-406,1999.

Hazey JW, Melvin WS (2004): Robot-assisted general surgery. *Semin Laparosc Surg. Jun;* 11(2): 107-12

Hidalgo DA (1998): Aesthetic refinement in breast reconstruction: complete skin-sparing mastectomy with autogenous tissue transfer. *Plast Reconstr Surg Jul;*102(1):63-7.

Ivens D, Hoe AL, Podd TJ, et al (1992): Assessment of morbidity from complete axillary dissection. *Br J Cancer Jul;* 66(1):136-8.

Kuehn T, Santjohanser C, Grab D, Klauss W, Koretz K, Kreienberg R (2001): Endoscopic axillary surgery in breast cancer. *Br J Surg May;* 88(5):698-703.

Maibenco DC et al (1999): Axillary lymph node metastases associated with small invasive breast carcinomas. *Cancer Apr 1;* 85(7):1530 -6.

Menon M, Hemal AK, Tewari A, Shrivastava A, Shoma AM, El-Tabey NA, Shaaban A, Abol-Enein H, Ghoneim MA (2003): Nerve-sparing robot-assisted radical cystoprostatectomy and urinary diversion. *BJU Int Aug;* 92(3):232-6.

Paepke S, Schwarz-Boeger U, Kiechle M, Jacobs VR (2003): Axillary dissection with access minimized: a new technique for lymph node dissection in conservative surgery for breast cancer. *Int J Fertil Womens Med Sep Oct;* 48(5): 232-237.

Recht A, Houlihan MJ (1995): Axillary lymph nodesand breast cancer: a review. *Cancer Nov 1;* 76 (9):1491-512

Schottenfeld D et al (1976): Ten year results of the treatment of primary operable breast cancer. *Cancer 1976;* 38:1001-7. Recht A, Houlihan MJ: Axillary lymph nodes and breast cancer: a review. *Cancer Aug;* 76(2):1491-1512.

Simmons RM, Hollenbeck ST, LaTrenta GS (2003): Areola-sparing mastectomy with immediate breast reconstruction. *Ann Plast Surg Dec;* 51(6):547-1.

Taylor KO (2004): Morbidity associated with axillary surgery for breast cancer. *ANZ J Surg. May;* 74(5): 314-7.

Tsangaris TN, Trad K, Brody FJ, et al (1999): Endoscopic axillary exploration and sentinel lymphadenectomy. *Surg Endosc Jan;* 13(1):43-47.

Undre S, Munz Y, Moothy K, Martin *S,* rockall T, Vale J, Darzi A (2004): Robot-assisted laparoscopic adrenalectomy: preliminary UK results. *BJU Int. Feb;* 93 (3): 357-9

Veronesi U et al (1994): Conservative approaches for the management of stage I/II carcinoma of the breast: Milan Cancer Institute trials. *World J Surg Jan-Feb;* 18(1):70-5.

Veronesi U, Paganelli G, Viale G, et al (2003): A randomized comparison of sentinel node biopsy with routine axillary dissection in breast cancer. *N Engl J Med Aug 7,* 349(6):546-53.

18

Robotic-assisted Laparoscopic Renal and Adrenal Surgery

Yves Caumartin, Jeffrey Warren and Patrick P.W. Luke
London Health Sciences Centre, CSTAR, The University of Western Ontario, Schulich School of Medicine
Canada

1. Introduction and Historical Perspective

The worldwide evolution of robotic surgery continues to advance at a staggering pace. In less than 20 years, the technology has grown exponentially from theoretical military application to daily use in operating rooms around the globe. In fact, the overwhelming success of robotic surgery with regards to invention, innovation, and adaptation is an excellent example of collaboration between surgeons, industry, and government. While the first robotic device to be used clinically dates back to computerized tomography-guided stereotactic neurosurgery by Kwoh *et al* in 1988 [1], the first urological application in a human was not described until Davies *et al*[2] used a modified industrial robotic arm to perform a transurethral resection of the prostate three years later. The first commercial application in laparoscopy did not come until the Automated Endoscopic System for Optimal Positioning (AESOP™) was FDA approved in the United States in 1993[7]. Originally designed by the U.S. military, the table-mounted device could precisely guide a laparoscope and was later put into production by Computer Motion Inc. (Santa Barbara, California).[3] Computer Motion Inc. would later introduce the ZEUS™ robotic system onto the U.S. market in 1998, just months after the unveiling of another surgical robot, the da Vinci® (Intuitive Surgical, Sunnyvale, California). The da Vinci® system was born out of technology designed by NASA, also originally intended for use by the U.S. military, but quickly adopted for civilian use. In 2003, Intuitive Surgical took over Computer Motion Inc., thereby paving the way for the da Vinci® robot, along with it's newly FDA approved EndoWrist™, to dominate surgical robotic use worldwide.[3] Today, the vast majority of published literature on robotic-assisted renal surgery has employed the use of the da Vinci® system, and it is the only commercially available master-slave robotic system in production today.

Few studies have addressed the comparative performance and efficiency between the three most cited robotic platforms, namely AESOP, ZEUS and da Vinci®. Sung *et al*[4] initially looked at this question in a porcine model, and we later compared our results in a cohort of patients undergoing pyeloplasty for ureteropelvic junction obstruction (UPJO).[5] Both groups concluded that the da Vinci® system was superior in terms of shorter operative time, quicker anastomotic time, and flatter learning curve. We also found the majority of technical manoeuvering inherently more intuitive with the da Vinci® system compared to the ZEUS system. There does exist some earlier reports of experience with the ZEUS

Telesurgical System by ourselves[6] and others;[7,8] however, the vast majority of published data in recent years has focused almost exclusively on the da Vinci® system. And since the da Vinci® robot is the only master-slave robotic platform currently in production and available commercially, the focus of this chapter will center on this particular system as it applies to renal and adrenal surgical applications.
While the field of urology was not the first medical discipline to embrace robotic technology, it has adopted the technology with open arms. Through innovation and research, robotic-assisted surgery is quickly becoming a routine tool in the urologist's armamentarium. Currently, the majority of clinical indications for the da Vinci® system are for urological use. The majority of published research and clinical experience in the past has focused on robot-assisted radical prostatectomy.[3,9,10] However, the role of robotics in renal surgery continues to be defined. With the exception of robot-assisted laparoscopic pyeloplasty (RALP), the majority of literary publications consist of case series and reports. As such, the emphasis of this chapter will be on RALP. For most other applications, the true role of robot-assisted renal surgery is yet to be defined. Herein we focus on the indications, techniques, and surgical experiences described in the literature to date as it applies specifically to robotic-assisted laparoscopic renal surgery.

2. Nephrectomy and Nephroureterectomy

Robot-assisted extirpative renal surgery has been described as a useful minimally invasive technique for both malignant and benign conditions. While a standard laparoscopic approach is usually employed for nephrectomy and at most centers today, robot-assisted technique are attractive to surgeons with minimal laparoscopic experience. In contrast, most surgeons facile with basic laparoscopic skills have difficulty justifying the use of robotics for what is considered by many a relatively straightforward procedure. Also, the da Vinci® system is not compatible with multi-fire clip appliers or standard endovascular stapling devices required for renovascular ligation and division, further discouraging routine use in the extirpative kidney surgery setting.[9]
Following induction of general anesthesia, the patient is placed in a modified 60° lateral decubitus position with the affected side elevated. Patients are placed on a clear fluid diet 48 hours before surgery and receive an oral mechanical bowel prep the day before. All pressure points are adequately padded and the patient fully secured to the operating table. Using standard laparoscopic techniques, intraperitoneal access is achieved with a 12-mm port for the laparoscope at the level of the umbilicus along the pararectus border on the affected side. Two additional trocars are placed for docking the robotic arms in a typical triangle configuration as per standard laparoscopic nephrectomy (Figure 1). A fourth port is placed at the umbilicus for the surgical assistant, to facilitate instrument exchanges, provide suction-irrigation, insert and remove suture material, and apply clips to the renal vessels [10]. The entire dissection is carried out robotically with the surgeon positioned at the remote console. Once the specimen is completely dissected, hemostasis is achieved with vascular staplers or clips. The specimen is removed via extension of the most inferolateral trocar site or Pfannenstiel incision after endoscopic entrapment in a bag.
A 12-mm camera port is placed just lateral to the rectus at the level of the umbilicus. Technique varies depending on surgeon preference. Additional ports are placed after pneumoperitoneum is established. Two 8-mm robotic arm ports are then positioned

equidistant (approximately 8 to 10 cm or a handwidth) from the camera port at right angles to each other. The surgical area of interest should falls in the center of the triangle created. A 12-mm assistant port is placed at the umbilicus. An extra port can be placed subxiphoid as needed (ie. for liver retraction). These recommendations may need adjustment on a case-by case-basis depending on patient body habitus and clinical scenario.

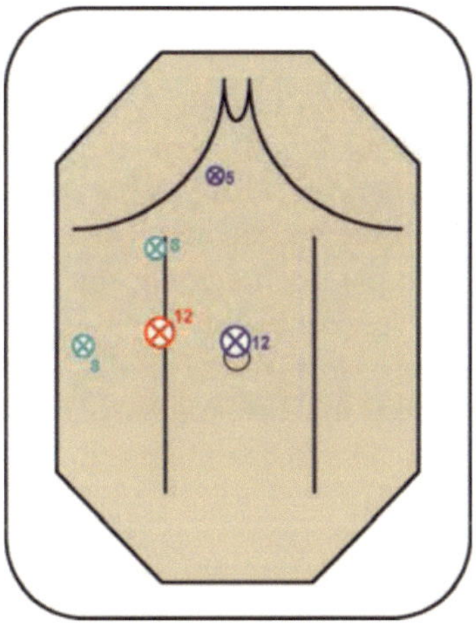

Figure 1. Recommended port placement for transperitoneal robot-assisted laparoscopic nephrectomy and adrenalectomy

While Gill *et al* was the first to report the feasibility of robotic-assisted nephrectomy in a porcine model in 2000[11], the first published report in a human was described by Guillonneau *et al*[12] the following year. The patient was a 77-year-old woman with a hydronephrotic non-functioning kidney secondary to ureteropelvic junction obstruction (UPJO). The ZEUS robotic surgical system was employed with total operating time of 200 minutes and blood loss of less than 100 mL. There were no peri-operative complications. Recently, Storm *et al*[13] presented on 100 cases of robot-assisted laparoscopic nephrectomy. Sixty-six were for suspicious renal masses and non-functioning kidneys, and the remaining 34 were live donors. Median operative time was 170 minutes, estimated blood loss 100 mL, and length of hospital stay was 48 hours. Peri-operative complications occurred in five patients and included atelectasis, pancreatitis, wound infection, bowel injury, and a post-operative death. There were 2 conversions: one to hand-assisted laparascopic nephrectomy and the other to open nephrectomy. The authors concluded robotic-assisted laparoscopic nephrectomy is safe, efficacious, and compares favorably with other minimally invasive techniques. The authors did not comment on cost.

While the need for robotic-assistance in simple and radical nephrectomy is questionable, reports employing the da Vinci® system in more complicated cases continue to be published. Recently, Finley *et al*[14] described combined robot-assisted nephroureterectomy with a hand-assist port followed by robot-assisted radical prostatectomy in a 57-year-old man. Ureteric mobilization and excision of a cuff of bladder was performed robotically followed by standard robotic prostatectomy. Lastly, nephrectomy was performed using a hand-assisted laparoscopy. Total operative time 6.5 hours, blood loss was 200cc, and the post-operative course was uneventful. Nanigian *et al*[15] similarly describe a case serie of ten patients of robotic-assisted distal ureterectomy with a cuff of bladder and pure laparoscopic nephrectomy for a case of upper tract transition cell carcinoma. These reports highlight the potential benefits of combining pure laparoscopic, hand-assisted laparoscopic, and robot-assisted laparoscopic techniques in complex cases.

Employing a retroperitoneal technique, Rose *et al*[16] described robot-assisted nephroureterectomy in two patients - one for a distal ureteric urothelial tumor and the other for a poorly functioning kidney with primary obstructed megaureter. With a mean operative time of 182.5 minutes, blood loss of 75 mL, and no post-operative complications, the authors concluded this is a feasible approach in select patients.

The observation that there have been limited published series in the literature on robot-assisted laparoscopic radical or simple nephrectomy since the initial report by Guillonneau in 2001[12] underscores the tenuous role for robotics in this setting. As experience with more complex combined upper and lower tract procedures are reported in the literature, the role for robotic-assistance in these settings will become further defined.

3. Live Donor Nephrectomy

The greatest experience with extirpative robot-assisted renal surgery involves live donor nephrectomy. While some centers still consider open live donor nephrectomy the "gold standard"[17], experience with laparoscopic donor nephrectomy, both purely laparoscopic and hand-assisted, continues to gain popularity. Advantages of a minimally invasive approach include less post-operative pain, shortened hospital stay, and a quicker return to regular daily activities.[18-20] Minimally invasive live donor nephrectomy is believed to have increased the donor pool by decreasing morbidity compared to open live donor nephrectomy.[21] However, the technically demanding nature of laparoscopic live donor nephrectomy has made it an attractive candidate for robotic assistance. Docking of the robotic arms, laparoscope, and assistant port is identical to that described for nephrectomy for other indications. Special considerations include maximal preservation of renal vessel length, a Pfannenstiel extraction incision, and immediate cold flush on ice with an appropriate preservation solution.[11]

Evidence exists that robotic-assisted live donor nephrectomy (RALDN) is safe, feasible, and with results equivalent to both open and other minimally invasive techniques. Experience from four independent series is summarized in Table 1. The first reported and most extensive series in the literature comes from the group at The University of Chicago. Horgan *et al*[22] described their first 13 cases in 2002 and updated their data on 273 consecutive RALDNs using a hand-assisted technique through April 2006.[23] Their results from both donor and recipient perspectives are similar to other published live donor nephrectomy series and the authors acknowledge the evolution of their own surgical technique over time. Talimini *et al*[24] included their first 15 RALDNs in an early analysis of 211 robotic-assisted surgeries, noting the safety, feasibility, and quick recovery associated with the da Vinci® robotic system. Renoult and colleagues[25] compared their initial 13 cases of RALDN with 13 matched open donor nephrectomies. The only statistically significant differences between the groups were longer warm and cold ischemia times and longer operative times in the RALDN arm; however, the absolute differences were unlikely to be clinically significant. Nonetheless, this does highlight the fact that a learning curve still exists with robotic-assisted techniques.

Author	Year	N	Mean OR time (min)	Mean WIT (sec)	Mean LOS (days)	Allograft outcome	Complications
Horgan [22]	2002	12	166	79	1.9	No DGF	C.diff colitis in 1 pt; wound infection in 1 pt
Talamini [24]	2003	15	143	--	1.0	Not commented on	None
Renoult [25]	2006	13	185	430	5.8	POD 5 Mean ClCr = 62 mL/min	DVT in 1 pt
Horgan [23]	2007	273	150	98	2.3	Mean Cr = 1.4 mg/dL at 6 mos	Overall 9 "major"; 1 death unrelated to OR

WIT = warm ischemic time. LOS = length of stay in hospital. DGF = delayed graft function. POD = post-op day. ClCr = creatinine clearance. DVT = deep venous thrombosis

Table 1. A summary of published surgical series on robot-assisted live donor nephrectomy

4. Partial Nephrectomy

In an era when the majority of renal tumors are discovered incidentally via abdominal imaging for an unrelated indication,[26] these tumors are frequently amenable to nephron-sparing extirpative techniques. Patients with exophytic lesions less than 4 cm are ideal candidates for partial nephrectomy in the elective setting.[27] These techniques are further justified in patients with baseline compromised renal function, the potential for future renal deterioration, or a solitary kidney.[28,29] In recent years, there has been an explosion of reports describing minimally invasive laparoscopic techniques for partial nephrectomy.[30-34] However, purely laparoscopic partial nephrectomy is technically challenging, and strategies to simplify resection and reconstruction while minimizing ischemic time have been sought. Theoretically, the enhanced ability to adjust resection angles facilitate intracorporal suturing with the EndoWrist™ instruments has made robot-assisted partial nephrectomy (RALPN) an especially attractive alternative.

To our knowledge, the first published feasibility report of RALPN was by Gettman *et al* in 2004.[35] Several authors have since described their technique and a number of these publications are summarized in Table 2. All authors have used the da Vinci® surgical robotic system with a transperitoneal approach. Some authors have advocated performing the initial dissection with standard laparoscopic or hand-assisted laparoscopic techniques, reserving the robot to facilitate resection of the tumor and reconstruction after hilar clamping. Use and technique of intra-operative ultrasound, intra-operative frozen sections, argon beam coagulation, and adjuvant hemostatic agents differ between reports. In Gettman's series of 13 cases from the Mayo clinic, 8 cases employed an intra-renal artery occlusion balloon catheter for infusion of cooling solution. The authors report the angiocatheter provided effective arterial occlusion and prevented venous backflow in all cases. However, others have questioned the cost, necessity, and invasiveness of this strategy in the absence of well-controlled prospective series looking at functional renal outcomes.[36]

Author	Year	N	Mean lesion size (cm)	Mean OR time (min)	Hilar clamp time (min)	EBL (mL)	Mean LOS (days)	Complications
Gettman [35]	2004	13	3.5	215	22	170	4.3	1 post-op ileus
Stifelman [105]	2005	1	2.0	230	32	150	2.0	None
Phillips [37]	2005	12	1.8	265	26	240	2.7	2 open conversions for bleeding; 1 conversion for robot malfunction; 1 post-op urine leak
Caruso [36]	2006	10	1.9	279	26	240	2.6	2 conversions for bleeding, poor visualization; 1 post-op urinary retention
Kaul [38]	2007	10	2.0	158	21		1.5	None commented on

EBL = estimated blood loss. LOS = length of hospital stay.

Table 2. Summary of published reports of robot-assisted partial nephrectomy with the da Vinci® system

Phillips *et al*[37] described their initial experience with 12 RALPNs. They highlighted the need for conversion in 3 patients (one of each to standard laparoscopy, hand-assisted laparoscopy, and open) and summarized advantages and disadvantages of robotic assistance in this setting. Specifically, the six degrees of freedom offered by the da Vinci® EndoWrist™, 3-D stereoscopic visualization, movement scale-down, negation of tremor, and console surgeon comfort were notable benefits. Purported disadvantages included cost, set-up time, equipment malfunction, need for robotic training, lack of haptic feedback, and dependence on the table-side assistant at many critical points during the procedure. Caruso *et al*[36], in evaluation of their first 10 RALPNs, found no convincing advantages of the robot over standard laparoscopic partial nephrectomy in experienced hands. They no longer perform RALPN at their institution, but instead emphasize the need for a randomized study in this population. Similarly, Kaul *et al*[38] summarized their initial 10 cases of RALPN at the Vattikuti Institute in Detroit. Their results were similar to other small series in the literature with no conversions and no positive margins. They also noted the need for larger evaluation in multi-center trials and recommended RALPN be performed by surgeons facile in advanced laparoscopy and robotics in order to minimize patient morbidity during the learning phase.

While experience with robotic-assisted renal surgery continues to expand, the exact role of RALPN has yet to be defined. Larger prospective studies with adequate follow-up are necessary to delineate whether or not a robotic approach is safe and effective compared to the "gold standard" open partial nephrectomy. We must also keep in mind that all minimally invasive surgical techniques in this setting are still considered experimental at many centers.

5. Adrenalectomy

The adrenal gland is particularly well suited for a laparoscopic surgical approach. Most adrenal lesions are small but often require a large incision for open surgical access. Since the first laparoscopic adrenalectomy by Gagner in 1992[39,40], a paradigm shift has taken place in favor of laparoscopic adrenalectomy versus the previous standard open approach. Similar to laparoscopic renal surgery, adrenalectomy has immeasurably improved the post-operative recovery in these patients. Objective benefits have been proven regarding shorter hospital stay, reduced pain scores, and faster return to regular activities.[41-45] To date, however, the robotic experience in this population is limited and the role for robotic-assisted adrenalectomy is not yet clear.

Gill *et al*[11] reported the first experience with robot-assisted laparoscopic adrenalectomy in a porcine model. An inferior vena cava injury was repaired via intracorporal suturing without the need for conversion. Young *et al*[46] later performed a robotic-assisted adrenalectomy (RAA) for an incidental left adrenal mass in a patient being evaluated for a widened mediastinum. Final pathology revealed an adrenal oncocytoma. In 2002, Bentas *et al*[47] reported on four robotic-assisted transperitoneal adrenalectomies. There were no complications or conversions. Similarly, Desai *et al*[48] described their experience with two robot-assisted adrenalectomies, including one for pheochromocytoma. There were no peri-operative complications and the patients were discharged home on post-op days 2 and 3, respectively. In an interesting case report, St. Julien and colleagues[49] recently reported a robot-assisted cortical-sparing adrenalectomy in an 18-year old male with Von Hippel-Lindau disease. The patient had presented with a metachronous pheochromocytoma of his remaining solitary adrenal. There were no peri-operative complications and the patient did not require adrenal cortical replacement medication at follow-up. Lastly, Winter *et al*[50] recently published the largest series of robotic-assisted laparoscopic adrenalectomy to date. The series of 30 patients had a median operative time of 185 minutes. They reported a 7% complication rate, including one patient with a prolonged ileus post-op and a brief episode of hypoxemia on the ward in another. There were no open conversions and operative time decreased with increasing surgeon experience. Mean length of hospital stay was 2 days. According to their cost analysis, laparoscopic adrenalectomy was more economical compared to an open approach primarily because of shorter hospitalization, with only a slight difference in favor of standard laparoscopic versus robotic-assisted techniques ($11,599 versus $12,977, respectively).

There are two reports in the literature comparing standard laparoscopic adrenalectomy and robotic adrenalectomy. Brunaud *et al*[51] evaluated their results of 14 robotic-assisted adrenalectomies with 14 standard laparoscopic adrenalectomies. They found an overall longer mean operative time in the robotic arm (111 versus 83 minutes), but a progressive decrease with increasing experience. They concluded no significant advantages to the robotic approach. However, they did highlight that an increased body mass index did not adversely affect the technique of robotic-assisted adrenalectomy, suggesting a possible benefit in larger patients. The same group reported a one-year follow-up quality of life study that did not show any difference between the two groups.[52] Morino *et al*[53] reported their experience with 10 robotic-assisted adrenalectomies (two for pheochromocytoma) and compared them with 10 standard laparoscopic adrenalectomies. Operative time was significantly longer in the robotic group (mean 107 versus 82 minutes) and there were no adverse peri-operative complications. However, four of the robotic cases were converted to standard laparoscopy for technical reasons. Furthermore, cost was strongly in favor of the standard laparoscopic approach ($2,737 versus $3,467). Publications about RAA are summarized in Table 3.

Author	Year	Comparison	N	Median OR time (min)	Complications (%)	Conversion (%)	LOS (day)	Comments
St. Julien [49]	2006		1		0	0	NA	Partial adrenalectomy on VHL patient
Winter [50]	2006		30	185	7	0	2	RAA $12, 997 LA $11, 599 OA $14, 600
Morino [53]	2004	LA	10	82	0	0	5.4	$2, 737
		RAA	10	107	20	40 to LA	5.7	$3, 467
Brunaud [51]	2003	LA	14	83	21	7		Similar Q of L [52]
		RAA	14	111	21	7		
D'Annibale[106]	2004		1	110	0	0	2	
Desai [48]	2002		2	135	0	0	2.5	
Bentas. [47]	2002		4	220	0	0	5	
Young [46]	2002		1	100	0	0	1	

LA = laparoscopic adrenalectomy. RAA = robot-assisted adrenalectomy. OA = open adrenalectomy. LOS = length of stay in hospital. Q of L = quality of life. NA = non available

Table 3. Summary of published reports of robot-assisted adrenalectomy with the da Vinci® robotic system

6. Pyeloplasty

Open dismembered pyeloplasty is the gold standard treatment for adult ureteropelvic junction obstruction (UPJO) with published success rates consistently over 90%.[54,55] However, the morbidity of an open flank incision led to experimentation with other less invasive modalities such as endopyelotomy and laparoscopic techniques. Following the first description by Schuessler *et al*[56], modern laparoscopic pyeloplasty series consistently demonstrate equivalent success rates to open series with improved postoperative convalescence.[57-62] The need for complex intracorporeal reconstruction has limited the widespread application of standard laparoscopic pyeloplasty, thereby paving the road for a robotic-assisted approach. The da Vinci® surgical robotic platform offers features that simplify intracorporeal reconstruction and suturing, thereby shortening the learning curve for residents, clinical fellows, and other novice laparoscopists alike.

Sung and colleagues[4,63] were the first to explore the feasibility of robotic-assisted laparoscopic pyeloplasty (RALP) in pigs. Guillonneau[64] later confirmed the technical feasibility and safety of a robotic approach in an animal model. The first clinical experience in humans was reported in 2002 by Gettman *et al*,[65,66] and provided satisfactory short-term results in a small number of patients. Since then, several other groups have reported their experience with robotic-assisted laparoscopic pyeloplasty. These reports are summarized in Tables 4 and 5.

Diagnosis of UPJO is based on clinical presentation (ie. renal colic, febrile urinary tract infection) and imaging studies. Traditional diagnostic investigations include excretory urogram, renal ultrasound, and CT, classically revealing hydronephrosis with a non-dilated ureter and no obvious cause for obstruction (ie. stone or tumor). Functional obstruction is typically confirmed by furosemide-nuclear renogram, providing information on the degree of obstruction and split renal function. It also serves as a baseline if surgical intervention is planned. In select cases, if a primary endoscopic treatment is planned, the presence of a crossing vessel can be established usisng CT [67], Magnetic Resonance Imaging (MRI) [68] or contrast-enhanced Doppler ultrasonography.[69-71]
The indications for RALP are the same as standard laparoscopic or open pyeloplasty. RALP has been performed safely and effectively in patients with primary UPJO or secondary UPJO following a failed previous repair.[72-75] RALP in pelvic and horseshoe kidneys has been reported with good results.[72,74,76] Also, the robotic approach can be used to successfully manage concomitant renal stones at the time of the surgery.[74,76-78] Contraindications to RALP are the same as standard laparoscopic pyeloplasty and include poor renal function, poor surgical candidate, uncorrected coagulopathy, abdominal wall infection, and bowel obstruction.
The technique for RALP has been well described in a number of reports. At our center, all patients receive a full mechanical bowel preparation the day before surgery. Prophylactic antibiotics are administered 30-60 minutes before the initial incision and deep venous thrombosis prophylaxis is routinely employed based on patient risk stratification (sequential compression device or thrombo-embolic stockings +/- subcutaneous heparin).

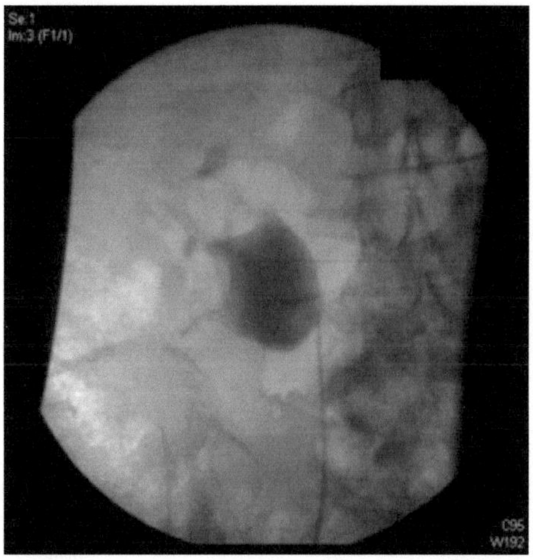

Figure 2. Pre-operative retrograde pyelogram demonstrating findings consistent with a right ureteropelvic junction obstruction

The use of an indwelling ureteral stent is recommended, but the timing and method of placement is based on surgeon preference. At our institution, after induction of general anesthesia we perform a retrograde pyelogram with the patient supine to confirm the diagnosis (Figure 2). The UPJ is localized and the overlying skin is marked for future reference and as a guide for port-placement. A double-"J" ureteral stent is then inserted under fluoroscopic guidance.[74,79-81] A 3-way bladder catheter is inserted and connected to a 1-litre bag of sterile normal saline with methylene blue. Some authors prefer an indwelling 5-French open-ended ureteral catheter prepped in the surgical field. This can later be used to exchange for a double-"J" stent with a guide wire under laparoscopic visualization.[77,82,83] Finally, others prefer to insert a double-"J" stent antegrade over a guidewire through the assistant port[72,76,84] or through a large-bore angiocath directly through the abdominal wall in a subcostal position.[85] With these latter strategies, it is recommended to confirm proper placement of the distal end of the stent intra-operatively by filling the bladder and observing for reflux laparoscopically. Alternatively, cystoscopy can be performed intra-operatively or placement confirmed with a single abdominal film in the recovery room.

Once the double-"J" stent placement is confirmed, the patient is placed and secured in a modified 60° lateral decubitus position with a beanbag and tape. We do not routinely flex the table and we ensure that all pressure points are padded appropriately. An orogastric tube is useful to decompress the stomach and increase the working spaces for left-sided procedures. Figure 3 give an overview of the operating room setup. Pneumoperitoneum is achieved with a Veress needle or Hasson trochar and the initial 12-mm port is placed at the umbilicus. Most authors use this port for the laparoscope. Two additional 8-mm robotic arm ports are then placed so as to form an isosceles triangle with the base facing laterally (Figure 4). Depending on surgeon preference, a 12-mm assistant-port is placed either subxyphoid, inferior to the camera port, or just caudal to McBurney's point on the ipsilateral side. This port can be used for suction-irrigation, to help with retraction, introducing and removing suturing material, and placement of a double-"J" stent. Nephroscopy and basket stone extraction can also be performed through this port as needed. Some authors, especially in the pediatric setting, use only 3 ports altogether.[74,85,86]

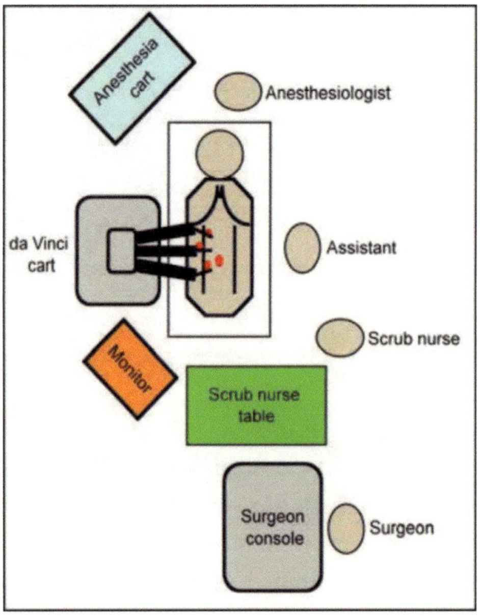

Figure 3. Operating room setup for robotic-assisted laparoscopic pyeloplasty

The patient is placed in a 60° lateral decubitus position. After port placement, the da Vinci® system is positioned over the patient's ipsilateral flank. The primary surgeon is seated at the remote surgical console. The surgical assistant is situated on the contralateral side across from the robot. A scrub nurse is near the foot of the bed. A monitor is positioned in view of the surgical assistant and scrub nurse. The anesthesiologist is at the head of the table.

A 12-mm camera port is placed at the umbilicus. Two robotic arm ports are then placed to create a triangle with the base facing laterally. A 12-mm assistant port can be placed as per surgeon preference -- subxyphoid, just medial to the camera port, or caudally in the vicinity of McBurney's point.

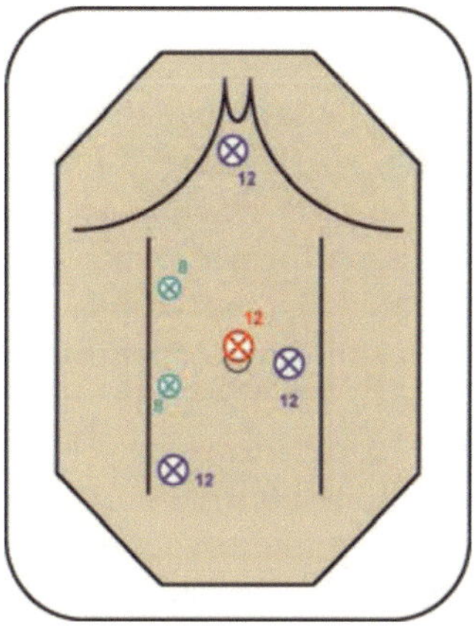

Figure 4. Port placement for transperitoneal robot-assisted laparoscopic pyeloplasty, as usually described in the literature

Our own technique is a somewhat different. We use a 12-mm umbilical port for the assistant. The laparoscope is placed at the skin marker previously set during retrograde pyelography. This point usually lies along the anterior axillary line. We then place two additional 8-mm robotic arm ports to create an isosceles triangle with the base facing medially (Figure 5). We feel this technique allows more freedom for the assistant to maneuver. The subxiphoid position is often constrained by the patient's arm and a too-medial position often is restricting due to nearby loops of bowel.
A 12-mm port is inserted at the umbilicus as described by Hassan and pneumoperitoneum is established. This serves as the assistant's. A second 12-mm camera port is placed lateral at the estimated location of the UPJ. Lastly, two robotic arm ports are placed medial to camera port so as to create a triangle with the base facing medially.

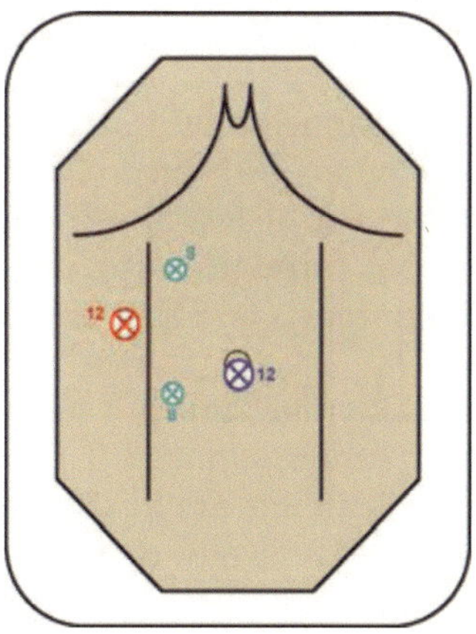

Figure 5. Port placement for transperitoneal robot-assisted laparoscopic pyeloplasty as per Luke's modification

Using the da Vinci® platform, all steps of traditional Anderson-Hynes dismembered pyeloplasty, Y-V plasty and Fenger-plasty can be performed.[65,72,74,77,87] We usually employ a dismembered technique as we believe this provides the best results in open and standard laparoscopic pyeloplasty. It also allows versatility in almost all clinical scenarios, including crossing vessels, renal calculi, a large pelvis that needs to be reduced, and secondary repairs.[88] A standard set of laparoscopic instruments is required in addition to the robotic ones, namely monopolar hook cautery, forceps, needle drivers and scissors.

Some authors described a hybrid approach whereby the initial dissection of the colon, renal pelvis and proximal ureter is performed using standard laparoscopic techniques, reserving the robot for the ureteropelvic anastomosis.[74,77,83,84,89] We routinely perform the entire procedure robotically to minimize operative time changing and exchanging instruments. The robot is positioned on the ipsilateral side of the patient, angled over their exposed flank and the three robotic arms are engaged with the working ports and the camera port (Figure 6). For right-sided UPJO, the line of Toldt is incised and the hepatic flexure is retracted medially to identify Gerota's fascia. For left-sided UPJO, the standard approach similarly involves incision of the line of Toldt and medial mobilization of the descending colon to expose Gerota's fascia. In thin or pediatric patients with left-sided UPJO, an alternative transmesenteric approach has been described.[72,74,85,86,90] The ureter is identified distally and followed cephalad to the UPJ. The UPJ itself and any associated crossing vessels are then dissected free. If renal calculi are present,[74,76-78] a small pyelotomy incision is made at the UPJ and flexible nephroscopy and stone extraction are performed through the assistant port. Stones are removed via basket extraction or placed in an extraction bag, depending on size and number. Next, the UPJ is transected, the stenotic segment is excised, and the ureteral end is spatulated laterally. The proximal end of the stent is removed from the renal pelvis and, if necessary, the pelvis is reduced by a diamond-shape excision. If an anterior crossing vessel is present, the renal pelvis is transposed anterior to the vessel and the posterior aspect of the anastomosis is performed with a running 5-0 polydioxanone suture, cut to 15 cm in length. The proximal end of the stent is then replaced into the renal pelvis. The anterior wall of the anastomosis is completed with a second running suture. Occasionally there is some redundancy of the proximal renal pelvis necessitating a third running suture for adequate closure. We then fill the bladder with the methylene blue saline solution to assess for reflux and ensure the anastomosis is watertight. Any obvious leak is corrected with additional suture. Once hemostasis is achieved and confirmed at low insufflation pressure, a 7-mm Jackson-Pratt close-suction drain is inserted through one of the 8-mm ports once the robot is undocked. The fascia of the 12-mm ports and skin are re-approximated as per surgeon preference.

Postoperative management is usually uneventful. The bladder catheter is removed in 1-2 days. The close-suction drain is then removed if there is no significant increase in output with spontaneous voiding. Patients are discharged home on post-operative day 1 or 2 pending no complications. We typically remove the ureteral stent 4 weeks post-op. A follow-up furosemide-nuclear renogram is performed at approximately 10 weeks and 6 months post-operatively. Follow-up ultrasound is obtained in pediatric patients, reserving a renogram for select cases or surgeon preference. Some authors prefer repeat imaging on an annual basis. In the context of normal post-operative imaging and no symptoms we usually stop follow-up at 6 months, recognizing that late recurrence in this setting is rare.[61]

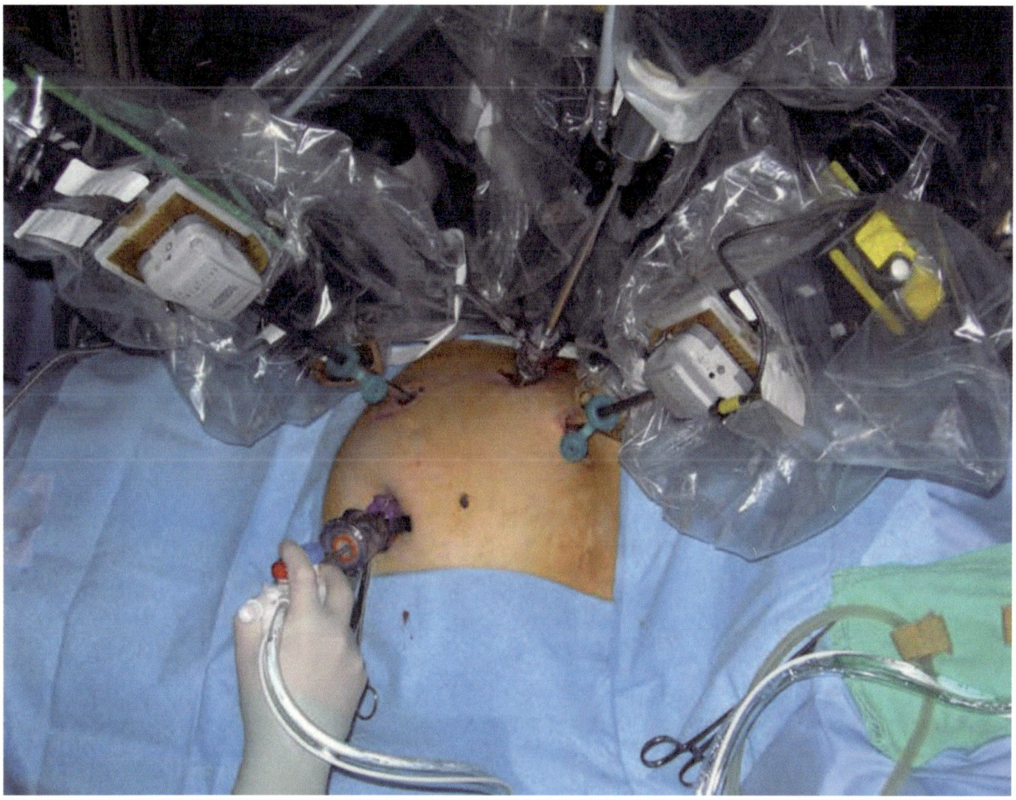

Figure 6. Port placement and robot docking position for a patient undergoing a right robotic pyeloplasty

There is an expanding body of literature on RALP, a summary of which is presented in Table 4. Comparative studies between RALP and open or standard laparoscopic pyeloplasty are summarized in Table 5. Schwentner *et al*[72] reported on the largest series of RALP with a relatively long median follow up of 39 months. All 92 patients underwent Anderson-Hynes dismembered RALP. Twelve patients had secondary UPJO and 2 patients had a horseshoe kidney. There were no intra-operative complications and no open conversion. Anterior crossing vessels were found in 45 patients (49%). The mean operative time was 108 minutes, including time to dock and undock the robot. As similarly reported by many other authors,[72,74,77,84,87,90,91] their operative time decreased significantly with increased experience of the surgical team and the technical staff. The mean anastomotic time was only 25 minutes and the average blood loss was less than 50 ml. There were three notable post-operative complications: one patient developed clot colic requiring stent exchange and percutaneous nephrostomy; another patient bled into the collecting system that was managed non-operatively; and one patient developed a prolonged urine leak managed conservatively. The mean hospital stay was 4.6 days and the overall success rate was 96.7%.

Author	Gettman [66]	Bentas [91]	Yohannes [89]	Peschel	Atug [78]	Atug [83]	Mendez-Torres [77]	Palese [84]	Patel [87]	Siddiq [74]	Atug [73]	Chammas [76]	Kutikov [85]	Schwentner [72]
Year	2002	2003	2003	2004	2005	2005	2005	2005	2005	2005	2006	2006	2006	2007
N	9	11	1	49	8	7	32	38	50	26	44	3	9	92
Mean f-up (months)	4.1	21	NA	7.4	12.3	10.9	8.6	12.2	11.7	6	13.1	21	6	39.1
Mean age (years)	NA	NA	73	NA	39.5	12	31.2	39.3	31	34.5	33.6	44.6	5.6 months	35.1
Crossing vessel (%)	NA	36	100	NA	25	43	44	26	30	42	41	0	0	49
Secondary UPJO (%)	22	0	0	19	NA	0	9	5	10	15	16	0	0	13
Associated calculi (%)	NA	NA	0	NA	100	NA	23	5	NA	23	NA	66	NA	NA
Horseshoe or pelvic kidney (%)	NA	NA	0	NA	NA	NA	NA	2.5	NA	4	NA	100	NA	2
OR time (min)	139	197	300	124	275	184	300	226	122	245	229 (primary UPJO 219 vs secondary UPJO 280)	148	123	108
Suturing time (min)	62	NA	45	NA	54	40	NA	64	20	47	NA	NA	60	25
Blood loss (ml)	< 50	50	150	50	48	31	50	77	40	69	50	<100	NA	<50
Complications (%)	11 (leak requiring reintervention)	0	0	2 (leak requiring open repair)	0	0	6 (1 UTI, 1 stent migration)	10.5 (3 UTI, 1 gluteal compartment syndrome)	0	11 (1 UTI, 1 leak, 1 hernia)	0	33 (1 UTI)	0	3 (1 leak, 1 hemorrhage, 1 clots in urine)
LOS (days)	4.7	5.5	4	NA	1.1	1.2	1.1	2.9	1.1	2	1.1	7.6	1.4	4.6
Success (%)	100	100	NA	100	100	100	94.4	94.7	100	95	100	100	100	96.7

UPJO = ureteropelvic junction obstruction. LOS = length of stay in hospital. UTI = urinary tract infection. NA = non available

Table 4. Summary of published reports of robot-assisted pyeloplasty with the da Vinci® system

Author	Gettman [65]				Bernie [81]		Lee [86]		Link [80]		Weise [82]		Yee [75]	
Year	2002				2005		2006		2006		2006		2006	
Comparison	LP		RALP		LP	RALP	OP	RALP	LP	RALP	LP	RALP	OP	RALP
Surgical technique	DM	FP	DM	FP	DM	DM	DM	DM	DM	DM	Combined	Combined	DM	DM
N	4	2	4	2	7	7	33	33	10	10	14	31	8	8
Mean f-up (months)	NA	NA	NA	NA	24	10	20	10	NA	NA	10	6	53.2	14.7
Mean age (years)	NA	NA	NA	NA	34	32	7.6	7.8	38	46.5	24.5	26	9.8	11.5
Crossing vessel (%)	NA	NA	NA	NA	86	57	45	33	NA	NA	50	74	NA	NA
Secondary UPJO (%)	NA	NA	NA	NA	0	0	0	0	0	0	7	0	0	12.5
OR time (min)	235	100	140	78	312	324	181	219	81	123	299	271	248	363
Suturing time (min)	120	28	70	13	NA	NA	NA	NA	NA	NA	NA	60	NA	NA
Blood loss (ml)	50		50		40	60	15	3	NA	NA	<100	<100	59	13
Complications (%)	0	0	0	0	28 (2 leak)	14 (1 UTI)	0	3 (1 missed crossing vessel)	0	10 (1 leak)	14 (1 port hernia, 1 hematoma)	6 (1 leak, 1 UTI)	0	12.5 (1 ileus)
LOS (days)	4		4		3	2.5	3.5	2.3	NA	NA	2.6	2.1	3.3	2.4
Success (%)	NA		NA		100	100	100	94	100	100	100	97	86	100
Cost									RALP 2.7X the cost of LP. 1.7X if they exluded robot depreciation					

DM = dismembered. FP = Fenger-plasty. UPJO = ureteropelvic junction obstruction. LOS = length of stay in hospital. UTI = urinary tract infection. LP = laparoscopic pyeloplasty. RALP = robot-assisted laparoscopic pyeloplasty. OP = open pyeloplasty. LOS = length of stay in hospital. Q of L = quality of life. NA = non available

Table 5. Summary of published reports comparing robot-assisted pyeloplasty with the da Vinci® system to standard laparoscopic pyeloplasty or open pyeloplasty

Patel *et al*[87] published a series of 50 patients with a median follow up of 11.7 months. There were no post-op complications and most patients went home on post-operative day one. Ninety-six percent had both objective and subjective improvement. As shown in Table 4 and in a recent publication by Shah and colleagues,[79] most series report operative times between 108 to 300 minutes and estimated blood loss from 30 to 100 ml. Complications ranged from 0 to 11% and include urine leak, urinary tract infection, stent migration, port site hernias, hemorrhage and hematoma. One group[92] reported a gluteal compartment syndrome in an obese patient following a long procedure at the beginning of their experience. Another group[86] reported missing a crossing vessel during a retroperitoneal RALP in a child. A second transperitoneal RALP was performed successfully. Most authors considered subjective improvement in symptoms and improved drainage on furosemide-nuclear renogram as markers for success. Reported success rates vary from 94 to 100%. Subgroup analysis by some authors reported comparable results for high-risk patients including secondary UPJO, UPJO in a horseshoe kidney, concomitant pelvicalyceal calculi, and infants less than 3 months old.[75,83,85,86,93] In an interesting case report Yee and colleagues described a robot-assisted reconstruction of a post-traumatic urteropelvic junction disruption. The procedure was performed one month after the injury with a satisfactory result.[94]

Based on these and other publications directly comparing RALP with open or standard laparoscopic pyeloplasty, we conclude that the robotic approach appears safe and effective (see Table 5). Intermediate-term results are slowly accumulating in the literature and compare favorably with open pyeloplasty results. Unfortunately, as with other applications of robotic-assisted surgery, the biggest drawback and criticism centers on the purported lack of cost-effectiveness compared to other less expensive modalities.[80,95-97]

7. Other Applications of Robotic-assisted Renal Surgery

There are numerous case reports and a few case series in the literature describing novel and innovative applications of surgical robots. A few examples of these applications have been described specifically pertaining to renal surgery.

Luke *et al*[98] described a technique of robotic-assisted renal artery aneurysm resection and reconstruction using the da Vinci® sytem. The patient was a 54-year-old male with a serially expanding 2.5-cm incompletely calcified saccular renal artery aneursym on the left side (Figure 7). Using a 5-trochar technique, the entire dissection, resection and end-end anastomotic reconstruction was carried out robotically (Figure 8). A saphenous vein interposition graft was harvested but not needed during the reconstruction. Total operative time was 360 minutes, warm ischemic time was 59 minutes, and arterial anastomotic time was 10.5 minutes. The estimated blood loss was 650 mL and the post-operative course was uneventful. At 2 months follow-up split renal function on renal scan was 55:45 for right and left, respectively. Follow-up CT-scan performed two years after surgery showed complete absence of aneurysmal dilatation and prompt, complete uptake of contrast by the kidney (Figure 9).

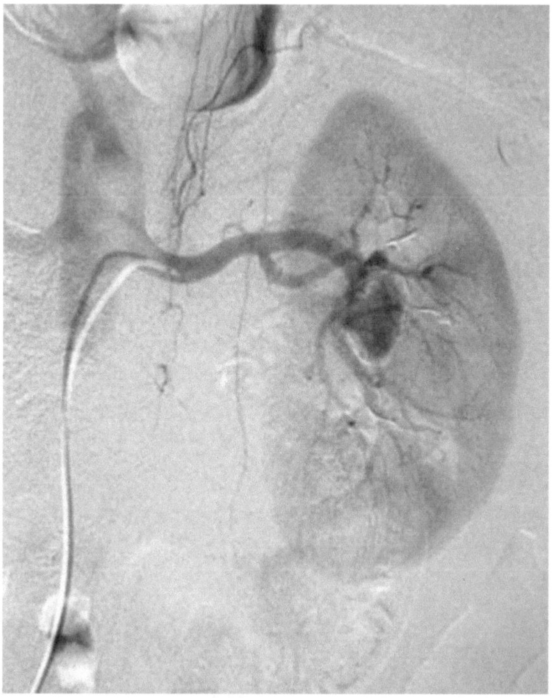

a)

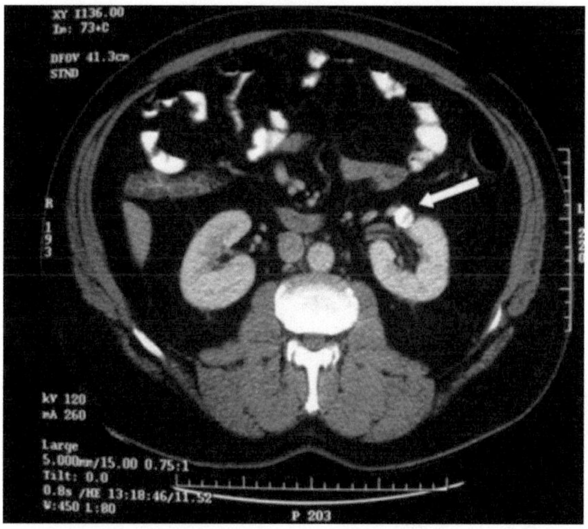

b)

Figure 7. a) Preoperative renal angiography demonstrates a calcified 2.5 cm left-sided saccular aneurysm. b) Preoperative abdominal CT scan shows the hilar location of the renal aneurysm (white arrow)

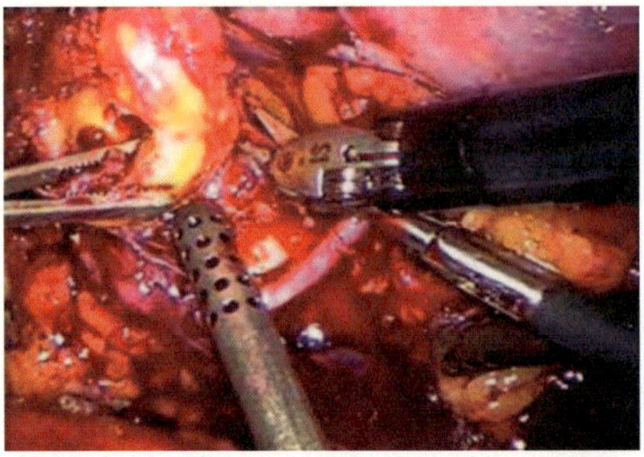

a)

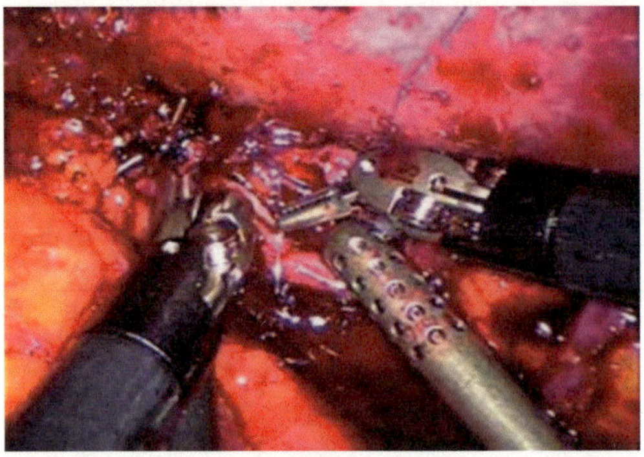

b)

Figure 8. a) Videoscopic view of the renal artery aneurysm during its excision with the laparoscopic scissors. b) Videoscopic view during robotic-assisted reconstruction of the anterior wall of the renal artery

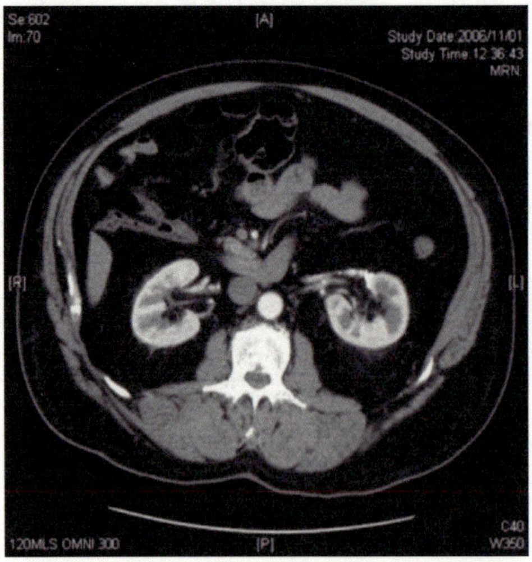

Figure 9. Follow-up abdominal CT scan performed 30 months postoperatively, confirming resolution of the aneurysm and prompt arterial flow to the left kidney

Hoznek *et al*[99] have described a robotic-assisted kidney transplant. The recipient was 26-year-old male with end-stage renal disease secondary to focal segmental glomerulosclerosis and a prior rejected transplant. The allograft was a right kidney with inferior vena cava reconstruction from a heart-beating cadaveric donor. The surgical assistant made a left lower quadrant Gibson incision, developed the retroperitoneal working space, positioned the retractor, provided cautery hemostasis, and placed vascular clamps. The external iliac arterial and venous dissections and the vascular anastomoses were performed entirely by the console surgeon. A Lich-Gregoir ureteroneocystostomy was also performed robotically. Cold ischemia time was over 26 hours, operative time was 178 minutes, and anastomotic time was 57 minutes. Delayed graft function secondary to acute tubular necrosis resolved after one week and there was satisfactory graft function at two months.

Orvieto *et al*[100] described robotic-assisted reconstruction of a strictured tranplant ureter. The patient was a 35-year-old recipient of a combined kidney-pancreas transplant. An extensive allograft ureteric stricture was diagnosed following recurrent urinary tract infections and an episode of urosepsis. The da Vinci® robot was employed for pyeloureterostomy from the allograft renal pelvis to the native ureter. The initial right lower quadrant dissection was performed with the Harmonic Scalpel® (Ethicon Endo-Surgery Inc.) and standard laparoscopic techniques. Total operative time was 320 minutes, estimated blood loss was 20 mL, and the patient was discharged home on post-operative day 4. Allograft function remained stable, radiographic resolution of obstruction was documented, and there were no recurrent episodes of infection at 12-month follow-up. The authors concluded that robotic assistance allowed for efficient complex reconstruction without sacrificing the benefits of a minimally invasive approach.

The above case reports highlight the potential role for robotic-assisted surgery in complex renal reconstructive procedures. And while certainly none of these techniques will become routine practice in the foreseeable future, pushing the boundaries of current technology will undoubtedly help form the basis for future innovation. Furthermore, exercises such as these will help define the collaborative role of open, laparoscopic, and robotic surgery in the future.

8. Future Considerations

Robotic surgery is still in its infancy. The fields of urology, cardiac surgery, neurosurgery, orthopedics, and fetal surgery have already embraced this new technology with the ambition of advancing medical frontiers and application. The goal of applied surgical robotics is improved patient care. Through active clinical and laboratory experimentation, applications specific to robotic renal surgery will hopefully advance in parallel with other disciplines.

Future invention and innovation with regards to surgical robotic technology currently evolves around a number of spheres. At the forefront is improved visualization technology in the form of augmented reality and image guided surgery. Enhanced real-time imaging has been proposed for the next generation surgical robot.[101] Robotic ultrasound and acoustic holography may soon provide real-time imaging that can predict normal from abnormal tissues intraoperatively. Robotic-enhanced haptic and temperature sensors may someday solve the problem of lack of haptic feedback with current surgical robots, and will likely mimic human tactile feeling with greater sensitivity and precision.[102] Diagnostic sensors engaged on robotic arms may preclude the need for biopsy and pathological analysis to detect cancer. Lastly, collaboration between nanotechnology and microbiology may someday permit "DNA-assembly robots" to perform "surgery" on the molecular level analogous to the console surgeon with the da Vinci® system today. A detailed synopsis on the future of robotic surgical technology is beyond the scope of this chapter.[102]

The current status of any new or developed discipline can quickly be gleaned from the number of students trying to learn it. The interest in acquiring laparoscopic skills, in general, and robotic skills, in particular, is evidenced by dramatic shifts in residency training programs. In a survey of American and Canadian urology residents on laparoscopic and robotic surgery, 54% of respondents reported robotic surgery was being performed at their center. Twenty-two percent of resident respondents had been trained in robotic surgery and 34% anticipated performing robotic surgery upon completion of residency. Questions in the survey addressed both robotic prostatectomy and pyeloplasty.[103] In contrast, results of a similar survey of residents and practicing urologists published just two years prior did not even address robotic surgery.[104] This observation highlights the shift in attitudes towards robotic surgery in urology in contemporary times.

Although the future role of robotics in renal surgery is still unclear, robotic-assisted surgery in urology as it pertains to prostatectomy appears here to stay. As a niche for robotic-assisted pyeloplasty and partial nephrectomy continues to be carved out, interest in radical extirpative renal surgery appears to have waned in recent years. And while there may be a role for robotic-assistance in complicated renal reconstructive procedures, this role has yet to be defined and for the time being consists solely of enlightening case reports. Nonetheless, these are interesting times in the collaborative fields of both urology and robotics, and the next decade of research and exploration will likely clarify some of these issues as robotic technology continues to mature. Hopefully, through further education, technological advancement and commercial competition, surgical robotics will become more accessible to the majority of practicing urologists and their patients in the near future.

9. References

Kwoh YS, Hou J, Jonckheere EA and Hayati S: A robot with improved absolute positioning accuracy for CT guided stereotactic brain surgery. *IEEE Trans Biomed Eng.* 35: 153-60, 1988.[1]

Davies BL, Hibberd RD, Ng WS, Timoney AG and Wickham JE: The development of a surgeon robot for prostatectomies. *Proc Inst Mech Eng* [H]. 205: 35-8, 1991. [2]

Eichel L: Robotics in urologic surgery: risks and benefits: *AUA Update Series*, 2005, vol. 24, pp 106-112. [3]

Sung GT and Gill IS: Robotic laparoscopic surgery: a comparison of the DA Vinci and Zeus systems. *Urology.* 58: 893-8, 2001. [4]

Nguan C, Kwan K, Al Omar M, Beasley KA and Luke PP: Robotic pyeloplasty: experience with three robotic platforms. *Can J Urol.* 14: 3571-6, 2007. [5]

Luke PP, Girvan AR, Al Omar M, Beasley KA and Carson M: Laparoscopic robotic pyeloplasty using the Zeus Telesurgical System. *Can J Urol.* 11: 2396-400, 2004. [6]

Miyake O, Kiuchi H, Yoshimura K and Okuyama A: Urological robotic surgery: preliminary experience with the Zeus system. *Int J Urol.* 12: 928-32, 2005.[7]

Lorincz A, Knight CG, Kant AJ, Langenburg SE, Rabah R, Gidell K, Dawe E, Klein MD and McLorie G: Totally minimally invasive robot-assisted unstented pyeloplasty using the Zeus Microwrist Surgical System: an animal study. *J Pediatr Surg.* 40: 418-22, 2005. [8]

Kaul S and Menon M: Robotics in laparoscopic urology. *Minim Invasive Ther Allied Technol.* 14: 62-70, 2005. [9]

Hoznek A, Hubert J, Antiphon P, Gettman MT, Hemal AK and Abbou CC: Robotic renal surgery. *Urol Clin North Am.* 31: 731-6, 2004. [10]

Gill IS, Sung GT, Hsu TH and Meraney AM: Robotic remote laparoscopic nephrectomy and adrenalectomy: the initial experience. *J Urol.* 164: 2082-5, 2000. [11]

Guillonneau B, Jayet C, Tewari A and Vallancien G: Robot assisted laparoscopic nephrectomy. *J Urol.* 166: 200-1, 2001. [12]

Storm D, Fulmer B, Danella J, Sumfest J and Rukstalis D: Robotic-assisted laparoscopic nephrectomy: experience with 100 cases. Abst.#697. *The Journal of Urology.* 177: 234, 2007. [13]

Finley DS, Melamud O and Ornstein DK: Combined robot-assisted laparoscopic nephroureterectomy and radical prostatectomy. *J Endourol.* 21: 411-4, 2007. [14]

Nanigian DK, Smith W and Ellison LM: Robot-assisted laparoscopic nephroureterectomy. J *Endourol.* 20: 463-5; discussion 465-6, 2006. [15]

Rose K, Khan S, Godbole H, Olsburgh J and Dasgupta P: Robotic assisted retroperitoneoscopic nephroureterectomy -- first experience and the hybrid port technique. *Int J Clin Pract.* 60: 12-4, 2006. [16]

Najarian JS, Chavers BM, McHugh LE and Matas AJ: 20 years or more of follow-up of living kidney donors. *Lancet.* 340: 807-10, 1992. [17]

Tooher RL, Rao MM, Scott DF, Wall DR, Francis DM, Bridgewater FH and Maddern GJ: A systematic review of laparoscopic live-donor nephrectomy. *Transplantation.* 78: 404-14, 2004. [18]

Novotny MJ: Laparoscopic live donor nephrectomy. *Urol Clin North Am.* 28: 127-35, 2001. [19]

Leventhal JR, Deeik RK, Joehl RJ, Rege RV, Herman CH, Fryer JP, Kaufman D, Abecassis M and Stuart FP: Laparoscopic live donor nephrectomy--is it safe? *Transplantation.* 70: 602-6, 2000. [20]

Lee BR, Chow GK, Ratner LE and Kavoussi LR: Laparoscopic live donor nephrectomy: outcomes equivalent to open surgery. *J Endourol.* 14: 811-9; discussion 819-20, 2000. [21]

Horgan S, Vanuno D, Sileri P, Cicalese L and Benedetti E: Robotic-assisted laparoscopic donor nephrectomy for kidney transplantation. *Transplantation.* 73: 1474-9, 2002. [22]

Horgan S, Galvani C, Gorodner MV, Jacobsen GR, Moser F, Manzelli A, Oberholzer J, Fisichella MP, Bogetti D, Testa G, Sankary HN and Benedetti E: Effect of robotic assistance on the "learning curve" for laparoscopic hand-assisted donor nephrectomy. *Surg Endosc,* 2007. [23]

Talamini MA, Chapman S, Horgan S and Melvin WS: A prospective analysis of 211 robotic-assisted surgical procedures. Surg Endosc. 17: 1521-4, 2003. [24]

Renoult E, Hubert J, Ladriere M, Billaut N, Mourey E, Feuillu B and Kessler M: Robot-assisted laparoscopic and open live-donor nephrectomy: a comparison of donor morbidity and early renal allograft outcomes. *Nephrol Dial Transplant.* 21: 472-7, 2006. [25]

Pantuck AJ, Zisman A, Rauch MK and Belldegrun A: Incidental renal tumors. *Urology.* 56: 190-6, 2000. [26]

Herr HW: Partial nephrectomy for unilateral renal carcinoma and a normal contralateral kidney: 10-year followup. *J Urol.* 161: 33-4; discussion 34-5, 1999. [27]

Lau WK, Blute ML, Weaver AL, Torres VE and Zincke H: Matched comparison of radical nephrectomy vs nephron-sparing surgery in patients with unilateral renal cell carcinoma and a normal contralateral kidney. *Mayo Clin Proc.* 75: 1236-42, 2000. [28]

Fergany AF, Hafez KS and Novick AC: Long-term results of nephron sparing surgery for localized renal cell carcinoma: 10-year followup. *J Urol.* 163: 442-5, 2000. [29]

Beasley KA, Al Omar M, Shaikh A, Bochinski D, Khakhar A, Izawa JI, Welch RO, Chin JL, Kapoor A and Luke PP: Laparoscopic versus open partial nephrectomy. *Urology.* 64: 458-61, 2004. [30]

Simon SD, Ferrigni RG, Novicki DE, Lamm DL, Swanson SS and Andrews PE: Mayo Clinic Scottsdale experience with laparoscopic nephron sparing surgery for renal tumors. *J Urol.* 169: 2059-62, 2003. [31]

Ogan K and Cadeddu JA: Minimally invasive management of the small renal tumor: review of laparoscopic partial nephrectomy and ablative techniques. *J Endourol.* 16: 635-43, 2002. [32]

Haber GP and Gill IS: Laparoscopic partial nephrectomy: contemporary technique and outcomes. *Eur Urol.* 49: 660-5, 2006. [33]

Guillonneau B, Bermudez H, Gholami S, El Fettouh H, Gupta R, Adorno Rosa J, Baumert H, Cathelineau X, Fromont G and Vallancien G: Laparoscopic partial nephrectomy for renal tumor: single center experience comparing clamping and no clamping techniques of the renal vasculature. *J Urol.* 169: 483-6, 2003. [34]

Gettman MT, Blute ML, Chow GK, Neururer R, Bartsch G and Peschel R: Robotic-assisted laparoscopic partial nephrectomy: technique and initial clinical experience with DaVinci robotic system. *Urology.* 64: 914-8, 2004. [35]

Caruso RP, Phillips CK, Kau E, Taneja SS and Stifelman MD: Robot assisted laparoscopic partial nephrectomy: initial experience. *J Urol.* 176: 36-9, 2006. [36]

Phillips CK, Taneja SS and Stifelman MD: Robot-assisted laparoscopic partial nephrectomy: the NYU technique. *J Endourol.* 19: 441-5; discussion 445, 2005. [37]

Kaul S, Laungani R, Sarle R, Stricker H, Peabody J, Littleton R and Menon M: da Vinci-assisted robotic partial nephrectomy: technique and results at a mean of 15 months of follow-up. *Eur Urol.* 51: 186-91; discussion 191-2, 2007. [38]

Gagner M, Lacroix A, Prinz RA, Bolte E, Albala D, Potvin C, Hamet P, Kuchel O, Querin S and Pomp A: Early experience with laparoscopic approach for adrenalectomy. *Surgery.* 114: 1120-4; discussion 1124-5, 1993. [39]

Gagner M, Lacroix A and Bolte E: Laparoscopic adrenalectomy in Cushing's syndrome and pheochromocytoma. *N Engl J Med.* 327: 1033, 1992. [40]

Thompson GB, Grant CS, van Heerden JA, Schlinkert RT, Young WF, Jr., Farley DR and Ilstrup DM: Laparoscopic versus open posterior adrenalectomy: a case-control study of 100 patients. *Surgery.* 122: 1132-6, 1997. [41]

Stanford A, Upperman JS, Nguyen N, Barksdale E, Jr. and Wiener ES: Surgical management of open versus laparoscopic adrenalectomy: outcome analysis. *J Pediatr Surg.* 37: 1027-9, 2002. [42]

Schell SR, Talamini MA and Udelsman R: Laparoscopic adrenalectomy for nonmalignant disease: improved safety, morbidity, and cost-effectiveness. *Surg Endosc.* 13: 30-4, 1999. [43]

Janetschek G: Surgical options in adrenalectomy: laparoscopic versus open surgery. *Curr Opin Urol.* 9: 213-8, 1999. [44]

Brunt LM: The positive impact of laparoscopic adrenalectomy on complications of adrenal surgery. *Surg Endosc.* 16: 252-7, 2002. [45]

Young JA, Chapman WH, 3rd, Kim VB, Albrecht RJ, Ng PC, Nifong LW and Chitwood WR, Jr.: Robotic-assisted adrenalectomy for adrenal incidentaloma: case and review of the technique. *Surg Laparosc Endosc Percutan Tech.* 12: 126-30, 2002. [46]

Bentas W, Wolfram M, Brautigam R and Binder J: Laparoscopic transperitoneal adrenalectomy using a remote-controlled robotic surgical system. *J Endourol.* 16: 373-6, 2002. [47]

Desai MM, Gill IS, Kaouk JH, Matin SF, Sung GT and Bravo EL: Robotic-assisted laparoscopic adrenalectomy. *Urology.* 60: 1104-7, 2002. [48]

Julien JS, Ball D and Schulick R: Robot-assisted cortical-sparing adrenalectomy in a patient with von hippel-lindau disease and bilateral pheochromocytomas separated by 9 years. *J Laparoendosc Adv Surg Tech A.* 16: 473-7, 2006. [49]

Winter JM, Talamini MA, Stanfield CL, Chang DC, Hundt JD, Dackiw AP, Campbell KA and Schulick RD: Thirty robotic adrenalectomies: a single institution's experience. *Surg Endosc.* 20: 119-24, 2006. [50]

Brunaud L, Bresler L, Ayav A, Tretou S, Cormier L, Klein M and Boissel P: [Advantages of using robotic Da Vinci system for unilateral adrenalectomy: early results]. *Ann Chir.* 128: 530-5, 2003. [51]

Brunaud L, Bresler L, Zarnegar R, Ayav A, Cormier L, Tretou S and Boissel P: Does robotic adrenalectomy improve patient quality of life when compared to laparoscopic adrenalectomy? *World J Surg.* 28: 1180-5, 2004. [52]

Morino M, Beninca G, Giraudo G, Del Genio GM, Rebecchi F and Garrone C: Robot-assisted vs laparoscopic adrenalectomy: a prospective randomized controlled trial. *Surg Endosc.* 18: 1742-6, 2004. [53]

Tan BJ and Smith AD: Ureteropelvic junction obstruction repair: when, how, what? *Curr Opin Urol.* 14: 55-9, 2004. [54]

O'Reilly PH, Brooman PJ, Mak S, Jones M, Pickup C, Atkinson C and Pollard AJ: The long-term results of Anderson-Hynes pyeloplasty. *BJU Int.* 87: 287-9, 2001. [55]

Schuessler WW, Grune MT, Tecuanhuey LV and Preminger GM: Laparoscopic dismembered pyeloplasty. *J Urol.* 150: 1795-9, 1993. [56]

Zhang X, Li HZ, Ma X, Zheng T, Lang B, Zhang J, Fu B, Xu K and Guo XL: Retrospective comparison of retroperitoneal laparoscopic versus open dismembered pyeloplasty for ureteropelvic junction obstruction. *J Urol.* 176: 1077-80, 2006. [57]

Winfield HN: Management of adult ureteropelvic junction obstruction--is it time for a new gold standard? *J Urol.* 176: 866-7, 2006. [58]

Inagaki T, Rha KH, Ong AM, Kavoussi LR and Jarrett TW: Laparoscopic pyeloplasty: current status. *BJU Int. 95 Suppl 2*: 102-5, 2005. [59]

Munver R, Sosa RE and del Pizzo JJ: Laparoscopic pyeloplasty: history, evolution, and future. *J Endourol.* 18: 748-55, 2004. [60]

Jarrett TW, Chan DY, Charambura TC, Fugita O and Kavoussi LR: Laparoscopic pyeloplasty: the first 100 cases. *J Urol.* 167: 1253-6, 2002. [61]

Janetschek G, Peschel R and Frauscher F: Laparoscopic pyeloplasty. *Urol Clin North Am.* 27: 695-704, 2000. [62]

Sung GT, Gill IS and Hsu TH: Robotic-assisted laparoscopic pyeloplasty: a pilot study. *Urology.* 53: 1099-103, 1999. [63]

Guillonneau B, Rietbergen JB, Fromont G and Vallancien G: Robotically assisted laparoscopic dismembered pyeloplasty: a chronic porcine study. *Urology.* 61: 1063-6, 2003. [64]

Gettman MT, Peschel R, Neururer R and Bartsch G: A comparison of laparoscopic pyeloplasty performed with the daVinci robotic system versus standard laparoscopic techniques: initial clinical results. *Eur Urol.* 42: 453-7; discussion 457-8, 2002. [65]

Gettman MT, Neururer R, Bartsch G and Peschel R: Anderson-Hynes dismembered pyeloplasty performed using the da Vinci robotic system. *Urology.* 60: 509-13, 2002. [66]

El-Nahas AR, Abou-El-Ghar M, Shoma AM, Eraky I, El-Kenawy MR and El-Kappany H: Role of multiphasic helical computed tomography in planning surgical treatment for pelvi-ureteric junction obstruction. *BJU Int.* 94: 582-7, 2004. [67]

Wang DS, Stolpen AH, Bird VG, Ishigami K, Rayhill SC and Winfield HN: Correlation of preoperative three-dimensional magnetic resonance angiography with intraoperative findings in laparoscopic renal surgery. *J Endourol.* 19: 193-9, 2005. [68]

Veyrac C, Baud C, Lopez C, Couture A, Saguintaah M and Averous M: The value of colour Doppler ultrasonography for identification of crossing vessels in children with pelvi-ureteric junction obstruction. *Pediatr Radiol.* 33: 745-51, 2003. [69]

Frauscher F, Janetschek G, Klauser A, Peschel R, Halpern EJ, Pallwein L, Helweg G, zur Nedden D and Bartsch G: Laparoscopic pyeloplasty for UPJ obstruction with crossing vessels: contrast-enhanced color Doppler findings and long-term outcome. *Urology.* 59: 500-5, 2002. [70]

Frauscher F, Janetschek G, Helweg G, Strasser H, Bartsch G and zur Nedden D: Crossing vessels at the ureteropelvic junction: detection with contrast-enhanced color Doppler imaging. *Radiology.* 210: 727-31, 1999. [71]

Schwentner C, Pelzer A, Neururer R, Springer B, Horninger W, Bartsch G and Peschel R: Robotic Anderson-Hynes pyeloplasty: 5-year experience of one centre. *BJU Int,* 2007. [72]

Atug F, Burgess SV, Castle EP and Thomas R: Role of robotics in the management of secondary ureteropelvic junction obstruction. *Int J Clin Pract.* 60: 9-11, 2006. [73]

Siddiq FM, Leveillee RJ, Villicana P and Bird VG: Computer-assisted laparoscopic pyeloplasty: University of Miami experience with the daVinci Surgical System. *J Endourol.* 19: 387-92, 2005. [74]

Yee DS, Shanberg AM, Duel BP, Rodriguez E, Eichel L and Rajpoot D: Initial comparison of robotic-assisted laparoscopic versus open pyeloplasty in children. *Urology.* 67: 599-602, 2006. [75]

Chammas M, Jr., Feuillu B, Coissard A and Hubert J: Laparoscopic robotic-assisted management of pelvi-ureteric junction obstruction in patients with horseshoe kidneys: technique and 1-year follow-up. *BJU Int.* 97: 579-83, 2006. [76]

Mendez-Torres F, Woods M and Thomas R: Technical modifications for robot-assisted laparoscopic pyeloplasty. *J Endourol.* 19: 393-6, 2005. [77]

Atug F, Castle EP, Burgess SV and Thomas R: Concomitant management of renal calculi and pelvi-ureteric junction obstruction with robotic laparoscopic surgery. *BJU Int.* 96: 1365-8, 2005. [78]

Shah KK, Louie M, Thaly RK and Patel VR: Robot assisted laparoscopic pyeloplasty: a review of the current status. *Int J Med Robot.* 3: 35-40, 2007. [79]

Link RE, Bhayani SB and Kavoussi LR: A prospective comparison of robotic and laparoscopic pyeloplasty. *Ann Surg.* 243: 486-91, 2006. [80]

Bernie JE, Venkatesh R, Brown J, Gardner TA and Sundaram CP: Comparison of laparoscopic pyeloplasty with and without robotic assistance. *Jsls.* 9: 258-61, 2005. [81]

Weise ES and Winfield HN: Robotic computer-assisted pyeloplasty versus conventional laparoscopic pyeloplasty. *J Endourol.* 20: 813-9, 2006. [82]

Atug F, Woods M, Burgess SV, Castle EP and Thomas R: Robotic assisted laparoscopic pyeloplasty in children. *J Urol.* 174: 1440-2, 2005. [83]

Palese MA, Munver R, Phillips CK, Dinlenc C, Stifelman M and DelPizzo JJ: Robot-assisted laparoscopic dismembered pyeloplasty. *Jsls.* 9: 252-7, 2005. [84]

Kutikov A, Nguyen M, Guzzo T, Canter D and Casale P: Robot assisted pyeloplasty in the infant-lessons learned. *J Urol.* 176: 2237-9; discussion 2239-40, 2006. [85]

Lee RS, Retik AB, Borer JG and Peters CA: Pediatric robot assisted laparoscopic dismembered pyeloplasty: comparison with a cohort of open surgery. *J Urol.* 175: 683-7; discussion 687, 2006. [86]

Patel V: Robotic-assisted laparoscopic dismembered pyeloplasty. *Urology.* 66: 45-9, 2005. [87]

Klingler HC, Remzi M, Janetschek G, Kratzik C and Marberger MJ: Comparison of open versus laparoscopic pyeloplasty techniques in treatment of uretero-pelvic junction obstruction. *Eur Urol.* 44: 340-5, 2003. [88]

Yohannes P and Burjonrappa SC: Rapid communication: laparoscopic Anderson-Hynes dismembered pyeloplasty using the da Vinci robot: technical considerations. *J Endourol.* 17: 79-83, 2003. [89]

Lee RS and Borer JG: Robotic surgery for ureteropelvic junction obstruction. *Curr Opin Urol.* 16: 291-4, 2006. [90]

Bentas W, Wolfram M, Brautigam R, Probst M, Beecken WD, Jonas D and Binder J: Da Vinci robot assisted Anderson-Hynes dismembered pyeloplasty: technique and 1 year follow-up. *World J Urol.* 21: 133-8, 2003. [91]

Palese MA, Stifelman MD, Munver R, Sosa RE, Philipps CK, Dinlenc C and Del Pizzo JJ: Robot-assisted laparoscopic dismembered pyeloplasty: a combined experience. *J Endourol.* 19: 382-6, 2005. [92]

Estrada CR and Passerotti CC: [Robotic surgery in pediatric urology]. *Arch Esp Urol.* 60: 471-9, 2007. [93]

Yee DS, Klein RB and Shanberg AM: Case report: robot-assisted laparoscopic reconstruction of a ureteropelvic junction disruption. *J Endourol.* 20: 326-9, 2006. [94]

Eden CG: Minimally Invasive Treatment of Ureteropelvic Junction Obstruction: A Critical Analysis of Results. *Eur Urol,* 2007. [95]

Badwan K and Bhayani S: Robotic pyeloplasty: a critical appraisal. *Int J Med Robot.* 3: 20-2, 2007. [96]

Bhayani SB, Link RE, Varkarakis JM and Kavoussi LR: Complete daVinci versus laparoscopic pyeloplasty: cost analysis. *J Endourol.* 19: 327-32, 2005. [97]

Luke P, Knudsen BE, Nguan CY, Pautler SE, Swinnimer S, Kiaii R and Kapoor A: Robot-assisted laparoscopic renal artery aneurysm reconstruction. *J Vasc Surg*. 44: 651-3, 2006. [98]

Hoznek A, Zaki SK, Samadi DB, Salomon L, Lobontiu A, Lang P and Abbou CC: Robotic assisted kidney transplantation: an initial experience. *J Urol*. 167: 1604-6, 2002. [99]

Orvieto MA, Chien GW, Shalhav AL, Tolhurst SR, Rapp DE, Galocy RM and Harland RC: Case report: robot-assisted laparoscopic pyeloureterostomy in a transplanted kidney with ureteral stricture. *J Endourol*. 20: 31-2, 2006. [100]

Cleary K and Nguyen C: State of the art in surgical robotics: clinical applications and technology challenges. *Comput Aided Surg*. 6: 312-28, 2001. [101]

Pandya A and Auner G: Robotics technology: a journey into the future. *Urol Clin North Am*. 31: 793-800, x, 2004. [102]

Duchene DA, Moinzadeh A, Gill IS, Clayman RV and Winfield HN: Survey of residency training in laparoscopic and robotic surgery. *J Urol*. 176: 2158-66; discussion 2167, 2006. [103]

Wang DS and Winfield HN: Survey of urological laparoscopic practice patterns in the midwest. *J Urol*. 172: 2282-6, 2004. [104]

Stifelman MD, Caruso RP, Nieder AM and Taneja SS: Robot-assisted laparoscopic partial nephrectomy. *Jsls*. 9: 83-6, 2005. [105]

D'Annibale A, Fiscon V, Trevisan P, Pozzobon M, Gianfreda V, Sovernigo G, Morpurgo E, Orsini C and Del Monte D: The da Vinci robot in right adrenalectomy: considerations on technique. *Surg Laparosc Endosc Percutan Tech*. 14: 38-41, 2004. [106]

19

Robin Heart - Perspectives of application of mini invasive tools in cardiac surgery

Zbigniew Nawrat[1,2], Pawel Kostka[1,3]
Foundation for Development of Cardiac Surgery, Zabrze Poland,
Medical University of Silesia, Katowice,
Silesian University of Technology, Gliwice,
Poland

1. Introduction

Robot invented for less, minimally invasive cardiac surgery is a computer-controlled device, located between surgeon's hands and the tip of a surgical instrument. Basic requirements for this device are first of all high reliability, stable operative field of view, direct surgeon control and high level of precision.

The Robin Heart® is a Europe's first heart surgery robot system with whole, original Polish design. Precise and optimally adapted to the surgeon's manual dexterity, it also helps him make the right decisions. Around 4 million minimally-invasive surgeries are performed in the world every year. The procedures are performed by means of special instruments inserted through small incisions in the patient's body. The aim is to limit the operative field and protect surrounding tissue, which could be damaged if a traditional surgical technique was used. The number of endoscopic procedures, less invasive than traditional surgery, performed through natural orifices in the patient's body, or through special openings called ports, is on the rise.

The success of the procedures largely depends on the instruments used. Unfortunately, typical endoscopic (laparoscopic) instruments reduce precision and make the surgery more difficult because they add to hand tremor and almost completely eliminate the natural sense of touch. Additionally, the surgeon does not have a direct view of the operative field-a camera inserted into the body through a third opening transmits the image to a display. So the surgeon's task is not easy. An ideal non-invasive surgery can be compared to the house renovation through a keyhole without disturbing the household members. Across the world, physicians and engineers are working to develop increasingly effective instruments to enable surgery with the use of the latest technology. But how can one enhance instrument precision and maneuverability, which are so important in the case of surgery on the beating heart, for instance? Surgical robots provide such capabilities.

In Poland, an interdisciplinary team led by Prof. Zbigniew Religa already introduced modern devices to clinical practice to save the lives of heart patients. An artificial heart, prosthetic heart valves and recently a surgical robot are the results of projects carried out by the Biocybernetics Laboratory of the Heart Prosthesis Institute, a research center run by the

Foundation for Cardiac Surgery Development in Zabrze. This is the only one research center of such a kind in Poland.
Works on building a prototype of a remote-controlled robot for performing and assisting heart surgeries and other surgical procedures was initiated in 2000. At the starting point of RH project the mutlidisciplinary team from several scientific centers in Poland was setup. The group of basic constructors both of mechanical and electronic part was mounted (fixed) consists of Leszek Podsedkowski, Krzysztof Mianowski and the authors of presented paper. The robot, or actually a "tele-manipulator," is the first ever tool capable of assisting a surgeon by providing the capability to directly use surgery simulation and planning methods. Several models of the robot have been developed, differing in control and mounting systems. The Robin Heart 0 and Robin Heart 1 have an independent base and are controlled via an industrial computer (with VME type bus) and author's software written in OS9 real time operating system. The Robin Heart 2 is fixed to the operating table and has two arms, on which one can fix various surgical instruments. The control system is implemented based on the Digital Signal Processor (DSP) as a central unit and net of motor regulators, created on specialized microcontrollers. The latest model, known as the Robin Heart Vision, will become the surgeon's partner in the operating room next year. It will replace a human assistant who usually holds the "telescope" of the video channel to enable the observation of the operative field of laparoscopic instruments. As a result, the surgeon will be able to perform part of the surgery unaided by other people. The Robin Heart Vision is easy to use and install, and can be conveniently carried in a suitcase. The Polish heart surgery robot is an original design. Thanks to its modular structure, it can be adjusted for surgery of different types. Work is under way to introduce a "tele-collaboration" (Robin EXPERT) system to be used during surgery. It will contain the real image from the camera, diagnostic data and surgery simulation data. The surgeon will be able to use the "tele-collaboration" program at any moment as it will be voice-activated and voice-controlled. New instruments and applications for the robot are also being developed. There are plans to use the robot for implanting artificial organs, prostheses and ventricular assist devices (*AOROBAS* project).
Results of works carried out in the range of RH project realisation were given under a public evaluation during annual Surgery Robotic Conference, started in 2001, in FCSD (Zabrze, Poland). Mentioned above conference - Medical Robots Conference, currently achieved the status of international platform for participant's projects presentation, exchange of experiences and is also occasion for polish Robin Heart system testing. Promotion action conducted from the beginning of the project realisation as well as fact, that the big group of young scientists and students were involved in it was the reason, that this pioneer project became an initial sparkle of huge wave of interest in medical robotic systems in polish universities. Currently several polish technical and also medical universities created autonomous faculties of medical robotics and run the lectures from this disciplines. Now there is a enormous and encouraging perspective for the development of surgical robotics in Poland - while all began from the short conversation between physics (dr Zbigniew Nawrat (ZN)) and famous cardiac surgeon (prof. Zbigniew Religa (ZR)):

ZN: We call it Robin Heart, Professor !

ZR: OK! When will I be able to operate with it?

1.1 Short historical review of surgery robotics

Robotic surgery was born out of microsurgery and endoscopic experience. Minimally invasive interventions require a multitude of technical devices: cameras, light-sources, high-frequency and insufflations. The mobility of instruments is decreased (from seven, natural for human arm, to four degrees of freedom DOF) due to the invariant point of insertion through the patients wall. Many companies worked on methods for doctors to do heart surgery through small holes in the patient's chest but with a computer controlling the movements of the long sticks.The surgery is a complex procedure requiring precise control of position and force. Conventional open-heart surgery requires full median sternotomy, which means cracking of ribs, compromising pulmonary function and considerable loss of blood.The basic advantages of minimally invasive robot-aided surgery are safe, reliable and repeatable operative results with less patient pain, trauma and recovery time.

The milestones of video-enhanced telescopes (laparoscopes) and tele-manipulators:

- 1805 Bozzini - first use a vision system in the body (urethra stones)
- 1912 Jacobeus - laparoscopy examination the abdomen
- 1945 Goertz - first modern tele-manipulator (applicated to space investigation, undersea exploitation, nuclear industry, medical therapy … .)
- 1960s Semm et al. - developing of laparoscopic instrumentation
- 1983 Semm - first laparoscopic appendectomy
- 1987 Mouret - first laparoscopic cholecystectomy
- 1993, 1994 Green et al. - developing the telepresence surgery (master and slave units were connected via a short cable to perform surgical actions such as grasping and cutting)
- 1993 Rovetta et all - first experimental robotic telesurgery by means of satellites network (USA -Italy)
- 1994 - first FDA-cleared robot for assisting surgery (Automated Andescopic System for optimal Positioning AESOP produced by Computer Motion)
- In 1995, Intuitive Surgical was founded
- 1998 Carpentier&Loulmet performed first in the world endoscopic operation of single bypass graft between left internal thoracic artery and left anterior descending (LITA - LAD) and 1998 first operation inside the heart - mitral valve plastic and atrial septal defect closure was performed (da Vinci)
- 1998 Mohr & Falk bypass surgery and mitral valve repairs in near endoscopic technique (da Vinci)
- 1999 D.Boyd - first totally endoscopic Zeus-based coronary artery bypass graft (E-CABG)
- 1999 - 250 robotically assisted operations performed worldwide among which 80 have been cardiac procedures 100 heart operations using da Vinci (Intuitive Surgical, Mountain View, CA) were performed.
- In 2000, da Vinci Surgical System became the first robotic surgical system cleared by the FDA for general laparoscopic surgery
- 2000 - Start polish project Robin Heart

In 2003, the Intuitive Surgical acquired its principal competitor, Computer Motion, strengthening its intellectual property holdings. While Intuitive Surgical supports Computer Motion's former customers, most hospitals and institutions that had Computer Motion's ZEUS® MicroWrist™ Robotic Surgical System for minimally invasive surgical procedures have chosen to participate in a trade-in program and now have da Vinci Surgical Systems. Intuitive Surgical continues to sell some AESOP® Robotic Endoscope Positioners, but primary focus remains the da Vinci Surgical System (www.intuitivesurgical.com).

In 2005, a total of 2984 cardiac procedures were performed worldwide using the da Vinci system. This includes totally endoscopic coronary artery bypass grafting (TECAB), mitral valve repair (MVR) procedures, ASD closure and cardiac tissue ablation for atrial fibrillation (Jacobs et al., 2006). In 2003, the number stood at a modest 3.4%. In 2004, the number climbed to 10% and then doubled to 20% the following year. For 2006, the figure is expected to come in around 35%. An estimated 36,600 robotic procedures will be performed this year—from heart-bypass surgeries to kidney transplants to hysterectomies. That's up nearly 50 percent from last year, and analysts predict the figure will nearly double in 2006 to more than 70,000 procedures. Since the da Vinci was approved by the Food and Drug Administration in July 2000 (the only robotic system to get the FDA nod), about 350 of the units have been purchased, including 30 in the last quarter alone, at about $1.3 million apiece (after J. Barrett, Newsweek, Dec. 4, 2005).

2. Asumptions and initial steps of Robin Heart project

The Foundation of Cardiac Surgery Development (FCSD) in Zabrze began in 2000 the grant for realization of the prototype of a robot useful for cardiac surgery. The multidisciplinary team including specialist in medicine and techniques during three years prepared families of robot prototypes named Robin Heart (Fig.1).

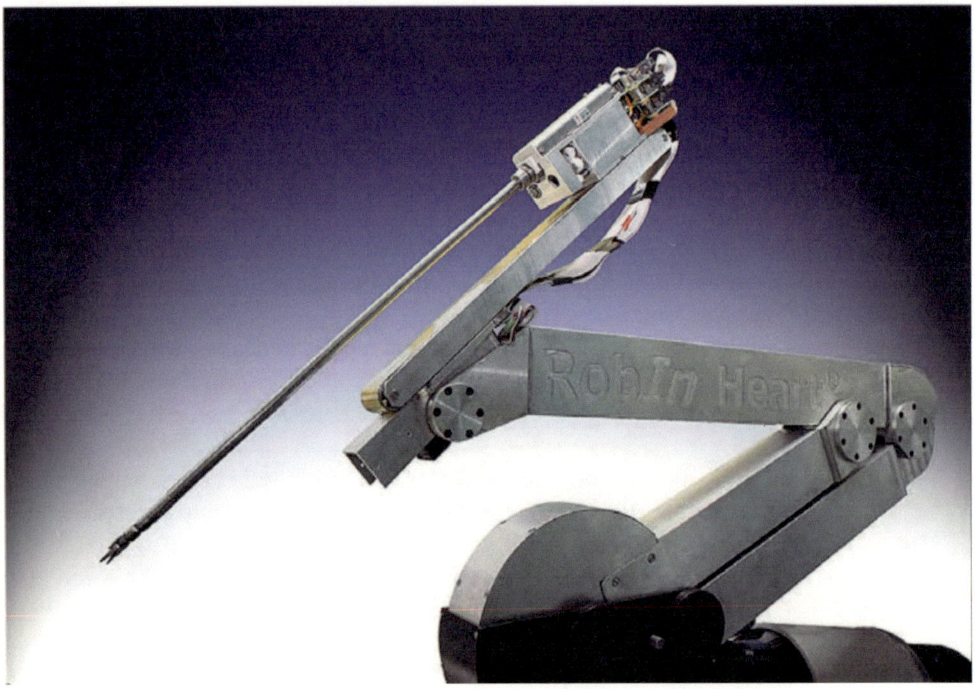

Figure 1. The Robin Heart 1

The goals of the project was:

- Safe, reliable and repeatable operative results with less patient pain, trauma and recovery time
- Healthcare costs decreasing
- Support the technology breakthrough - significant increase of the number and type of minimally invasive procedures available to patients.
- Friendliness guarantee both for the patient and surgeon.

Design criteria & problems:

Man-Machine interface – the design of surgeon user interface. We worked out many models of suitable for surgeon contact systems, using the experiences of centres designing the artificial hand and HAPTIC systems. Master tool similar to traditional laparoscope with sensors, solutions based on PC like joystick, head movement interface (for RH Vision endoscopic arm), foot pedal control and voice commands.

Safety - checking the quality of device execution, working on the multi-type sensor systems including the arm sensors and image processing information

The advisory systems – supporting the operation planning. Using the experiences of our Bio-Cybernetics Lab. FCSD in cardiac surgery procedures simulations we work on the system for recognizing the object, comparing it with diagnostic image from data base and advising the surgeon the optimal solution.

Surgical tools - working out of series of universal and specialised small, elastic, adaptive control and easy to operate, tools for performing the concrete activities during the cardiac procedure. The experience in clinical beating heart cases has demonstrated the importance of small instrumentation to successfully complete these procedures. The space in the chest when performing a beating heart case is limited to about 3 cm between the chest wall and the target vessel. The working tips of microsurgery instruments must be smaller than 5 mm to not obscure the small endoscopic field of view and efficient maneuver in the small space within the chest. The bigger instruments are not able to effectively articulate due to the wide space that is swept out when articulating, thus negating any benefit articulation might afford. We plan the usage of micro-engines, elastic grabbers matching their properties to the object shape and application the new materials – alloys with shape memory, diamonds facing etc.

The testing and training stands – every part of robot, before introducing to the further designing stage will be tested by physicians on special prepared stands

Small invasive placing the artificial organs – we work out the ways of valves, heart assist pumps and pacemakers fixing etc. Especially the semiautomatic tools for caniula implantation is designed.

Assistant - the assistant in beating heart cases can provide counter traction for the arteriotomy, facilitate suturing during the anastomosis and must be able to effectively integrate amongst the robotic arms to use a mister/blower to clear the field.

Port - optimal port location is necessary to provide a significant benefit to the patient, ensures patient safety and minimizes any pain at the port site. For surgery planning, optimal port location and robot's arm navigation the virtual reality technology was used.

Sterility – the robot system have to be easy configured for the sterile field. The arms are draped.

According to assumptions Polish cardiac surgery robot was to be an original construction with segment type structure to allow the combination of its parts for different type of surgery operation.

2.1 Minimally Invasive cardiac Surgery (MIS) description

The minimally invasive cardiac surgery may be performed manually using classic, modified semi-classic tools or in robotic supported way. Currently several techniques are used. The most important application of MIS is the coronary artery bypass grafting CABG.

2.1.1 CABG MIS description

Coronary bypass surgery is common (about 800 000 people undergo the procedure every year worldwide) but the operation is expensive and risky. Grafting bypasses onto the heart typically involves attaching between three and five vessels to existing arteries so that blood flow through the bypasses will circumvent blockages. Surgeons can use either arterial grafts (arteries, mostly, left internal mammary artery (LIMA), redirected from the vicinity of the heart) or venous grafts (vein segments taken from the leg).
Full sternotomy means that surgeons must open the chest (sternum must be split with a saw and the chest cavity spread open). Next, they must stop the heart and the patient must be put on heart-lung machine, which artificially circulates blood and supplies the body's tissues with oxygen until doctors restart the heart. In the mid-1990s new surgical techniques emerged that signal a revolution in coronary bypass surgery.
We have to explain a meaning of few medical abbreviations used in field of MIS:
MIDCAB - minimally invasive direct coronary artery bypass grafting done through a left anterolateral minithoracotomy. The surgery is performed by a beating-heart approach (10% of this kind operation) and a pressure stabilizer is used. It is applicable, for the most part, only single vessel disease on anterior surface of the heart.
MIS require special techniques for connection circulatory system for artificial perfusion.
Port Access Surgery - this is the method for cardiopulmonary bypass system using in case of coronary bypass grafting through a limited access incision on an arrested heart.
OPCAB - off-pump coronary artery bypass grafting. The surgery (multi-vessel disease) is performed through a small sternotomy approach on beating heart using stabilizers. In many centers in Europe and in the United States, greater than 90% of all CABG is now performed by OPCAB techniques, because of its ability to multi-vessel surgery and allowing access to the posterior circulation of the heart without significant hemodynamic compromise.
TECAB - Totally Endoscopic Coronary Bypass Surgery - the surgery performed without of sternotomy using only observation via endoscopic camera.
AORobAS -- Based on Robin Heart project development, currently our team works on system AORobAS - Artificial Organs Robotically Assisted Surgery artificial organs implantation, services, repair, exchange, removing.
Endoscopic microsurgery is difficult to carry out with standard hand held instruments. This due primarily to the poor ergonomic position that results when a surgeon stands at the table using standard endoscopic instruments to perform a complex surgical task. Robot is intended to keep the surgeon in the most comfortable, dexterous and ergonomic position for the entire procedure. In most assisted by robot surgery procedures, only part of heart procedure are made using robot, for instance mammary artery harvests. The first ever in US closed-chest totally endoscopic coronary artery TECAB bypass procedure was performed (Argenziano& Craig in New York) using the da Vinci System from start to finish only in January 2002. The first robot assisted operation inside the heart was also mitral valve plastic and atrial septal. Currently the application of cardio-robots is developed in wider range of

surgery procedures. For us, Institute of Heart Prostheses FCSD the most interesting is surgery connecting to artificial organ implantation.

2.2 Preliminary tests creating the base for surgery robot assumptions

Cardiac surgery is carried out on soft tissues.

Results connected with surgical action analysis allowed to determine the maximum values of forces needed for typical procedures performed in heart area, with the usage of different type tools. This can be the basis for cardiac surgery robot design assumptions, in the field connected with controlling of robot tools movements.

The penetration of soft tissue requires such action as cutting, slicing, inserting a needle, knotting etc. The difficulty with soft tissue consist in fact, that it deforms and changes shape. As our result of basic mechanical properties of typical surgical actions the map of force resistance during pricking for left and right heart chamber was obtained. For example the maximal force value of heart muscle right ventricle equalled 30[G] (1[cm] depth) and 90[G] (2[cm] depth) for Dexon 2/0 surgical needle, while for Prolene 3/0 type 40[G] and 140 [G] respectively. This same needle Prolen during pricking through papillary muscle reached the max. load, up to 150 [G]. During scalpel cutting procedure for left ventricle (the mitral valve ring) the measured load value equalled 200[G] (2[cm] depth). For sewing tests - the knot tying using Prolen needle: up to 200[G], with 0.1 [mm/s] test speed.

2.3 Consideration toward Robin Heart construction

Basic idea of the manipulator Robin Heart consists of mechanisms realizing fixed in space "constant point", consists of two closed kinematics' chains (Nawrat et al., 2003). The first loop is in fact a typical parallelogram mechanism, used as a transmission mechanism coupled with the second one realized inverse mechanism. By special connection of two rotations coupled by constant angle internal link, the mechanism can change external angle to approximately 150 degrees. In the version Robin Heart 0 shown in Fig.2, the first DOF is driven by electric, brushless motor integrated with Harmonic Drive gear. The second (range up to 150 degrees doubled system of parallel mechanisms) and third DOFs (the parallel mechanisms eliminates the necessity of using a linear slideway) are driven by brushless motors, roller screws and system of strings. The construction makes possible fast and not complicated disconnection the drive part of the bunch from the manipulating part.

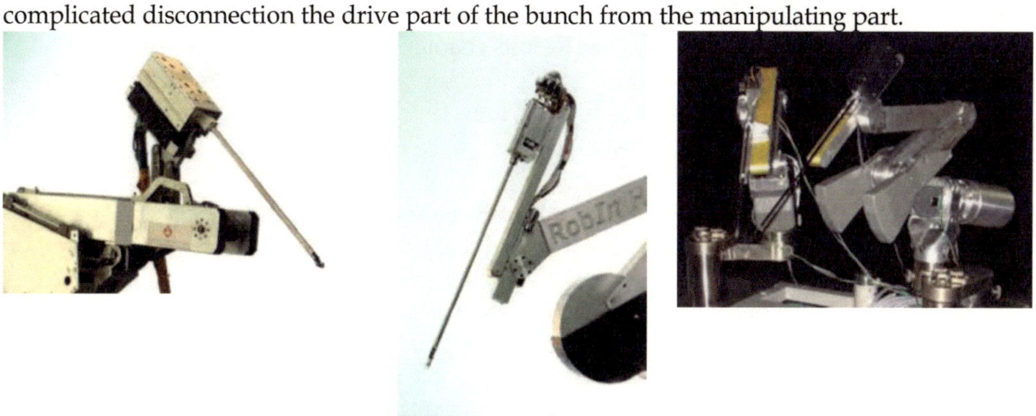

Robin Heart 0 Robin Heart 1 Robin Heart 2

Figure 2.

The separable part does not contain any elements requiring lubrication. In the bunch part five independent drives and the string drive were applied gives 3 DOFs enable to obtain any orientation in the workspace. The fourth DOF makes possible opening and closing the jaws of the tool, the fifth one (called "the elbow") is redundant and increases manoeuvrability, enables avoiding obstacles and operating "backwards". In the pre-prototype version the diameter of the bunch is 10mm. For driving, the servomotors with DC electric motors and no-clearance gears have been used.
Presented above preliminary prototype (number 0) have been tested and the new prototype have been designed. In prototype Robin Heart 1 (Fig.2) diminution of mass and size of tools driving block, enlargement of stiffness of arm and arrangements of carriage of drive were introduced. As a results driving block has dimensions 46 x 48 x 90 mm and five times smaller mass (0,4 of kg). Additionally project of so-called „penknife", universal possessing ending more than one working tool element was executed. In Robin Heart 1 the diameter of the bunch was decreased to 8mm (Nawrat et al., 2003).
In addition, we decided to perform also, competing model of robot arms: relatively light construction mounted directly to the operating table. In construction Robin Heart 2 (Fig.2) compact versions modules of parallelogram mechanism were placed inside compactly to them of well-fitting elements consist of rectangular pipes. Advantage of this solution is straight, aesthetical, compact and tight construction presenting high functionalities in operating action. Manipulator is driven by DC servomotors. The arms is mounted to the table using special folding console from two passive arms and columns.
The Robin Heart 2 manipulator has very good and relatively large working space, in which surgeon can select small subspace with very good isotropic kinematics' properties for manipulating of objects with good position accuracy. Each of models are under testing program provided in Bio-Cybernetics Laboratory.

2.4 Robin Heart Vision (RHV) chosen technical and functional assumptions.

RHV telemanipulator is a youngest member of RH family designed as a robotic holder for endoscopic camera, so it is equipped with special socked for quick endoscope fixing.
Based on RH0&RH1 constructions the set of technical assmuptions was created as well (Nawrat & Kostka, 2007):

- Four degrees of freedom (DOF)
- Relatively large working space (see Results chapter for detail info).
- Resolution less or equall 0.5 mm

As a one surgery robotic arm RHV is adapted to be fixed both directly to operation table and to stand on autonomous column next to it.

2.5 Operation field and techniques analysis for robotic supported cardiac surgery.

The main assumption that makes Robin Heart 1 useful, is construction of double closed loop, which provides point constancy between laparoscope instrument and patient tissue. To optimize this type of construction, Robin Heart structure was based on a double closed loop mechanism, which provides constancy of a point outside the robot structure. In this way only one reliable servomotor is used with a simple steering algorithm.
To identify the 'constant kinematics point' and to explain the necessity and the principle of working this type of structure, a separate simplified model was created in a CAD program.

Overlapping all final position of the Robin Heart 3D model, the geometric position surface of laparoscopic instrument was described in geometry and dimensions.
To provide all necessary functionality of modern laparoscopic devices, robot Robin Heart gives user a three degrees of freedom to orientate in space, fourth one is responsible for opening and closing jaws of the tool and the fifth one increases the manipulation skills to avoid obstacles, or like Robin Heart allows to work "backwards". Standard laparoscopic device has got a limited mobility and do not offer very sophisticated types of movement that are provided by a robotic systems. To see the differences in a mobility between two various Robin Heart instruments, a tool workspace was calculated for a robot equipped with a standard laparoscopic device and a more advanced robotic instrument (Fig.3.). Having a workspace sphere calculated for all of the robot instruments it is very easy to verify the goal of using a suitable device for a proper surgery treatment. Combining this workspace with a geometric position surface we were able to calculate the total range of movement for both robotic instruments inside the patient body (Fig.4.).

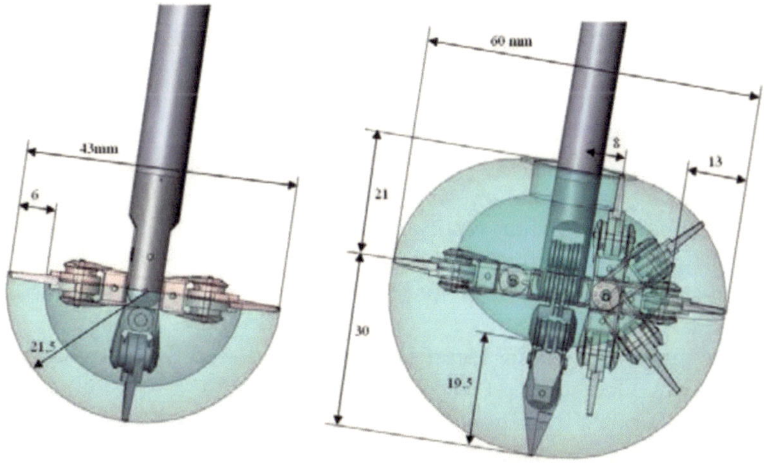

Figure 3. Instrument workspace: a.) standard laparoscopic tool, b.) Robin Heart 1 instrument. (*performed by Kozlak&Nawrat*)

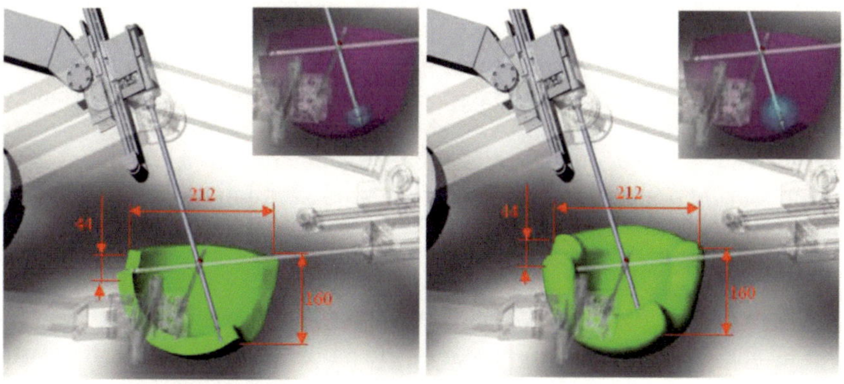

Figure 4. General rage of robot mobility equipped with: a.) standard laparoscopic tool, b.) Robin Heart 1 instrument (*performed by Kozlak&Nawrat*)

2.6 Virtual Reality modeling

To be up to date the part of Robin Heart system research and the modeling work is using a Virtual Reality latest technology. Nowadays in a RiH project this technology is implemented in a three different areas that cooperate together in creating an advanced computer system for a surgery planning. In this manner a Virtual Reality equivalent of surgery scene (Fig.5,6) was created including: - three separate Robin Heart robots that can be manipulated realistically with all of their functionality; - a human model with basic organs; - surgery room and all the basic equipment. This type of intuitive understanding of virtual objects was used by FCSD to create a several training station that helps us better to see the benefits of robotic surgery and how to use a robotic system during the surgery treatment. All of the virtual Robin Heart robots were connected to the native wireless controllers, so having a true joysticks in your hands user can manipulate and stand next to the robots that actually do not exist. Virtual copy of those robot prototypes are able to perform all of the movements and provides the same behavior as the origin Robin Heart. Possibility of interaction between all of the three robots and the surrounding virtual objects is a great chance of an advanced training for young surgeons but also gives an opportunity to plan (or even practice) surgery procedures that have to be perform in the real world by a professionals.

Efficiency of using a robotic equipment in an endoscope procedures significantly depends both on a precise tools manipulation and a proper surgery procedure planning. Accurate arrangement of setting up the robots arm with reference to surgery table, positioning the trocars location and right choice of a correct tools, makes the surgery procedure much more safe and harmless. Using a virtual reality technology, based on EON Reality interactive software, we plan all those important steps, increases an effectiveness in noninvasive surgeons training and helps to verify the benefits of using robotic systems in a various surgery treatments.

To be up to date the part of Robin Heart system research and the modeling work is using an EON Reality Virtual Reality latest technology. Because VR is a very intuitive solution this type of modeling gets much more popular nowadays helping surgeons and even patients to understand very complex procedures much more clear and efficient. Nowadays in a RiH project VR technology is implemented in four different areas:

- as a training station in surgeon education process,
- as a tool used for a surgery treatment procedure planning with a step by step briefing, - in an advisory voice operated system with an external database,
- to verify a different construction versions in aspect of ergonomic and functionality.

FCSD has used a Virtual Reality technology to create several training station that helps user better to understand the benefits of robotic surgery and how to use a robotic system during the surgery treatment. The total impression of immerse in a computer world was emphasized by using a special active stereoscopic projector and a shutter glasses. The total Virtual Reality scene was completed with a three separate Robin Heart robots that can be manipulated realistically with all of their functionality; endoscope camera viewport displayed in a PIP technology (picture in picture), human model with basic organs which might be exchanged to ones from a patient CT or NMR; surgery room with a surgery table, lamps and all the basic equipment. Prepared VR model and also a Robin Heart training system was created in a EON Professional, and fully supports real time rendering with advanced graphic effects, contact between the objects, friction, gravity and a mass properties. Foundation for Cardiac Surgery Development is using virtual model: to verify the choice of using a specific instrument inside the surgery area by comparing the size and the shape of the different workspaces; to plan and simulate the surgery treatment with step by step instructions; for a surgery room choreography optimizing the position of each robot arm for different procedures; to set the correct trocar ports between the patient ribs; to educate how to use an endoscope camera during the surgery procedure.

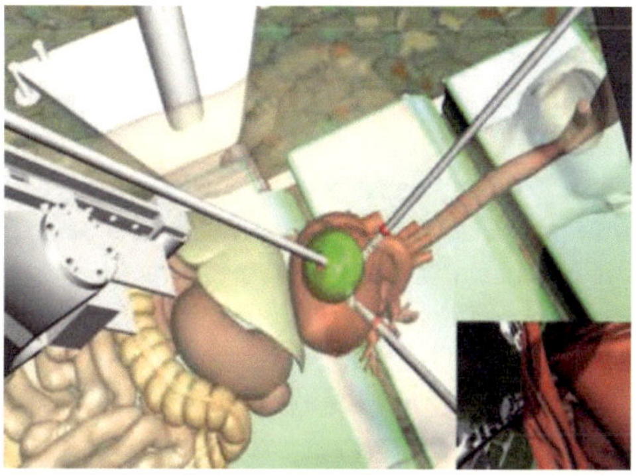

Figure 5. Robin Heart surgery scene planning inside the patient body

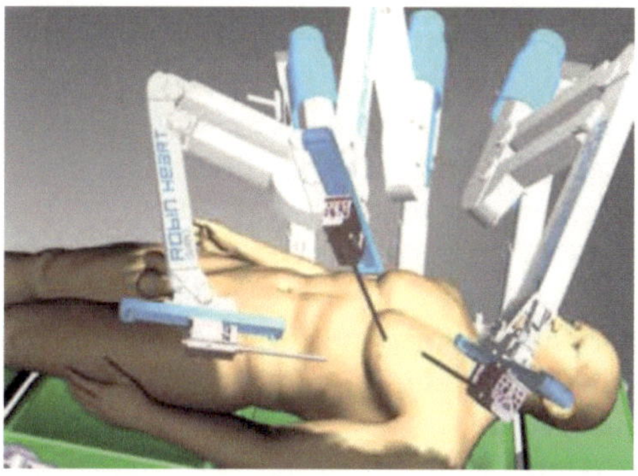

Figure 6. Robots choreography planning and training (*performed by Kozlak&Nawrat*)

2.7 Planning of robot assisted cardiac surgery

Pre-operation planning means several researches using computer and physical models, performed to reach optimisation surgery effect by optimisation of methodology, materials, devices and techniques of surgery.

Modern medical imaging methods like computer tomograhy (CT), nuclear magnetic resonance (NMR) enable the surgeon to view very precise a representation of internal anatomy from pre-operative scan modalities. Scan can be combined with an anatomical atlas producing 3-D patient model and the model of devices like artificial heart or valve can be add for treatment planning prior the operation. For surgery robots (telemanipulator) the following distinct phases can be recognised:

- pre-operative planning: The optimal strategy is defined based on 3-D computer model.
- robot assisted intervention: A calibration routine brings robot, patient and image system to common frame of reference – e.g by anatomical (or artificial)landmarks.
- feedback and re-planning: The robot stars the to work under supervision of surgeon. Sensor information assure that the anatomy is as expected and stored by a model in

computer. If deviations occur the surgeon asked for a revised strategy, or for permission to continue.

The image - guided surgery is easy to implement for orthopedic surgery, where fiators are commonly used to fix bones, and also for neurosurgery, where the stereotactic helmet, mounted on the patient's head, is quite popular to provide absolute matching between pre-operative and intra-operative reference frames. Vision - based surgery may be viewed as a robotic CAD-CAM system where diagnostic images (from CT, NMR, US, etc.) are used for off-line planning of the intervention. The robot is used as a tools-machine for precise cutting, milling, drilling ..(for instance bone milling for hip implant). The geometrically precision of the surgical planning often greatly exceeds that of surgical execution that the solve is partnership between humans and computers and robots. For example, Robodoc (ISS Inc., Sacramento, CA,USA) is it industrial system currently used in human trials for implant of hip prostheses. The architecture of the hip replacement surgery system consist of a CT-based presurgical planning sub-system. The surgical procedure includes manual guiding to approximate positions of pins, pre-operatively inserted into bones and automatic tactile search for each pin. Robots controller computes the appropriate transformation to machine out the implant cavity. Then, the pins are removed and the surgeon proceeds in the manual procedure. Robodoc include checking and monitoring of cutter force. Similar techniques adapted to different scenarios have been developed for the cases of total knee arthoplasty, spine surgery, neurosurgery, prostate and eye surgery.

For medical application very important are matching procedures between diagnostic images and off-line intervention planning and real execution. Many problems still remain for soft tissue surgery where deformations may occur. The navigation and guidance of the instruments highly depends on the surgeon's skill who has to combine his intra-operative views with the information extracted from the pre-operative images. System currently developed in our laboratory allows for parallel displaying, four pictures on monitor taken from independed sources (e.g. one real from operation field, next - diagnostic images or pre-operation simulation results).

To plan the whole surgery procedure by means of physical and mathematical models, particular objects belonging to field of operation should be characterized in this domain.

We propose an original solution of remote-control manipulator for cardiac surgery with computer based advisory system. Information gathered in prepared database may be use by surgeon as on-line expert system to support him in decision making. A first step is to prepare the robot-assisted surgery relates to both computer and physical models of particular operation type. Based upon pre-operation cardiac surgery simulations the optimisation of cardiac surgery procedures can be established. The implementation of in vitro simulation for surgery procedure has been performed. As a results of a physical and computer simulations (ProEng®, Fidap® systems) surgery modification of biological system effectiveness with the different surgery techniques usage is studied. As a result of research connected with operation planning the optimisation of port location and choreography of robot arm for this cases is performed. Based on this works effects, the control algorithm for cardiac surgery robot will be proposed.

Currently used cardiac surgery robots fulfil the function of manipulators, which main task is to detect and scale up or down the surgeon hand motions and precisely translate them to the movements of robot's arm equipped in appropriated tools. The basic advantages of cardio-robots are safe, reliable and repeatable operative results with less patient pain, trauma and recovery time.

The main issues of computer simulation support of surgery robot:

1. The operation planning - Based on diagnostic data (images, pressure and flow signals, etc.) computer and physical models can be created. In vitro simulations performed on them, may be used to find the optimal way of operation (the joint point localization, the graft selection). Prepared report can be presented to surgeon as a hint for robot choreography planning. This stage also should include: input port localization on patient skin, the type of tools and the way of taking and preparing the graft branch.
2. Advisory and control system - During the operation, diagnostic image from various sources (data base, diagnostic device) can be called by surgeon and superimposed on real operating image to localise the optimal place for CABG connection. Also the simulated or real taken from previous operation recorded in database effect of particular way of connection could be obtained.

The introduction of robots to cardiac surgery gave as the possibility of direct and practical use of surgery procedures simulation results to the robot information system.

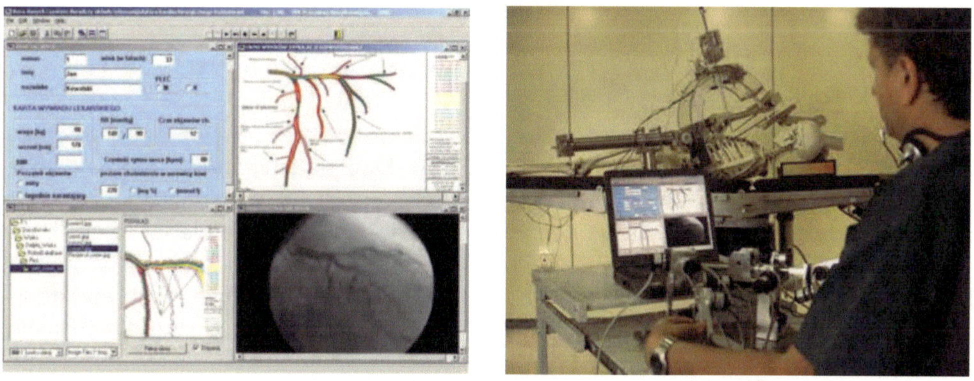

Figure 7. Intelligent voice control Database and Advisory System

3. Mechanical Construction of Robin Heart. Comparison with commercial surgery robots.

3.1 Robin Heart 0&1&2

Mechanics of existing cardiosurgical robots constructions consist of mechanical arm with replaceable laparoskopic tools specialisated for different functions: cutting, sewing, removing of tissues etc. Introduced to the patient body tools can possess different number of degrees of freedom (DOF). Suitable number of DOF of tool wrist makes possible executing of different types of operation. In described constructions this as follows: in robot da Vinci (DV) bunch about diameter 8,5 mm possesses 3 DOF, in robot Zeus (Z) dependent on model: for diameter 3,9 mm we have 2 DOF, and for diameter 4,9 mm - 3 DOF. Both Rob*In* Heart 0 and 1 (RH) has 4 DOF including additional joint for working backwards. In RH 0 diameter of tool carries out 10 mm, when in new RH1 already 8 mm. For RH 2 currently is performed simply 2 DOF tools, this model is dedicated especially as a base for endoscopic camera (Nawrat et al., 2003).

Second element of telemanipulator is the arm assure possibility of translocating of working ending of tool inside body of patient at maintenance of one constant point - passage through skin of patient body (so-called port). In described constructions two methods: kinematic passive of constant point creation in working space are applied. Passive method is modeled based on classic laparoscopy solution. Point of passage of tool through patient body (point of support of tool) treats itself how joint of 4 class - with 2 DOF. To fix all of 6 tool DOFs, the robot arm should have 4 DOF. Three of them are achieved by positioning of the external end of the tool. In the Zeus arm it is realized using SCARA type of manipulator construction. To obtain proper maneuverability it is necessary to use two not driven joints (kind of Cardan universal joint) in the place of connection of robot arm with the tool. Next DOF responsible for turning of the tool in relation to its axis is usually driven by motor. The disadvantage of this solution is loading of tissue near the port as a result of tools support during action. Flexibility of tool grows up also. In summary, the Z arms possesses 3 DOF which together with tools DOF gives us 5 or 6 DOF, depending on kind of the tool used. In telemanipulator DV, RH0, RH1 and RH2 for realization the constant point condition of work kinematics solution was used. In robot DV entire number of degrees of freedom carries out 6 DOF. In RH0, RH1 this is 7 DOF because of tool with one additional joint. Separate problem is range of arm movement what, in some situations, can limit possibilities of robot usage. Parallelogram mechanism of RH1 work correctly in range to 120°, in RH 0 range of movement is 150 ° (Nawrat et al., 2003).

The next important problem is a power transmission into tools. In presented constructions it is realized using strings or followers. In DV each of DOF is driven via strings. Range of movement of individual joints of tool is considerable – usually ± 90 ° for every joint. Strings pass through rollers along whole arm of telemanipulator. Motors are placed on base, what in considerable degree discharge construction of arm. Due to considerable length of thin lines and its extensions the continuous inspection and trickery before every operation is required. If strings breaks, arm is not useful for further manipulation, what is disadvatage of this type construction.

Used in Zeus robot follover type of transmission has limited possibilities of drive of large number of successive degrees of freedom. Fundamentally two movements can be obtained: pitch of tool and its closing or opening. Strongly limited is also range of movement: ± 40 ° for pitch and 20° for opening of tool. It possesses however some undeniable advantages: small diameter of tool (3.9 of mm) and high reliability.

In preliminary prototype RH0 string drive were used, similarly to DV, however for not so long sections. The strings are only 40 cm. Because endoscopic tool part is separable, eventually their breaking down of driven strings does not cause immobilizing of robot. The change of tool on new one will permit to finish operations with robot. The increase of mechanical properties and durability of this element was reached in RH 1. In this model the hybrid drive, follower - strings are applicated. The longest of strings were shortened to about 10 cm.

New compact construction of arm together with smaller motors is the reason, that the new arms are lighter and occupy smaller area above operating field. The most space occupies robot DV, in which 3 settled arms are on common massive column (Nawrat et al., 2003).

3.2 Robin Heart Vision for endoscope holding.

Mechanical construction of RH Vision (Fig. 8) is based on the prototype surgery telemanipulator Robin Heart, especially Robin Heart 1, developed and tested in FCSD between 2000-2005 (Fig.1).

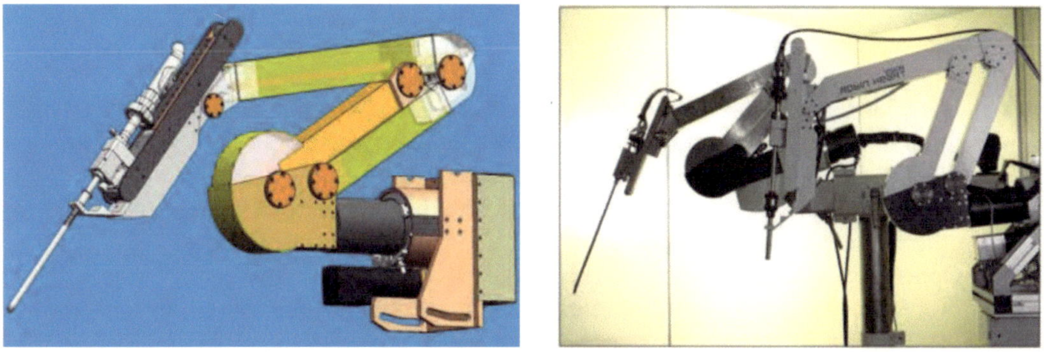

Figure 8. The Model of Robin Heart Vision (a) and the picture of real arm RHVision in the foreground together with Robin Heart prototype in background (b).

Its construction and driven system is an effect of modification of previous models based on their examinations. The main difference is the replacing of the AC motor with harmonic gear used for DOF_1 in RH0&RH1 systems with the electric, brushless motor integrated with planetary gear. The second (range up to 120 degrees doubled system of parallel mechanisms) and third DOFs (the parallel mechanisms eliminates the necessity of using a linear slideway) are driven by brushless motors, roller screws and system of strings. All four DOFs uses Maxon® DCBL motors with hall sensors and digital encoders as a control loop position sensor. The construction makes possible fast and not complicated disconnection the drive part of the bunch from the manipulating part (Nawrat & Kostka, 2007).

4. Control System of Robin Heart Tele-manipulator

4.1 General assumptions of Robin Heart telemanipulator control system

The main idea of control system is common for all described cardio-surgical systems (including Zeus and daVinci systems). The main task of Master-Slave teleoperator is reliable mapping of surgeon hand movements (setting of position/velocity/acceleration of other physical quantity) onto the movements of tool arm, through calculation of control signals for its motors.

Technical requirements of Robin Heart surgical tele-manipulator control system could be listed below:

- frequency of updating signals in the main control loop for translating the Master arm commands into the Slave arm movements, which ensures fluent work should be at least 1000 [Hz],
- satisfactory precision of surgery procedures, taking into account the small sizes of anatomical objects (e.g. 1 mm diameter of coronary vessels) should be guaranteed by the positioning accuracy and resolution equals at least 0.1 [mm],
- delay between Master and Slave arm movement shoul be lower then acceptable limit : $T_{DEL\_MIN} < 100\ [ms]$

- possibility of scaling the movements between the operator and the arm with surgical tool,
- an introduction apart from position surgeon commands (by means of master arm) also other forms of communication with system (e.g. voice control), to increase the comfort of the user interface,
- elimination of surgeon hands tremor,
- optional possibility of the "mirror" movements effects reduction.
- Hardware and software movement limit detection on particular axis
- Communication with host computer (RS, Ethernet) to change work parameters and monitor current state of the system
- Optionally, introduction of force feedback with the possibility of scaling of the force (or others: audio-visual, termical or mechanical - vibrations) sense, passing to operator.
- Optionally, software implementation of movement sets, realizating base surgery procedures in semi-automatic mode (commanded and supervised by surgeon) is planned.

A few different concepts of hardware and software were analyzed to obtain the best result: a system easy to develop and debug, and reliable during normal operation. Two technical solutions were designed, developed and put into practice during the project realization:

System based on VME bus and specialized cards for motor control (PEP® Modular Computers, OS9) (Nawrat et al., 2003).

Systems of regulators working in net, base on DSP and microcontrollers specialized for motor control – this type of hardware/software solution were also applied in Zeus and daVinci system.

4.2 Control System Implementation based on VME bus (RH0&RH1).

A specialised computer system based on VME (VersaModule Eurocard) bus, employing Motorola processor on the main board and working under real time operating system OS-9 was built. VMEbus is widely used in industrial, commercial, medical and military applications with over 300 manufacturers of products worldwide. The proposed control system has a few very important features:

- modular structure,
- industrial mechanical (19" wide and 3U high case) and electrical standard,
- wide range of specialized measurement, communication and control cards,
- open and scalable structure of hardware and software,
- real time operating system working on target controller and comfortable development software working on MS Windows platform.

Fast serial communication has been employed for synchronization and collision avoidance of three arms of robot. The main processor card VM62 based on Motorola MC68060 microprocessor communicates with other measurement and control cards through VME bus and with PC computer through Ethernet link. Specialized position control cards (VIMC) realize the low level regulation of drives with feedback provided by incremental encoders. Quadrature counters (CNT2) and D/A and A/D converters are used to connect haptic device described in the previous section (Nawrat et al., 2003).

4.3 Control System Solution based on Specialized Digital Signal Processors – DSP (RH2).

4.4 Robin Heart 2 solution.

Due to huge technological progress in microcontrollers and microprocessors in last years, units with very high computational power as well as with peripherial specialized for motor control accessible on the market, were used to create telemanipulator control system. Digital Signal Processor (DSP) (tested solutions: Sharc ADSP-2106x Analog Device® oraz TMS 320xxx Texas Instruments®, dsPIC family, Microchip®, ARM uC) is the heart of the system, which performs the task connected with kinematics computation and task sharing / synchronization. Set of N (number of motors) - control units, consisted of PID regulator (specialized microcontroller PIC® Microchip®), optional 10-12 bit D/A converter and power driver, realize the control commands of particular motor.
The surgeon tool is connected to the system through the set of M interface modules, sending information from sensors activated by surgeon hands.
Thanks to assumed hardware solutions control system can be flexible, easy prepared for development and improvement and relatively low cost.
In system Zeus endovision camera is steered by voice (AESOP), while in robot DV foot clutch permits interchangeable starting of camera or tools onto using. In Vinci system electronic control system consist of 4 DSP gives the computational power of 250 millions' floatingpoing operation per second (250 Mflops) and 300 million of operation for second execute to inspect movement of 48 engines with sampling frequency f_S = 1500 [Hz] (http://www.intusurg.com) exactly. Calibrating of movement is to 5:1, often it complies 3:1. Filter of palm tremble removing in DV is typical set on 6 [Hz]. In our system RobInHeart, we test arrangement of limitation now on level 10 Hz.

4.5 Robin Heart Vision solution.

Control system of RHV system for reading and processing the data from Master tool must create the output signals for set driving motor (Maxon DCBL motors, EC&ECPowerMax family), which drivers net has a distributed structure. Every motor unit assigned to particular DOF has its control PID unit with very advanced communication and safety systems (EPOS® , Maxon) placed next to it. All driver units are connected in serial CAN bus. Mentioned above assumptions were fulfilled in implemented control system based on digital signal processor (DSP) specialized for motor control, working as central unit. Main parts of Robin Heart Vision control system are following:
Master tool interface. Depending of type of Master tool (see below) signals from digital encoder sensors (A,B,I) or analogue voltage output (anal. gyroscopes) are translated to common, universal SPI serial bus. In case of Master tools cooperating with PC (joystick and voice recognition system) USB bus is used as a communication channel to system
Central unit. Input signals acquired and translated from Master tool are processed, where several control algorithms are implemented:

- forward kinematics of Master tool
- options: scaling, tremour removing, others
- inverse kinematics of Slave arm

Communication unit. Control system is an autonomous module working in real time system. Communication with host industrial PC realized by USB or Ethernet protocol is applied only for system parameter changing and monitoring (Nawrat & Kostka, 2007).

5. Tests for Robin Heart examination and evaluation.

The main idea of various tests started from first Robin Heart 0 prototype arm is to reveal potential weak points both of construction and control system to correct it and improve in the next model. The goal of surgery robot testing program is evaluation of whole system efficiency. Some parts of Robin Heart testing procedure include classical examination of telemanipulators with additional requirements for medical devices (Fig.9). After preliminary tests and elimination of mechanical and control defects we are preparing to perform tests on animals in condition of operational room and as a last step clinical application is planned.

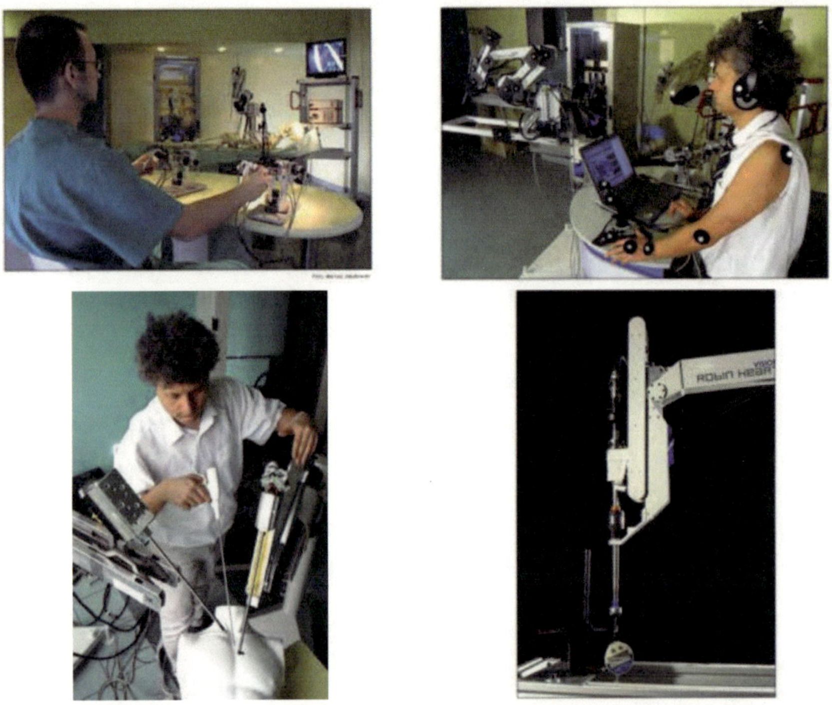

Figure 9. The testing and measurement stands.

On the initial stage of mechanical system assumptions the analysis of maximal forces needed for standard surgery procedures was performed. During tests carried out by means of dynamometric stand on fresh pig hearts from basic surgery acitions like:

- sewing
- cutting
- knot tying

The maximal force (18 N) was applied in case of scalpel cutting. Based on these results the load for robot arm tool tip was designed.

For the robot tests standarization, we tried to replace the operation on real tissues into actions into simulation environment, which consist of electromechanical system, which is able to create load conditions in the range and dynamics of natural material. The control system for this sophisticated testing stand is built based on analysis of real data and modeling the interactions which appear during surgery. Currently we test this system for 1 degree of freedom, but we plan to extend it to 3 D system in Cartesian coordinates.
The procedure of arm test is following:

- the tool tip is fixed to the modeled object (during crash tests only touch
- definition of tested object character (e.g. aorta) by choosing appropriate procedure
- definition of robot task
- the analysis of test results

Thanks to this procedure we are able to compare robots and their particular parts (mechanics, control system, force feedback) in repeatable, standardize tests.
For different testing procedures several testing stands and systems were created:

- environment for monitoring and recording the given (user handle), commanded for motor and real motor position/velocity/current
- stand for hystheresis and repeat tests for both arms (RH0&RH1)
- external trajectory measurement for verification of theoretical settings.
- the usage of technological top semiconductor accelerometer and gyroscope sensors for acceleration and angle velocity measurements opened the new field of robot dynamic properties study. It allowed to record temporal velocity and acceleration values and to analyze and evaluate many phenomena's like e.g. vibration propagation with its frequency domain spectral analysis, angular movements (after integration of input signals)

5. 1 Tests of Robin Heart 0&1&2 systems

Mechanical system examinations.

Mechanical tests included:

- study of the arm stiffness with tool mounted
- repeat tests of tool tip positioning for chosen directions
- measurements of forces between tool tip and surrounding tissues
- tests of tool tip velocity for different movement directions
- tests of absolute accuracy of tool tip positioning in the coordinates of arm base
- hystheresis tests of tool tip positioning

Practically verified resolution of tool tip for every directions is $\pm$ 0.02 mm. The accuracy of operator tool trajectory mapping is about 0.3 mm. Preliminary examinations showed the mechanical hystheresis equal 0.03 mm (for RH1) and 0.02 (for RH2). Stiffness coefficient in this configuration was about $4.85 * 10^3$ N/m (RH0), $2.86 * 10^4$N/m (RH1) and $5.5 * 10^3$ N/m (RH2).

Tests of control and driving systems.

During test phase of project realisation following basic preliminary assumptions were positively verified:

- basic function of telemanipulator like mapping of user interface tool movements into arms movements with such options like scaling and low pass filtering was implemented and tested (Fig.10).

Tests of control systems computational efficiency acknowledged the algorithm sampling frequency F_S equal or above the 1 kHz. (T_S <= 1ms):

- F_S = 1kHz for Robin 0&1
- F_S = 1.4 kHz for Robin 2 robot.

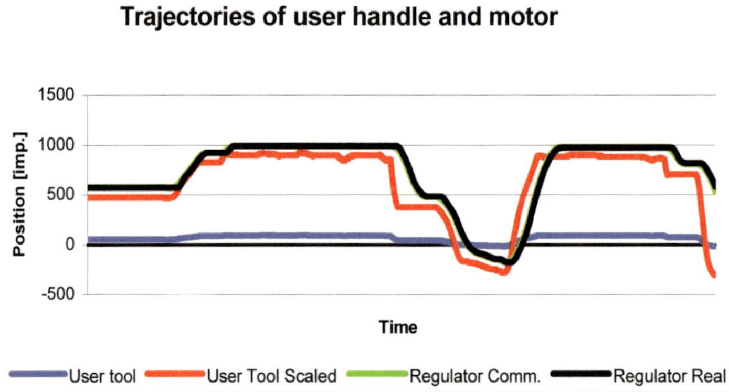

Figure 10. Trajectory of operator handle (original and scaled) and trajectory of corresponding motor (commanded and real). Movement scaling as well as the effect of low pass filtering (trajectory smoothening)

Analysis by means of technological top semiconductor accelerometer and gyroscope sensors for acceleration and angle velocity measurements.

These new sensor opened the new field of robot dynamic properties study. It allowed to observe and evaluate many phenomena's like e.g. vibration propagation with its frequency domain spectral analysis, which allowed to find the maximum vibration at frequency equal to 5 [Hz] for RH0 and more advanced analysis carried out for RH1, where gyroscope and accelerometer signal processing results are presented on time-frequency plane correlated with motor trajectory Time-frequency plane of vibration energy distribution allows to observe the spectral components with its localization also in time domain (Fig.11).

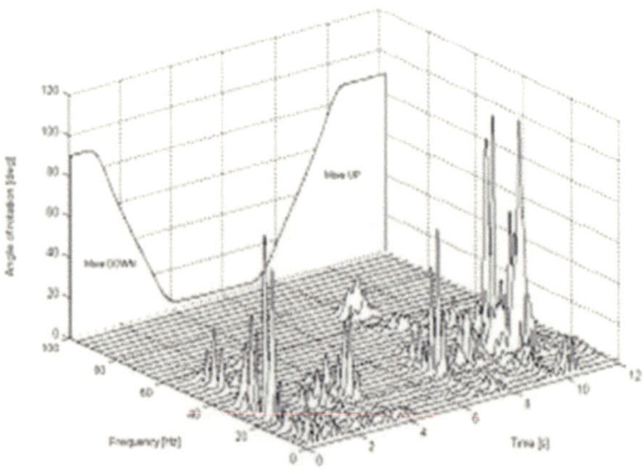

Figure 11. Results of Time-Frequency analysis of gyroscope sensors signals recording during 2nd DOF of Robin Heart 1 up and down movement. Main vibration moved toward higher frequencies (20-35 Hz) can be observed in acceleration and deceleration phase of trapeizodal trajectory. 3D time-frequency distribution

Summary of RH0&RH1&RH2 test results.

Test type / Parameter	RobIn Heart 0 (RH0)	RobIn Heart 1 (RH1)	RobInHeart 2 (RH2)
Arm stiffness coefficient [N/m]	$4.85 * 10^3$	$2.86 * 10^3$	$5.50 * 10^3$
Mechanical hystheresis	-	0.03	0.02
Main control loop refresh frequency [Hz]	1000	1000	1400
Max. vibration amplitude on tool tip [mm]	4	1	0.5
Frequency range of vibrations [Hz]	4-6	20 - 35	30-35

Table 1. Chosen, the most important test results for RobIn Heart systems family.

5.2 Examinations of Robin Heart Vision System.

Basic tests for project assumptions verification.

Technical evaluation of Robin Heart Vision by means of digital micrometer fixed to prepared testing stand.

Verification of the movement range for particular DOFs:

Range of movement	DOF1 [deg]	DOF2 [deg]	DOF3 [mm]	DOF4 [deg]
	187	117,5	Effect. range :165 Max. range :400	350

The assessment of arm positioning resolution:

	DOF1 [mm]	DOF2 [mm]	DOF3 [mm]	DOF4 [mm]
Resolution	0.2	0.2	0.1	0.1

The test of arm precision during the repeat test – registration of the real external trajectory for every of n=100 constant position movements.

	DOF1	DOF2	DOF3	DOF4
Max [mm]	12,486	8,672	9,844	3,157
Min [mm]	12,466	8,625	9,791	3,024
Mean [mm]	12,473	8,668	9,820	3,109
Std. dev. [mm]	0,0054	0,0075	0,013	0,021

Histheresis test

Consecutive n movements with incremented (1.phase) and decremented (2.phase) commanded position (x_i) during "forward" and "backward" phases (1):

$$x_i = x_0 + i * step \ ; \ i = \{1..n..1\} \ ; \ x_0, step \in Z \qquad (1)$$

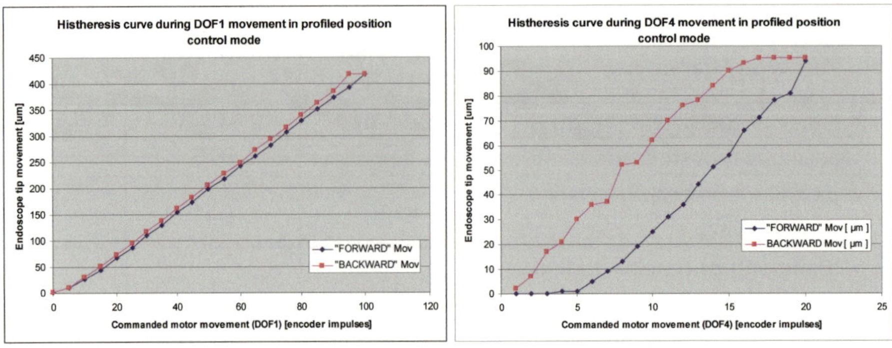

Figure 12. Results of histheresis tests for chosen DOFs: DOF1 & DOF4 (Nawrat & Kostka, 2007).

Visualization tests

The goal of this group of tests is to measure robot performance by objective real, external trajectory measurement by means of specialazed image recording and analysis method.

The measuring system consists of:

- two digital cameras A602fc-2 Basler 100 [Hz];
- computer with motion analysis system APAS;
- set of reflective markers stuck on tested object;
- two sources of light;
- calibration cube.

System of three digital cameras synchronize record the movement of robotic system with special markers fixed to its characteristic points (mainly joints and linear movement parts) (fig.6). Trajectories recorded from different cameras are combined and analyzed in specific image analysis software to compute real external trajectory of robot arm.

Synchronize recording of 'Slave' arm movements, reflecting operator command movement using head movement interface was also performed and trajectories for both 'Master' and 'Slave' tools are presented (Fig.9).

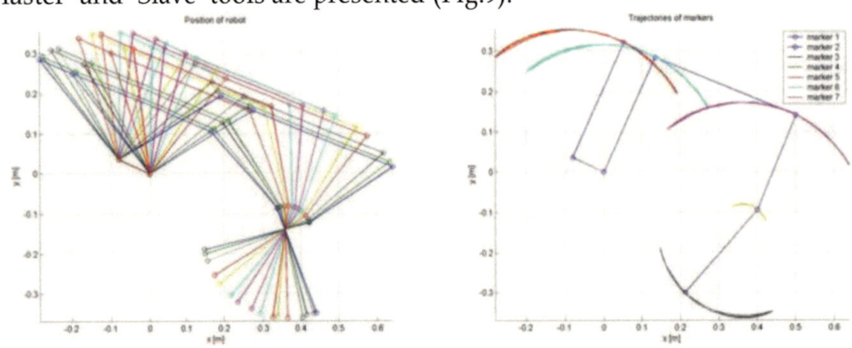

Figure 13. Positions of markers at the following moments of time (Michnik et al 2007)

The motions of reflective markers puted on: upper limb of surgeon, laparoscope master tool manipulator, robot arm (in axises of rotationat kinematic pairs) and operation tool were recorded by two cameras. The movies were transmited to laptop through video

card. After synchronization of movies from two cameras in Digitize module of the APAS system, the kinematic analyses were performed (Michnik et al., 2007)
The Apas system allows to determine automatically trajectories of markers. Linear displacements, velocities and accelerations of markers as well as angular displacements, velocities and accelerations of individual segments of robot arm (Fig.13), upper limb of surgeon, laparoscope master tool manipulator LMTM (angular and linear) and operation tool were obtained in this way.
The results enable verification of three values, which have a significant influence on MASTER-SLAVE systems:
values of determined delays **T** beetwen motions of MASTER and SLAVE parts;
coefficients of scale of displacements **k**;
mapping of adequate motions beetwen laparoscope master tool manipulator (LMTM) and robot arm with operating tool.
Experimental scientific research and kinematics' analysis were performed for motions of robot in three degrees of freedom:
1 DOF - angular motion of SLAVE around axis of 1 DOF;
2 DOF - angular motion of SLAVE around axis of 2 DOF;
3 DOF - linear motion of operating tool ;

Modal examination by means of PCB accelerometers.

To verify the correctness of surgical robot supporting structure, a detailed modal examination was performed and the result data was analyzed. Experiment examination was performed as a first step to compare a different version of surgical prototype structure. The received data was used to estimate a natural frequencies of different robot constructions and to obtain a vibroacustic signal shape from acceleration sensors during a programmed robot move. Stability of an analyzed system was verified in aspect to find the most unsafe robot position which might lead to loose a movement accuracy. This type of knowledge will be necessary in planning a surgery procedure choreography and a Robin Heart position in reference to a surgery table.
Measuring set consists of (Kozlak et al., 2007):

- Signals analyser: SigLab 20-42 DSPT Technology,
- One axis accelerometer sensor: 333B31 made by PCB,
- Modal hammer symbol 086C20, with the force sensor, range: 1 kHz,
- PC + Matlab\SigLab\Vioma software.

As a result in the frequency range up to 500 [Hz], based on stabilizing diagram 12 frequencies of self vibrations were identified for the chosen robot arm position. For example for DOF2 (in max angle) the lowes frequency = 15.3 [Hz] was observed with the 41% smother, next 58 [Hz] with the smother 9.3% (Kozlak et al., 2007).

The animal experiment exam

The last pre-clinical robot examination will be the animal test performed in the specific conditions of operation room. At the end of 2003 our team received the Permission from the Etics Committee of Silesian Medical Academy to perform the first series of in vivo experiments of Robin Heart.
The first stage of tests will include following surgery procedures:

- Robot assisted surgery in abdominal cavity (ganadectomy , bladder excision)
- Bypass implantation on bitting heart by means of surgery robot

- Extracorporal circulatory procedure using Robin Heart (artificial heart valve replacement)

In near future after specialized tools preparation, the operation of ventricular assist device implantation by means of Robin Heart is planned.

7. Conclusion

Currently there are two different robotic systems designed for a cardiac surgery: clinically working daVinci® offered by Intuitive Surgical (since 1998) and a Polish prototype Robin Heart (RH). Both daVinci and the Robin Heart systems are computer-controlled tools, located between surgeon's hands and the tip of a surgical instrument. Polish system named Robin Heart was constructed as a result of work on several prototypes. The project was carried out by a wide area of specialist (Technical Universities from Lodz, Warszawa, Gliwice) under the leadership of Foundation for Cardiac Surgery Development (FCSD) in Zabrze. Launching of the first clinical Robin Heart application is planed by 2009.

Endoscopic microsurgery is difficult to perform with standard hand held instruments but till now robotically assisted did not solve all the problems. In most surgery procedures assisted by robots, only part of these kind of operation are carried out using robot. In this connection the strategy of RH project plans to prepare the family of robotic or semi-automatic surgical tools, which usage could be planned according to required functionality. RH clients will be able to chose both Master tool interface and expert system efficient and comfortable for them. The surgery planning can be carried out using 3D virtual operation room.

Efficiency of using a robotic equipment in an endoscope procedures significantly depends both on a proper tools geometry optimization and a correct surgery procedure planning. Accurate arrangement of setting up the robots arm with reference to an surgery table, positioning the trocars location in a patient body and right choice of a correct tools, makes the surgery procedure much more safe and harmless. Using a virtual reality technology to plan all those important steps, increases efficacy of a noninvasive surgery methods and helps to verify a benefits of using robotic systems in a various surgery treatment.

The FCSD future plans include to carry out the robotically assisted less invasive procedures to implant pumps and valve and mini-invasive service of temporary applicated artificial organs (AORobAS project). In our team the first work on the assumption for heart pump and valve special for robot & MIS (Minimally invasive Surgery) application is done and special tools of robot is constructed.

Efficiency and development of robots usage fields requires searching for the most optimal cardiac robots application range, building the strategy of its usage, simulation the operation results issue and creating the knowledge base supporting the robot's arm navigation and cardiac surgeon decision making, studying of image processing methods for optimal robot's arm navigation

The education and training influences the achievement of success. Next point is cost effectiveness. Currently used robot is to expensive. The investment and maintenance costs still represent the major problem of the da Vinci robot working in about 300 hospitals worldwide. Due to the high cost several clients resigned from continuing robotically assisted practice. To make robotically-assisted surgery wider acceptable the

operation have to be more easier and more attractive for the end user - surgeon (new tolls, pre-planning, advisory system) and less expensive for hospital owner. The lack of rapid improvement and the time consuming procedure led to frustration and many centers did not proceed. We hope that the family robots Robin Heart is good answer for this postulate and create alternative opportunity for currently used technology.
To summarize the current state of polish Robin Heart project realization we can state, that several prototypes of Robin Heart robot for usage in cardiac surgery has been prepared both surgery tool arms as well as RH Vision for camera channel holding. The development of simulation methods for advisory system was reached. The research included:

- strategy planning
- on-line control
- expert and advisory systems for cardiac surgery robot.

We plan that our robot will be more friendly for surgeon, as well as more safety for patient. Our activity in this subject is directed towards two sides: voice control advisory system and interface system.
We plane the first animal test of our robot in autumn of 2007. The first clinical application of endocamera Robin Heart Vision robotically controlled in 2009, the first operation performed by Robin Heart in 2011.
To summarize, on this stage of project realisation the multidiscyplinary team was set up, many students and young researches were included and the construction works go according to plan.

8. Acknowledgement

The research is suppported by State Committee for Scientific Research (KBN 8 T11E 001 18) and Foundation of Cardiac Surgery Development. Warmly thank we fold workers KBN and sponsors for engagement into our project, our numerous collaborators: L.Podsędkowski, K.Mianowski, Z.Małota & Z.Religa and considerable group of students of some universities, which wrote qualifying works, graduate and participated in occupations of scientific wheel.

9. References

Jacobs, S., Falk, V., Holzhey, D., Mohr, F.W. (2006), Perspectives in endoscopic cardiac surgery. *Comp. Biol. Med.* (2006), doi: 10.1016/j.compbiomed.2006.11.007

Kozlak, M., Myk, A., Kciuk, S., (2007), Analiza drgań prototypu robota medycznego Robin Heart. XV *KBiB (Biocybernetics and Bioengineering Conference),* Wroclaw, September 2007, Proceedings in press,

Michnik, R., Ilewicz, G., Jurkojć, J., Tejszerska, D., Nawrat, Z., (2007) Controlling of the operating tool displacement of Master-Slave system of cardiosurgical telemanipulator. Modelling and Optimization of Physical Systems 6, *Zeszyty Naukowe Katedry Mechaniki Stosowanej,* no 6, pp.117-122,Gliwice 2007 Wydawnictwo Katedry Mechaniki Stosowanej, ISBN 9788360102266

Nawrat, Z., Podsędkowski, L., Mianowski; K., Kostka, P., Wróblewski, P., Małota, Z. (2003) Robin Heart - Actual project state of polish telemanipulator dedicated for cardiac surgery. *The Journal of Artificial Organs*. Vol 26/no.12,2003/pp.1115-1119

Nawrat. Z, Kostka, P.,(2007) The Robin Heart Vision, telemanipulator for camera holding preliminary test results. *Journal of Automation, Mobile Robotics & Intelligent Systems, volume1, No. 1, April 2007,* str.48-53

20

Robot Assisted Laparoscopic Surgery for Aortoiliac Disease; a systematic review

Jeroen Diks[1], Denise Nio[1], Willem Wisselink[3] and Willem Bemelman[2]
[1] Department of Surgery, Spaarne Hospital, Hoofddorp,
[2] Department of Surgery, Academic Medical Center, Amsterdam
[3] Department of Surgery, Vrije Universiteit Medical Center, Amsterdam
The Netherlands

1. Abstract

Robotic systems have been used to overcome the technical difficulties in laparoscopic aortoiliac surgery. In this chapter the outcomes of clinical and experimental studies using a robotic surgical system for treatment of aortoiliac disease are reviewed.

1.1 Methods

A computerized search was conducted in the medical databases Medline (from January 2000 to July 2007), Embase (from January 2000 to July 2007) and the Cochrane Database of Systematic Reviews. Operative times, ICU-stay, clamping time, blood loss, anastomosis time, time to resume to solids, hospital stay, mortality and conversion rates were described. Experimental studies reporting on the creation of an aortic anastomosis with the robotic system were included.

1.2 Results

Experimental studies on vascular anastomoses showed equal results when compared to laparoscopy using the Zeus system, whereas the da Vinci robot showed better anastomosis-times and more precise anastomoses when compared to laparoscopic surgery.
Five clinical studies were identified, with in total 70 patients. Operative time varied from 188 to 480 minutes, anastomosis time was 27 to 40.8 minutes. Total hospital stay differed between 4 and 7.3 days. An overall conversion rate of 7 (10%) was reported.

1.3 Conclusion

Little data on robotic assisted laparoscopic surgery exist and the available data are of low quality. The application of robotic systems is feasible and safe, but no robust conclusions can be drawn with respect to comparison with conventional laparoscopic techniques or its cost effectiveness. Robotic assistance might facilitate an endoscopic vascular anastomosis and enhance laparoscopic surgery for aortoiliac disease, but comparative studies are necessary to support this hypothesis.

2. Introduction

Conventional aortoiliac surgery for either occlusive disease or aneurysm repair is accompanied by significant surgical trauma. Minimal invasive surgery reduces the tissue trauma and might result in reduced morbidity and mortality of aortoiliac surgery. Dion et al. pioneered towards the first total laparoscopic approach of the aortoiliac tract in 1993, by performing a laparoscopy assisted aortobifemoral bypass (Dion et al., 1993). Several open minded surgeons followed into his footsteps and several techniques for a total laparoscopic approach of aortoiliac disease were developed (Ahn et al., 1997; Alimi et al., 2000; Kolvenbach et al., 2001; Coggia et al., 2002). One-and-a-half decade later minimally invasive surgery of the aortoiliac vessels is performed only in a few centers around the globe. The slow implementation of laparoscopic assisted aortoiliac surgery can be explained by the technical difficulties encountered embarking on this kind of surgery. The most demanding parts of the total laparoscopic approach for aortoiliac disease are the creation of sufficient and stable exposure, and suturing of the aortic anastomosis. Various techniques are described to approach the abdominal aorta, such as a retro-peritoneal approach, use of the "apron" technique (a peritoneal 'flap' which is used to suspend the bowel), or a total transabdominal approach with extreme lateral rotation of the patient (Ahn et al., 1997; Alimi et al., 2000; Wisselink et al., 2000; Kolvenbach et al., 2001; Coggia et al., 2002; Dion et al., 2003).

Creation of the anastomosis requires a lot of skill, exercise and dexterity. Various authors reported to have been practicing for several months before gaining sufficient proficiency to implement vascular laparoscopy into everyday practice (Coggia et al., 2004; Olinde et al., 2005).

Robotic surgical systems have been developed to facilitate advanced laparoscopic procedures particularly suturing anastomosis as in aortoiliac laparoscopic surgery (Wisselink et al., 2002; Killewich et al., 2004; Desgranges et al., 2004; Kolvenbach et al., 2004; Ruurda et al., 2004; Nio et al., 2004; Nio et al., 2005a; Nio et al., 2005b; Stadler et al., 2006; Ishikawa et al., 2006; Mehrabi et al., 2006; Diks et al., 2007; Diks et al., submitted).

This chapter reviews the use of robotic assistance in laparoscopic surgery of the aortoiliac vessels and its potentially additional value.

3. Methods

A computerized search was conducted in the medical databases Medline (from January 2000 to July 2007), Embase (from January 2000 to July 2007) and the Cochrane Database of Systematic Reviews, using the keywords "robot AND vascular surgery". The results were extended using a combination of the following Medical Subject Heading (MeSH) terms: robotics, aortoiliac disease, arterial occlusive disease, abdominal aneurysm, laparoscopy, robotic assistance, abdominal, experimental.

After identifying relevant titles, the abstracts of these studies were read to decide if the study was eligible. The full article was retrieved when the information in the title and/or abstract appeared to meet the objective of this review. A manual cross-reference search of the bibliographies of relevant articles was conducted to identify studies not found through the computerized search. The "related articles" feature of Pubmed was simultaneously used. Only articles in English language were included.

All experimental studies in which a robotic surgical system was utilized to perform an anastomosis of the aorta are included, evaluated and results described.
All clinical studies describing the use of a robotic surgical system for operating on the abdominal aorta were evaluated. Only papers describing the original patient group were selected. When duplicate material was reported in consecutive articles, the last publication - describing the largest patient group - was included. Data on operation time, ICU stay, clamping time, blood loss, anastomosis time, time to resume oral diet, total hospital stay, mortality and complication rate were identified and evaluated.

4. Results

Experimental studies:
Five experimental studies were included in which a laboratory setup model was used to perform a vascular anastomosis. These studies included two training box models (Nio et al., 2004; Nio et al., 2005b), one human cadaver study (Ishikawa at al., 2006), two porcine models (Ruurda et al., 2004; Mehrabi et al., 2006) and one rat model (Mehrabi et al., 2006). Either the Zeus (Nio et al., 2004; Nio et al., 2005b) - or the daVinci surgical system (Ruurda et al., 2004; Mehrabi et al., 2006; Ishikawa et al., 2006) was used.
In the training box models, the Zeus robotic system (n=40) was compared with a conventional laparoscopic approach (n=40) to conduct a vascular anastomosis. Results showed no significant benefit of the use of the Zeus robotic system in operative time, surgical efficacy and learning curve.
The human cadaver case study described replacement of the thoracic aorta with assistance of the daVinci surgical system (n=1). It reported the feasibility of a thoracic aortal tube replacement with both the proximal and distal anastomoses being conducted in less than 20 minutes each.
In the porcine model, the da Vinci surgical system was used to compare robotic assisted with totally laparoscopic abdominal aortic tube replacement (n=20 vs n=20). The authors concluded that robotic assistance is superior to conventional laparoscopic techniques, because of shorter anastomotic- and clamping times and less blood loss (respectively 22 vs 40 min, $p<0.01$; 63 vs 106 min, $p<0.01$ and 55 vs 280 ml, $p<0.01$). At autopsy the robotic anastomoses showed to be more precise, with less space between consecutive stitches (> 3 mm space between stitches was found in 0/20 vs 12/20 anastomoses).
In a porcine/rat model, the learning curve of an aortic anastomosis using the daVinci surgical system was described. The authors used a training module (n=4) in which an aortic tube replacement was performed in a pig, subsequently in four rats and finally in another pig. The first aortic tube replacement was compared to the last one and a learning curve in the rat model was described. They demonstrated that after training the time to perform an aortic anastomosis was significantly reduced (25:19 vs 12:29 min:sec, $p<0,05$). The authors concluded from this study that robotic assistance has a steep learning curve for conducting an aortic anastomosis.
Patient series:
Five clinical studies were identified (total number of patients: n=70). These studies included one case-report (Killewich et al., 2004), one small case-series (n=5) (Desgranges et al., 2004) and three larger series from Kolvenbach (n=10), Stadler (n=30) and Wisselink (n=24) (Kolvenbach et al., 2004; Stadler et al., 2006; Diks et al., submitted). Of one series earlier results were reported in separate papers (Nio et al., 2005a; Diks et al., 2007). In these studies,

either the Zeus (Computer Motion, Santa Barbara, CA, USA) (n=15) or the daVinci surgical system (Intuitive Surgical, Sunnyvale, CA, USA) (n=55) was used to construct aortic anastomoses in surgery for aortoiliac occlusive - or aneurysmal disease (Table 1).

	Number of patients	Indication for surgery	Robotic system	Conversion (n)	Operative time (minutes)	Anastomosis time (minutes)	Clamping time (minutes)	Blood loss (ml)	ICU stay (days)	Resume diet (days)	Hospital stay (days)
Killewich	1	AOD	dV	0/1	480	X	65	500	X	2	4 (po)
Desgranges	5	AOD	dV	1/5	188	X	75 (± 28)	540	X	X	8 (po) (± 2.4)
Kolvenbach	10	AAA	Z	2/10	242.5 (± 40.5)	40.8 (± 4.1)	95.9 (± 21.6)	X	2.1 (± 1.0)	1.3 (± 0.6)	7.3 (± 2.4)
Stadler	30	AOD/AAA	dV	0/30	236 (180-360)	27 (20-60)	54 (40-120)	320 (100-1500)	1.8 (1-5)	2.5 (2-4)	5.3 (4-10)
Diks	24	AOD	Z / dV	4/24	355 (225-589)	40 (21-110)	77.5 (25-205)	1000 (100-5800)	1 (1-16)	3 (1-4)	5 (3-57)

dV: da Vinci, Z: Zeus, AOD: Aortoiliac Occlusive Disease, AAA: Abdominal Aortic Aneurysm, X: not reported, po: post operative

Table 1. Operation requirement

Operative times varied from 188 to 480 minutes. ICU-stay, reported only in some of the cases, varied from 1 to 2.1 days. Clamping time was reported from 54 to 95.9 minutes. Blood loss varied between 320 and 1000 milliliters. Anastomosis time is reported inconsistently, but when reported it varied from 27 to 40.8 minutes. The time to resume a normal diet varied between 1.3 and 3 days. Total hospital stay varied from 4 to 7.3 days. One of the 70 reported patients died postoperatively. Seven of the 70 patients were converted to open surgery (10%). Reasons for conversion were either technical difficulties with the robotic system (n=4) or an unstable operative field (n=3). The technical difficulties with the robotic system consisted of failure of the robotic system and interference of the robotic arms outside the patient (Desgranges et al., 2004; Kolvenbach et al., 2004; Diks et al., submitted).

Some of the studies described patient selection criteria for robot assisted laparoscopic surgery. Patients with replacement of infected prostheses, with prior abdominal surgery, with redo-surgery of occluded prostheses and with class 4 ASA (American Society of Anesthesiologists) were generally excluded (Diks et al., 2007).

5. Discussion

Two contradictory conclusions emerge from the experimental studies. When the Zeus robotic system was used, no additional value in creating a vascular anastomosis was observed. However, the Zeus system, which was used in these experiments, was not equipped with microwrist instruments yet. In studies where the da Vinci robotic system was used, all authors concluded robotic assistance to be helpful. They noted operation times to be significantly shorter and the anastomoses to be significantly more precise when compared to conventional laparoscopy. A conclusion that the da Vinci robot would be superior to the Zeus could be speculated. This is consistent with results found in other experimental studies which compared the Zeus with the da Vinci robotic system (Sung & Gill, 2001; Dakin & Gagner, 2003). This observation is irrelevant, since the Zeus robot is no longer commercially available.

Only a few patient series were identified. The number of reported patients was small and the study quality of most series was low. Inclusion criteria, study population and individual patient data were poorly described. Since a variety of surgical procedures was performed, patient data could not be pooled to one large series. For this reason no robust conclusions can be made with respect to patient outcomes of robotic assisted aortoiliac surgery compared to conventional laparoscopic surgery.

This review shows that robot assisted laparoscopic surgery (RALS) is an under-explored technique when it comes to minimally invasive treatment for aortoiliac disease. Where RALS has been used in various fields of surgery, such as cardiac-, general-, gynecologic-, thoracic-, and urologic surgery, vascular surgery remains an area in which robotic surgery has yet to establish its current role.

Reported series show that RALS is a feasible and safe procedure, with operative- and clamping times which are comparable to larger series of totally laparoscopic aortoiliac surgery (Coggia et al., 2004; Dion et al., 2004; Olinde et al, 2005). Conversion rate was less when compared to some smaller series in laparoscopic vascular surgery (Barbera et al., 1998; Rouers et al., 2005; Dooner et al., 2006). Outcome parameters e.g. post operative pain and incidence of incisional hernias were not studied, so no conclusions can be made.

An alternative minimally invasive approach, viz. endovascular therapy, is gaining rapidly in popularity in vascular surgery. The implementation of endovascular therapy has been broadened over the last decade and it has shown good results in patient outcome. Nevertheless, long-term results of endovascular treatment still do not surpass those of surgical bypass (Rzucidla et al., 2003). For aneurysm repair, the promising early results favouring endovasculair compared to open repair are not sustained in time. The applicability of endovascular therapy is also limited by the extension of occlusive lesion in aortic occlusive disease and the anatomic suitability in aneurismal disease. Since (robot assisted-) laparoscopic surgery is less bound by vascular anatomy and the same reconstruction is obtained as in open surgery, the solid and durable results of open repair are likely extrapolated to the laparoscopic approach.

The advantages of robotic systems consist of a 3D view and articulating instruments, providing increased degrees of freedom of movement over conventional laparoscopic instruments. These aspects seem helpful when performing complex endoscopic procedures such as suturing a vascular anastomosis. Furthermore, RALS has shown to overcome a long learning curve which is associated with laparoscopic vascular surgery (Coggia et al., 2004). Even with few numbers of patients, clamping - and anastomosis time reduced significantly after only eight patients (Diks et al., 2007). These results show that robotic assistance can help conventional vascular surgeons to start up laparoscopic surgery, even without prior extensive laparoscopic experience.

The use of a robotic system does not obviate training and exercise in advanced laparoscopic techniques. (Laparoscopic) surgical proficiency is established by education and training. A robotic system must be considered as a tool to improve the performance of the surgeon, not be a means to obviate education and training. Several laparoscopic vascular surgeons have shown to suture vascular anastomoses with great proficiency (Coggia et al., 2004; Kolvenbach et al., 2004).

So far, no totally robotic vascular procedures have been described. Robotic systems were only used to create the aortic anastomosis, while conventional laparoscopic techniques were used to approach the aortoiliac vessels. The larger part of the operation however, consists of conventional laparoscopic aortic dissection. Criticasters might argue that since the robotic system is merely used to create the vascular anastomosis, the time advantage compared to conventional laparoscopic suturing is limited. It has to be established whether the purchase of robotic systems and the use of extremely expensive disposables is cost effective compared to laparoscopic suturing of the anastomosis. A benefit of using robotic systems for the total operation has not been evaluated.

Otherwise it has to be considered that if the case volume is insufficient for maintaining these specific endoscopic skills, a robotic system, when available, might be useful to ensure a high quality vascular anastomosis.

It has been shown that RALS for aortoiliac disease is still in a very early stage. Operative times, although comparable to conventional laparoscopic series (Nio et al., 2007), still surpass those of open surgery by far. Furthermore, no research has been done to investigate the cost-effectiveness of a robotic surgical system. It is the task of dedicated centers to answer this research question, ideally in the setting of a randomized clinical trial, in order to provide scientific evidence for the additional value of robotic assistance in laparoscopic vascular surgery.

Meanwhile, with new developments at the horizon - such as an intravascular stapler (Shifrin et al., 2007) - it is yet to see whether this bridging technology has a future in the field of minimally invasive treatment for aortoiliac disease.

6. References

Ahn SS, Hiyama DT, Rudkin GH, Fuchs GJ, Ro KM, Concepcion B (1997). Laparoscopic aortobifemoral bypass. *J Vasc Surg* 26, 1 (Jul 1997) 128–132.

Alimi YS, Hartung O, Orsoni P, Juhan C (2000). Abdominal aortic laparoscopic surgery: retroperitoneal or transperitoneal approach? *Eur J Vasc Endovasc Surg*, 19, 1 (Jan 2000) 21-26.

Barbera L, Mumme A, Metin S, Zumtobel V, Kemen M (1998). Operative results and outcome of twenty-four totally laparoscopic vascular procedures for aortoiliac occlusive disease. *J Vasc Surg*, 28, 1 (Jul 1998) 136–142.

Coggia M, Bourriez A, Javerliat I, Goeau-Brissonniere OA (2002). Totally laparoscopic aortobifemoral bypass: a new and simplified approach. *Eur J Vasc Endovasc Surg* 24, 3 (Sep 2002) 274–275.

Coggia M, Javerliat I, Di Centa I, Colacchio G, Leschi JP, Kitzis M, Goeau-Brissonniere OA (2004). Total laparoscopic bypass for aortoiliac occlusive lesions: 93-case experience. *J Vasc Surg* 40, 5 (Nov 2004) 899–906.

Dakin GF, Gagner M (2003). Comparison of laparoscopic skills performance between standard instruments and two surgical robotic systems. *Surg Endosc* 17, 4 (Apr 2003) 574-579.

Desgranges P, Bourriez A, Javerliat I, Van Laere O, Losy F, Lobontiu A, Melliere D, Becquemin JP (2004). Robotically assisted aortofemoral bypass grafting: lessons learned from our initial experience. *Eur J Vasc Endovasc Surg*, 27, 5 (May 2004) 507–511.

Diks J, Nio D, Jongkind V, Cuesta MA, Rauwerda JA, Wisselink W (2007). Robot-assisted laparoscopic surgery of the infrarenal aorta : The early learning curve. *Surg Endosc*, (Mar 2007) [Epub ahead of print]

Diks J, vd Vijgh R, Nio D, Jongkind V, Yeung KK, Cuesta MA, Wisselink W (2007). Robot Assisted Laparoscopic vs Open Aortoiliac Reconstruction; A Case Control Study. *submitted*

Dion YM, Katkhouda N, Rouleau C, Aucoin A (1993). Laparoscopy-assisted aortobifemoral bypass. *Surg Laparosc Endosc* , 3, 5 (Oct 1993), 425–429.

Dion YM, Thaveau F, Fearn SJ (2003). Current modifications to totally laparoscopic "apron technique." *J Vasc Surg* , 38, 2 (Aug 2003) 403–406.

Dion YM, Griselli F, Douville Y, Langis P (2004). Early and mid-term results of totally laparoscopic surgery for aortoiliac disease: lessons learned. *Surg Laparosc Endosc Percutan Tech* 14, 6 (Dec 2004) 328–334.

Dooner J, Lee S, Griswold W, Kuechler P (2006). Laparoscopic aortic reconstruction: early experience. *Am J Surg*, 191, 5 (May 2006) 691–695.

Ishikawa N, Sun YS, Nifong LW, Ohtake H, Watanabe G, Chitwood WR Jr (2006). Robotic replacement of the descending aorta in human cadaver. *Artif Organs*, 30, 9 (Sep 2006) 719-21.

Killewich LA, Cindrick-Pounds LL, Gomez G (2004). Robot assisted laparoscopic aortic reconstruction for occlusive disease. *Vasc Endovascular Surg*, 38, 1 (Jan-Feb 2004) 83–87.

Kolvenbach R, Ceshire N, Pinter L, Da Silva L, Deling O, Kasper AS (2001). Laparoscopy-assisted aneurysm resection as a minimal invasive alternative in patients unsuitable for endovascular surgery. *J Vasc Surg*, 34, 2 (Aug 2001) 216–221.

Kolvenbach R, Schwierz E, Wasilljew W, Miloud A, Puerschel A, Pinter L (2004). Totally laparoscopically and robotically assisted aortic aneurysm surgery: a critical evaluation. *J Vasc Surg*, 39, 4 (Apr 2004) 771–776.

Mehrabi A, Yetimoglu CL, Nickkholgh A, Kashfi A, Kienle P, Konstantinides L, Ahmadi MR, Fonouni H, Schemmer P, Friess H, Gebhard MM, Buchler MW, Schmidt J, Gutt CN (2006). Development and evaluation of a training module for the clinical introduction of the da Vinci robotic system in visceral and vascular surgery. *Surg Endosc*, 20, 9 (Sep 2006) 1376-1382.

Nio D, Balm R, Maartense S, Guijt M, Bemelman WA (2004). The efficacy of robot-assisted versus conventional laparoscopic vascular anastomoses in an experimental model. *Eur J Vasc Endovasc Surg*, 27, 3, (Mar 2004) 283-286.

Nio D, Diks J, Linsen MA, Cuesta MA, Gracia C, Rauwerda JA, Wisselink W (2005a). Robot-assisted laparoscopic aortobifemoral bypass for aortoiliac occlusive disease: early clinical experience. *Eur J Vasc Endovasc Surg* 29, 6 (Jun 2005) 586–590.

Nio D, Bemelman WA, Balm R, Legemate DA (2005b). Laparoscopic vascular anastomoses: does robotic (Zeus-Aesop) assistance help to overcome the learning curve? *Surg Endosc*, 19, 8 (Aug 2005) 1071-1076.

Nio D, Diks J, Bemelman WA, Wisselink W, Legemate DA (2007). Laparoscopic vascular surgery: a systematic review. *Eur J Vasc Endovasc Surg*, 33, 3 (Mar 2007) 263-271.

Olinde AJ, McNeil JW, Sam A, Hebert SA, Frusha JD (2005). Totally laparoscopic aortobifemoral bypass: a review of 22 cases. *J Vasc Surg*, 42, 1 (Jul 2005) 27–34.

Rouers A, Meurisse N, Lavigne JP, Francart D, Quaniers J, Desiron Q, Limet R (2005). Potential benefits of laparoscopic aorto-bifemoral bypass surgery. *Acta Chir Belg*, 105, 6 (Nov-Dec 2005) 610–615.

Ruurda JP, Wisselink W, Cuesta MA, Verhagen HJ, Broeders IA (2004). Robot-assisted versus standard videoscopic aortic replacement. A comparative study in pigs. *Eur J Vasc Endovasc Surg*, 27, 5 (May 2004) 501-506.

Rzucidlo EM, Powell RJ, Zwolak RM, Fillinger MF, Walsh DB, Schermerhorn ML, Cronenwett JL (2003). Early results of stent-grafting to treat diffuse aortoiliac occlusive disease. *J Vasc Surg*, 37, 6 (Jun 2003) 1175–1180.

Shifrin EG, Moore WS, Bell PR, Kolvenbach R, Daniline EI (2007). Intravascular stapler for "open" aortic surgery: preliminary results. *Eur J Vasc Endovasc Surg*, 33, 4 (Apr 2007) 408-411.

Stadler P, Matous P, Vitasek P, Spacek M (2006). Robot-assisted aortoiliac reconstruction: A review of 30 cases. *J Vasc Surg*, 44, 5 (Nov 2006) 915-919.

Sung GT, Gill IS (2001). Robotic laparoscopic surgery: a comparison of the Da Vinci and Zeus systems. *Urology*, 58, 6 (Dec 2001) 893-898.

Wisselink W, Cuesta MA, Berends FJ, van den Berg FG, Rauwerda JA (2000). Retroperitoneal endoscopic ligation of lumbar and inferior mesenteric arteries as a treatment of persistent endoleak after endoluminal aortic aneurysm repair. *J Vasc Surg*, 31, 6 (Jun 2000) 1240–1244.

Wisselink W, Cuesta MA, Gracia C, Rauwerda JA (2002). Robot-assisted laparoscopic aortobifemoral bypass for aortoiliac occlusive disease: a report of two cases. *J Vasc Surg*, 36, 5 (Nov 2002) 1079-1082.

21

Basic Study of Appropriate Knot-tying Force in the Gastrointestinal Tract for Development of Haptic Surgical Robot

Junya Oguma, Soji Ozawa, Yasuhide Morikawa, Toshiharu Furukawa, Yuko Kitagawa, Masakazu Ueda, Kouhei Ohnishi[1] and Masaki Kitajima
Department of Surgery, School of Medicine, [1]Department of System Design Engineering, Keio University
Japan

1.Introduction

While endoscopic surgery has frequently been performed as minimally invasive surgery in recent years, it is more difficult to perform than open surgery. Our experience with endoscopic surgery using the latest surgical robot daVinci at our hospital has shown that robotic surgery is beneficial in terms of the safe and easy performance of difficult surgical techniques, however, one of its drawbacks use of the robot does not impart a feeling that the surgeon's hands are touching the tissues, making meticulous procedures rather difficult (Anthony et al., 2004).

In ordinary open surgery or endoscopic surgery, surgeons apply knot-tying force spontaneously based on their experience and the feel of the tissues being handled. In robotic surgery, on the other hand, the force exerted is decided on the basis of visual information alone, such as the tautness of the thread and degree of deformation of the tissue. We therefore thought that objective data should be obtained to determine the optimal knot-tying force to apply when suturing during robotic surgery.

To achieve this goal we developed forceps for robotic surgery whose tips have six degrees of freedom (Matsuhira et al., 2003) and a new system at our hospital that displays information about force at the tip of the forceps measured by a sensor to the surgeons on monitor or via auditory signals. No studies have ever been conducted to investigate the relationship between knot-tying force and the efficiency of wound healing in the operated tissue, or to estimate the optimal knot-tying force for tissues. We thought that knowing the optimal knot-tying force for tissues in terms of the efficiency of wound healing would make it possible to tie knots based on the information concerning the force at the tip of the forceps displayed during robotic surgery, and to provide basic data in vivo for the development of robotic forceps that impart a feeling that the surgeon's hands are touching the sutures and tissues. The purpose of this study was to estimate the optimal knot-tying force by investigating the relationship between the force applied assessed on the basis of the information displayed on the surgeon's monitor and the efficiency of wound healing in the gastrointestinal tract in canine models.

Wound healing in the gastrointestinal tract may be closely related to angiogenesis (Frank et al., 1991), and various growth factors may be involved in the process of wound healing (Glenn et al., 1992). Some studies have indicated that basic-fibroblast growth factor (bFGF) may be involved in the repair of epithelial cells, especially in the stomach and intestine (Dignass et al., 1992). In this study we examined angiogenesis and growth factor expression in the area of ligation as wound healing parameters to estimate the optimal knot-tying force for gastrointestinal tissues during suturing. We also attempted to determine the minimal knot-tying force that causes tissue ischemia by making real-time measurements of local blood flow (Oguma et al., 2007).

2.Methods

2.1 Canine models and suture and ligation methods

Twelve male Beagles were fasted for 24 hours before the start of the experiment. The animals were anesthetized by intravenous injection of sodium pentobarbital, and a laparotomy was performed through an upper abdominal midline incision. We cut by 1 cm length and then sutured by 1 cm length and full-thickness the stomach and jejunum by using different magnitudes of knot-tying force ranging from 0.5 N to 5.0 N (N: Newton). As a control ligation was performed without suturing under the same conditions and using the same knot-tying forces. The abdominal wound was closed, and on postoperative days (PODs) 4, 7, 11, and 14, a second laparotomy was performed to remove the stomach and jejunum. The specimens were stained immunohistochemically (anti-bFGF antibody) and with hematoxylin and eosin.

2.2 Local blood flow in the area of ligation

The knot-tying force that caused ischemia was determined by measuring local blood flow in the area of ligation. The wall of the stomach and jejunum was sutured and ligated using a series of knot-tying forces that ranged from 0.5 N to 5.0 N. Local blood flow at the site of first ligature was measured by laser Doppler velocimetry.

3. Results

3.1 Relation between the knot-tying force and local blood flow

There was an inverse correlation between knot-tying forces of 1.5 N and under and local blood flow. At forces of 2.0 N and over, local blood flow was slow and constant. (Fig. 1)

3.2 Relation between knot-tying force and microvessel density

On POD 7 in the stomach (Fig. 2), and on PODs 7 and 11 in the jejunum (Fig. 3), microvessel density in the submucosa at the sites that had been cut and sutured was highest at the knot-tying force of 1.5 N whereas there were no significant differences in microvessel density at any force used at the sites of ligation alone on any of the PODs. Nor were there any significant differences in microvessel density in the mucosa at the sites of cutting and ligation at any force used on any of the PODs. Microvessel density in the submucosa was low on the day of the operation. There were no significant differences in microvessel density in the mucosa or submucosa at the sites of ligation alone at any force used on any of the PODs.

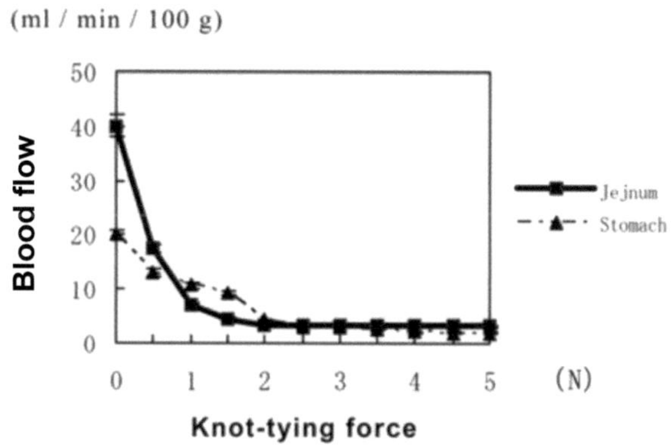

Figure 1. Relation between knot-tying force and local blood flow in the stomach and jejunum

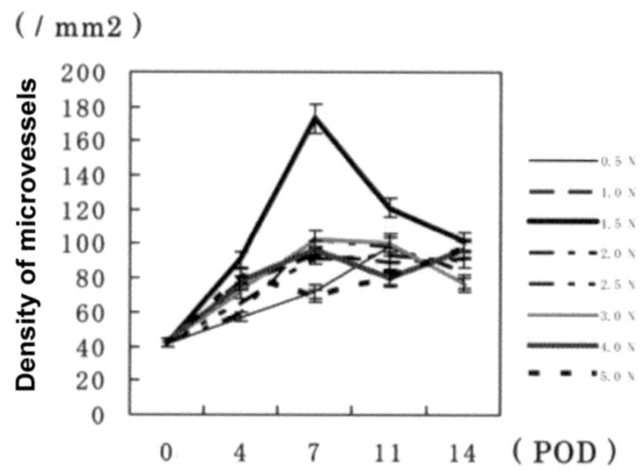

Figure 2. Relation between knot-tying force and microvessel density in the submucosa of the stomach

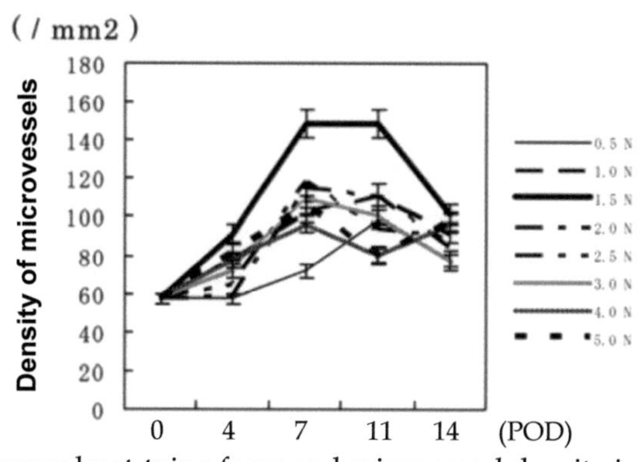

Figure 3. Relation between knot-tying force and microvessel density in the submucosa of the jejunum

3.3 Relation between knot-tying force and expression of bFGF

On PODs 4 and 7 in the stomach and on POD 11 in the jejunum, the density of bFGF-positive cells in the mucosa at the sites of cutting and ligation was highest at the knot-tying force of 1.5 N. There were no significant differences in the density of the bFGF-positive cells in the submucosa at any force used on any of the PODs (Fig. 4, 5).

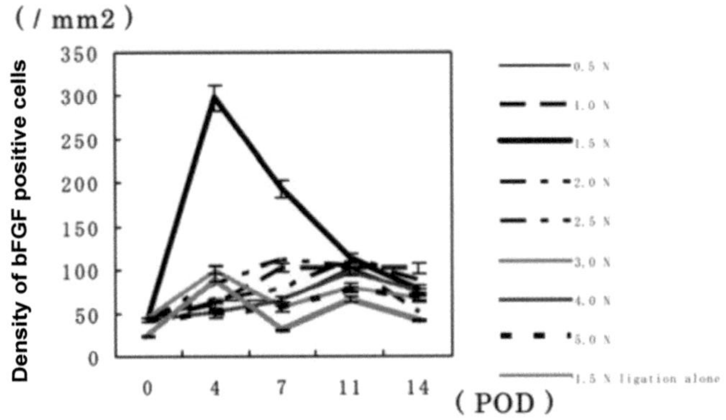

Figure 4. Relation between the knot-tying force and density of the bFGF positive cells in the mucosa of the stomach

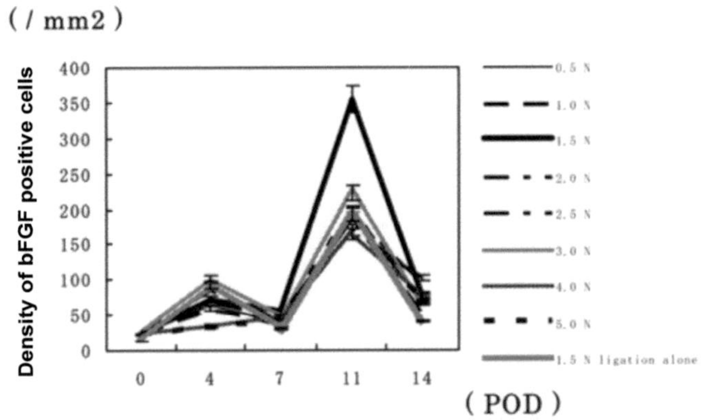

Figure 5. Relation between knot-tying force and density of the bFGF positive cells in the mucosa of the jejunum

4. Discussion

Assessment of the efficiency of wound healing in terms of the extent of angiogenesis and expression of growth factor at the wound sites in this study revealed that a knot-tying force of 1.5 N may be the most appropriate for optimal wound healing in the gastrointestinal tract of the Beagle model.

Wound healing can be evaluated on the basis of physical parameters and histological parameters. The physical parameters include shear stress and tensile strength, and some reports have suggested relationships between these parameters and wound healing (Thijs et al., 1990). Angiogenesis is one of the most important parameters for measuring wound healing, including the healing of wounds in the gastrointestinal tract (Seifert et al., 1997), where it has been suggested that the angiogenesis that occurs during the wound healing process is mainly in the submucosa (Peter et al., 1989). Since application of tension or pressure at the repair site following anastomosis of the gastrointestinal tract is rare in actual clinical practice, we decided that a good histological parameter was more suitable to accurately evaluate wound healing in this situation. In this study we mainly evaluated angiogenesis as the most suitable parameter for assessing wound healing. No previous studies have investigated the relationship between the force applied when placing the sutures and the efficiency of wound healing in the tissue that was sutured, or estimated the optimal force to use when placing sutures in gastrointestinal tissues. In this study we estimated the most appropriate force to use when placing sutures to obtain optimal wound healing in the gastrointestinal tract by assessing the efficiency of wound healing in terms of the extent of angiogenesis as a histological parameter, and we adopted tissue microvessel density as one of the parameters to measure angiogenesis in this study.

Because microvessel density at the sites of ligation alone was lower than that at the sites of cutting and ligation the increase in microvessel density in the submucosa of the stomach and jejunum at the sites of cutting and ligation at the knot-tying force of 1.5 N appeared to be attributable to angiogenesis associated with wound healing and not to inflammation secondary to local tissue damage. Therefore, based on microvessel density in the submucosa we were able to objectively estimate that 1.5 N was the optimal knot-tying force for wound healing in the gastrointestinal tract of the Beagles.

We thought that wound healing would not occur at knot-tying forces less than 1.5 N, because agglutination of the edges at the sites of cutting and ligation was incomplete and the angiogenesis and fibrosis associated with the wound healing process were prevented. While some reports have suggested that local blood flow is important for wound healing (Chung et al., 1987), no previous studies have investigated the relationship between knot-tying force and local blood flow. The results of this study suggest that knot-tying forces greater than 1.5 N would make the tissue ischemic and prevent efficient wound healing.

To select the range of knot-tying forces to test in our study, three surgeons were blindfolded and asked to place several sutures manually, and we measured the knot-tying force used in each instance. The forces applied during tying ranged from 0.8 N to 2.0 N, although there were a few differences among the three surgeons. We therefore selected 0.5 N to 5.0 N as the range of knot-tying forces to test in our study.

It has been reported that bFGF may be related to acceleration of angiogenesis, formation of granulation tissue, and proliferation of fibroblasts (Spyrou et al., 2002). In this study we measured the expression of bFGF at the sites of cutting and ligation as a diachronic study and investigated the relationship between knot-tying force and expression of bFGF. The increase in expression of bFGF in the mucosa of the jejunum at the sites of cutting and ligation was observed later than the increase in microvessel density in the submucosa. In the stomach, the expression of bFGF in the mucosa preceded the increase in microvessel density in the submucosa. It has been reported that bFGF is the major contributor to the formation of granulation tissue and increase in number of fibroblasts in the intestine during the process of wound healing, and that angiogenesis is also induced mainly by bFGF. The timing of the expression of bFGF in the stomach differed from the timing of the expression in the jejunum, and the role of bFGF in wound healing would seem to differ in different organs.

In recent years the development and application of robotic surgery has progressed to such an extent that the poor flexibility of the tips of forceps, which was one of the drawbacks of endoscopic surgery, has been overcome, making telesurgery possible, and suturing and ligation can now be performed more smoothly (Cadiere et al., 2001). On the other hand, since a sense of touching the tissue is not imparted to the surgeon's hands from the tip of the forceps, use of appropriate force during ligation has been difficult. We developed a system that displays information concerning the force at the tip of the forceps to the surgeon on a monitor or via auditory signals, and based on the results of this study the system appeared makes it possible to apply appropriate force during suturing and ligation in the gastrointestinal tract. We are now planning to develop a system in which the force at the tip of the forceps that directly imparts a sense of touch to the surgeon's hands. We need to program information on variable senses of touch to this system to create a database. We believe that the results of our study will serve as useful data for surgery on live beings and contribute to the development of robotic forceps with a sensor of touch in the future.

5. References

Anthony RL, Andres EC, Jaydev PD, William CM: Robotic Surgery. *Ann Surg* 2004; 239: 14-21, doi: 10.1097/01.sla.0000103020.19595.7d

Matsuhira N, Jinno M, Miyagawa T, Sunaoshi T, Hato T, Morikawa Y, Furukawa T, Ozawa S, Kitajima M, Nakazawa K: Development of a functional model for a master-slave manipulator for laparoscopic surgery. *Advanced Robotics* 2003; 17: 523-539

Frank A, David CW: Angiogenesis in wound healing. *Pharmac Ther* 1991; 52: 407-422.

Glenn FP, John ET, Donna Y Thomas AM, Gary MF, Arlen T: Platelet-derived growth factor (BB homodimer), transforming growth factor-β1, and basic fibroblast growth factor in dermal wound healing. *Am J Pathol* 1992; 140: 1375-1388.

Dignass AU, Tsunekawa S, Podolsky DK: Fibroblast growth factors modulate intestinal epithelial cell growth and migration. *Gastroenterology* 1994; 106: 1254-1262.

Oguma J, Ozawa S, Morikawa Y, Furukawa T, Kitagawa Y, Ueda M, Kitajima M: Knot-tying Force during Suturing and Wound Healing in the Gastrointestinal Tract J Surg Res 2007; 140: 129-134, doi:10.1016/j.jss.2006.12.008

Thijs H, Walter JBM: Healing of experimental intestinal anastomosis. *Dis Colon Rectum* 1990; 33: 891-901.

WF Seifert, AAJ Verhofstad, T Wobbes, W Lange, PFJW Rijken, AJ van der Kogen, T Hendriks: Quantitaion of angiogenesis in healing anastomoses of the rat colon. *Exp Mol Pathol* 1997; 64: 31-40.

Peter B, Matti L, Seppo R: Changes in the connective tissue composition of the submucosal layer of clonic anastomosis. *Acta Chir Scand* 1989; 155: 413-419.

Chung RS: Blood flow in colonic anastomoses. *Ann Surg* 1987; 206: 335-339.

GE Spyrou, IL Naylor: The effect of basic fibroblast growth factor on scarring. *Br J Plast Surg* 2002; 55: 275-282, doi: 10.1054/bjps.2002.3831

Cadiere GB, Himpens J, Germey O, Izizaw R, Degneldre M, Vandromme J, Capelluto E, Bruyns J: Feasibility of robotic laparoscopic surgery: 146 cases. *World J Surg* 2001; 25: 1467-1477, doi: 10.1007/s00268-001-0132-2

22

Robotic Gastrectomy with Lymphadenectomy for Gastric Cancer

Casandra Anderson, Joshua Ellenhorn and Alessio Pigazzi
City of Hope , Duarte, California
USA

1. Introduction

Minimally invasive surgical approachs to early stage gastric cancer have been employed as a means to improve postoperative outcomes in patients undergoing gastrectomy for gastric cancer. However, conventional laparoscopic techniques have not gained wide acceptance due to the inherent difficulty in performing a laparoscopic gastric lymph node dissection (D2). Although laparoscopic D2 lymphadenctomy has been described and found to be feasible by experienced laparoscopic surgeons (Uyama et al. 1999, Tanimura et al. 2006 Pugliese et al. 2006), it is technically challenging and can be associated with significant bleeding during dissection around the hepatic, celiac, and splenic arteries. With increasing evidence supporting that D2 dissections can be performed with low morbidity (Wu et al. 2006, Roukos et al. 1998 Hartgrink et al 2004), we employed robotic technology to help facilitate a minmally invasive approach to gastric lymph node dissection.
This chapter will review our operative method for performing a robotic-assisted gastrectomy with lymph node dissection. In this description, advantages and disadvantages of robotic technology will be reviewed. Our short-term post-operative and oncologic outcomes will be discussed and compared with other laparoscopic and robotic series.

2. Operative Method

Positioning and room set-up

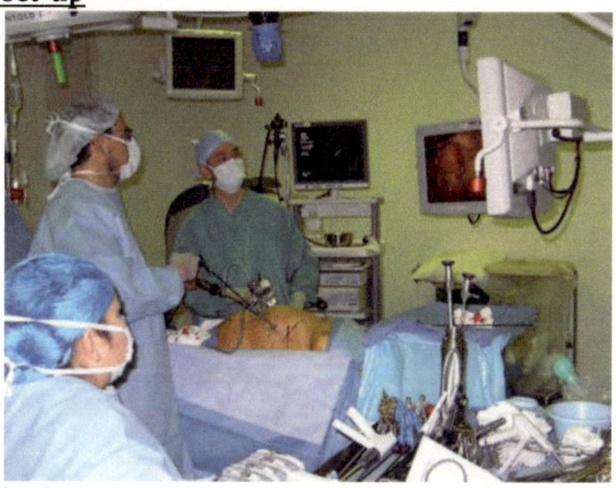

Figure 1. Room set-up for laparoscopic portion of the procedure

The procedure is performed under general anesthesia. An operating surgeon and one assistant perform this procedure. The patient is placed in a 30 degrees reverse Trendelenburg supine position. The first part of the operation which entails an complete omentectomy and gastric mobilization is performed laparoscopically. Robotic technology is then used to perform the lymphadenectomy and gastrointestinal reconstruction. The laparoscopic room set-up is illustrated in figure 1 with the monitors placed above the patient's head.

Port Placement

A pneumoperitoneum to 15 mmHg is established using a Veress needle technique, after which a 10-mm supra-umbilical camera port is placed. Four additional ports are placed under direct visualization: three 8-mm robotic trochars, 2 in the upper abdomen bilaterally at the midclavicular line, one in the right anterior axillary line for liver retraction, and a 10-mm assistant's port between the left robotic port and the camera port. (Fig 2).

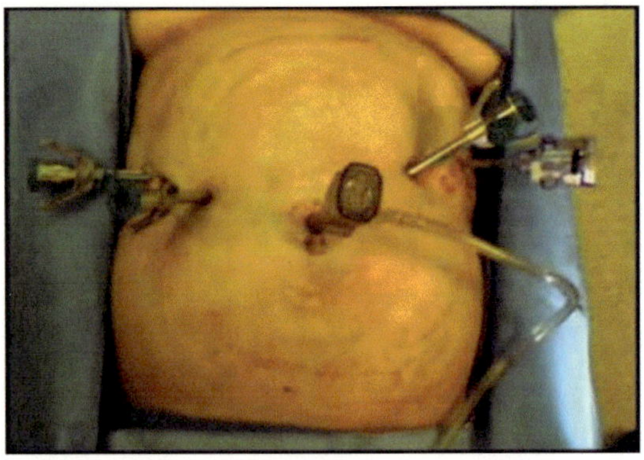

Figure 2. Port site placement

Laparoscopic Portion of Procedure

The abdomen is explored for metastatic disease, an then an on-table endoscopy is performed to identify and mark the tumor if it cannot be seen laparoscopically.

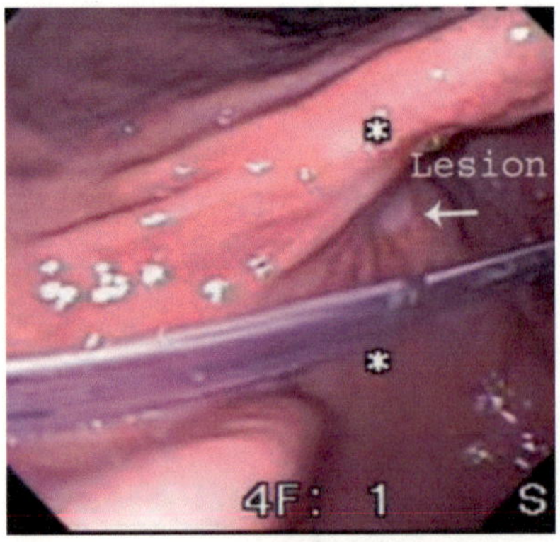

Figure 3. Intraoperative EGD

Using a harmonic scalpel an omentectomy is performed. Once completed, the lesser sac is entered and the posterior attachments of the stomach are divided. Next, the right gastroepiploic vessels are identified and divided using a vascular stapler, clips or the ultrasonic shears. (Fig 3)

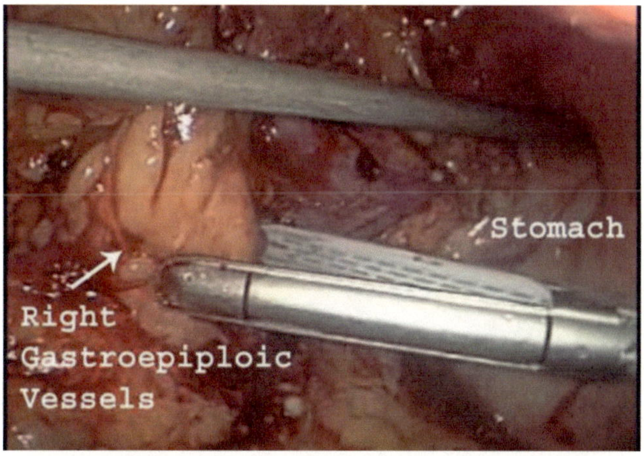

Figure 3. Staple Ligation of gastroepipolic vessels

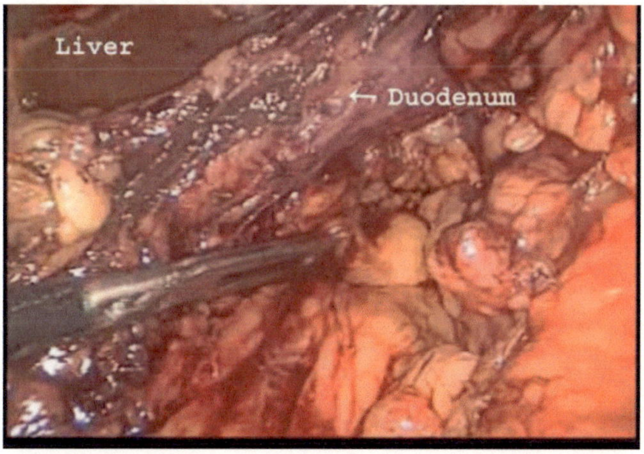

Figure 4a. Mobilized Duodenum

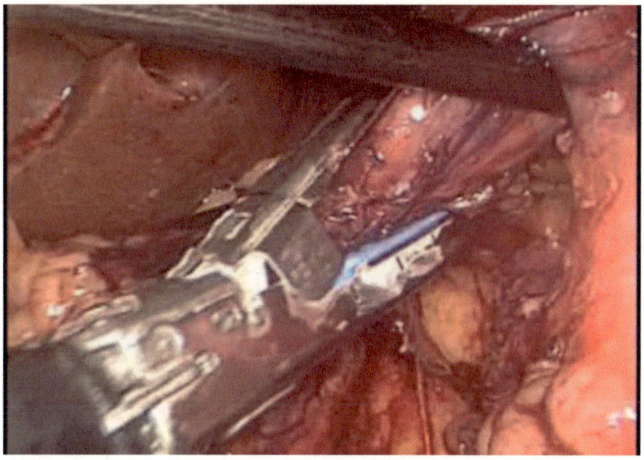

Figure 4b. Stapling of Duodenum (Blue- 3.5 mm staples)

The post pyloric duodenum is subsequently circumferentially dissected and transected using an endo-GIA stapler. (Fig 4) Infraduodenal lymph nodes are dissected and are included with the specimen during the division of the duodenum.

Robotic Portion of Procedure

A four-arm da Vinci robotic system is used. The left most lateral arm is used for liver retraction, the left midclavicular arm holds a bipolar dissector and the right robotic arm carries a fine hook cautery. A 30-degree robotic scope is used. The surgeon moves to the console and the assistant to the patient's left side. (Fig 5)

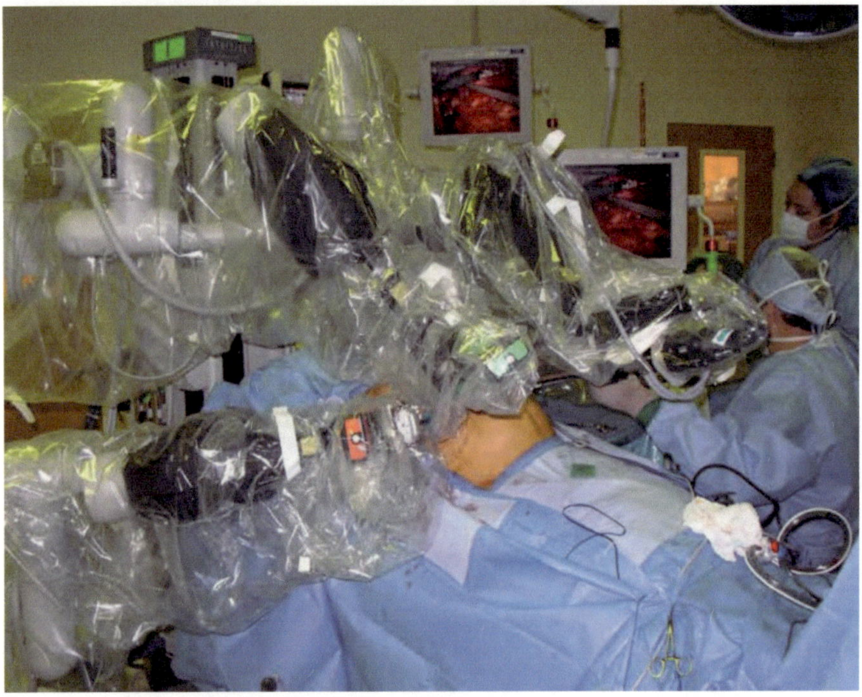

Figure 5. Robotic room-setup

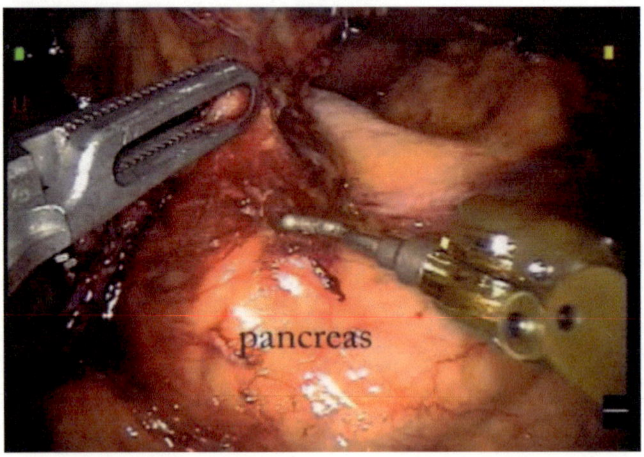

Figure 6. Beginning of lymphadenectomy

Based upon the Japanese guidelines for D2 lymphatic dissecion for middle and lower gastric tumors, the following lymph node stations are harvested: stations1- right paracardial, 3- lesser curvature, 4- greater curvature, 5- suprapyloric, 6-infrapyloric, 7- left gastric, 8- common hepatic, 9- celiac, 11- splenic, and 12- hepatoduodenal ligament. The lymphadenctomy is begun by identifing the gastroduodenal and common hepatic arteries at the superior border of the pancreas. (Fig 6)

Using hook cautery an extensive lymphadenctomy is carried out along the common hepatice artery. During this dissection the right gastric vessels are divided using endo-clips.(Fig 7) The dissection continues to the hepatic helium until the proper hepatic artery has been completely skeletonized anteriorly. Once this has been completed the dissection continues along the common hepatic artery to the celiac trunk.(Fig 8) The left gastric vessels are ligated at their origin using either endo-clips or ties.(Fig 9) Next, the right paracardial nodes are dissected towards the specimen.(Fig 10) Subsequently, the splenic artery is skeletonized of lymphatic tissue from its origin to the splenic helium. (Fig 11) The lymphadenectomy is completed by stipping the lesser curvature nodes of the stomach. (Fig 12)

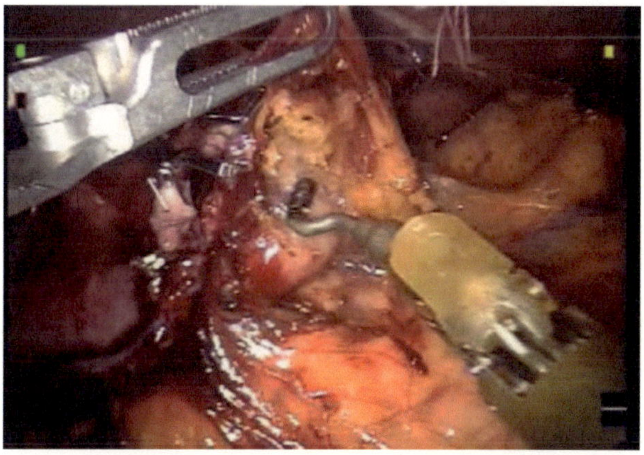

Figure 7. Right gastric artery ligated, proper hepatic artery dissected with hook cautery

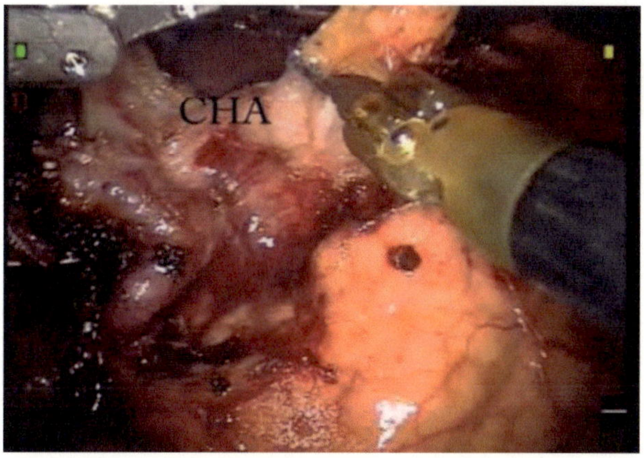

Figure 8. Dissection continuing towards celiac trunk

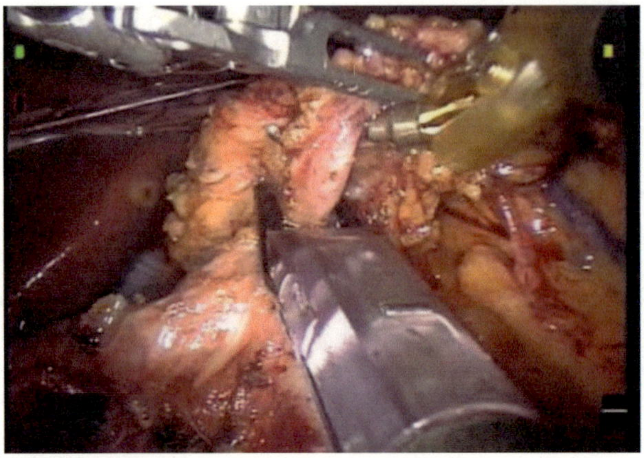

Figure 9. Left gastric artery ligation

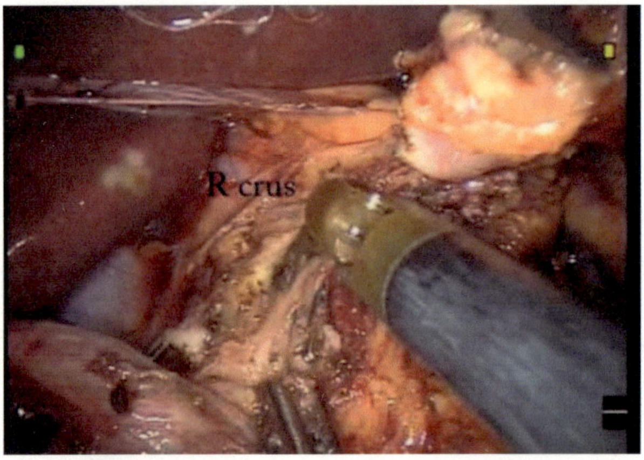

Figure 10. Right paracardial node retreival

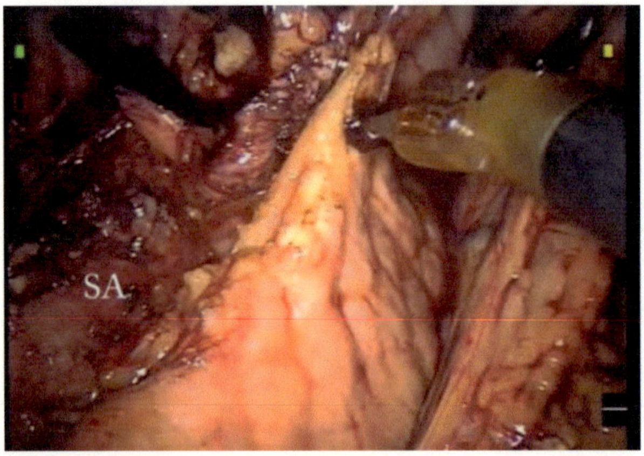

Figure 11. Splenic artery nodes

The resection is completed by dividing the stomach using a endo-GIA stapler (blue or green loads). This manuever is performed by the assistant from the patient's left side. The entire specimen is placed into a large endocatch bag and removed through a suprapubic minilaparotomy incision. Gastrointestinal continutity is restored by performing a partially stapled/partially handsewn anti-colic, side-to-side gastrojejunostomy. An endo-GIA 60 stapler (blue load), is again fired from the assistant's port, creating the anastomosis. The common enterotomy is closed in a two layer hand sewn fashion with 3-0 vicryl using two robotic needle holders. Methylene blue (300ml) is injected into the stomach to test the integrity of the anastomosis.

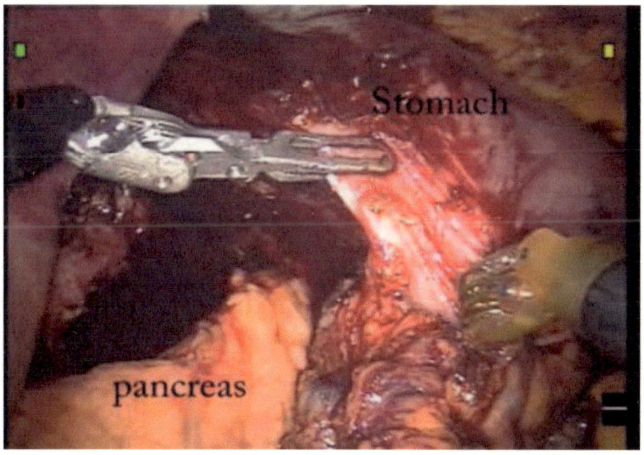

Figure 12. Lesser curature nodes

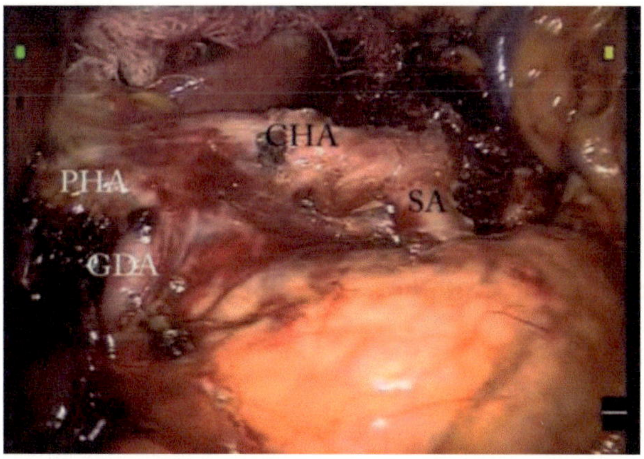

Figure 13. Completed Lymphadenctomy

3. Results

Between 7/05-2/07 ten patients with early stage gastric cancer were treated with this approach. The operative and short-term outcomes are listed in table 1.

Results	
Operative time (mins)	430 (390-459)
Estimated blood loss (ml)	300 (100-850)
# of nodes harvested	27 (17-41)
Size of tumor	1.3 (.3-3.4)
Length of Hospital stay	
Total	5 (3-9)
Intensive Care Unit	1 (0-2)
Return to diet	
Liquid	1.5 (1-6)
Solid	4 (2-8)

Table 1. Operative and short-term outcomes

The 30-day morbidity and mortality was 20%and 0% respectively. Post-operative complications included; one patient with a port site hematoma requiring transfusion, and another patient that required overnight readmission for dehydration. Additionally two patients developed deep venous thrombosis more than thirty days postoperatively.

4. Discussion

The main advantages of robot technology over conventional laparoscopy include; 3-D stereoscopic vision, the ability to tremor filter and scale motions, and the internally articulated instruments that are controlled by the robotic masters that transfer the surgeon's hand movements to the tip of the instruments in an intuitive manner. All of these features enhance the surgeon's ability to perform precise fine dissection. The disadvantages of the current robotic technology include the lack of tactile feedback, and difficulty operating in multiple abdominal quadrants with heavy abdominal structures. Some of these concerns may be resolved with the newest robotic model. (DaVinci S, Intuitive Surgical Inc, Sunnyvale, CA)

Table 2 lists comparative data for subtotal gastrectomies performed either laparoscopically or robotically. The largest robotic series for gastric cancer is reported by Giulianotti (Giulianotti et al., 2003). Their results are similar to those found in this report. Additionally, there are two important laparoscopic trials; one published by Lee (Lee et al., 2006) which is a large retropsective series, and the second by Huscher (Huscher et al., 2005) which is a prospective randomized trial comparing laparoscopic distal gastrectomies to open. Our robotic series compares favorable in terms of shorter hospital stays, quick return to diet, and low mortality. However, robotic operative time is longer.

Author (number of pts)	Giulianotti[2] (21)	Lee[1] (136)	Huscher[1] (30)	Current Series[2] (10)
Operative time (mins)	365	158	196	430
Lymph nodes retreived	-	31	30	27
Length of Hospital stay	9	8	10	5
Return to diet	-	4	5	4
Morbidity	9%	8.%	23%	20%
Mortality	9%	-	3%	0%

[1] laparoscopic, [2] robotic

Table 2. Comparative trials for subtotal gastrecomies

5. Conclusion

There is still limited data to support robotic surgery for management of gastric cancer. It appears to be safe and feasible technology that allows for adequate lymph node retrieval with a low morbidity and short hospital stay. If this novel therapy allows surgeons to more easily perform complex oncologic resections, then potentially this will allow more patients with gastric cancer to be managed with a minimally invasive approach.

6. References

Giulianotti P, Coratti A, Angelini M, Sbrana F, Cecconi S, Balestracci T, Caravaglios G (2003) Robotics in general surgery. *Arch Surg*, 138,7, (July 2003) 777-784, 0004-0010

Hartgrink H, Van de Velde C, Putter H, Bonenkamp J, Kranebarg E, Songun I, Welvaart K, van Krieken J, Plukker J, van Elk P, Obertop H, Gouma D, van Lanschot J, Taat C, deGraaf P, von Meyenfeldt M, Tilanus H, Sasako M. (2004) Extended lymph node dissection for gastric cancer: who may benefit? Final results of the randomized dutch gastric cancer group trial. *J Clin Oncol*, 22,11, (June 2004) 2069-77, 1527-7755

Hashizume M, Keizo Sugimachi (2003) Robot-assisted gastric surgery. *Surg Clin N Am*, 83,6, (Decemeber 2003) 1429-1444, 0039-6109

Hashizume M, Shimada M, Tomikawa M, Ikeda Y, Takahashi I, Abe R, Koga F, Gotoh N, Konishis K, Maehara S, Sugimachi K (2002) Early experiences of endoscopic procedures in general surgery assisted by a computer-enhanced surgical system. *Surg Endosc*, 16,8, (August 2002) 1187-1191, 1432-2218

Pugliese R, Maggioni D, Sansonna F, Scandroglio I, Ferrari G, DiLernia S, Costanzi A, Pauna J, DeMartini P (2007) Total and subtotal laparoscopic gastrectomy for adenocarinoma. *Surg Endosc* 21,1 (January 2007) 21-27, 1432-2218

Roukos D, Lorenz M, Encke A (1998) Evidence of surivival benefit of (D2) lymphadenectomy in Western patients with gastric cancer based on a new concept: A prospective long-term follow-up study. *Surgery*, 123,5, (May 1998) 573-8, 0039-6060

Tanimura S, Higashino M, Fukunaga Y, Osugi H (2003) Laparoscopic distal gastrectomy with regional lymph node dissection for gastric cancer. *Surg Endosc,* 17,5, (May 2005) 58-62, 1261-8942

Uyama I, Sugioika A, Fujita J,Komori Y, Matsui H, Soga R, Wakayama A, Okamota K, Ohyama A, Hasumi A (1999). Completely laparoscopic extraperigastric lymph node dissection for gastric malignancies located in the middle or lower third of the stomach. *Gastric Cancer,* 2,3,(November 1999) 186-190, 1436-3305

Wu C, Hsiung C, Lo S, Hsieh M, Chen J, Li A, Lui W, Whang-Peng J (2006) Nodal dissection for patients with gastric cancer: a randomised controlled trial. *Lancet Oncol,* 7,4,(April 2006) 309-15, 1470-2045

23

Robotic Rectal Cancer Surgery

Minia Hellan, Joshua Ellenhorn and Alessio Pigazzi
City of Hope, Duarte, California
USA

1. Introduction

Minimally invasive surgery has influenced the approach used in a variety of operations. Laparoscopic surgery is an accepted modality for the treatment of colon cancer, resulting in superior short term functional outcome and equivalent survival when compared with open surgery (Veldkamp et al., 2004; Nelson et al., 2004). However, minimally invasive rectal cancer surgery is still a matter of great debate. The concept of a sharp total mesorectal excision (TME) has become standard of care for the treatment of rectal cancer with the lowest recurrence rates published in literature (Heald et al., 1998). TME includes the routine excision of the intact mesorectum by precise sharp dissection of the areolar tissue between the visceral and parietal layers of the fascia. Multiple authors have shown that this approach can be carried out laparoscopically offering the patient the advantages of minimally invasive over open techniques (Morino et al., 2003; Leroy et al., 2004; Leung et al., 2004). However, there is little doubt that laparoscopic TME is technically very challenging with a steep learning curve. We therefore began using robotic technology to facilitate the dissection in the pelvis, a confined space requiring precise movements, thus taking advantage of the enhanced dexterity of the robot.
This chapter will review our operative technique of robotic-assisted total mesorectal excision for low rectal cancer as well as advantages and disadvantages of this technology.

2. Operative Technique

2.1 Positioning of the patient

We prefer a "hybrid" technique with laparoscopic mobilization of the splenic flexure and robotic-assisted TME. After induction of general anesthesia, the patient is moved to a modified lithotomy position with the legs 30-45° apart to ensure room for the robot, which will be brought in between the legs at a later time. The patient is kept in a steep Trendelenburg position during the whole procedure in order to remove the small bowel from the pelvis. During the laparoscopic mobilization a 20-30° right lateral rotation aids in better exposure of the ligament of Treitz and vessel dissection. Both the assistant and the surgeon stand on the patient's right side throughout the procedure.

2.2 Port placement

Pneumoperitoneum is created with the Verres needle technique, and the abdomen is insufflated to 15 mm Hg. A 12 mm camera port C is placed halfway between the umbilicus and the xiphoid. During the laparoscopic dissection a 30° 10-mm telescope is used, which is subsequently replaced with the 0° standard 12-mm robotic laparoscope. Under direct vision two 8 mm robotic trocars (R1, R2) are placed in the midclavicular line approximately 12-14 cm from the symphysis to reach the pelvic floor. The robotic ports themselves need to be at least 10 cm apart from each other in order to avoid collision of the arms. The third robotic port, which is used for retraction, is placed after the robot is docked to find the most suitable position lateral and superior to the anterior superior iliac spine (ASIS). The laparoscopic ports L1 and L2 (5-mm ports) are placed each 10 cm above the other in the midclavicular line. Finally a 10-mm laparoscopic port is inserted just lateral and superior to the ASIS to be used for staplers and the ligasure device.

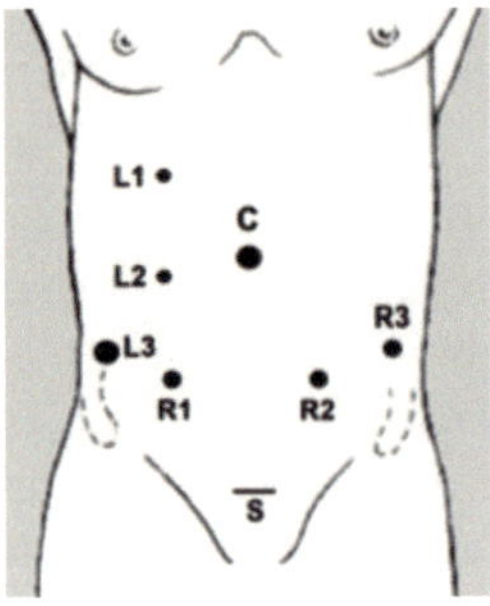

Figure 1. Port site placement

2.3 Laparoscopic mobilization of splenic flexure and left colon

During the laparoscopic portion of the operation the surgeon uses R1 and L2, while the assistant holds the camera and uses L1. Both are standing on the patient's right side. We routinely carry out a medial-to-lateral mobilization of the left and sigmoid colon. After inspection of the abdominal cavity for metastatic disease, the inferior mesenteric vein (IMV) is identified and used as initial anatomic landmark. To expose the IMV the ligament of Treitz and the loose attachments between the proximal jejunum and the descending mesocolon may have to be divided sharply so that the small bowel can be retracted towards the right upper quadrant (Fig. 2).

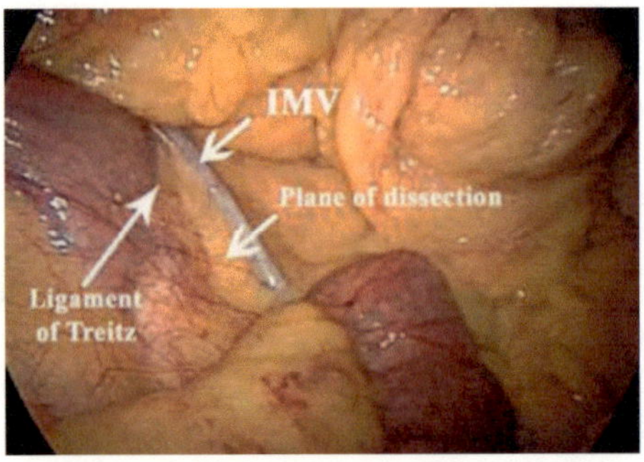

Figure 2. Exposure of the inferior mesenteric vein (IMV)

Next, the peritoneum just under the vein is incised, and the space between mesocolon and Toldt's fascia is developed toward the abdominal wall; ureter and gonadal vessels are identified. In order to avoid traction injuries we recommend early division of the IMV near its insertion posterior to the pancreas where the IMV is azygous, traveling without a paired artery. More distally, the IMV runs parallel to the upward traveling left colic artery (LCA). Therefore the IMV/left colic artery pedicle should be followed inferiorly and freed from its posterior attachments to the aorta until the origin of the inferior mesenteric artery (oIMA) is encountered (Fig.3)

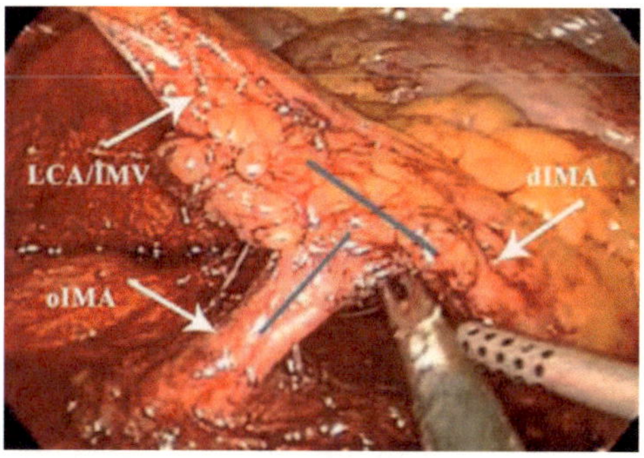

Figure 3. Identification if inferior mesenteric artery

The IMA can now be divided at the origin or distal to the left colic artery depending on the particular case. Division of these vessels can be carried out with an endoscopic linear stapler device or clips inserted trough the L3 port. The medial-to-lateral dissection is completed as far laterally as possible, the white line of Toldt is incised and the colon freed from its attachments to the abdominal wall. If necessary the splenic flexure is taken down after the omentum is divided from the transverse colon.

2.4 Robotic Total Mesorectal Excision

A four-arm DaVinci robotic system is used. With the patient remaining in a steep Trendelenburg position, the DaVinci robotic system is brought into the field in between the patient's legs.

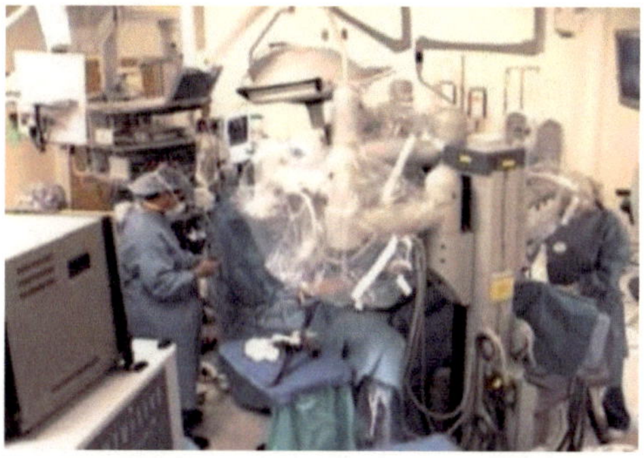

Figure 4. Position of the DaVinci robot

The three arms are docked to ports C, R1 and R2. These are the working arms usually carrying a grasper on the left connected to bipolar cautery and a hook with monopolar cautery on the right. Now the port for the fourth robotic arm is placed laterally and docked. A Cadiere grasper is used through this port to help with anterior retraction of the bladder or rectum during part of the dissection. The assistant remains on the right side. He/she uses ports L2 and L3 for suctioning and additional retraction of the sigmoid colon/rectum out of the pelvis. The rectosigmoid mesentery is elevated superiorly and anteriorly. The plane between the fascia propria of the rectum and the presacral fascia is identified and entered (arrow, Fig. 5).

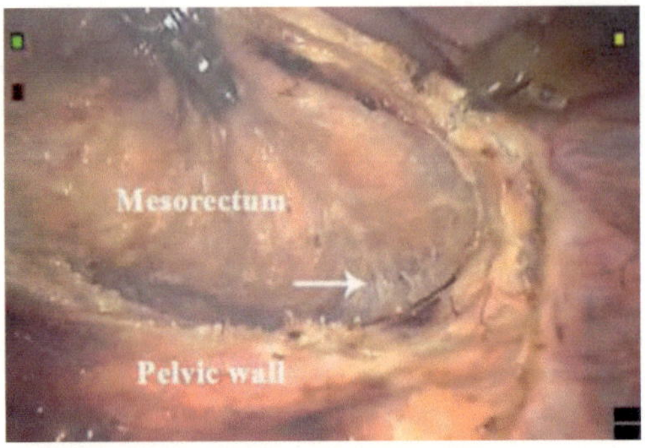

Figure 5. Entering the plane posterior to the mesorectum

This plane consists of fine areolar tissue that can be divided sharply with the electric hook cautery. The ureters on both sides are identified and remain lateral to the dissection. The hypogastric nerve plexus lies posterior to the presacral fascia and should not be injured if the dissection is continued along the correct plane. The dissection continues circumferentially around the rectum. Anteriorly the peritoneal reflection is incised and the anterior dissection is continued along the rectovaginal septum in women or the rectovesical/retroprostatic (Denonvilliers) fascia in men (Fig.6).

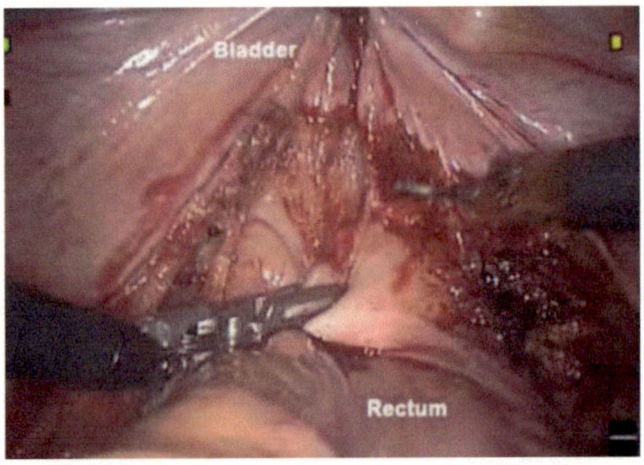

Figure 6. Anterior dissection

This posterior dissection is carried out all the way to the pelvic floor by dividing the rectrosacral fascia (Waldeyer's fascia) thus ensuring a total mesorectal excision (Fig.7)

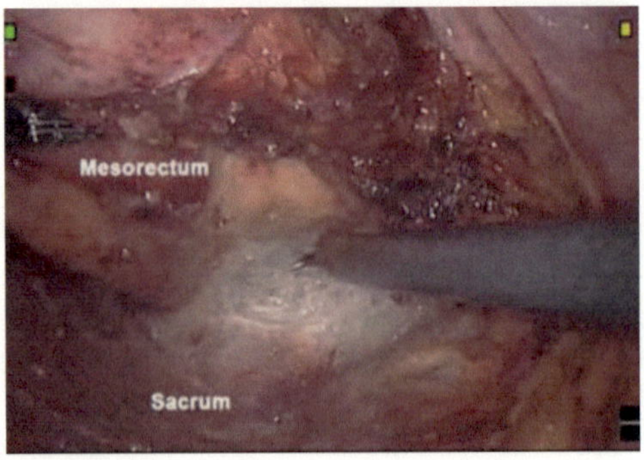

Figure 7. Posterior dissection

At completion of the TME the pelvic floor muscles should be clearly visible. The muscle fibers of the puborectalis sling are divided around the rectum for full mobilization (arrow, Fig. 8).

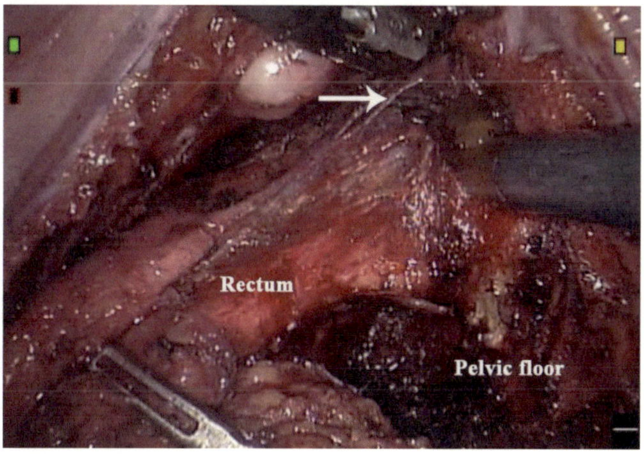

Figure 8. Full mobilization of rectum to pelvic floor

Before dividing the rectum, one member of the team performs a digital rectal exam under direct visualization to assess the distal margin. A margin of at least 1 cm is targeted.

2.5 Creation of Anastomosis

The distal rectum is divided by the assistant with multiple loads of a reticulating 30-mm linear stapler (blue load) (Fig. 9).

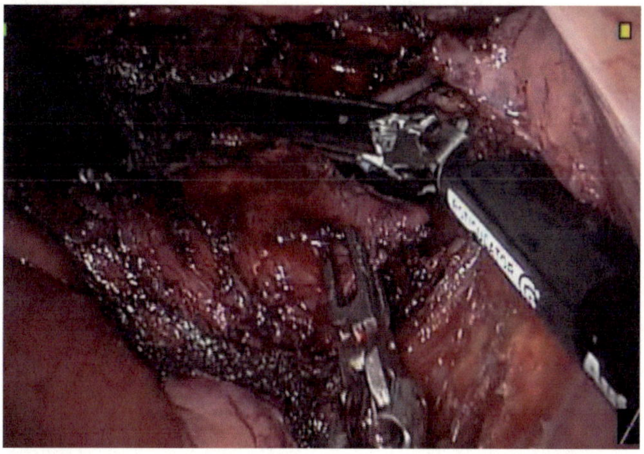

Figure 9. Division of rectum

The specimen is extracted by creating a 4-cm suprapubic mini-laparotomy covered with a plastic wound protector. The proximal bowel is divided and an anvil is introduced into the proximal stump. The bowel is dropped back into the abdomen, the incision closed and the pneumoperitoneum reinsuflated. The anastomosis is now created with a circular stapler under direct laparoscopic visualization. Care is taken to assure that no tension is exerted on the anastomosis (Fig.10).

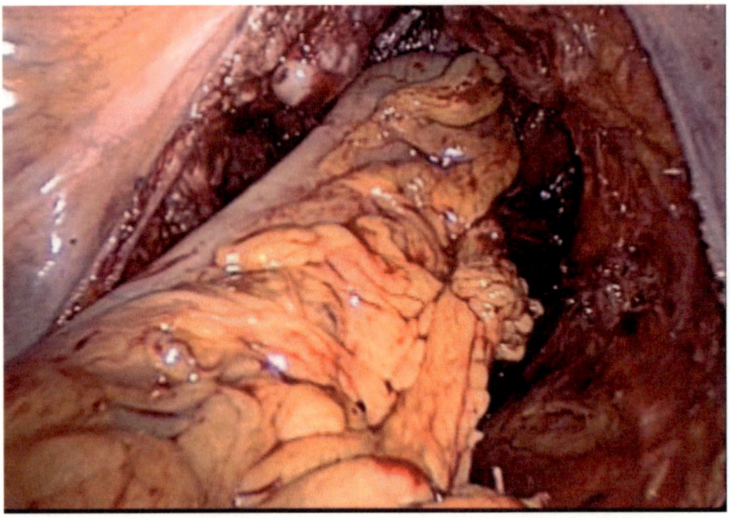

Figure 10. Completed anastomosis

In case of a very low rectal cancer the dissection can be continued along the intersphincteric plane with the robot. The mucosa is then divided from below just above the dentate line, the intersphincteric plane is entered, and the specimen pulled through the anus and divided. A hand-sewn coloanal anastomosis is then created in the standard fashion. We usually perform a diverting ileostomy when the anastomosis is at 5 cm from the anal verge or fewer.

2.6 Full robotic approach

Full robotic approaches are described for resection of the lower rectum. Two robotic positions may be used as described by D'Annibale et al (2004). For the left colon and splenic flexure mobilization the robot is positioned beside the patient's left shoulder. The DaVinci system is then moved down between the patient's legs for the rectal dissection. To avoid moving the robotic cart a compromise in the setup is necessary to achieve completion of a left flexure mobilization, TME and rectal resection. In this setting the robotic cart comes from the left thigh of the patient. However due to the limited reach of the robot this setup is only feasible for short and average build patients. The use of the new DaVinci S system may eliminate some of these problems as a larger range of motion will be possible with the robotic arms.

3. Results

Since November 2004 a total of 37 patients underwent robotic-assisted laparoscopic rectal resection with total mesorectal excision for primary rectal cancer. The operative and short-term outcomes are listed in Table 1. Low anterior resections were performed in 22 patients, 10 patients had intersphincteric and 5 abdominoperineal resections (APR). There was only one conversion to open surgery in a morbidly obese patient (conversion rate 2.7%). A total of four patients experienced anastomotic leaks (12.5% leak rate). One patient experienced severe hemorrhage during an APR as consequence of the perineal resection. A total mesorectal excision with negative circumferential and distal margins was accomplished in all patients.

Results	
Operative time (min)	285 (180-540)
TME time (min)	60 (35-135)
Estimated blood loss (ml)	200 (25-6000)
# nodes harvested	13 (7-28)
Distal margin (cm)	2.75 (0.2-6.4)
Time to clear liquid diet (days)	2 (1-11)
Length of stay (days)	4 (2-22)

Table 1. Operative and short-term outcomes (median values)

4. Discussion

Major pitfalls of laparoscopic rectal surgery are the technical and anatomic complexity in the narrow pelvis where some maneuvers are difficult to perform with non-articulating instruments. Because of the potential advantages of robotic assistance in the pelvis, we started to assess the utility of the DaVinci system for total mesorectal excisions. We found that telerobotic surgery facilitates several aspects of the pelvic dissection in the confined pelvic space, and that the three-dimensional imaging gives excellent view of the pelvic anatomy.

Early experiences with different robotic-assisted colorectal procedures such as colectomies (Rawlings et al., 2006; D'Annibale et al., 2004), rectopexy (Munz et al., 2004) and anterior resections (D'Annibale et al., 2004, Anvari et al., 2004) are described in recent literature including our previous early report of robotic-assisted TMEs (Pigazzi et al., 2006). These studies found no difference in specimen length, number of lymph nodes retrieved, estimated blood loss, recovery of bowel function or hospital stay between laparoscopic and robotic colorectal resections. Our data showing no positive circumferential or distal margins support these findings. Additionally our leak rate of 12.5% is comparable to a leak rate of 13-19% seen in laparoscopic TME series (Morino et al., 2003; Leroy et al., 2004). Our operative times of 180-540 minutes also compare favorable to reported operative times (88-600 minutes) for laparoscopic rectal surgery (Morino et al., 2003; Leroy et al., 2004; Leung et al., 2004). However, increased operative times due to robotic and operating room set-up have been reported (D'Annibale et al., 2004, Anvari et al., 2004). The low conversion rate of 2.7% and high success rate of TMEs suggest that the advantage of the robot system may translate in better patient outcome.

Nevertheless, there are some drawbacks to current robotic systems. The most significant disadvantage is the inability of the robotic arms to self-adjust around the bed to allow the surgeon to gain access to more than one quadrant of the abdominal cavity at any one time. Another criticism of current robotic systems includes a lack of adequate instruments for bowel surgery such as staplers and suction devices necessitating the use of additional laparoscopic ports.

5. Conclusion

In conclusion we can confirm that robotic surgery for rectal cancer is safe and feasible. Rectal cancer surgeons without extensive laparoscopic colorectal experience who wish to transition from open to minimally invasive TME may benefit from this modality. Future studies are necessary to determine the long-term oncologic outcomes of robotic assisted total mesorectal excision.

6. References

Veldkamp, R. ; Gholghesaei, M. ; Bonjer, HR. ; Meijer, DW.,Buunen, M. ; Jeekel, J. ; Anderberg, B. ; Cuesta, MA. ; Cuschier, A. ; Fingerhut, A. ; Fleshman, JW. ; Guillou, PJ. ; Haglind, E. ; Himpens, J. ; Jacobi, CA. ; Jakimowicz, JJ. ; Keockerling, F. ; Lacy, AM. ; Lezoche, E. ; Monson, JR. ; Morino, M. ; Neugebauer, E. ; Wexner, SD. & Whelan, RL. (2004). Laparoscopic resection of colon cancer. Consensus of the European Association of Endoscopic Surgery (EAES). *Surg Endosc*, 18, 8, Aug. 2004, 1163-1185, 0930-2794

D'Annibal, A. ; Morpurgo, E. ; Fiscon, V. ; Trevisan' P. ; Sovernigo, G. ; Orsini, C. & Guidolin, D. (2004). Robotic and laparoscopic surgery for treatment of colorectal diseases. *Dis Colon Rectum*, 47, 12, Dec. 2004, 2162-2168, 0012-3706

Nelson, H. ; Sargent, DJ. ; Wieand, HS. ; Fleshman, J. ; Anvari, M. ; Stryker, SJ. ; Beart, RW. ; Hellinger, M. ; Flanagan, R. ; Peters, W. & Ota, D. (2004). A comparison of laparoscopically assisted and open colectomy for colon cancer. *N Engl J Med*, 350, 20, 2050-2059, 0028-4793

Heald, RJ. ; Moran, BJ. ; Ryall, RD. ; Sexton, R. & MacFarlane, JK. (1998). Rectal Cancer : the Basingstoke experience of total mesorectal excision, 1978-1997. *Arch Surg*, 133, 8, Aug. 1998, 894-899, 1591-1063

Leung, KL. ; Kwok, SP. ; Lam, SC. ; Lee, JF. ; Yiu, RY. ; NG, SS. ; Lai, PB. & Lau WY. (2004). Laparoscopic resection of rectosigmoid carcinoma : prospective randomised trial. *Lancet*, 363, 9416, April 2004, 1187-1192, 0140-6736

Morino, M. ; Parini, U., Giraudo, G.,Salval, M., Contul, RB. & Garrone, C. (2003). Laparoscopic total mesorectal excision: a consecutive series of 100 patients. *Ann Surg*, 237, 3, March 2003, 335-342, 0003-4932

Leroy, J., Smith, M., Rubino, F., Mutter, D., & Marescaux, J. (2004). Laparoscopic total mesorectal excision (TME) for rectal cancer surgyer: long-term outcomes. *Surg Endosc*, 18, 2, Feb. 2004, 281-289, 0930-2794

Munz, Y., Moorthy, K., Kudchadkar, R., Hernandez, JD., Martin. S., Darzi, A. & Rockall, T. (2004). Robotic assisted rectopexy. *Am J Surg*, 187, 1, Jan. 2004, 88-92

Pigazzi, A., Ellenhorn, JD., Ballantyne, GH. & Paz, IB. (2006). Robotic-assisted laparoscopic low anterior resection with total mesorectal excision for rectal cancer. *Surg Endosc* 20, 10, Oct. 2006, 1521-1525, 0930-2794

Rawlings, AL., Woodland, JH. & Crawford, DL. (2006). Telerobotic surgery for right and sigmoid colectomies: 30 consecutive cases. *Surg Endosc* 20, 11, Nov. 2006, 1713-1718

Anvari, M., Birch, DW., Bamehriz., F., Gryfe, R. & Chapman T. (2004). Robotic-assisted laparoscopic colorectal surgery. *Laparosc Endosc Percutan Tech* 14, 6, Dec. 2004, 311-315, 1530-4515

24

Efficient Non-Invasive Registration with A-mode Ultrasound in Skull Surgery

Aleksandra Popovic[1], Stefan Heger[1], Axel Follmann[1], Ting Wu[1], Martin Engelhardt[2], Kirsten Schmieder[2] and Klaus Radermacher[1]
RWTH Aachen University, Ruhr-University Bochum
Germany

1. Introduction to Neuronavigation

Surgical navigation is an interactive localization technique to establish a relation between surgical instruments, patient's anatomy, and additional data (e.g. preoperative or intraoperative patient images or atlases).

The first attempt to localize structures within the brain using orientation points on the skull surface and a standardized brain atlas was done at the beginning of 20th century (1908) by Sir Victor Horsley and Robert H. Clarke (Tan & Black 2002). They used a rigid frame (Horsley-Clarke apparatus) designed to measure salient points on the skull in Cartesian 3D coordinate system and transform them to the coordinate system of a brain atlas. Coordinate system computations allowed a surgeon to position a tool to a desired position within the skull. Findings of Horsley and Clarke were followed by further improvements in frame design, coordinates computations, and brain atlases. However, the major breakthrough was achieved as imaging technologies emerged, Computed Tomography (CT) in 1973 and Magnetic Resonance Imaging (MRI) during 1980s. Three-dimensional brain images allowed an extension of stereotactic computation to the entire intracranial space. Until the end of 1990s, stereotaxy has been the most common localization technique in the neurosurgery (Grunert et al. 2003). Frameless navigation emerged as an alternative to conventional stereotactic surgery, in order to decrease invasiveness and to improve localization and targeting. The main objective of image-guided surgery is to track surgical instruments in relation to the patient images. To achieve this, a geometric transformation between physical and image space has to be established in a registration procedure. First attempts to avoid invasive stereotactic frames in neurosurgical navigation emerged at the end 1980s with neuronavigator arms (Watanabe et al. 1987, Watanabe 1996, Laborde et al. 2002), six-dimensional mechanical digitizers performing point-based registration of the patient and image space and computer-based arm tracking. The main disadvantage of those systems is the need for repeated registration after each repositioning of the patient's head (Schiffbauer 1992). Further development of digitalization system introduced magnetic (Tan et al. 1993) and optical localizers (Zamorano et al. 1992;1993) in the neuronavigation, able to interactively track instruments and patient position. Although optical tracking devices have a disadvantage of requiring permanent line-of-sight during tracking, they are currently state-of-the-art technique in surgical navigation due to a better localization accuracy compared to the magnetic systems. Commercially available optical neuronavigation systems include StealthStation© (Medtronic, USA) and Vector Vision©cranial (BrainLab, Germany). The technique in which an operator freely moves tracked surgical instruments is referred to as a free-hand navigation. Although image-guidance combined with a preoperative planning allows a better spatial orientation through the position feedback, the positioning accuracy is restrained by human factors, such as hand-eye coordination. For some deep brain targeting applications requiring high precision, frame-based stereotaxy is still preferred to free-hand image-guidance (Spivak and Pirouzmand 2005). An alternative approach is to use a robotic system, providing a high spatial accuracy, an ability to perform time-lasting repetitive movements, and high movement predictability (Nathoo 2005). In recent years, research efforts have been made to introduce robotic systems in the neurosurgical practice (Bai et al. 2001, Federspil et al. 2003, Federspil and Plinkert 2004, Handini et al. 2004, Bast et al. 2006).

2. Motivation – CRANIO System for Robot and Computer Aided Neurosurgery

Osseous tumors of the calvaria are rare diseases presented with various histological and imaging findings (Arana 2004, Engelhardt 2006). The majority of calvarial tumors encountered in the field of neurosurgery are either meningiomas or metastases. They are usually treated by a total or subtotal recision followed by a removal of the tumorous tissue.
The CRANIO system for computer and robot assisted craniectomy (Bast et al. 2006) is being developed for the surgical treatment of patients suffering from calvarial tumors, accompanied by preoperative design and manufacturing of individual implants for immediate cranial reconstruction, also called cranioplasty (Wu et al. 2006). Clinical motivation for the robotic craniectomy (removal of a cranial tumor) is twofold:

- A robotic removal of the cancerous bone is significantly more time-efficient than manual procedures. Laboratory experiments showed 50%-70% milling time reduction in comparison to the manual micro-milling (Bast et al. 2003). This might lead to a decrease in operating time with benefits to patient's health and cost reduction. Furthermore, the operating surgeon is relieved from a tenacious instrument holding.
- In order to preoperatively manufacture an individual implant and perform cranioplasty immediately following a tumor ablation, the resection geometry has to be known prior to the operation and has to be accurately reproduced during the operation. Free-hand neurosurgical milling, even with a navigational help, cannot meet the accuracy requirements.

To achieve these objectives, all aspects of the computer aided surgery have to be addressed: segmentation (Popovic et al. 2006), resection planning, milling path generation and simulation (Popovic et al. 2003), implant planning and manufacturing (Wu et al. 2006), intraoperative navigation and robot control (Popovic et al. 2003, See Figure 1). Intraoperatively, a geometrical relation between patient's physical space and preoperative data (e.g. the resection path in coordinate system of the CT scanner) has to be established in the process of an intraoperative registration (see section 2.3.1). Accuracy of execution of the preoperative plan intraoperatively depends on three factors:

1. Patient registration accuracy, i.e. transformation accuracy of the planed milling path from the coordinate system of the model data to the *in situ* coordinate system of the patient.

2. Robot registration accuracy, i.e. transformation accuracy of the planed milling path from the coordinate system of patient to the robot coordinate system.
3. Robot accuracy, i.e. the positioning accuracy of the robot.

Due to the mechanical precision and reproducibility of the robotic system, the patient registration is the most accuracy-critical part of the system. Apart from accuracy requirements, time efficiency, reliability and intuitiveness of the registration process are crucial for application of the system in clinical routine. The problem of simultaneous accuracy improvement and invasiveness reduction can be solved using A-Mode Ultrasound (AUS) based registration.

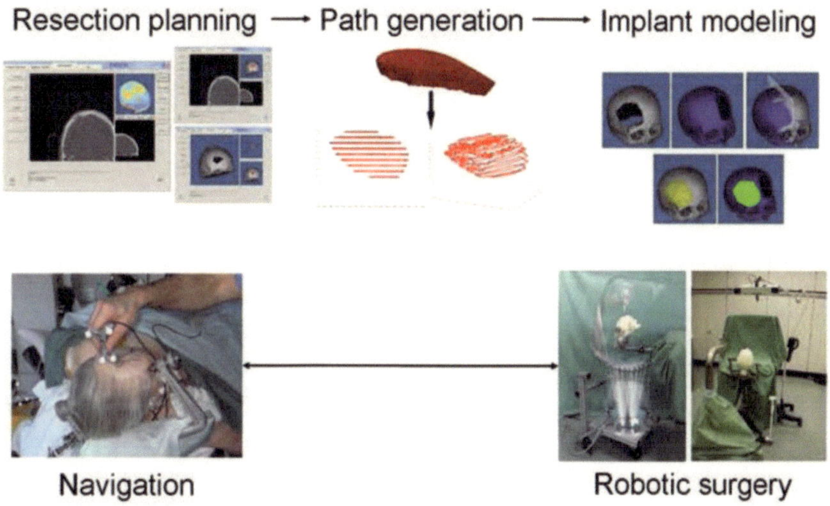

Figure 1. The concept of the CRANIO system

3. Registration algorithms

The process of patient registration involves finding a transformation relating the patient's physical space with the coordinate system(s) of preoperative and/or intraoperative acquired images. The registration procedure is an optimization method searching for an optimal transformation between the points in patient's physical space, i.e. measurement points $\{\vec{m}_i\}$ and points in image space, i.e. data points $\{\vec{d}_i\}$. Therefore, the transformation is represented as:

$$T : \vec{m} \mapsto \vec{d} \Leftrightarrow T(\vec{m}) = \vec{d}\,, \tag{1}$$

where $\vec{m}$ is a measurement vector with $\vec{m} = [\vec{m}_0 ... \vec{m}_{N-1}]^T, \vec{d} = [\vec{d}_0 ... \vec{d}_{N-1}]^T$ a data vector and N the number of points. If T is a linear, rigid transformation, it represents a rotation and a translation of the points:

$$T(\vec{m}_i) = R \cdot \vec{m}_i + \vec{t}\,, \tag{2}$$

where R is a 3x3 rotation matrix and t is a 3x1 translation vector.

3.1 Point based registration

Point based registration refers to problems of finding a transformation between two coordinate systems using pairs of points in both systems, i.e. if the number of measurement and data points is the same and there exists a unique correspondence between the points. Those points are referred to as homologous markers to point out pair wise point correspondence. In a general case, the transformation may include a scaling. However, since the goal of registration for neurosurgical navigation is a registration between the images and the patient's space for the same patient, a linear, rigid transformation is assumed.

Point based registration is an instance of the orthogonal Procrustes optimization problem. As mentioned above, the objective is to minimize the transformation error. A first step is to replace the points with their demeaned values:

$$\vec{m}^m = \frac{1}{N}\sum_{i=0}^{N-1}\vec{m}_i \tag{3}$$

$$\vec{d}^m = \frac{1}{N}\sum_{i=0}^{N-1}\vec{d}_i \tag{4}$$

$$\vec{m}_i^m = \vec{m}_i - \vec{m}^m \tag{5}$$

$$\vec{d}_i^m = \vec{d}_i - \vec{d}^m \tag{6}$$

The demeaned measurement and data points can be arranged in two NxD matrices, **M** and **D** respectively, N being the number of points and D being the dimension of data. The DxD correlation matrix:

$$K = M^T D \tag{7}$$

represents the goodness of prediction of the data points from the measurement points. Using the Singular Value Decomposition (SVD), the matrix K can be represented as:

$$K = U \cdot \Sigma \cdot V^T \tag{8}$$

Where U and V are DxD orthogonal matrices and Σ is a DxD diagonal matrix.

Finally, the rotation matrix representing a rotation of measurement points in the coordinate system of the data points is:

$$R = V \cdot \Delta \cdot U^T, \tag{9}$$

where

$$\Delta = diag(1,1,\det(VU^T)), \tag{10}$$

The translation is computed as a vector of distance between centres of mass of measurement and data points:

$$t = \vec{d}^m - R\vec{m}^m \tag{11}$$

If the number of points is three (N=3), the SVD is uniquely defined. For N>3, the system is over-defined and the singular value decomposition is not a trivial task.

3.2 Surface based registration

Surface based registration uses a surface representation of at least one of the initial sets (measurement or data points). In the neurosurgical registration with CT images, a natural way to represent data points is a bone surface extracted from the 3D-CT images of the patient. Intraoperativelly, using the A-mode US probe, a significantly fewer number of bone surface points can be obtained. Therefore, the surface registration problem for this application is *de facto* a surface to points matching. The iterative closest point (ICP) is a widely used algorithm for this kind of matching issues. The ICP was proposed by Besl and McKey for the registration of 3D shapes (Besl and McKey 1992). The algorithm works with different surface representations. For this application, a point set surface representation is assumed.

The ICP is an iterative procedure with two phases: detection of closest point on the surface and least squares registration. If *D* is a bone surface from CT images, the closest point from a measurement point m_i is:

$$d_i(\vec{m}_i, D) = \min_{\vec{x} \in D}\left(\left\|\vec{x} - T_0(\vec{m}_i)\right\|\right) \tag{12}$$

where T_0 is an initial transformation. As the result, N pairs of associated points $\{m_i, d_i\}$ are obtained, where N is the number of measurement points. Afterwards, a point based least squares registration is performed, as described in section 3.1. The iterations are repeated until one of the following conditions is met: a convergence is reached or the number of iterations exceeded the predefined maximal iterations number. An obvious advantage of the ICP algorithm is that a correspondence between the measurement and the data points is computed. This is a particularly important issue influencing total registration time in the operating theatre. Therefore, if the ICP algorithm is used, the number of points (N) can be significantly higher than in the case of point based matching.

3.3 Registration errors

The goal of the registration is to find an optimal transformation T, such that the transformation error between the two coordinate systems is minimal. In an ideal case, a transformation maps the measurement points exactly to the data points. Otherwise, the registration error is:

$$FRE = \sqrt{\frac{1}{N}\sum_{i=0}^{N-1}(T(\vec{m}_i) - \vec{d}_i)^2} \tag{13}$$

This error is usually referred to as the Fiducial Registration Error (FRE). For the most clinical applications, a more relevant error is the Target Registration Error (TRE) showing the error in remote surgical target points. The TRE depends on FRE and on the position of a target in relation to the data points. According to the statistical analysis from (Fitzpatrick 1998), TRE is proportional to the distance between the target point and the principal axis of the points and reverse-proportional to distance between the fiducial points and their axes. From these considerations, heuristics considering selection of the points can be drawn. The configuration of fiducials should follow a regular pattern with isometric axes, e.g. a tetrahedron, in order to avoid a large deviance between the target and the principal axes. This conclusion can be applied to both Procrustes point based registration and ICP surface based registration. In further text, as the registration error, TRE will be assumed.

3. Registration techniques

The essential factor influencing accuracy of a neuronavigational system is the type and the position of the used markers. Implantable bone screws (BS) offer high precision, since their identification in CT-images and operating site is trivial. However, this approach implies significant additional efforts for the clinical team concerning the clinical work flow (including an additional operation and anaesthesia) as well as discomfort for the patients, skull or skin infection including postoperative pain. Adhesive skin markers (SM) are a more convenient alternative and are widely used (overview in Steinmeier et al. 2000 and Bernardete et al. 2001), although they induce a decreased accuracy through the skin shift, especially due to the immobilization of the patient with a clamp (Wolfberger et al. 2002). Furthermore, the placement of both types of markers requires trained personnel and partial shaving of the patient. (Wolfsberger et al. 2002) proposed a set of anatomical landmarks (AL) for point to point registration, and reported an error of 3.2 ± 1.1mm using five anatomical landmarks.
In contrast, surface based methods may be inaccurate as far as registration is restricted to the very limited bone surface area of the surgical approach. Using a transcutaneous A-mode ultrasound (US) registration of anatomic landmarks and surface areas underneath the soft tissue may be a solution overcoming displacement problems without increasing the invasiveness (Mauerer 1999 et al., Heger et al. 2005). Furthermore, the ultrasonic registration avoids the need for the preoperative segmentation of the markers. The approach to achieve a time efficient and robust registration by a combination of an optimized man-machine-interaction strategy, signal processing and different registration techniques has been reported in detail in (Heger et al. 2005). Its application in skull surgery is presented here. A clinical protocol is developed for US-based registration, namely concerning the selection of adequate numbers and positions of points to be palpated.

Technique/ Feature	Bone Screws (BS)	Adhesive Skin Markers (SM)	Anatomical Landmarks (AL)	Surface points
Accuracy	++	-	-	+
Invasiveness	---	+	+	+
Patient discomfort	---	+-	+	+
Palpation area	+	+	+	--
Additional Training of the OP staff	-	-	+-	+

Table 1. Cross-comparison of the clinical and technical features

4. Registration approaches

Three registration approaches have been investigated: point-to-point matching, direct surface-based matching and US-based surface matching. The tests are performed in the following modes:

- Mode I
  (a) Point based registration with implanted markers
  (b) Point based registration with skin adhesive markers

- Mode II
  (a) Point based registration with anatomical landmarks, followed by
  (b) Surface-based registration, directly on the bone surface
- Mode III
  Point based registration with anatomic landmarks, followed by transcutaneous surface-based matching, using the US probe

Surface-based registration (IIb) is done by palpating points in skull convexity and facial structures and fitting them to the 3D model obtained from CT imaging study of the patient. Surface based registration is done using a pre-registration with anatomical landmarks followed by the ICP algorithm. Combining the ICP algorithm with different registration techniques (SM or BS) would not address the issue of invasiveness reduction and is therefore omitted.

For AL registration, using both previous experience and guidelines from the literature (Wolfsberger et al. 2002), following anatomical landmarks are used: the most posterior point in the root of the nose, the most anterior point at the nose tip, and the most anterior part of frontozygomatic suture (left and right). Surface palpated points were defined as follows: three lateral left, three lateral right, four on the frontal skull convexity, four on the forehead, and four periorbital, summing up to total 18 surface points for the ICP algorithm.

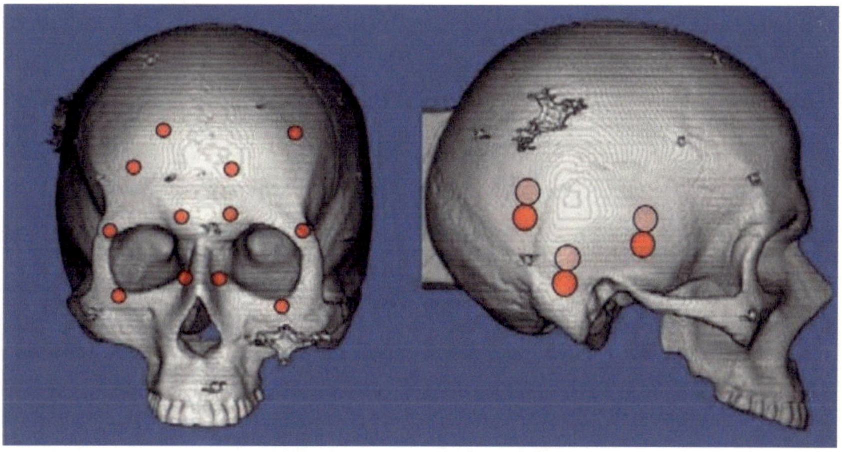

Figure 3. Surface registration protocol with 18 points

The palpation protocol is shown in Figure 3. A limiting factor for the selection of palpation surfaces is patient fixation in a Mayfield-clamp. A pre-evaluation of standard fixation techniques and postures has been performed prior to the registration trials, in order to detect unapproachable structures. This analysis resulted in a palpation protocol excluding posterior and caudal cranium. Furthermore, although highly distinctive, the jaws were omitted, since the jaws are normally not scanned in a standard radiological protocol for neurosurgery.

5. Experimental setup

The registration approaches described in section 4 have been evaluated in three settings:

- Phantom laboratory trials with a Sawbone® solid foam model.
- Anatomical laboratory trials with a formalin fixed cadaver skull.
- Patient clinical trials.

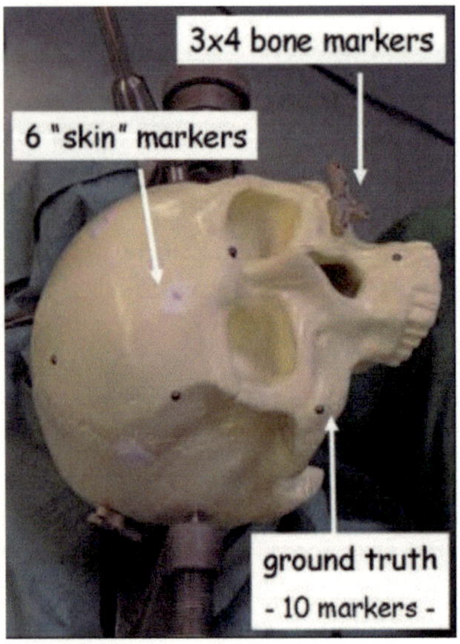

Figure 3. The laboratory set-up for phantom trials. Twelve bone markers (3x4 BS) have been used for point based matching with implanted markers (Mode Ia). Further 10 markers have been used as the Ground Truth

The setup for the laboratory phantom trials is shown in Figure 3. The phantom was equipped with six adhesive skin markers, using the same placement procedure as in a standard neurosurgical patient preparation at Clinic for Neurosurgery, Ruhr-University Bochum. Three sets of four bone markers have been implanted for Mode Ia registration. Additional ten spherical bone markers (ø 4mm) served as the Ground Truth. The phantom skull was fixed in a standard Mayfield-clamp.

The cadaver skull was prepared with similar sets of four bone markers, implanted prior to the scanning (Figure 4). The same markers have been used for both, fiducial point based registration and ground truth, due to difficulties to implement further markers. Adhesive skin markers have been omitted for the reasons given in the further text. The cadaver skull was fixed in the Mayfield-clamp.

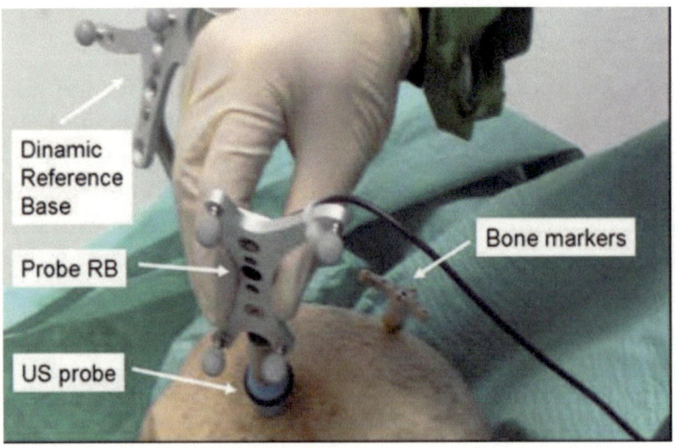

Figure 4. The laboratory set-up for cadaver trials

For the clinical trials, a standard clinical procedure was utilized (Figure 5). Registration tests have been performed prior to intervention, after patient fixation and before sterilization, without interfering with the standard procedure.

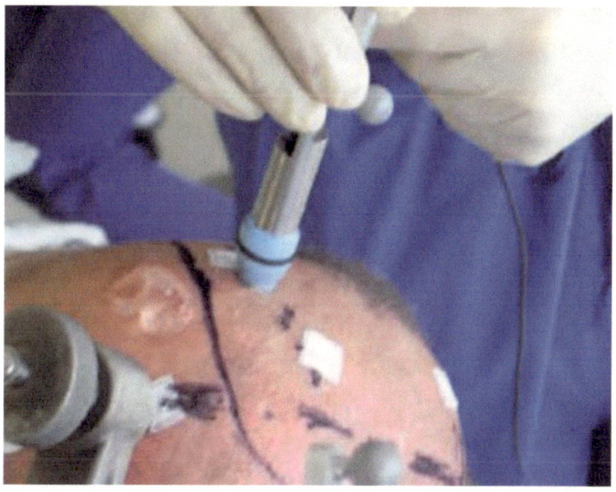

Figure 5. A clinical trial set-up

For all trials, the same radiological protocol has been used: slice thickness = 2 mm, slice distance 2 mm, pixel size 0.42 mm.

5.1 Ground Truth

In order to evaluate the registration accuracy, titanium bone markers have been used. Due to a high contrast between the markers and the bone and high Hounsfield values of titanium, an automatic segmentation of titanium spheres is a trivial task. It was followed by an automatic sphere clustering and detection of centre of mass (i.e. geometrical centre) of each bone marker in the coordinate system of the CT scanner. Centre of each spherical marker is g_i^{CT}. After the registration, a transformation T_R, which maps points from the patient space to the coordinate system of the CT scanner, is obtained. The position of markers in patient's space coordinate system (g_i^P) can be detection with a pointer, as described in 5.4. Therefore, the TRE in the i-th marker is:

$$TRE_i = \left\| g_i^{CT} - T_R(g_i^P) \right\| \tag{14}$$

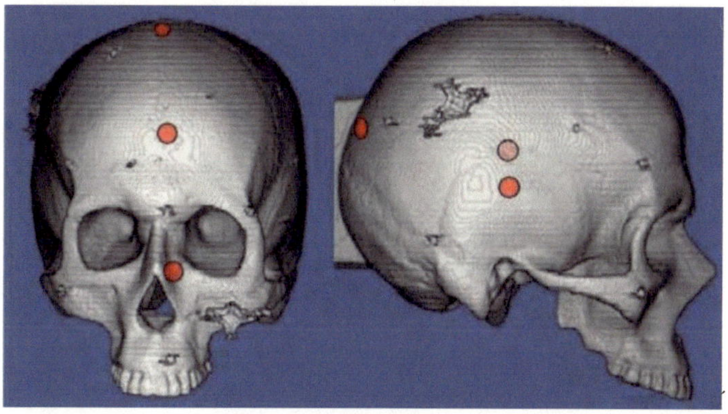

Figure 6. Points for the plausibility test (das Bild sieht aus, als wären da 6 Punkte)

5.2 Plausibility test

Due to ethical reasons, to avoid discomfort to patients, no bone markers have been implanted for the clinical trials. In absence of fiducial bone markers, an alternative accuracy test (*plausibility test*) was performed. After a registration, bone surface points have been transcutaneously digitized at five uniformly distributed locations (Figure 6) using the US probe and subsequently have been transformed into the coordinate system of the CT dataset. The error was computed as the shortest distance to the closest point on the surface of the 3D model. This kind of error cannot account for different displacements of the transformation. However, the plausibility test might indicate a large registration error.

5.3 Ultrasound system

A-Mode ultrasound systems in general utilize single element transducers using a single channel pulser and receiver. The most common scanning method used for medical applications is the pulse-echo technique. Short pulses are sent into the tissue; a reflection profile, due to interfaces or small scatters, is received usually by the same transducer element. After amplification and digitization, the recorded A-Line can be further processed and analyzed. Interfaces are characterized by different acoustic impedance values, e.g. between bone and soft tissue. For a transcutaneous US-based registration, the objective is to detect a bone-soft tissue (skin) interface, in order to transcutaneously digitize the skull surface. The reflectivity of field intensity in case of the bone and soft tissue, assuming perpendicular sound incidence, is about 45%. The distance between a transducer and a bone layer is calculated as $d = ½\, t \cdot v$, where t is the delay of the US wave propagation through the tissue and v is sound velocity in soft tissue (1450-1630 m/s (Heger et al. 2005)).
In this study a 5 MHz, non-focused, heavily damped transducer with 5 mm element size is used. Based on the wavelength in water the measured focal distance for pulse excitation is approximately 17 mm. The nominal -6dB beam width of the focus area is 1.2 mm, which is equal to the theoretical lateral resolution.

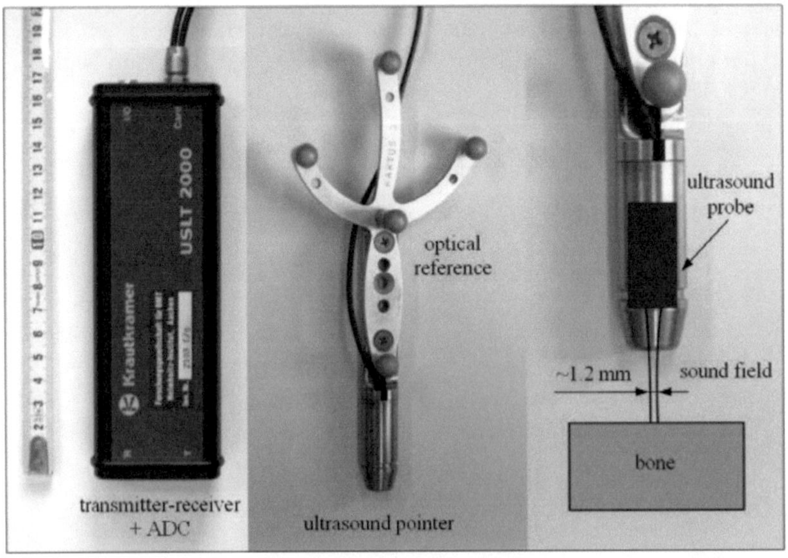

Figure 7. Portable single channel transmitter/receiver and ADC (left), A-mode Ultrasound pointer with optical reference (mid) and larger view of pointer and probe (right)

A portable pulser/receiver hardware including analog to digital conversion (USLT 2000, Krautkramer, Germany) is used for the signal generation and basic signal processing (band pass filtering, signal amplification). A special autoclavable forerun is used to adapt the probe's working range to the typical thickness of skin tissue (Fig. 7). In order to receive a reliable ultrasound echo reflected at the bone tissue interface the beam axis of the transducer element has to be approximately perpendicular to the reflecting surface area. However, due to non-invasive palpation it is not possible for the user to see the local bone surface. Therefore, a perpendicular alignment of the ultrasound probe conventionally is difficult and time consuming, as reported by (Maurer 1999). For this reason a computer based guiding tool and a man-machine interaction algorithm has been developed to support the interactive alignment of the ultrasound transducer (Heger 2005). In order to simulate the intraoperative situation during the US registration on the phantom, i.e. the presence of the skin tissue, a piece of fresh meat is used to uncouple the probes' forerun and the phantom surface. In cadaver and patient studies, the forerun was applied directly to skin surface. The US probe was tracked using a 6-DOF optical tracking system.

5.4 Tracking system

A NDI Polaris System® for 6-DOF optical tracking of passive wireless rigid bodies has been used in a standard pyramid volume. Four different tools have been tracked: US probe, a pointed tool for AL, SM and surface-based registration, a Dynamic Reference Base (DRB) fixated at the Mayfield-clamp providing a dynamic coordinate system and allowing movement of the clamp during the registration, and a tool with a spherical tool-tip (ø 4mm) pivoted to the centre of the sphere, used for the Ground Truth. The rigid bodies have been equipped with at least four reflecting spheres. The rigid body at the US probe was optically pivoted to the surface of US transducer, along the central line of the probe. The probe with the rigid body is shown in Figure 7.

6. Results

6.1 Accuracy

For each mode in the phantom study, fifteen consecutive registrations were performed to assess the accuracy and robustness of the registration method. Each accuracy test was done by palpating ten accuracy markers. The mean accuracy is computed as follows:

$$TRE_m = \frac{1}{N_t}\sum_{i=1}^{N_t}\left(\frac{1}{N_m}\sum_{j=1}^{Nm} TRE_i^j\right) \tag{15}$$

where TRE_i^j is the TRE in the i-th marker during the j-th trial, N_m is the number of markers (ten) and N_t is the number of trials. Standard deviation of TRE is computed as:

$$TRE_{SD} = \frac{1}{N_t}\sum_{i=1}^{N_t}\sqrt{\left(\frac{1}{N_m}\sum_{j=1}^{Nm} TRE_i^j - TRE_m\right)^2} \tag{16}$$

Table 2 shows the values achieved in the phantom study with ten repeated tests.

	Mode Ia	Mode Ib	Mode IIa	Mode IIb	Mode III
TRE_m [mm]	0.58	1.78	2.78	1.38	1.37
TRE_{SD} [mm]	0.23	0.39	1.20	0.35	0.51
TRE_{max} [mm]	1.01	2.52	5.91	2.06	2.27
TRE_{min} [mm]	0.28	1.15	1.34	1.12	0.86

Table 2. Accuracy values achieved in the phantom trial for different registration modes

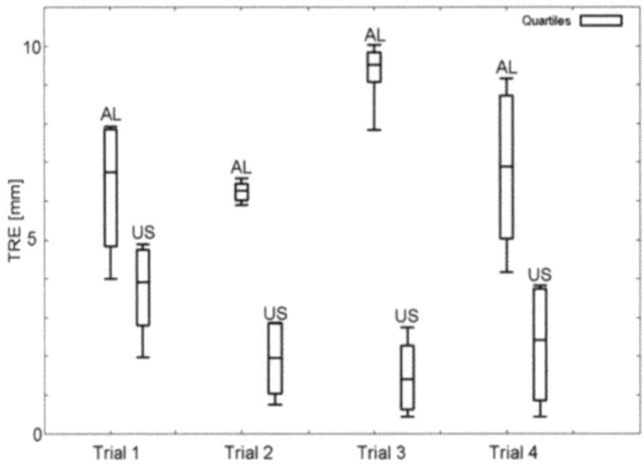

Figure 8. Box-Whisker-plot of four cadaver trials. A pre-registration with anatomical landmarks (AL) is refined with an US surface-based registration

The accuracy using the adhesive skin markers in the phantom study (Table 2, column Ib) was significantly worse than surface-based registration (Table 2, columns IIb and III). Cadaver study is performed in modes Ia, IIa and III. A viable assumption is that accuracy of SM would decline if a cadaver is used, due to the presence of displaceable skin. Therefore, registration with SM in the cadaver study was omitted. Accuracy in mode Ia was similar as in the phantom study (TRE_m = 0.51, TRE_{SD}=0.18, TRE_{max} = 0.97, and TRE_{min} = 0.26). Results of AL and US-based registration for four cadaver trials are shown in Figure 8. It is important to notice that a pair of AL and US registration is subsequently performed (AL registration is used as a pre-registration for US surface-based matching). The US part of the plot is repeated in Figure 9 with a better resolution in y-axis.

PATIENT	Trial	P1 [mm]	P2 [mm]	P3 [mm]	P4 [mm]	P5 [mm]
A	1	0.24	1.04	1.93	0.15	0.56
	2	2.88	1.91	1.75	1.34	0.87
B	3	0.78	0.63	1.43	0.33	1.02
C	4	1.32	1.89	2.15	2.11	1.67

Table 3. Plausibility test in five salient points (P1-P5) for three patients (A-C)

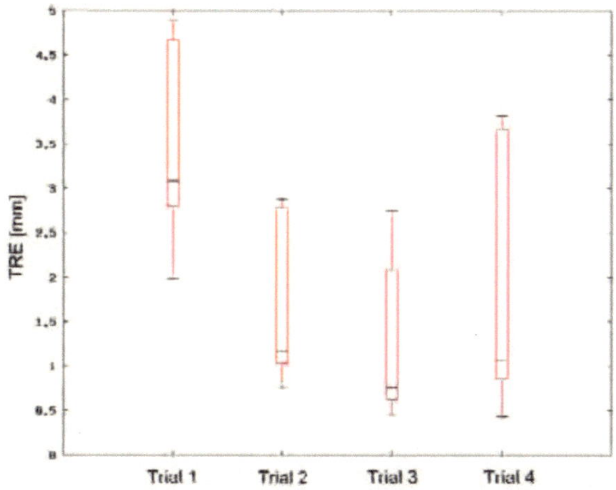

Figure 9. Box-Whisker-plot (quartiles) for four cadaver trials with A-mode US surface based registration

As mention before, in patient studies (three trials) the ground truth was not available, due to invasiveness of bone implantable markers. Therefore, a plausibility test, as described by the protocol in section 5.2 has been performed (Table 3). In order to analyse the results of the plausibility test, the Figure 10 shows a relation of accuracy and plausibility in the cadaver study.

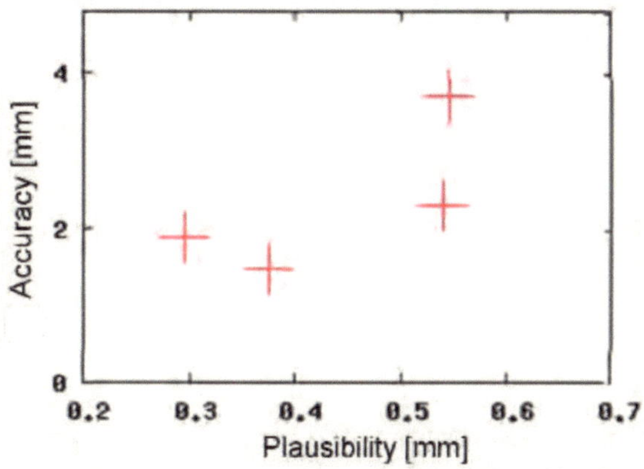

Figure 10. Relation between the plausibility and the accuracy in four cadaver trials

6.2 Time efficiency

The overall mean registration time using A-mode ultrasound (mean = 389s, SD 63s) is acceptable and smaller then the ones reported in the literature (15 min, Maurer 1999). The pre-registration with anatomical landmarks is less time critical (Figure 11) since it does not involve the US probe orientation. The ideal probe orientation is estimated from the 3D-CT model. During a registration, the user is supported with a graphical interface (Figure 12) showing an angular position of the probe to the surface normal vector. The majority of the time needed for US cadaver registration was spent for palpating the periorbital areas, due to significantly stiffer formalin-fixated soft tissue.

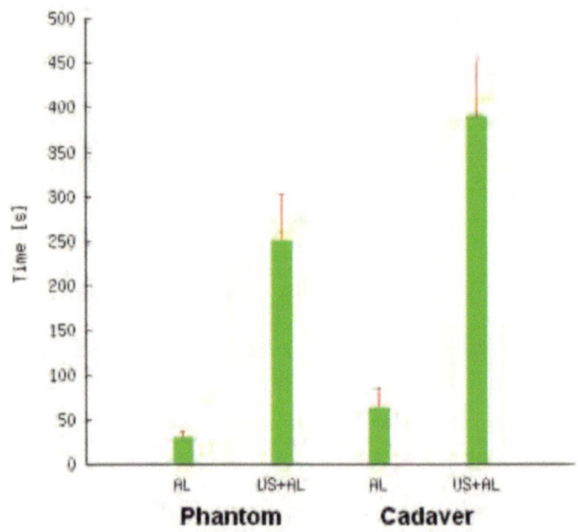

Figure 11. Time efficiency of the registration procedure

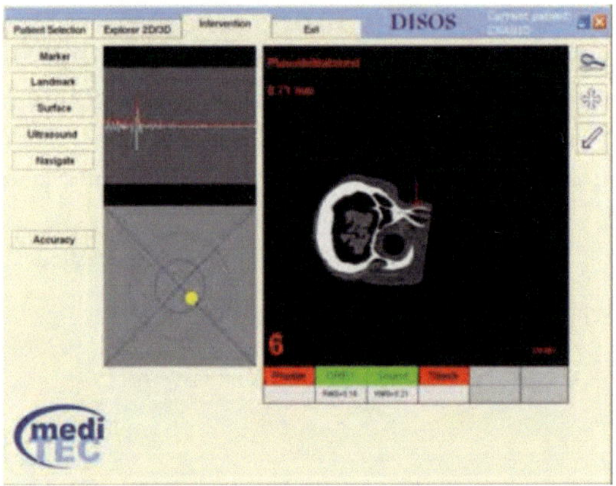

Figure 12. A screenshot of tool adjustment dialog

7. Discussion

The laboratory phantom tests have shown a significant correlation in error results between direct surface palpation and US-based registration indicating that the latter can be used in cases when direct palpation is not possible, e.g. in the presence of skin. The main limitation of surface based registration in neurosurgery is that only a small portion of bone is exposed during the operation. Therefore, the distribution of points can not follow a defined pattern, as described in section 2. The A-mode US transcutaneous registration offers two major improvements: palpation of a pervasive area of the skull surface and registration prior to sterilization (prior to skin opening). In comparison with anatomical landmarks, US-based surface registration has shown a significantly better accuracy (1.37±0.51 mm vs. 2.78±1.20 mm). The result of AL registration was similar to those previously reported (e.g. (Wolfsberger et al. 2002)). Registration with adhesive skin markers has also shown poorer accuracy than US registration. As expected, registration with bone markers has shown an excellent accuracy in the range of CT pixel size (0.58±0.23 mm), but, as discussed previously, this technique requires an additional intervention prior to the surgery causing discomfort, possible skull infection and postoperative pain as well as additional costs.

Cadaver trials have shown a similar output as the phantom study. A significant improvement of the registration accuracy, if an US-based surface registration is used subsequently to AL registration, is shown (Figure 8). It is interesting to notice that the AL pre-registration accuracy is not significantly influencing the final result. For example, the worst AL registration accuracy has been observed in Trial 3. However, the final accuracy resulting from US surface-based matching, has shown the best performance in comparison with other trials. These results suggest that moderate pre-registration might be sufficient. However, a precaution in defining the palpation protocol should be taken, due to the local nature of the ICP algorithm.

Accuracy of the cadaver US-registration study has shown a promising mean and minimal values (1.97 and 0.63 mm, respectively) with a strong standard deviation and poor maximal value (1.76 and 4.78 mm, respectively). These results indicate that an acceptable registration with US-based technique is feasible; however, it should be done with a great care. A reason for inaccuracies in the cadaver study is an unusual ultrasound signal damping in the formalin-fixated soft tissue. Signal processing algorithms have been previously trained and tested on the normal tissue.

Due to lack of bone markers posing the ground truth, accuracy in patient studies could not have been assessed. The plausibility test was used as an indicator of registration goodness rather than an accuracy test. As Figure 10 indicates, there is a large discrepancy between the plausibility and accuracy. Therefore, although widely used, plausibility is of a questionable validity.

The overall mean registration time using A-mode ultrasound (mean = 389s, SD 63s) appear to be tolerable and smaller than the ones reported in the literature. The computer assisted alignment tool provides efficient support for US-based registration in cranial surgery. In vivo tests of US signal detection in regions where palpation was intended were more successful then in cadaver test, due to the stiffness of formalin-fixated soft tissue. Therefore, the majority of the time needed for US cadaver registration was spent for palpating the periorbital areas.

8. Conclusions and Further Work

In the first part of this chapter, theoretical background and practical considerations for the rigid registration of a patient dataset and a patient space in the operating theatre are given. Based on these, a surface palpation protocol has been developed and evaluated in three trials: phantom, cadaver and patient study.

The results have shown that A-mode US surface-based registration has a potential to be used in the clinical practice, due to its non-invasive nature and a better accuracy in comparison with other low invasive techniques (skin markers and anatomical landmarks). A user interface for computer guided probe orientation has shown time efficiency improvement, reducing total registration time to below seven minutes.

The major issue that needs to be address in the future is accuracy. Although registrations with acceptable accuracies have been demonstrated, the robustness remains questionable. It was shown that pre-registration plays a minor role in the overall accuracy. Therefore, the future work should focus on improving the palpation protocol and surface matching algorithms. Random ICP algorithm has shown promising results in both phantom and

cadaver studies (Fieten et al. 2007). Furthermore, further development of the US signal processing is necessary to account for unusual tissue composition.
The registration techniques presented herein have been used in the CRANIO-System tests (Bast et al. 2006, Popovic et al. CARS 2007)

7. References

Arana, E., Martí-Bonmatí, L., Bautista, D., and Paredes, R (2004). Qualitative diagnosis of Calvarial metastasis by neural network and logistic regression. *Academic Radiology,* 11 (1):pp. 45–52, Jan 2004.

Bai, S., Teo, M., Ng, W., and Sim, C (2001). Workspace analysis of a parallel manipulator with one redundant DOF for skull-base surgery. In: *Proceedings of the IEEE RSJ International Conference on Intelligent Robot and Systems,* Outrigger Wailea Resort, Maui, Hawaii, USA. IEEE, 2001, pp. 1694–1699.

Bast, P., Engelhardt, M., Lauer, W., Schmieder, K., Rohde, V., and Radermacher, K. (2003) Identification of milling parameters for manual cutting of bicortical bone structures. *Computer Aided Surgery,* 8 (5):pp. 257–263, 2003.

Bast, P., Popovic, A., Wu, T., Heger, S., Engelhardt, M., Lauer, W., Radermacher, K., and Schmieder, K (2006). Robot- and computer-assisted craniotomy: resection planning, implant modelling and robot safety. *The International Journal of Medical Robotics and Computer Assisted Surgery,* 2 (2):pp. 168–178, June 2006.

Bernardete EA, Leonard MA, Weiner HL (2001). Comparison of frameless stereotactic systems: Accuracy, precision, and applications. *Neurosurgery* 2001;49:1409–1416.

Besl and McKay (1992): A method for registration of 3-D shapes. *IEEE Trans. Pattern Anal. Mach. Intell.,* vol. 14, pp. 239–256, 1992.

Engelhardt, M., Bast, P., Jeblink, N., Lauer,W., Popovic, A., Eufinger, H., Scholz, M., Christmann, A., Harders, A., Radermacher, K., and Schmieder, K (2006). Analysis of surgical management of calvarial tumours and first results of a newly designed robotic trepanation system. *Minimal Invasive Neurosurgery,* 49 (2):pp. 98–103, April 2006.

Federspil, P. A., Geisthoff, U. W., Henrich, D., and Plinkert, P. K (2003). Development of the First force-controlled robot for otoneurosurgery. *Laryngoscope,* 113 (3):pp. 465–471, Mar 2003.

Federspil, P. A. and Plinkert, P. K (2004). Robotic surgery in otorhinolaryngology. *Otolaryngol Pol,* 58 (1):pp. 237–242, 2004

Fieten, L., Heger, S., Pasalic, L., Engelhardt, M., Schmieder, K., Radermacher, K. (2007) Registration of Cranial CT Images with A-Mode-Ultrasound Data Using the Random-ICP Algorithm -- A Cadaver Study, Proc. *Biomedizinische Technik* 2007

Fitzpatrick, M., West, J., Maurer, C. (1998) Predicting Error in Rigid-Body Point-Based Registration. *IEEE Trans. on Medical Imaging,* 17(5):694-702, 1998

Grunert, P., and J. Espinosa, K. D., and Filippi, R (2003). Computer-aided Navigation in Neurosurgery. *Neurosurg Rev,* 26:pp. 73–99, 2003.

Handini, D., Teo, M., and Lo, C (2004). System integration of NeuroBot: A skull-base Surgical robotic system. In: *Proceedings of the IEEE Conference on Robotics, Automation and Mechatronics.* December 2004, volume 1, pp. 43–48.

Heger, S., F. Portheine, Jörg A. K. Ohnsorge, E. Schkommodau, K. Radermacher (2005). User Interactive Registration of Bone with A-Mode Ultrasound. *IEEE Engineering in Medicine and Biology Magazine (M-EMB)* March/April 2005; 85-95

Hill Derek and Philippe Batchelor (2005). Registration Methodology: Concepts and Algorithms. In Book: Medical Image Registration, CRC Press Inc., 2005

Laborde, G., Gilsbach, J., Harders, A., Klimek, L., Moesges, R., and Krybus, W (1992). Computer assisted localizer for planning of surgery and intra-operative orientation. *Acta Neurochir (Wien)*, 119 (1-4):pp. 166–170, 1992.

Maurer, C., Jr. Ronal P. Gaston, D. L. G. Hill, M. J. Gleeson, M. G.Tayler, M. R. Fenlon, P. J. Edwards, D. J. Hawkes (1999). AcouStick: A Tracked A-Mode Ultrasonography System for Registration in Image-Guided Surgery. *Proceedings MICCAI, Lecture Notes in Computer Science*, 1679. (1999) 953-962

Nathoo, N., Cavusoglu, M. C., Vogelbaum, M. A., and Barnett, G. H (2005). In touch With robotics: neurosurgery for the future. *Neurosurgery*, 56 (3):pp. 421–33; discussion 421–33, Mar 2005.

Popovic, A., Engelhardt, M., Wu, T., Portheine, F., Schmieder, K., Radermacher, K (2003). CRANIO - Computer Assisted Planning for Navigation and Robot-assisted Surgery on the Skull. *Computer Assisted Radiology and Surgery, Proceedings of the 17th International Congress and Exhibition, International Congress Series*, 1256:1269-1276. Elsevier, June 2003.

Popovic, A., Wu, T., , Engelhardt, M., Radermacher, K (2006). In Medical Image Computing and Computer Assisted Intervention -- MICCAI 2006, Lecture Notes in Computer Science, 4191: 864-871. Springer, 2006.

Popovic, A., Wu, T., Follmann, A., Cunha Cruz, V.C.S., Schröder, K., Ibach, B., Engelhardt, M., Schmieder, K., Radermacher, K (2007). Cranio system for robot and computer assisted removal of calvarial tumors. In Computer Assisted Radiology and Surgery, Proceedings of the 19th International Congress and Exhibition (CARS 2007. International Journal of Computer Assisted Radiology and Surgery. Supp1 Vol 1 2007.

Radermacher K. (2006). Modeling of Intensity Priors for Knowledge-Based Level Set Algorithm in Calvarial Tumors Segmentation.

Schiffbauer H. (1999). Neuronavigation in brain tumor surgery Clinical beta-phase of the Oulu Neuronavigator System. Ph.D. thesis, Faculty of Medicine, University of Münster, 1999.

Spivak, C. J. and Pirouzmand, F. (2005) Comparison of the reliability of brain lesion localizationwhen using traditional and stereotactic image-guided techniques: a prospective study. *J Neurosurg*, 103 (3):pp. 424–427, Sep 2005.

Steinmeier R, Rachinger J, Kaus M, Gansalndt O, Huk W, Fahlbusch R (2002). Factors Influencing the application accuracy of neuronavigation systems. *Stereotact Funct Neurosurg* 2000;75: 188–202.

Tan TC, Black PM (2002). Sir Victor Horsley (1857-1916): pioneer of neurological surgery. *Neurosurgery*. 2002 Mar; 50(3):607-11

Tan, K. K., Grzeszczuk, R., Levin, D. N., Pelizzari, C. A., Chen, G. T., Erickson, R. K., Johnson, D., and Dohrmann, G. J (1993). A frameless stereotactic approach to neurosurgical planning based on retrospective patient-image registration. Technical note. *J Neurosurg*, 79 (2):pp. 296–303, Aug 1993.

Watanabe (1996). *Computer-integrated surgery: technology and clinical applications*, MIT Press, Chapter: The neuronavigator: a computer-controlled navigation system in neurosurgery, pp. 319–327. 1996.

Watanabe, E., Watanabe, T., Manaka, S., Mayanagi, Y., and Takakura, K (1987). Three dimensional digitizer (neuronavigator): new equipment for computed tomography-guided stereotaxic surgery. Surg Neurol, 27 (6):pp. 543–547, Jun 1987.

Wolfsberger, S., K. Rössler, R. Regatschnig, K. Ungersböck (2002). Anatomical land-marks For image registration in frameless stereotactic neuronavigation. *Neurosurg Rev* 2002, Vol. 25, pp. 68–72

Wu T., Engelhardt M, Fieten L., Popovic A., Radermacher K.: Anatomically Constrained Deformation for Design of Cranial Implant: Methodology and Validation. In R. Larsen, M. Nielsen, and J. Sporring, editors, Medical Image Computing and Computer-Assisted Intervention (MICCAI 2006), vol. 4190 of Lecture Notes on Computer Science, pp. 9–16. Springer, 2006.

Zamorano, L., Kadi, A. M., and Dong, A (1992). Computer-assisted neurosurgery: simulation and automation. *Stereotact Funct Neurosurg*, 59 (1-4):pp. 115–122, 1992.

Zamorano, L. J., Nolte, L., Kadi, A. M., and Jiang, Z (1993). Interactive intraoperative Localization using an infrared-based system. *Neurol Res*, 15 (5):pp. 290–298, Oct 1993.

25

Camera Holding Robotic Devices in Urology

Sashi S Kommu[1] and Abhay Rané[2]
[1]*The WPU-SIMISAD Group, Surrey*
[2]*The Department of Urology, East Surrey Hospital, Redhill, United Kingdom*

1. Introduction

The efficacy of an operating surgeon in Laparoscopic Urological Surgery (LUS) is dependent on a two dimensional view seen on a monitor or projection device. The role of the camera driver is central to the procedure and the operating surgeon has usually had to constantly indicate exactly where he wants his assistant to focus to help optimise tissue exposure and handling during the procedure. The realization that the camera holder need not necessarily be a human and that a given task could be completed by devices under the direct or indirect control of the operating surgeon has led to the objective and subjective evaluation of several devices. Ideally, the surgeon should have full control of all instruments required that are directly required for conducting a given procedure. This includes surgical operative instruments and control of the operative field. The purpose of non-human camera holders is to return camera-control to the surgeon and to stabilize the visual field during minimally invasive procedures. As such, active and passive camera holders have been developed in a bid to offer the surgeon an alternative and better tool for control of the operating surgeon's direct visual field. Herein we describe the current Camera Holding Robots in surgery focusing on voice activated i.e. AESOP® (automated endoscopic system for optimal positioning) (Unger et al., 1994) and motion controlled robots i.e. EndoAssist® Camera Holding Robot (Kommu et al., 2007). We also look at camera holding elements of other robotic surgical systems including the da Vinci® and ZEUS® Surgical Systems.

2. Types of Camera Holding Robots

There are predominantly two type of robots, namely motion controlled and voice activated. Motion controlled camera holders currently in use are the EndoAssist® Camera Holding Robot, The camera arm of the da Vinci® Robotic System and Zeus® Surgical System. The Voice activated device currently in use is the AESOP® device.

2.1 Motion controlled camera holding robots – The EndoAssist® Camera Holding Robot

Ideally, the surgeon should have optimal control of all instrumention that is directly required for conducting a given procedure including surgical operative instruments and control of the operative field. The purpose of non-human camera holders is to return camera-control to the surgeon and to stabilize the visual field. As a result of this, active and passive camera holders have been developed in a bid to offer the surgeon an alternative and potentially better tool for control of the operating surgeon's direct visual field. The published advantages include: [1] elimination of fatigue of the assistant who holds the camera, [2] elimination of fine motor tremor and small inaccurate movements and [3] delivery of a steady and tremor-free image (Allaf et al., 1998 & Nebot et al., 2003).

The EndoAssist® is a novel and unique robotic camera holder (EndoAssist®; Armstrong Healthcare, High Wycombe, Bucks, UK) (Fig. 1). that is controlled by simple head movement by the surgeon and enables complete autonomy over camera movement. Movement is executed by a head-mounted infrared emitter; the sensor is placed above the monitor and picks up any operator executed head movements (Fig. 2). The foot clutch ensures there is no unnecessary travel when movement is not required.

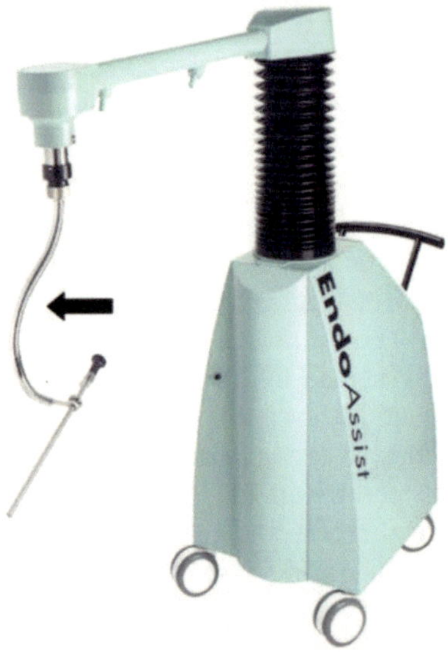

Figure 1. The *arrow* shows the camera driver of the EndoAssist®. [Copyright © *JORS* 2007]

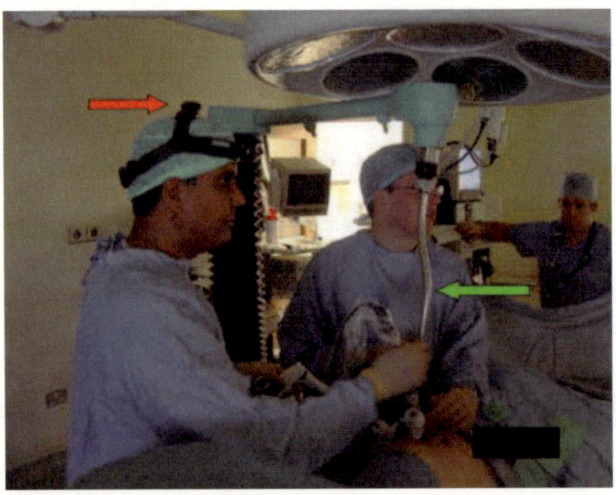

Figure 2. Head-mounted infra-red emitter (*red arrow*) and the camera driver being positioned (*green arrow*). [Copyright © *JORS* 2007]

We conducted a study using the EndoAssist® device in a total of 51 urological procedures (25 using the EndoAssist® device and 26 using a conventional human camera driver). The procedures studied were conducted by three experienced surgeons. Cases included nephrectomy (simple and radical), pyeloplasty, radical prostatectomy, and radical cystoprostatectomy. We used two separate groups, the Endoassist arm [E-Arm] and the conventional arm [C-Arm], which involves a human camera holder or driver. For the EndoAssist® arm, data were prospectively collected for 25 procedures. For the conventional arm, data for 26 cases were retrospectively collected from our database. The surgeon noted six parameters:

1 THE EXTENT OF BODY COMFORT AND MUSCLE FATIGUE IN EACH CASE, BY USING A MODIFIED BODY PART DISCOMFORT SCORE (BPDS), A SCORE OF 0 IMPLYING NO DISCOMFORT DURING THE PROCEDURE AND 10 BEING SUFFICIENT DISCOMFORT TO STOP THE TASK BEFORE RECOMMENCING

2 EASE OF SCOPE MOVEMENT OR USABILITY

3 NEED TO CLEAN THE TELESCOPE

4 TIME OF SET-UP AND EFFECT ON OVERALL OPERATIVE TIME

5 SURGICAL PERFORMANCE

6 WHETHER IT WAS NECESSARY TO CHANGE THE POSITION OF THE ARM DURING SURGERY

Ease of scope movement was graded on basis of the International Organization for Standardization (ISO) which defines usability as the extent to which goals are achieved with effectiveness, efficiency, and satisfaction. Each of these was graded on a linear scale of 1–5, from lowest to highest. The number of times the scope had to be cleaned was also recorded for each case in both the E-Arm and C-Arm. The time to set up the device was also tabulated as mean time in minutes ± standard deviation. The E-Arm data were collected prospectively whereas the C-Arm data was collected from database pool of retrospective data. For the renal surgery, a thirty-degree laparoscope was used. For the pelvic surgery, a 0° scope was used. The Harmonic® scalpel (Ethicon Endosurgery, Bracknell, UK), the Olympus SonoSurg (Keymed, Southend, UK), or the Lotus® (SRA Developments Ashburton, UK) were used to aid circumferential specimen mobilisation. Hem-o-lok® (Weck, High Wycombe, Bucks, UK) clips were used as appropriate for securing pedicles. Where statistical analysis was performed in this study, we used a Wilcoxon matched pairs signed-rank test and a result was deemed statistically significant if $P < 0.05$. All data were analysed by use of a preformed computer generated template of the variables of interest. Exclusion criteria were cases with major intraoperative complications including major bleeding or other factors which would have demanded additional haemostatic or reconstructive steps.

Findings with body comfort and muscle fatigue- all three surgeons felt comfortable with the E-Arm for each of the procedures studied, with no loss of autonomy. The surgeons were uncomfortable with use of the C-Arm for laparoscopic radical prostatectomy, and prompting for motion adjustment was required repeatedly for the cases studied. There was no reported difference between muscle fatigue for the two modes. The overall Modified BPDS (body part discomfort score) was 2.1 for the E-Arm and 2.2 for the C-Arm ($P = 0.2$) indicating no statistically significant difference between the two.

Findings with ease of scope movement and the need to clean the telescope-on average, the large arc generated whilst performing a nephrectomy led to more episodes of lens cleaning for the E-Arm group than for the C-Arm group. For laparoscopic nephrectomy, the EndoAssist port had to be relocated on several occasions whereas the C-Arm group did not require camera port relocation. Fewer problems were encountered while performing pelvic surgery or pyeloplasty. The grading for ease of scope movement was, on average, 3 for radical prostatectomy, 2 for pyeloplasty, and 1 for laparoscopic nephrectomy. There was a statistically significant difference between ease of scope movement, i.e. "usability", in favour of radical prostatectomy compared with simple or radical laparoscopic nephrectomy. For laparoscopic pyeloplasty the difference was statistically insignificant.

Findings of the time of set up (Tab. 1).- Set up time was greatest for laparoscopic radical cystectomy ([E-Arm] 6.8 ± 2.3; [C-Arm] 7.1 ± 1.9 min) and least for pyeloplasty ([E-Arm] 5.1 ± 1.8; [C-Arm] 5.3 ± 1.7 min) and there was no statistically significant difference between set up times for the E-Arm and C-Arm groups. The set-up time was < 8 mins in 100% of cases. Utility of EndoAssist had no effect on set up time compared with the conventional approach.

PROCEDURE	TOTAL NUMBER OF CASES USING ENDOASSIST [E]	TOTAL NUMBER OF CASES CONVENTIONAL [C]	MEAN SETTING UP TIME (MINS)	STATISTICALLY SIGNIFICANT [Y/N]
Nephrectomy	16	17	[E] 5.9 ± 1.2 Vs [C] 5.6 ± 1.3	N
Pyeloplasty	4	4	[E] 5.1 ± 1.8 Vs [C] 5.3 ± 1.7	N
Prostatectomy	3	3	[E] 5.8 ± 2.8 Vs [C] 5.6 ± 2.9	N
Cyctectomy	2	2	[E] 6.8 ± 2.3 Vs [C] 7.1 ± 1.9	N

Table. 1. Setting up times for EndoAssist® and for the conventional human driver template (mean time in minute ± standard deviation). [[Copyright © *JORS* 2007]

Findings of surgical approach – All three surgeons reported that the EndoAssist® device did not compromise surgical performance. They found that EndoAssist was a viable option and comparable with use of a human camera driver. There were no significant differences between complication rates or total operative time for procedures conducted with the EndoAssist® device or with a conventional human assistant.

Findings with need to clean scope – The need to clean the scope during the individual case depends on several factors, e.g. patient anatomy, the body mass index, the assistant's level of experience and inherent skill in driving the camera, and the exact type of surgery performed. We found this was not a useful tool for measuring the performance of the two arms because of the multiple confounding factors.

We have made several interesting observations. There are a number of advantages that are immediately apparent, primarily the intuitive positioning of the camera by the surgeon to optimise his operating field and, secondly, the potential reduction in cost without an assistant. There is a short learning curve but proficiency in the execution of the robotic movements is easily acquired over a few minutes. There was no neck or shoulder discomfort since the head mounted sensor weighs less than 10 grams and can easily be mounted onto a headband should the surgeon so decide. The BPDS showed no increased discomfort of one procedure over the other. The EndoAssist® allowed the surgeon to intuitively control his field of laparoscopic vision while co-ordinating movements of his instrumentation. Overall we found the EndoAssist® to be an effective and easy to use device for robotic camera driving. This could potentially reduce the constraint of having to have an experienced camera driver.

2.2 Motion controlled camera holding robotic elements – da Vinci® Robotic System

The advent and indeed propulsion of minimally invasive surgery over the last two decades has seen marked improvements in instrumentation. One of the main drawbacks of minimally invasive surgery is the use of a 2 Dimensional picture of the operative field fed to a monitor. The resulting elimination of natural depth of field significantly reduces the surgeon's initial ability to perform the task optimally in terms of speed and accuracy when compared to an open or 3 Dimensional view. This makes the learning curve for a given procedure suboptimal. The da Vinci® Robotic System represents a paradigm shift in our approach to minimally invasive surgery.

The Camera port is position and optic feedback is controlled by the surgeon with a default mechanism that is entirely under the operating surgeon's control. This can be classed as a form of camera holding robot [Fig 3]. The coupling of this control with the world's first robotic surgical system with 3D HD vision makes this system a very desirable platform for many surgeons. However, the use of this robotic system is different from conventional laparoscopic surgery in terms of instrumentation and the cost of running such a unit is highly restrictive in most units with overall purchase and maintenance costs in excess of $1,000,000 USD (2006).

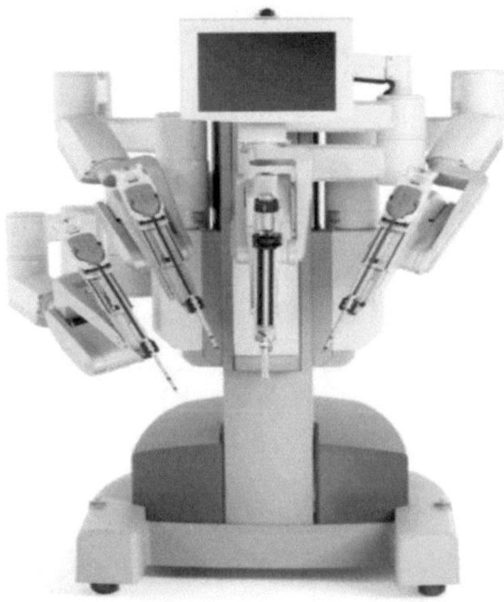

Figure 3. da Vinci® Robot. The Middle Arm represents the camera holder controlled by the operating surgeon

2.3 Motion controlled camera holding robotic elements – ZEUS® Surgical System

The ZEUS® Surgical System (Computer Motion and Medtronics) is a more recent addition to robotic surgery [Fig 4]. It is made up of an ergonomic surgeon control console and three table-mounted robotic arms. Two of these arms perform the surgical procedure. The third arm represents the endoscope with its camera providing either 2D or 3D visualization. The camera driver utilises an AESOP® Endoscope Positioner technology providing the surgeon with magnified, tremor free visualization of the internal operative field. The camera device can be operated either by voice activation or by non verbal command. One of the drawbacks of ZEUS® is its cost which has been estimated at $1,000,000 USD (2007 Cost).

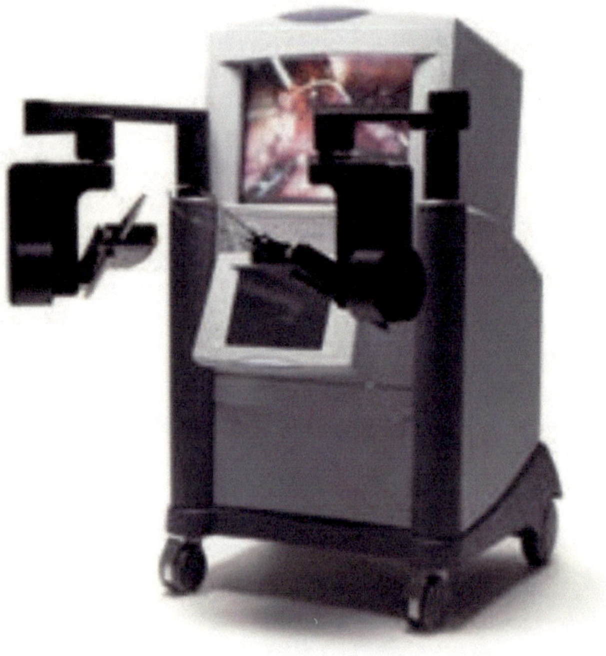

Figure 4. The ZEUS® Surgical System. The camera holder and driver is actually an AESOP derivative which uses AESOP® Endoscope Positioner technology

3. Voice activated camera holding devices

3.1 AESOP (Automated Endoscopic System for Optimal Positioning)

Since voice activation was recognised as a useful mode of direct communication with a mechanical tool to perform a preprogrammed task on verbal command, several devices have been developed mainly for commercial purposes. Surgical assist devices were among those develped at a later stage. The world's first surgical robot certified by the FDA in the USA was The AESOP® 1000 system (Intuitive Surgical, Inc., Sunnyvale, CA, USA) and was released in 1994. AESOP® stands for Automated Endoscopic System for Optimal Positioning. Later Computer Motion followed with AESOP® 2000 in 1996. The coupling of voice recognition technology with camera holding devices in surgery has seen the development of the AESOP® 3000 (in 1998) to control a robotic arm with seven degrees of freedom giving further flexibility in desired positioning of the endoscope [Fig 4].

Some of the shortcomings noted with master-slave design robots (e.g. Intuitive Surgical's da Vinci® Surgical System), such as excessive bulk or dimensions and high cost are were not similarly restrictive with AESOP®. This realisation led to the propulsion of several trials involving the use of AESOP® in minimally invasive surgery. The operating surgeon trains the device in simple commands for driving the camera holding tasks. The unique voice signature is then stored in a card which the surgeon can use at the time of surgery [Fig 5].

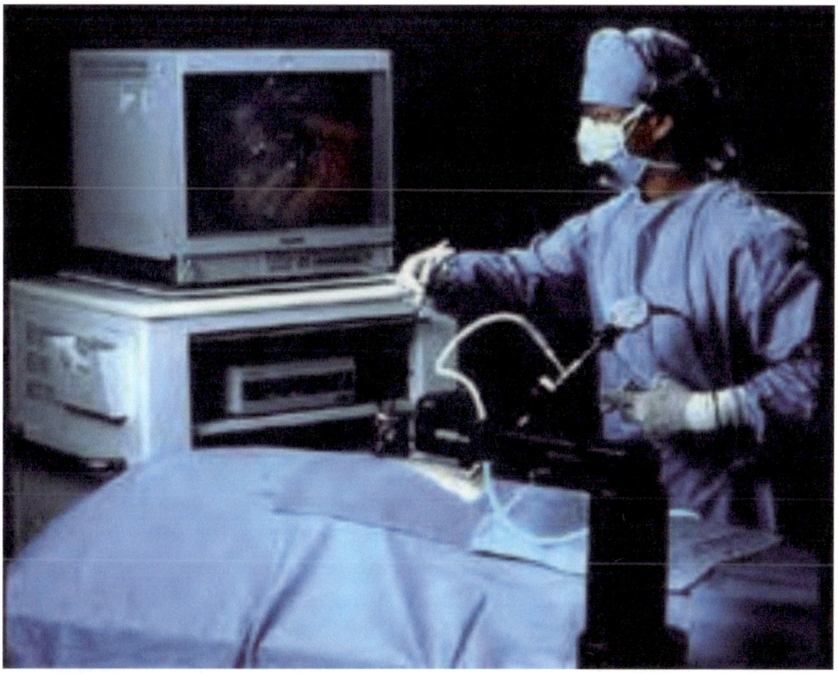

Figure 4. AESOP®. [Copyright JORS 2007]

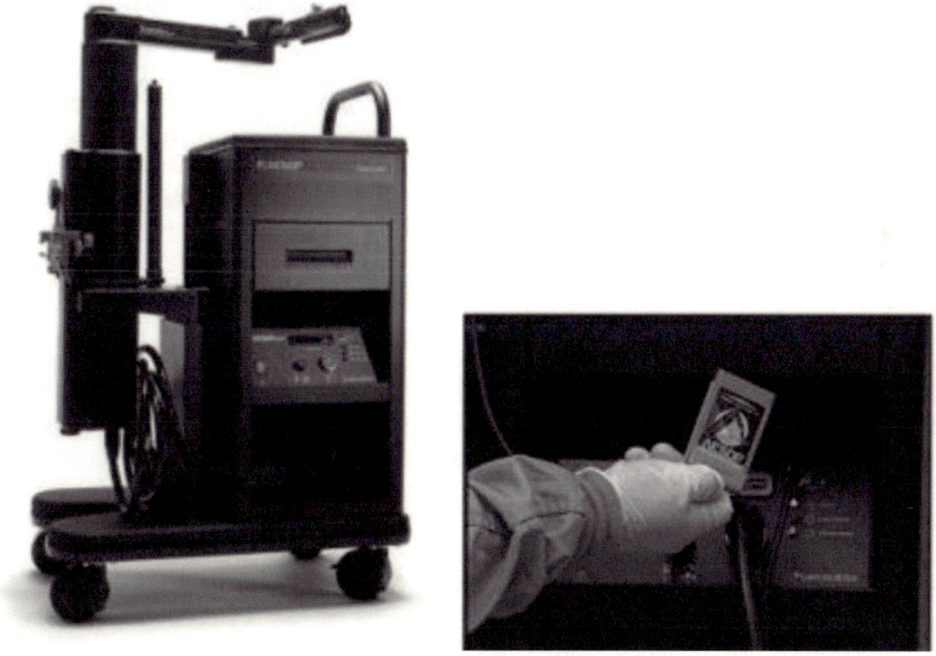

A B

Figure 5. (A) The AESOP® with its camera holding arm (B) The signature voice card. [Copyright © 2006 by Thieme Medical Publishers, Inc., 333 Seventh Avenue, New York, NY 10001, USA.]

AESOP can potentially eliminate the need for an assistant i.e. a member of the surgical team whose duty would conventionally be to physically manipulate the endoscope. Today in the USA approximately a third of all minimally invasive procedures incorporate AESOP. In Europe the uptake has been slower but is gradually increasing. The cost of AESOP is approximately $65,000 to $70,000 USD (in 2006).
Recently, a device called ViKy (endocontrol - medical, La Tronche, France) has been demonstrated, with both voice as well as foot pedal control. Publications regarding its efficacy and ease of use are awaited.

4. Discussion

In 1995, Kavoussi et al. (Kavoussi et al., 1995) reported their findings on their experience with the accuracy and use of a robotic surgical arm compared with a human assistant during LUS. They found that the positioning of the camera was significantly steadier with fewer unwanted or abberant movements when under robotic control when compared with the human counterpart. There was no significant difference, however, in the total operative times using the robot or human assistant. In a later study, by the same team looked at the use of surgeon-controlled robotic arms as a substitute for human assistants and found that simultaneous use of remote-controlled robotic arms as surgical assistants was feasible in minimally invasive surgery (Partin et al., 1995). They found that when the robotic arms were deployed, there was little increase in the total operating time. Furthermore, there was no difference in set up and breakdown times.
The quest for replacements to human assistants was not just confined to urologists alone. Several non urological surgeons explored the potential of alternative camera drivers. One team (Benin et al., 1995), explored the motions of the human camera operator and expressed them mathematically by use of a spherical displacement model. This led to the development of a revolving robotic arm with six degrees of freedom in close association with a camera. This was tested in animal models for cholecystectomy and other procedures. Another team (Geis et al., 1996) explored robotic arm enhancement and its effect on efficiency and resource optimisation in complex minimally invasive surgical procedures. They found that robotic arm enhancement reduced costs and minimized risk for patients. In their study of the actual general surgical cases, they found that versatility, safety and reduction in burden of resources had an overall beneficial advantage.
With health economics in mind, Turner (Turner et al., 1996) compared the cost-effectiveness of using a robotic versus a human assistant in a series of laparoscopic bladder neck suspension cases. His conclusion was that the overall cost of deploying and using the robotic arm was less than that of using a human assistant and that the former was a cost-effective mode for performing the procedures. In an analysis of several studies to determine whether the robotic arm can effectively provide the surgeon with complete control of the surgical field, and the impact of this device on overall cost, it was found that a robotic arm not only outperformed human camera assistants but also improved efficiency and cost savings (Dunlap & Wanzer 1998). The current price of the EndoAssist® and AESOP® devices are under $100,000 US. From a health economics point of view, these costs when balanced against use of man power and cost per hour of employing a human camera assistant, points in favour of the non-human-controlled camera devices.
The preliminary findings that robotic camera holders were economically and technically feasible led several groups to compare the actual devices in terms of different parameters of

functional efficacy. A team from Johns Hopkins (Allaf et al.,1998) evaluated the standard foot pedal for the AESOP® robot compared with a voice control interface and found that voice control was more accurate and had the advantage of not requiring the surgeon to look away from the operative field. However, voice control was slower and required more attention as an interface. The first direct comparison of EndoAssist® and AESOP® (Wagner et al., 2006) using the index procedure of laparoscopic radical prostatectomy, found that the EndoAssist was as efficient as AESOP® with regard to surgical performance. The advantages of the EndoAssist® included its accurate response and its ability to provide the surgeon with complete control of the desired operative view. The disadvantages of the EndoAssist were found to be its large size, the inability to mount it on the table, and its pedal activation dependance.

A review of published literature revealed that the advantage of the EndoAssist over AESOP is its seeming short response time. Furthermore, EndoAssist obviated the need for multiple surgeons to be trained in the use of the same robot and the need to generate different sound cards for each user. The disadvantages of the EndoAssist appear to be its reasonably large footprint (it cannot be mounted on the operating table). Additionally, EndoAssist's foot-operated clutch requires the surgeon to focus away from the operative field to search for the foot pedal from time to time. Further comparative studies using larger cohorts of procedures are currently under way.

Nguan et al. (Nguan et al., 2007) recently published a clinical comparison between three robotic surgical systems (Aesop, Zeus and da Vinci) in assisting laparoscopic pyeloplasty procedures, a technically challenging minimally invasive surgical procedure. They found that the da Vinci robot required significantly more time to set up initially than the AESOP platform but the time was similar to that for the Zeus robot. However, despite the startup time disadvantage, laparoscopic robotic pyeloplasties performed using the da Vinci robot was significantly faster than that for AESOP and Zeus. They concluded that procedures performed using the da Vinci robotic system resulted in decreased anastomotic and operating times. The exact role of the camera holding element in each of these procedures is difficult to quantify. Intuitively, a 3 D camera holding robot under complete autonomous control of the surgeon would be optimal. This could be one of the reasons, apart from differences in other instrumentations, why the camera holding and driving element of the da Vinci System is optimal.

5. Conclusion

The coherent blend between man and machine is now well established and has been taken to the next level. This is exemplified by the seeming symbiotic relationship between some surgeons and their robot assist devices during surgical procedures in ensuring optimal performance. The replacement of a camera holding human surgical assistant by camera holding mechanical robot devices is a testament to the advances in one area of surgical robotics made over the last two decades. The current role played by each camera holding device is likely to evolve in the near future; precision camera holding devices will become a matter of preference by individual surgeons in many instances with each individual device having its pros and cons. We are currently working on several concepts including the next generation of the EndoAssist that could help achieve the very exciting prospect of a near ideal camera holding device.

6. References

Aiono S, Gilbert JM, Soin B, Finlay PA, Gordan A (2002). Controlled trial of the introduction of a robotic camera assistant (EndoAssist) for laparoscopic cholecystectomy. *Surg Endosc* 16(9):1267-1270. Epub 2002 Jun 14.

Allaf ME, Jackman SV, Schulam PG, Cadeddu JA, Lee BR, Moore RG, Kavoussi LR (1998) Laparoscopic visual field. Voice vs foot pedal interfaces for control of the AESOP robot. *Surg Endosc* 12(12):1415-1418.

Begin E, Gagner M, Hurteau R, de Santis S, Pomp A (1995) A robotic camera for laparoscopic surgery: conception and experimental results. *Surg Laparosc Endosc* 5(1):6-11.

Dunlap KD, Wanzer L (1998) Is the robotic arm a cost-effective surgical tool? AORN J 68(2):265-272. Review. Erratum in: *AORN J* 68(3): pp. 368.

Geis WP, Kim HC, Brennan EJ Jr, McAfee PC, Wang Y. (1996) Robotic arm enhancement to accommodate improved efficiency and decreased resource utilization in complex minimally invasive surgical procedures. *Stud Health Technol Inform* 29: pp. 471-481.

Kavoussi LR, Moore RG, Adams JB, Partin AW. (1995) Comparison of robotic versus human laparoscopic camera control. *J Urol* 154(6): pp. 2134-2136. Erratum in: J Urol 1997 158(4):1530.

Kommu SS, Rimmington P, Anderson C, Rane A. (2007). Initial experience with The EndoAssist® Camera Holding Robot. *JORS*. Vol 1, No 2 (July 2007). Pp.1863-2483.

Nebot PB, Jain Y, Haylett K, Stone R, McCloy R (2003) Comparison of task performance of the camera-holder robots EndoAssist and Aesop. Surg Laparosc Endosc Percutan Tech 13(5): pp. 334-338.

Nguan C, Kwan K, Al Omar M, Beasley KA, Luke PP. (2007). Robotic pyeloplasty: experience with three robotic platforms. *Can J Urol.* Jun;14(3):3571-6.

Sackier JM, Wang Y. (1994). Robotically assisted laparoscopic surgery. From concept to development. *Surg Endosc.* 8(1): pp. 63-66.

Su LM, Link RE, Bhayani SB, Sullivan W, Pavlovich CP (2004). Nerve-sparing laparoscopic radical prostatectomy: replicating the open surgical technique. *Urology* 64(1): pp. 123-127.

Turner DJ (1996). Solo surgery—with the aid of a robotic assistant. *J Telemed Telecare.* 2(Suppl 1): pp. 46-48.

Unger SW, Unger HM, Bass RT. (1994). AESOP robotic arm. *Surg Endosc.* Sep;8(9): pp. 1131.

Wagner AA, Varkarakis IM, Link RE, Sullivan W, Su LM (2006). Comparison of surgical performance during laparoscopic radical prostatectomy of two robotic camera holders, EndoAssist and AESOP: a pilot study. *Urology* 68(1): pp. 70-74.

26

Telerobotic Surgery for Right and Sigmoid Colectomy

Arthur Rawlings, M.D., M.Div. and David Crawford, M.D.
University of Illinois College of Medicine at Peoria, Illinois
USA

1. Introduction

Surgery, unlike modern medicine, retains its link with ancient traditions. Human anatomy has not changed and the surgical approach to many diseases has remained the same for decades, even centuries. However, the techniques have evolved. For centuries, the sole approach to the disease was a large incision. Laparoscopic surgery ushered in a new era. Small incisions promised shorter hospital stays, less postoperative pain, better cosmesis, and a quicker return to normal activity. Patients now desire a minimally invasive surgical approach to their disease if at all possible.

The benefits to the patient were bought with the price of surgeons losing maneuverability in the operative field and having only a two-dimensional instead of a three-dimensional view. For many the transition was difficult. The learning curve was steep. In a short time, though, some procedures such as a laparoscopic cholecystectomy became the gold standard and basic laparoscopic skills were incorporated into general surgery training programs.

The next major advance in minimally invasive surgery was the development of telemanipulation systems, also referred to as robots. Originally spearheaded in the United States by the Department of Defense, these robotic devices were intended for surgeons to operate from a remote location. These systems restored pitch and yaw at the end of the instruments, the two degrees of freedom lost with the use of traditional laparoscopic instruments. They also added other benefits such as tremor reduction, motion scaling, surgeon camera control, comfortable ergonomics, and a three-dimensional view of the operative field.

The first robotic system approved for intraabdominal surgery in the United States by the Food and Drug Administration (FDA) was the AESOP (Automated Endoscopic System for Optimal Position) system in 1993 (Oddsdottir & Birgisson, 2004). AESOP (Computer Motion, Goleta, California) is a computerized robotic camera assistant for laparoscopic surgery. It has gone through several modifications since then and is still available today as a voice-activated, surgeon-controlled, camera assistant. It offers a stable camera platform but has no arm for direct manipulation or dissection of the tissues.

The first robotic system approved for intraabdominal surgery that did offer direct manipulation and dissection capabilities was the da Vinci system (Intitive Surgical, Inc., Sunnyvale, California). In 2000, the FDA approved the da Vinci system. Approval for a second system, ZEUS (Computer Motion, Goleta, California), quickly followed in 2001

(Marescaux & Rubino, 2004). Since then, the two companies have merged and ZEUS is no longer available. The da Vinci system is the only surgical platform available on the market that offers direct manipulation and dissection capabilities. Now, there are two generations of da Vinci robots in use: the da Vinci and the da Vinci S. These will be the systems focused on in this chapter.

2. The da Vinci System

The da Vinci system consists of three basic components: surgical cart, vision tower, and surgeon's console. The surgical cart is home to the three robotic arms. A fourth optional arm is also available. One arm is used for the camera, two arms are used for a variety of available surgical instruments, and the fourth optional arm is used mainly as an assistant for retraction. Laparoscopic surgery reduced the degrees of freedom in the abdomen to five: 1) in/out, 2) pitch (up/down), 3) yaw (left/right), 4) rotate, and 5) grasp. The robotic arms added 6) internal pitch and 7) internal yaw at the end of the instruments, restoring the full seven degrees of freedom available during an open abdominal case. The surgical cart to which the arms are attached is on rollers and can approach the operating table and be positioned over the patient from any direction necessary.

The surgeon's console consists of binocular monitors, foot pedals, and two hand-held masters used to manipulate the camera and surgical instruments. The binocular monitors can be switched during the case from a two-dimensional to a three-dimensional view with the press of a button. Having a three-dimensional view regains another component of open surgery that was lost with laparoscopic surgery. The surgeon sits at the console with his forearms and forehead resting on cushions, leaving his hands and feet free to operate the controls.

The vision tower contains the insufflator, light source, printer, camera, and computer hardware that generates the image. It also provides a stand for a monitor for the assistants in the room to watch during the case. The da Vinci S system also sports high definition vision in a panoramic 16:9 ratio along with an interactive video monitor called TilePro that allows a proctor to draw on the screen, thus giving visual direction to the person behind the surgeon's console.

3. Robotic Colectomy

The da Vinci system has been used for practically every intraabdominal procedure performed by general surgeons (Hanly & Talamini, 2004; Ballantyne, 2007). Our focus is on the use of the da Vinci system for a colectomy.

3.1 Our Background

The Peoria Surgical Group is a university-affiliated, community training program with the University of Illinois College of Medicine at Peoria. There are three general surgery residents per year and no fellowships within the program. In 2002, the Peoria Surgical Group became the first private practice owner of the da Vinci system. At that time, the fourth arm was not available. It has since been purchased, but is presently not used for a right or sigmoid colectomy. As of August 2005, the chief of minimally invasive surgery, Dr. Crawford, had performed 109 cases with the da Vinci system. He has performed 34 colectomies. The results of his first 30 colectomies have been published (Rawlings et al., 2006, 2007).

3.2 Patient Selection

Dr. Crawford's patients have the choice of three hospitals in Peoria, Illinois, two of which now have the da Vinci system. Robotic assistance is not discussed with the patients until they have chosen one of the robot's host hospitals. If a robot's host hospital is chosen, the patients are offered a choice between robotic and laparoscopic surgery if a minimally invasive approach is deemed appropriate. No patients are diverted to a robot's host hospital specifically for a robotic colectomy. Laparoscopic colectomies are performed at all three hospitals and on several occasions the second colectomy of the day at a robot's host hospital is performed laparoscopically instead of robotically because of staffing concerns expressed by the hospitals.

3.3 Robotic Right Colectomy

The patient is lying supine on a bean bag. The bag is positioned flush with the patient's right side, allowing excess bag on the left side with which to wrap the left side of the patient. The chest is secured circumferentially to the table with heavy tape at the level of the clavicles. The legs are secured at the thigh and calf with straps. Establishment of pneumoperitoneum, trocar placement (Figure 1), and initial exploration are performed in the supine position. The tattooed lesion or pathology is located and the planned point of transverse mesocolic division is marked based on the location of the right branch of the middle colic artery. The table is tilted to the left to allow the small intestine to fall off of the midline. The robot is then brought in over the right upper quadrant to dock with the camera port periumbilically and the right lower and left upper quadrant ports (See arrow, Figure 1). A five millimeter port is placed in the left lower quadrant and is used to grasp the ileocecal valve and to put the ileocolic vascular pedicle on tension. This pedicle is divided at the level of the duodenum with a vascular stapler that is brought in through the left-sided twelve millimeter port. The right mesocolon is mobilized off Gerota's fascia, the ureter is identified and then the ileal mesentery is divided with harmonic energy shears out to a point ten centimeters from the ileocecal valve. The mesocolic mobilization is then carried up to the duodenum and the transverse mesocolon. The transverse mesocolon is divided with harmonic shears, clips, and vascular staplers as needed. The transverse colon and ileum are then divided with a stapler from the left-sided twelve millimeter port. The colon remains attached to the right paracolic gutter to keep it from falling medially.

An isoperistaltic side-to-side anastomosis is then created between the ileum and transverse colon. A thirty centimeter long 2-0 silk suture on a Keith needle is used to join the distal transverse colon to the ileum six centimeters from the cut end. The Keith needle is then brought out through the abdominal wall in the right upper quadrant laterally and held with a hemostat. This keeps the anastomosis away from the camera and up in the air, making it easier to work on. The colon and ileum are also joined with suture near the cut end of the ileum. Harmonic shears are used to create an ileotomy and colotomy. Then a linear cutting stapler from the left-sided twelve millimeter port joins the bowel through these openings. The ileocolotomy is then sewn closed with running 2-0 Vicryl in two layers. The mesenteric defect is not closed. The suture holding the anastomosis up and to the right is cut, allowing the colon to fall medially out of the way. The right colon's lateral attachments are divided with cautery, and the specimen is extracted through the left-sided twelve millimeter port site after being converted to a small four centimeter muscle splitting incision (Solid line, Figure 1). This incision is protected from potential contamination with a short segment of a camera bag. Port sites are anesthetized and closed in the usual manner.

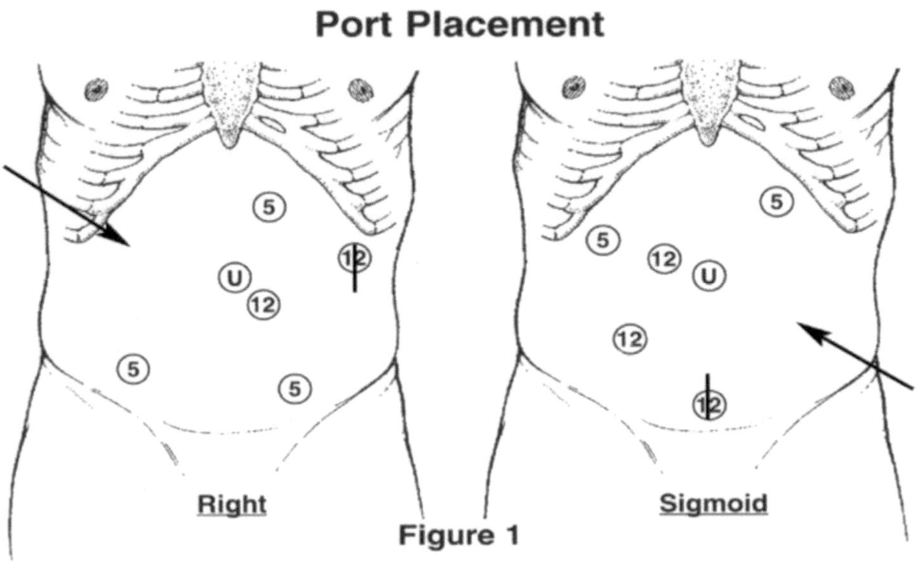

Figure 1. Port Placement for a Robotic Colectomy. The arrows show the angle of approach by the surgical cart. The number in the circle indicates to size of trocar. The "U" is the umbilicus. The solid line through the 12 mm trocar sites is the specimen extraction site

3.4 Robotic Sigmoid Colectomy

The patient is in supine lithotomy position with the anterior thighs in the same plane as the abdominal wall. The bean bag is embracing the patient's right side. The chest is secured circumferentially to the table with heavy tape at the level of the clavicles. Establishment of pneumoperitoneum, trocar placement (Figure 1), and initial exploration are performed in the supine position. The patient is tilted steeply to the right and the tattooed lesion or pathology is localized. Reverse Trendelenburg position is added to the right tilt and the surgical robot is brought up to the table in the left lower quadrant (See arrow, Figure 1). The robot's left arm goes in the left upper quadrant five millimeter port. The camera arm is in the periumbilical port. A five millimeter port remains on the robot's right arm and is inserted through the twelve millimeter suprapubic port. The splenic flexure is completely mobilized. All three arms are then adjusted as the patient is put into Trendelenburg position, along with the right arm and its five millimeter port being moved to the right lower quadrant twelve millimeter port. The inferior mesenteric artery is identified and isolated from a medial to lateral approach, and the left ureter is identified. All mobilization of the colon and mesorectal division is completed using electrocautery and harmonic energy. The robot is disengaged and endoscopic staplers are used to divide the inferior mesenteric artery and rectum. The specimen is externalized through the extended suprapubic port site that is protected from potential contamination with a short segment of a camera bag (Solid line, Figure 1). The specimen is resected, the stapler anvil introduced, and the proximal colon is dropped back in the abdomen. The fascia is closed and pneumoperitoneum reestablished. A standard end-to-end anastomosis is performed using conventional laparoscopy, and tested in the usual manner. Port sites are anesthetized and closed in the usual manner.

Port placement in males and females is identical. Initially, when only eight millimeter instruments were available for the da Vinci system, the ports were placed through twelve millimeter dilating trocars. This allowed the assistants at the table to advance or retract the robot trocars/arms to optimize instrument use with less fear of dislodging the robot trocar from the abdominal wall. The switch to five millimeter instruments took place November of 2004, when these instruments became available to us. The five millimeter instruments handle differently, but were easy to adjust to. Five millimeter instruments are now routinely used in order to minimize incision size. The only place that the trocar through a trocar technique is still used is in a sigmoid colectomy between the suprapubic and right lower quadrant sites. The scrub staff makes this exchange without the surgeon returning to the field.

3.5 Post Operative Care

The patients are placed on clear liquids the day of surgery and receive a single dose of Milk of Magnesia on the morning of postoperative day one. All robotic colectomies are placed on a hospital-wide activity protocol. All patients have a patient controlled analgesia pump for pain control that is discontinued when they tolerate liquids well. Patients are discharged when tolerating liquids well, voiding, moving their bowels, and having adequate pain control with oral analgesics.

4. Review of Literature

As stated earlier, the da Vinci system has been used for practically every intraabdominal procedure performed by general surgeons (Hanly & Talamini, 2004; Ballantyne, 2007). We will limit our discussion to colectomy.

4.1 Robotic Colectomy

Webber reported performing the first robotic colon resection in 2001 using the da Vinci system (Webber et al. 2002). Since then, at least fifteen other studies of robotic colectomy have been reported. The published series are listed in table 1. The difficulty in comparing one series to another is that a wide range of procedures are included in some series and the parameters reported vary from one study to another. For example, Giulianotti included abdominoperineal resections and ileocecal resections along with right and left hemicolectomies while Woeste reported only sigmoid colectomies (Giulianotti et al., 2003; Woeste et al., 2005). Delany reported times from anesthesia to incision and incision to extubation whereas we reported times from initial incision to robot engagement, from robot engagement to robot disengagement, and from robot disengagement to the end of the case. (Delany et al., 2003; Rawlings et al., 2006, 2007).

Among all of these studies are four that specifically compare a laparoscopic colectomy with a robotic colectomy (Anvari et al., 2004; D'Annibale et al., 2003; Delany et al., 2003; Rawlings et al., 2007). Since a laparoscopic colectomy is the only competition a robotic colectomy has if the patient wants a minimally invasive approach, we will focus on these four studies.

First Author	YEAR	Number	Operative Time*	Conversions
Weber	2002	2	284 (228-340)	0
Hashizume	2002	3	260 (180-335)	0
Delaney	2003	6	217 (170-274)	1
Giulianotti	2003	16	211 (90-360)	0
Vibert	2003	3	380 (330-450)	0
Ewing	2004	12	248 (180-350)	0
Hanly	2004	35	177 (NA)	5
Ayav	2004	5	265 (180-240)	0
Anvari ‡	2004	10	155 ± 14	0
D'Annibale	2004	53	240 ± 61	5
Hubens	2004	7	NA	0
Woeste	2004	4	237 ± 6	1
Braumann	2005	5	201 (80-300)	2
Ayav	2005	6	172 (45-280)	0
Anvari	2005	6	109 (90-160)	1
Rawlings	2006 &2007	30	226 (90-340)	2

* Average (Range) or ± Standard Deviation in Minutes, NA: Not Available
‡ The only study using the ZEUS system

Table 1. Robotic Colectomy Series Articles in Chronological Order of Publication

4.2 Robotic verses Laparoscopic Colectomy

Anvari used the ZEUS system to compare ten robotic and ten consecutive laparoscopic colectomies (Anvari et al., 2004). Although the ZEUS system is no longer available, the authors reported one definite advantage of the system for a colectomy that highlights one of the deficiencies of the da Vinci system. The ZEUS system integrated the robot and the operating room table so the patient could be tilted or rotated without any readjustment of the robotic arms. The da Vinci is not integrated with the operating room table. Rotating or tilting the patient is not impossible with the da Vinci system. It is just very inconvenient.

D'Annibale has the largest comparison to date of robotic and laparoscopic colectomies, with fifty-three consecutive robotic patients and fifty-three matched laparoscopic patients (D'Annibale et al., 2003). The authors reported no significant difference in operative time with 240 ± 61 minutes for robotic cases and 222 ± 77 minutes for laparoscopic cases. There was, however, a statistically significant difference in system and patient setup time. It took 24 ± 12 minutes to set up for a robotic case but only 18 ± 7 minutes for a laparoscopic case ($p = 0.002$). Their length of hospital stay for robotic cases averaged ten days and did not differ from a matched laparoscopic group. Though favorable toward the da Vinci system over traditional laparoscopy for specific stages of the procedure, they concluded their study stating that, "investigations are needed to evaluate the cost-effectiveness of this approach."

The third comparison study does include cost. In 2003, Delany published a comparison of six robotic operations with procedure matched control laparoscopic patients (Delany et al., 2003). Total hospital cost was higher for the robotic group, but this did not reach statistical significance. They attributed this to their small sample size. They stated that the operating room and equipment cost was approximately $350 higher for the robotic group, to cover the robotic instruments and sterile drapes. Their study did include disposable operating cost, but did not include the acquisition or maintenance costs of the da Vinci system, nor was cost a major focus of their publication.

In our comparison, the fourth published, we had a significant focus on cost, breaking it down into total hospital cost, operating room cost, operating room supply cost, and operating room personnel cost (Rawlings et al., 2007). All of our costs were adjusted to 2005 US dollars. We showed that each cost category was higher for the robotic group over the laparoscopic group (Tables 2 & 3). Despite our sample size being twice as large as Delany's sample size for right and sigmoid colectomy, a statistically significant increase in our study was lacking in several cost categories. For a right colectomy, there was a significant difference in all the operating room cost categories, but this did not result in a significant difference for total hospital cost. For a sigmoid colectomy, a significant difference was only reached in operating room personnel and supply costs. The remaining cost categories for a sigmoid colectomy did not reach statistical significance. This is undoubtedly due to our small sample size. To illustrate, the analysis of our total hospital cost had a power of only 6% for a sigmoid colectomy and 12% for a right colectomy in showing a statistically significant difference. Using our existing data set and assuming a similar ratio of robotic and laparoscopic cases, there would have to be a total of 1,616 sigmoid colectomy cases and 391 right colectomy cases to reach a desired power of 80% with a significant difference of $p < 0.05$ in total hospital cost. Needless to say, with these numbers, a randomized controlled trial comparing the cost of a laparoscopic with a robotic colectomy is well beyond the ability of any one institution in the near future.

Even though we had a significant focus on cost in our study, we did not include the acquisition and maintenance costs of the da Vinci system. In our setting, these costs cannot be directly passed on to the patient. We can, however, charge the patient for the robot disposables such as drapes and the robotic instruments that have a ten to twenty case lifetime. At our institution we are presently required to have two circulating nurses in all robotic cases instead of one, as we normally have in a laparoscopic case. This helps explain the difference in operating room personnel cost between robotic and laparoscopic cases. As far as the acquisition and maintenance costs go, they are presently viewed as capital expenses. They are not directly passed on to the patient undergoing a robotic procedure, in the same way we do not directly pass on the cost of the handicapped access ramp only to the patients who are wheelchair bound. To our knowledge, no one has studied and published the true cost-to-benefit ratio of the da Vinci system. This is a very complex economic issue, but could be a very fruitful area of investigation.

RIGHT COLECTOMY - COST ANALYSIS*			
	Laparoscopic (n=15)	**Robotic (n=17)**	***p* value**
Total Hospital Cost	$8,073 ± 2,805	$9,255 ± 5,075	0.430
Total OR Cost	$4,339 ± 867	$5,823 ± 907	< 0.000
OR Personnel Cost	$1,340 ± 402	$2,048 ± 309	< 0.000
OR Supply Cost	$1,841 ± 518	$2,950 ± 475	< 0.000
OR Time Cost	$990 ± 300	$1,521 ± 321	< 0.000

Table 2. Cost Analysis for a Right Colectomy: *Adjusted to 2005 US Dollars

SIGMOID COLECTOMY - COST ANALYSIS*			
	Laparoscopic (n=12)	**Robotic (n=13)**	***p* value**
Total Hospital Cost	\$10,697 ± 11,719	\$12,335 ± 12,162	0.735
Total OR Cost	\$4,974 ± 1,596	\$6,059 ± 1,225	0.068
OR Personnel Cost	\$1,621 ± 617	\$2,134 ± 432	0.024
OR Supply Cost	\$2,137 ± 905	\$3,159 ± 637	0.003
OR Time Cost	\$1,348 ± 681	\$1,500 ± 461	0.519

Table 3. Cost Analysis for a Sigmoid Colectomy: *Adjusted to 2005 US Dollars

In our study, the robotic and laparoscopic groups for a right and sigmoid colectomy were similar in gender, age, body mass index, and indications for surgery. The average case time for a robotic right colectomy was 219 minutes, which was 50 minutes longer than the 169 minute average for the laparoscopic group. This was statistically significantly longer ($p = 0.002$). Two factors contributed to a longer average case time in the robotic cases. Our first study showed that the robotic port setup time – the time from initial insufflation with a Veress needle until the surgeon sits at the robot's console – for a right colectomy averaged 30 minutes (Rawlings et al., 2006). Also, an isoperistaltic side-to-side anastomosis was performed intracorporeally with robotic assistance, whereas an extracorporeal bowel resection and anastomosis was performed in the laparoscopic cases. The port setup time and the variation in anastomotic technique accounts for the robotic cases requiring more time than the laparoscopic cases in a right colectomy. In contrast, the average case time for a robotic sigmoid colectomy was 225 minutes, which was 26 minutes longer than the 199 minute average for the laparoscopic group. This was not statistically significant ($p = 0.128$). The robotic and laparoscopic sigmoid colectomy cases were performed in similar sequence, and the additional time for the robotic cases is mainly attributed to the 30 minute port setup time for the robot (Rawlings et al., 2006).

Our length of stay did not differ between the two comparison groups. A laparoscopic right colectomy averaged 5.5 days and a robotic right colectomy averaged 5.2 days ($p = 0.862$). A laparoscopic sigmoid colectomy averaged 6.6 days and a robotic sigmoid colectomy averaged 6.0 days ($p = 0.854$). We also showed no difference in estimated blood loss between our comparison groups.

5. Reflections on the da Vinci for Colectomy

At least fifteen published series have demonstrated the technical feasibility of using the da Vinci system for performing a colon resection (Table 1). The use of this system for this procedure has definite advantages and disadvantages.

5.1 Colectomy: The da Vinci Advantages

There are several advantages of using the da Vinci system. The first is the enhanced visualization of the operative field. The da Vinci system allows the surgeon to choose between two-dimensional and three-dimensional representations of the operative field with its stereoscopic camera. The three-dimensional view is particularly helpful in depth of field and clarity of tissue planes during dissection. The camera also allows for a ten-fold magnification compared to the two-fold on standard laparoscopic cameras.

The second advantage is that the surgeon has control over the camera by toggling a switch with a foot pedal. This allows the surgeon to place the camera at the location he desires when he desires it, rather than depending on an assistant to anticipate his desired view or respond to a command.

The third advantage is the wristed instruments, which introduce two more degrees of freedom into the operative field. Traditional laparoscopic surgery reduced the maneuverability in the operative field to only five degrees: 1) in-out, 2) rotation of shaft, 3) pitch (up-down), 4) yaw (left-right), and 5) grasp. The robotic instruments add two more degrees of freedom: 1) internal pitch at the end of the wristed instruments and 2) internal yaw at the end of the wristed instruments. In essence, the robot restores the maneuverability available during an open case with the surgeon's hand in the operative field to a laparoscopic case. It is like having your hands back in the field. It should also be mentioned that the robotic software provides tremor reduction and motion scaling to the wristed instruments, both significant advantages in delicate dissection and fine suturing situations.

Another advantage is the reduction of the surgeon's fatigue. During the robotic portion of the case, the surgeon is sitting with her forearms resting comfortably on a pad and her head resting against the console. Fatigue is also reduced because the hand controls can be recentered while leaving the surgical instruments in their present location. In traditional laparoscopic surgery, the surgeon had to move her hands to whatever location is needed to position the surgical instruments at their proper locations. This, at times, requires some rather awkward movements and pushes the limits of one's flexibility and reach. With the recentering feature of the da Vinci system, the surgeon can relocate her hands back to a normal position and then resume working. It is like lifting up the computer mouse and putting it back to a comfortable spot while leaving the cursor at its present location on the computer screen.

Finally, it should be mentioned that using the da Vinci system in the present surgical climate in the United States does allow one to be promoted as a "regional Minimally Invasive Surgery (MIS) expert," which is often a unique marketing opportunity. This is another aspect of the total cost-to-benefit ratio that comes from an institution or surgical group owning the da Vinci system. The perception is that having the da Vinci system enlarges your referral base, but this would be very hard to demonstrate.

5.2 Colectomy: The da Vinci Disadvantages

There are several general disadvantages of using the da Vinci system that apply to its use for any case. These include loss of tactile sensation, difficult team communication with the surgeon sequestered behind the console away from the patient and staff, increased room size requirements to accommodate the equipment, and cost of the device.

There are three distinct disadvantages of using the da Vinci system for a colectomy. The first is the inconvenience of altering port placement of the camera and instruments during the case. In the traditional laparoscopic approach, one easily pulled the camera out and placed it in another port that would accommodate it if another perspective were desired. Changing which port the camera or instruments enter the patient is not impossible with the da Vinci system. It is just very inconvenient. This precludes taking a quick look around from another port site during the robotic portion of the procedure. It also keeps one from quickly shifting an instrument from one port site to another to gain a different angle of attack for dissection.

A second disadvantage is the difficulty encountered with working in the far lateral extensions of the operative field. For example, while working in the left lateral most aspect of the field (splenic flexure) the instrument in the right port (suprapubic) may reach its inner most limits before reaching the desired spot, and visa versa. Working with an instrument tip too close to the end of the port can also limit the ability of the instrument to function optimally. In traditional laparoscopic surgery, this is sometimes overcome by switching the camera and operating port for a portion of the case. That would be very inconvenient with the da Vinci system. Knowing this places a greater burden on proper port placement for the robotic case because the location determines how far laterally one may reasonably work in the surgical field. The port setup is the key aspect of any smoothly running robotic procedure. There are definite limits in movement with the robotic arm compared to the standard laparoscopic approach. For example, the robotic arm has a definite extension end point, whereas a few centimeters can be gained in traditional laparoscopic surgery by depressing the insufflated abdomen.

A third disadvantage in using the da Vinci system with this particular type of case is the inconvenience of rotating or tilting the patient. In minimally invasive procedures, the patients are sometimes tilted or rotated to allow gravity to help pull the organs that obstruct the operative field out of the way. Every change in the patient's position requires each arm of the robot to be reset to a new location. So, other forms of retraction must be implemented to compensate. Usually this entails another port for retraction. This assistant port can also be used to introduce objects into the field such as sutures, staplers, and measuring tapes. It is also used to remove the pathological specimen. This assistant port is usually not placed solely for retraction, but it will be used for retraction and the port will require surgical personnel to staff it.

6. Conclusion

The first reported robotic colectomy was performed in March, 2001. Since then, fourteen other studies have been published showing the safety and feasibility of using the da Vinci system for a colectomy and one study showed the safety and feasibility of using the ZEUS system. No robot specific complication has yet to be reported. There are definite advantages as well as disadvantages of using the da Vinci system for a colectomy. Though studies have been done comparing the cost of a laparoscopic colectomy with a robotic colectomy, more work needs to be done looking at cost from an even wider perspective than just cost per case. Is there any true marketing advantage to an institution having the da Vinci system? How does the cost of the robot as well as the cost of ongoing company support figure into the picture? The da Vinci system has been used for colectomy for less than a decade. We are optimistic that refinements in this system will make it even more attractive in the future for a right or sigmoid colectomy.

7. Acknowledgements

The surgical technique descriptions, figures, and the advantages and disadvantages discussion are used with kind permission from Springer Science and Business Media, Springer New York, Surgical Endoscopy, Vol. 20, No. 11, 2007, pp. 1713-1718, *Telerobotic Surgery for Right and Sigmoid Colectomies: 30 Consecutive Cases*, Rawlings, A.; Woodland, J. &

Crawford, D. and Surgical Endoscopy, Vol. 21, No. 10, 2007, pp. 1701-1708, *Robotic versus Laparoscopic Colectomy*, 2007, Rawlings, A.; Woodland, J.; Vegunta, R. & Crawford, D.

8. References

Anvari, M.; Birch, D.; Bamehriz, F.; Gryfe, R. & Chapman T. (2004). Robotic-assisted Laparoscopic Colorectal Surgery, *Surgical Laparoscopy, Endoscopy & Percutaneous Techniques*, Vol. 14, No. 6, (December 2004), pp. 311-315, ISSN 1530-4515

Anvari, M.; McKinley, C. & Stein, H. (2005). Establishment of the World's First Telerobotic Remote Surgical Service for Provision of Advanced Laparoscopic Surgery in a Rural Community. *Annals of Surgery*, Vol. 241, No. 3, (March 2005), pp. 460-464, ISSN 0003-4932

Ayav, A.; Bresler, L.; Brunaud, L. & Boissel, P. (2004). Early Results of One-Year Robotic Surgery Using the Da Vinci System to Perform Advanced Laparosopic Procedures. *Journal of Gastrointestinal Surgery*, Vol. 8, No. 6, (September 2004), pp. 720-726, ISSN 1091-255X

Ayav, A.; Bresler, L.; Hubert, J.; Brunaud, L. & Boissel, P. (2005). Robotic-Assisted Pelvic Organ Prolapse Surgery. *Surgical Endoscopy*, Vol. 19, No. 9, (September 2005), pp. 1200-1203, ISSN 0930-2794

Ballantyne, G. (2007). Telerobotic Gastrointestinal Surgery: Phase 2 - Safety and Efficacy. *Surgical Endoscopy*, Vol. 21, No. 7, (July 2007), pp. 1054-1062, ISSN 0930-2794

Braumann, C.; Jacobi, C.; Menenakos, C.; Borchert, U.; Rueckert, J. & Mueller, J. (2005). Computer-Assisted Laparoscopic Colon Resection with the Da Vinci System: Our First Experiences. *Diseases of the Colon and Rectum*, Vol. 48, No. 9, (September 2005), pp. 1820-1827, ISSN 0012-3706

D'Annibale, A.; Morpurgo, E.; Fiscon, V.; Trevisan, P.; Sovernigo, G.; Orsini, C. & Guidolin, D. (2004). Robotic and Laparoscopic Surgery for Treatment of Colorectal Diseases. *Diseases of the Colon and Rectum*, Vol. 47, No. 12, (December 2004), pp. 2162-2168, ISSN 0012-3706

Delaney, C.; Lynch, A.; Senagore, A. & Fazio, V. (2003). Comparison of Robotically Performed and Traditional Laparoscopic Colorectal Surgery. *Diseases of the Colon and Rectum*, Vol. 46, No. 12, (December 2003), pp. 1633-1639, ISSN 0012-3706

Giulianotti, P.; Coratti, A.; Angelini, M.; Sbrana, F.; Cecconi, S.; Balestracci, T. & Caravaglois, G. (2003). Robotics in General Surgery: Personal Experience in a Large Community Hospital. *Archives of Surgery*, Vol. 138, No. 7, (July 2003), pp. 777-784, ISSN 0004-0010

Hanly, E. & Talamini, M. (2004). Robotic Abdominal Surgery. *The American Journal of Surgery*, Vol. 188, No. 4A, (Supplemental to October 2004), pp. 19S-26S, ISSN 0002-9610

Hashizume, M.; Shimada, M.; Tomikawa, M.; Ikeda, Y.; Takahashi, I.; Abe, R.; Foga, F.; Gotoh, N.; Konishi, K.; Maehara, S. & Sugimachi, K. (2002). Early Experiences of Endocsopic Procedures in General Surery Assisted by a Computer-enhanced Surgical System. *Surgical Endoscopy*, Vol. 16, No. 8, (August 2002), pp. 1187-1191, ISSN 0930-2794

Hubens, G.; Ruppert, M.; Balliu, L. & Vaneerdeweg, W. (2004). What Have We Learnt After Two Years Working with the Da Vinci Robot System in Digestive Surgery? *Acta chirurgica Belgica*, Vol. 104, No. 6, (November 2004), pp. 609-614, ISSN 0001-5458

Marescaux, J. & Rubino, F. (2004). The ZEUS Telerobotic Surgical System, In: *Primer of Robotic & Telerobotic Surgery,* Ballantyne, G.; Marescaux, J. & Giulianotti, P. (Ed.), pp. 61-65, Lippincott Williams & Wilkins, ISBN 0-7817-4844-5, Philadelphia

Oddsdottir, M. & Birgisson, G. (2004). AESOP: A Voice-Controlled Camera Holder, In: *Primer of Robotic & Telerobotic Surgery,* Ballantyne, G.; Marescaux, J. & Giulianotti, P. (Ed.), pp. 35-41, Lippincott Williams & Wilkins, ISBN 0-7817-4844-5, Philadelphia

Rawlings, A.; Woodland, J. & Crawford, D. (2006). Telerobotic Surgery for Right and Sigmoid Colectomies: 30 Consecutive Cases. *Surgical Endoscopy,* Vol. 20, No. 11, (2006), pp. 1713-1718, ISSN 0930-2794

Rawlings, A.; Woodland, J.; Vegunta, R. & Crawford, D. (2007). Robotic versus Laparoscopic Colectomy. *Surgical Endoscopy,* Vol. 21, No. 10, (2007), pp. 1701-1708, ISSN 0930-2794

Vibert, E.; Denet, C. & Gayet, B. (2003). Major Digestive Surgery Using a Remote-Controlled Robot: The Next Revolution. *Archives of Surgery,* Vol. 138, No. 9, (September 2003), pp. 1002-1006, ISSN 0004-0010

Weber, P.; Merola, S.; Wasielewski, A. & Ballantyne, G. (2002). Telerobotic-Assisted Laparoscopic Right and Sigmoid Colectomies for Benign Disease. *Diseases of the Colon and Rectum,* Vol. 45, No. 12, (December 2002), pp. 1689-1696, ISSN 0012-3706

Woeste, G.; Bechstein, W. & Wullstein, C. (2005). Does Telerobotic Assistance Improve Laparoscopic Colorectal Surgery? *International Journal of Colorectal Disease,* Vol. 20, No.3, (May 2005), pp. 253-257, ISSN 0179-1958

27

Robotic Assisted Microsurgery (RAMS): Application in Plastic Surgery

Dr. Sanjay Saraf
Dept. of Plastic Surgery, NMC Specialty Hospital, Dubai
United Arab Emirates

1. Introduction

The essence of plastic surgery is to have innovative thinking, capacity to find new methods and to adopt newer technologies to its benefit. The development of medical robotic system to assist surgeons in various surgical specialties is a new advancement and is a growing field of telerobotic research. The Robotic Assisted Microsurgery (RAMS) represents one of the latest innovations of telerobotics in the microsurgical field and with the continuing success of Robotic Assisted Microsurgery in various surgical specialties, the plastic surgeons have started exploring its application for performing technically challenging, time consuming and physical exhausting micro-vascular procedures. RAMS represents an advanced application of telerobotic surgery and a possible answer to the surgeon's demand for ways to overcome the surgical limitations of microsurgery. Basically the RAMS system is a telerobot with mechanical arms which is controlled by a computer but operated by a surgeon. RAMS allows performing high dexterity microsurgical operations with the help of robotic arms and improves microsurgery through tremor filtration, articulation, motion scaling, and improved ergonomics. The surgeon actually does a better, more precise, dexterous and highly controlled microsurgical procedure under high magnification resulting into optimal microsurgical outcome. This chapter reviews various developments in the field of robotic microsurgery and discusses various aspects related to human versus robotic microsurgery and its potential use in plastic surgery.

2. History of telerobotics

A robot is defined as a sensor-based tool capable of performing precise, accurate and versatile actions on its environment. In medicine, robots have recently evolved into complex systems integrating perception (medical images and information) and action (precise spatial positioning and sensory feedback) by mechanically controlled systems and image-guided devices (Brady & Paul, 1984) resulting in their practical utility.
The telerobotic era started in the early 1990's when NASA's jet propulsion laboratory (JPL) began a project in telerobotics as part of its emergency response robotic program. The primary aim was to develop a robotic system (HAZBOT) to allow safe exploration of potentially dangerous sites (defusion of bombs, nuclear warfare, battle sites) and handling of hazardous materials (wastes from nuclear reactors)(Edmonds &Welch ,1993)(Figure-1). The concept was also looked at by the military strategists who envisioned a situation where

surgeons could operate remotely on casualties without ever having to enter the combat zone (Cubano et al, 1999) .The engineers from NASA and the JPL also intended this concept for telesurgery in space to enable surgeons on earth to operate on astronauts at the space station. The time lag, however, prevented this from becoming feasible. The development of telerobotic technology was subsequently accelerated by various concomitant advancements in computer and surgical related technology. However, for a long time, placing dexterity enhancing robotic systems in the operating room remained an elusive goal. The further evolution of the robotic surgical system culminated in the development of a different skill and advanced instrumentation resulting in feasibility of the concept.

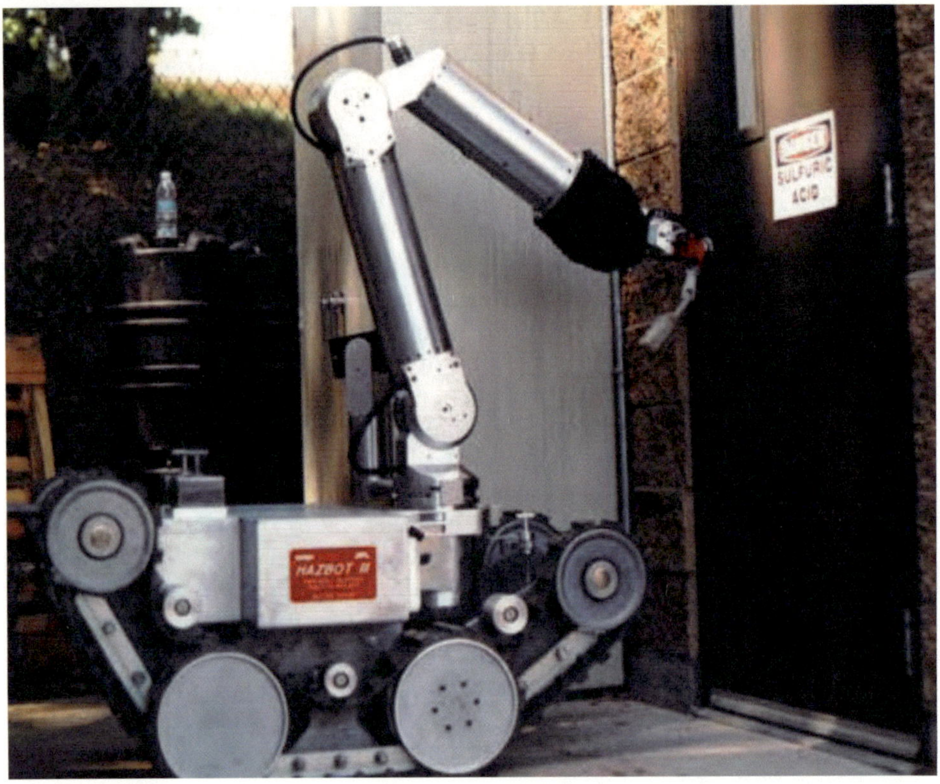

Figure 1. HAZBOT,"Courtesy NASA/JPL-Caltech"

3. Development of robotic surgical technology

In the mid 90's there was a sudden surge in the development of robotic surgical technology. The Computer Motion, a medical robotic company founded in 1989 played a pivotal role in developing early surgical robotic technology (Bushnell P,2001). Their first product was Aesop; a robotic system used for holding an endoscopic camera in minimal invasive laparoscopic surgery and became the first surgical visual aid robotic device certified by the FDA. Aesop 2000 was released in 1996 which used voice control, the Aesop 3000 was released in 1998 which added another degree of freedom in the arm, and the Aesop HR version was networked with other smart devices. The Zeus Robotic Surgical System with three robotic arms attached on the side of the operation table was developed as an extension of Aesop arms to control surgical instruments. The first prototype was demonstrated in 1995, tested in animal in 1996 with first tubal re-anastomosis and first CABG procedure carried out in 1998. After 2000, Micro-wrist and Micro-Joint were also added. Micro joints in Zeus were designed to hold 28 different instruments including scalpels, hooks to tie knots, scissors and dissector. The Zeus system got FDA approval in 2001. One of the major contributions of Computer Motion to the field of digital surgery was Zeus capability to digitally filter out human hand tremor making the robotic procedure more steady and reliable. The system was designed for minimally invasive microsurgery procedures, such as beating heart, endoscopic coronary artery bypass grafting and initiated more complex procedures like a mitral valve surgery (Robotic Surgery, 2005).

In 1992 Integrated Surgical Systems introduced RoboDoc for orthopedic surgery and first robot-assisted human hip replacement was successfully done on a 64-year-old man suffering from osteoarthritis.

In 1995 Intuitive Surgical, another company in the field of robotic surgery was formed based on foundational robotic surgery technology developed at Stanford Research Institute. In a short time the company collaborated with leading institutions and companies like IBM, Massachusetts Institute of Technology (MIT), Heartport Inc., Olympus Optical, Ethicon Endo-Surgery and came up with the da Vinci System. In 1997 da Vinci Surgical system got FDA approval for assisting surgery and in July 2000 the da Vinci Surgical system became the first laparoscopic surgical robotic system that got cleared by the FDA to perform surgery. (Figure-2). Then market forces dictated further innovations. The Computer Motion and Intuitive Surgical companies finally merged into a single company, Intuitive Surgical in 2003.

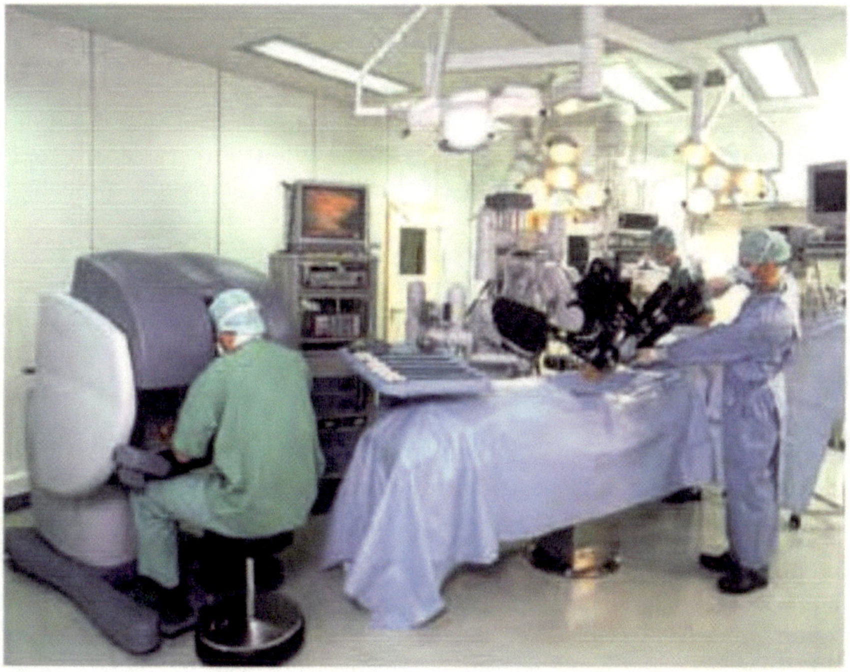

In the da Vinci system, the surgeon sits at a viewfinder (left) and remotely manipulates probes and instruments on actuator arms over the operating table

Figure 2. The da Vinci system, "Courtesy Intuitive Surgical"

With the release of the da Vinci System ,Intuitive's major contributions to the history of robotic surgery is the 'EndoWrist', a miniaturized hand, and the control system, reproducing the range of motion and dexterity of the surgeon's hand, providing high precision, flexibility and the ability to rotate instruments 360 degrees through tiny surgical incisions(Robotic Surgery,2005)(Figure-3). Later seven degrees of freedom were added which offered considerable choice in rotation and pivoting (Camarillo et al, 2004). The da Vinci Surgical System replicates the surgeon's movements in real time. It cannot be programmed, nor can it make decisions on its own to move in any way or perform any type of surgical maneuver.

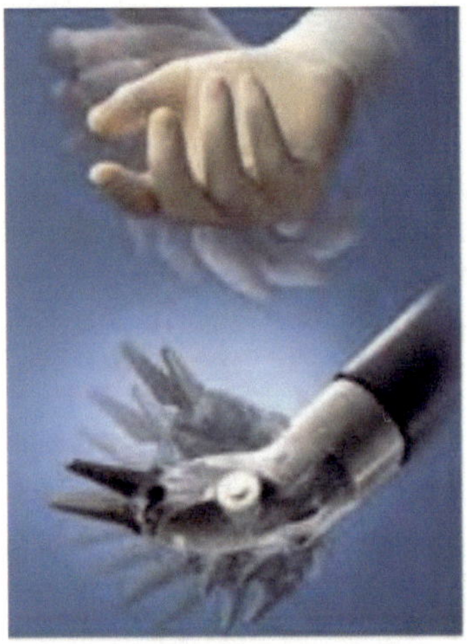

Figure 3. Endowrist,"Courtesy Intuitive Surgical"

The FDA cleared da Vinci Surgical system for use in performing many surgical procedures including general laparoscopic surgery, thoracoscopic (chest) surgery, laparoscopic radical prostatectomies, and thoracoscopically assisted cardiotomy procedures (Robotic Surgery, 2005).

The robotic arm is the end-effector of robotic systems and the continuing development of robotic arms remains the foundation of telerobotics research. This involves the integration and application of haptics, engineering neurobiology, cognitive science and computers (Le Roux et al, 2001). The ongoing research aims to evolve compact but more efficient, more dexterous, more maneuverable surgeon friendly robotic arms with more degrees-of-freedom.

4. Development of the Robotic Assisted Microsurgery (RAMS)

While the early writing on the new technology covered a variety of surgical procedures, special attention was given to cardiovascular procedures. In the mid nineties, Steve Charles, a vitreoretinal surgeon, originated the concept of a telerobotic system as a tool to assist the microsurgical procedures (Turner et al, 1997). Subsequently, in 1994-95 JPL engineers developed RAMS based on surgical requirements provided by Steve Charles using previously developed NASA telerobotics technology (Figure-4). It was a six-degrees-of-freedom surgical robot slave made up of a torso-shoulder-elbow body with a three-axis wrist. The robot manipulator was about 10 inches long and 1 inch in diameter.

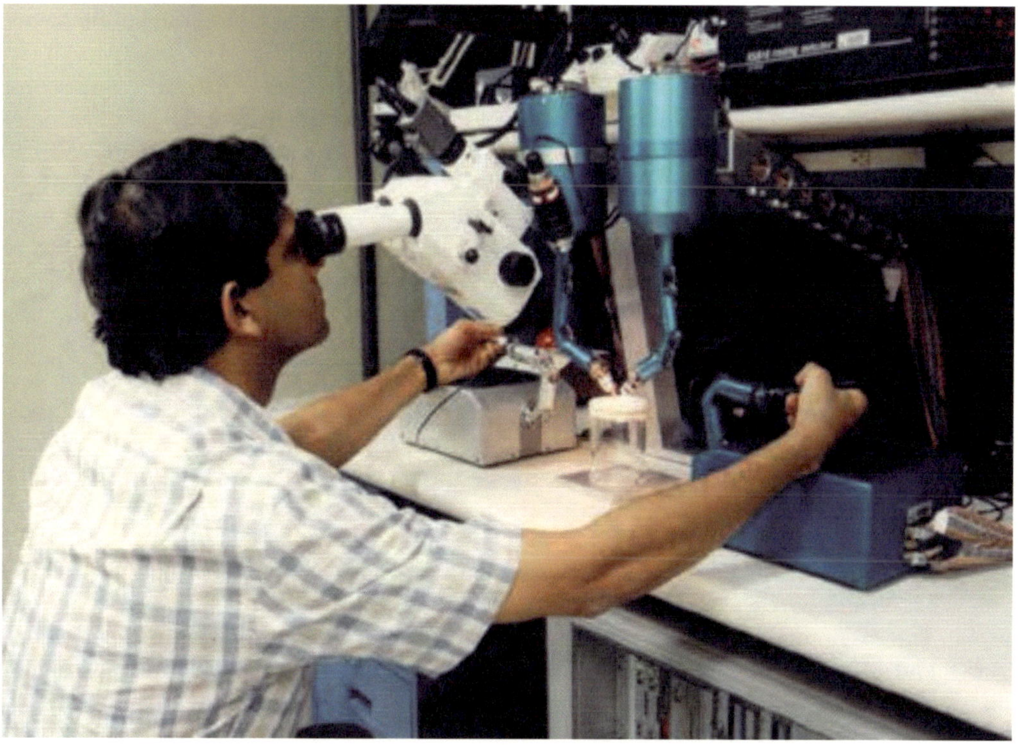

Figure 4. RAMS: Robot Assisted Microsurgery," Courtesy NASA/JPL-Caltech"

In 1998, a study by Stephenson first pointed out to the fact that coronary artery anastomoses are technically feasible with the use of robotic instruments(Stephenson et al,1998).An additional study done by the same group reported the successful use of this approach in a large animal trial(Schaff,2001). Further studies of the feasibility of endoscopic cardiac surgery was performed by various surgical teams verifying that robotic technology could be used to accomplish a completely endoscopic anastomosis (Le Roux et al,2001;Szymula et al,2001;Schiff et al,2005).

Additional studies involving cardiac procedures have also produced positive findings with regard to the clinical efficacy and benefits of robotic assisted anastomosis. In 1999, Schueler performed the world's first closed-chest multivessel cardiac bypass using the daVinci system (Stephenson et al, 1998). In September 24, 1999 Dr. Boyd performed the world's first robotically-assisted closed-chest beating heart cardiac bypass operation using the Zeus system.

Mohr et al first used the da Vinci Robotic system and the AESOP system for ITA harvesting and CABG surgery (Mohr et al,1999). On July 11, 2000, FDA approved the first completely robotic surgery device, the da Vinci surgical system from Intuitive Surgical to perform general surgical procedures while seated at a computer console and 3-D video imaging system across the room from the patient(Stephenson et al,1998). The da Vinci used technology that allowed the surgeon to get closer to the surgical site than human vision, and worked at a smaller scale than conventional surgery permitted. The da Vinci's Surgical System integrated 3D HD laparoscopy and state-of-the-art robotic technology to virtually extend the surgeon's eyes and hands into the surgical field. The da Vinci later incorporated

the latest advancements in robotics and computer technology to enable minimally invasive options for complex surgical procedures.
In 2000, a German study found out that using the daVinci system to perform endoscopic beating heart (single or double) bypass surgery is safe, causes significantly less trauma to the patient and allows for quicker recovery. In another study with a prototype RAMS, 10 carotid arteriotomies were created and closed using either the RAMS system or conventional microsurgical techniques. The precision, technical quality and error rate of telerobotic surgery were similar to those of conventional techniques but it was found to be associated with a twofold increase in the length of the procedure (Le Roux et al, 2001). Later, many studies were performed to evaluate the effectiveness of the Zeus system in performing complex, open, microsurgery tasks in various animal models. A study done in 2000 concluded that concurrent use of the RAMS as a microsurgical assistant is applicable in microsurgery, with the advantages of greater precision and more rapid microsurgical manipulation(Siemionow et al,2000).
An important comparative RAMS study was performed by several international scientific teams to analyze various features related to micro-vascular anastomosis. This comparative study was carried out between RAMS and surgeon performing anastomosis with 3-D endoscope. The mean total operative time per 3 mm robotic anastomosis, utilizing 9-0 suture using 2-D visual port was 29.5±15 minutes (excluding setting up and dismantling robotic arms). The mean total operative time per 3 mm surgeon anastomosis using 3-D endoscope was found to be 16.3±5 minutes. The inference was, though the robot took longer time for anastomosis, they performed high quality, tremor free precise microsurgery without any technological problem and intraoperative complications (Schenker et al, 2001).
In 2004, FDA cleared the marketing of a robotic-like system to assist in coronary artery by-pass surgery enabling the surgeon to perform heart surgery while seated at a console with a computer and video monitor.
A study done in 2005 compared the micro-vascular anastomoses performed with a robot-enhanced technique (31 anastomoses) with a standard hand technique (30 anastomoses) on 1-mm rat femoral arteries with interrupted 10-0 suture(Knight et al ,2005).They compared the anastomotic time, patency, and leak rates between traditional microsurgery techniques (by hand) and a robot-enhanced technique using the Zeus robotic surgery system. A remarkable degree of tremor filtration was observed in the robot-enhanced cases. All anastomoses from both groups were found patent, however, the anastomoses done by hand (mean time, 17.2 minutes) were significantly faster than those done with Zeus (mean time, 27.6 minutes). They concluded that the Zeus system is effective at performing complex, open, microsurgery tasks in vivo.
Another Japanese study in 2005 successfully demonstrated the closure of a partial arteriotomy and complete end-to-end anastomosis of the carotid artery in the deep operative field performed on 20 rats (Morita et al , 2005). A study was undertaken in 2005 to see the feasibility of doing free flap in a porcine model by surgical robot .The free flap was successfully performed. The advantages conferred by the da Vinci robot were found to be elimination of tremor, scalable movements, fully articulating instruments with six degrees of spatial freedom and a dynamic three-dimensional visualization system. The drawbacks included the cost and the absence of true microsurgical instruments (Katz et al, 2005).
A study conducted on canine tarsal and superficial femoral vessels at The Johns Hopkins University School of Medicine, Baltimore in 2006 demonstrated the success of da Vinci robot

to perform micro-vascular anastomoses (Katz et al 2006). A study conducted on pig models in 2006 also demonstrated the technical feasibility of performing a safe and efficient robotic-assisted microsurgical anastomosis but took longer anastomotic times with robotic assistance [Robot: 14.0 versus Freehand 14.8 minutes](Karamanoukian et al,2006).

Technical details of Surgical Robot The typical surgical robot architecture follows a classical mater/slave tele-operation set up. This set up consists of two modules: the surgeon console (master) and the robot (slave). The surgeon's console is both viewing and active computer controlled console having set of ergonomically designed handles along with integrated 3-D vision system and in some cases voice command components. High resolution optical encoder is selected for transmitting the command from master arm to slave arm. The surgeon, sitting at the control console analyze the 3-D images sent by the camera inside operating room. The robotic system interacting with the patient includes usually three robotic arms; two to manipulate the surgical instruments and a third to position the endoscopic camera at the optimal position. The surgeon controls the position of the robotic arms and in turn surgical instruments via joystick-like controls at the console and third endoscopic camera arm by voice command, providing the surgeon precise and stable view of the actual surgical field. Each time a joystick moves, computer transmits an electronic signal to the respective surgical instrument, which moves in complete synchronization with the movements of the surgeon's hands.

5. Configuration of RAMS system

Surgeon

- Surgeon's console (Master)
- Robotic arms (Slave)-2 arms
- Microsurgical instruments

Endoscopic camera

- Visualization of operating field

Robotic arm (voice activated)-3rd arm

- Endoscopic camera

Assistant/nurse

- For setting robotic arms
- For changing instruments

6. Robotic Assisted Surgery

The development of telerobotic system to assist surgeons is a growing field of research. The quickly expanding field of telerobotics with faster processors and new algorithms has lead to a significant paradigm shift from performing open surgeries to minimally invasive procedures. The robotic technology has started moving from the developmental phase to the application phase. Robots are becoming revolutionary tools for surgeons in a variety of clinical applications. Robots are increasingly being used in laparoscopic surgery(Marescaux et al, 2001), urological surgery (Hoznek et al, 2002; Menon, 2003, Menon et al, 2004) neurosurgery (Le Roux et al 2001; Zimmermann et al, 2002) and cardiac surgery with varying success (Schenker et al, 1994; Stephenson et al 1998; Tang et al 2001). They have also been successful employed in orthopedic surgery to perform total hip arthroplasty surgery (Taylor et al, 1994)). Robotic surgery offers many benefits over conventional surgery which includes reduced trauma, less blood loss, less post-operative pain, shorter hospital stay, faster recovery and early return to work.

The other exciting aspect of robotic technology is teleconsultation and tele proctoring. With the help of internet the robotic system can be linked to another surgeon with more expertise in another institute/country when one surgeon encounters difficulty or a more experienced surgeon can act as a preceptor for less experienced surgeon. The Telerobotic surgery will also be particularly suited to countries with a high technological and medical expertise possessing a number of remote communities who could be potential beneficiary of this technique (Dasgupta & Challacombe, 2005).

In robotic surgery, the robots are not independently automated opearators. They are highly advanced teleoperated systems which are under direct control of the surgeon (Cavusoglu et al, 2003). They work basically as manipulators, working on a master-slave principle and have nothing in common with the science fiction robots. Robots can be defined as "automatically controlled multitask manipulators, which are freely programmable in three or more spaces." The success of robots in surgery is based on their precision, lack of fatigue, and speed of action (Moran, 2003).

7. Robotic Assisted Microsurgery-Advantages

The term robotic surgery probably gives an impression of a Robot independently operating on a patient in operation theatre. This image is not correct as they do not replace the surgeon at all in the operation theatre. They only maneuver the surgical instruments necessary for surgery and are always under the direct, total control of the surgeon. The RAMS workstation is a precise tool and can assist the surgeon as a "second" or "third hand". It cannot entirely replace the microsurgical instruments held by the surgeon (Krapohl et al, 1999). As JPL's Tom Hamilton rightly commented "RAMS takes the most skilled surgeon and makes his or her skills better. RAMS can improve surgical techniques to allow faster and safer procedures" (Hamilton, 1997). This option of performing high precision surgery has sparked the potentially huge hope for its application in doing micro-vascular surgery in plastic surgery. Microsurgery is a specialized technique which requires many years of training to be proficient. In microsurgery, the instruments virtually become specialized extensions of the surgeon's hands. As the surgeons differ in hand steadiness, dexterity, maneuverability and technical quality, the outcome of microsurgery is limited by the individual surgeon's manual dexterity. Further, surgical performance varies during the procedure or throughout an individual surgeon's life time. The role of robotic automation is to standardize the procedure and the surgical robots can reduce the variations in the patient outcome among surgeons and for an individual surgeon.

During microsurgery the surgeon has to manipulate tissue with the instruments and the result is likely to be the affected by individual surgeon's dexterity. In addition, several factors such as lengthy period, time constraint and tremors during the procedure can adversely affect the surgeon's technical performance. As the current microsurgical practice is now challenging the limits of human dexterity, stamina and patience, the limiting factors basically arise due to undesired involuntary and inadvertent movement of the hand which creates an error component in hand motion (Riviere & Khosala, 1997). The most familiar source of undesired hand motion is physiological tremor which is an approximately rhythmic, roughly sinusoidal involuntary component inherent in all human motion (Elble, 1996). Low frequency errors or drift are also present in hand motions and are often longer than tremors (Riviere et al, 1997). Irregular high-frequency motions or jerk can also occur (Schenker et al, 1995). The results are that some movements are less precise than is desired and some desired movements cannot be done at all. Microsurgical practice would therefore benefit greatly from RAMS that enhance accuracy by compensating position error. RAMS is based on typical master slave tele-operation. Using RAMS, the surgeon sitting on the console orchestrates or commands the motions of the robotic arms to perform microsurgical procedures. The surgeons hand motions are transferred in a real-time through a computer system, where they are processed to automate the robotic movements. This process reduces the surgeon's movement at the tissue level and prevents tremor or inadvertent movement often associated with fatigue, anxiety, age related or other factors.

The following table (Table-1) compares the strengths and limitations of Humans and Robot (Howe & Matsuoka, 1999):

Humans	**Robots**
Strengths	Strengths
Strong hand-eye coordination	Good geometric accuracy
Dexterous (at human scale)	Stable and untiring
Flexible and adaptable	Can be designed for a wide range of scales
Can integrate extensive and diverse information	May be sterilized
Able to use qualitative information	Resistant to radiation and infection
Good judgment	Can use diverse sensors (chemical, force, acoustic, etc.) in control
Easy to instruct and debrief	
Limitations	Limitations
Limited dexterity outside natural scale	Poor judgment
Prone to tremor and fatigue	Limited dexterity and hand-eye coordination
Limited geometric accuracy	Limited to relatively simple procedures
Limited ability to use quantitative information	Expensive
Large operating room space requirement	Technology in flux
Limited sterility	Difficult to construct and debug
Susceptible to radiation and infection	

[a]Adapted from Taylor & Stulberg (75).

Table 1. The strengths and limitations of Humans and Robot

The advantages of RAMS are thus obvious. As hours of exacting work can tire anybody, superior ergonomics while seated at the console optimizes the surgeon's performance and dexterity. Any tremor in the surgeon's own hands and fingers is completely eliminated with the help of tremor filters and motion scalers leading to superior dexterity (Louw et al, 2004). Another important feature is that there is greatly increased precision due to scalability of movements which can be up to 1:6 scale, meaning that six mm movement of fingers will result in 1 mm movement of the instrument (Rosson, 2005). This increased precision is of great importance during microsurgery, with complete elimination of hand and finger tremors. These qualities allow an average surgeon to perform at par with the best surgeons and allow the skillful surgeons to perform at unprecedented levels of dexterity.

Another feature is that one can always find the perfect angle towards the vessel due to enhanced rotating ability of the camera and wrists of the robotic arm. RAMS also provides more range of motion and more degree of freedom than the human hand leading to easy maneuverability in difficult positions. It can virtually be viewed as a specialized extension of the surgeon's hands. Other added features like optimal magnification with 3-D visualization, superior resolution and 3-D spatial accuracy mark the characteristics of RAMS. This indefatigable nature of RAMS is likely to be of enormous help in performing vascular anastomosis especially in cases of free flaps, digital replantations, microneurorrhaphy and other similar demanding microsurgical procedures (Rosson, 2005).

It also has a potentially invaluable use during microsurgery involving high risk patients /patients with HIV, to protect the surgeon from virus transmission.

8. Robotic Assisted Microsurgery-Limitations

Despite of all mentioned advantages, there are some limitations too. Although reproducible in ex-vivo model, more clinical trials will be required to explore its full potential in clinical micro vascular practice. The initial capital cost ranging from one million to several million dollars is prohibitive for its free use. The average base cost of the da Vinci System is $1.5 million. However, multi-specialty utilization of robotic technology along with improvement in surgical outcome and more expeditious return to work will make this approach cost-effective, justifying investment in this technology. The use of the robots by many specialties will bring down the cost of investment and will make them more cost effective for use in micro vascular surgery. The improved accuracy in microsurgery will ultimately be reflected in improved surgical outcome thus justifying their use (Karamanoukian et al, 2006).

However the system has inherent limitations too. The present systems are cumbersome and there is potential interference between the robotic arms and loss of tactile feedback. The proper functioning of computer software component which is a “command central" for the device's operation is also essential for error proof working of the surgical robot. The other limitation is that there is no haptic feedback which often makes the surgeon feels detached from the patient and the procedure. However, high magnification of operative site negates this draw back(Rosson ,2005).There is also a learning curve but after dedicated training and some experience, one feels comfortable working with the instrumentation and doing the surgery without actually touching the patient. Surgeons may require surgical reeducation and familiarization with a whole new set of complex skills and recent studies are indicating that robotically assisted microanastomosis can be mastered equally well by surgical trainees and fully trained vascular surgeons and prior experience in performing microsurgery is not all that significant factor (Karamanoukian et al 2006). The time taken for the surgery is often more as compared to the conventional surgery. However, operating time is likely to reduce significantly with more familiarity and decreasing learning curve. Another current limitation in micro-vascular field is that the presently available instruments are not yet small and fine enough to perform delicate micro-vascular surgeries like free flaps, micro-neurorrhaphy and digital replantations with finesse. (Rosson, 2005).

Although it is proved beyond doubt the advantages of Robotic micro-vascular surgery, persuading surgeons to use robots for microsurgery from microscope will not be easy. The appearance of Robot in the operation room definitely forces new skills upon the surgeon. Not all micro vascular surgeons perceive that robotic assisted micro vascular surgery is going to bring a significant change in the outcome. Though majority of surgeons agree that robotic micro-vascular surgery is feasible but puts a question mark over its superiority over the conventional methods both from technical aspect and cost-effectiveness.

9. The Future

RAMS in near future is likely to change the outcome in micro-surgical procedures by transcending the human limitations such as tremor filtration, dexterity and precision .With further advancement and refinement in areas of 3-D video imaging and display systems, tele-operative controls, tele-manipulators, graphic planners and micro-instruments, surgeon's capabilities will be tremendously increased with much improved surgical outcome. These advances will certainly make microsurgeries easier to perform and in the longer run will prove to be a dependable associate of plastic surgeons. The future of RAMS seems to be promising and continuing advancement of this technology holds the key.

10. Summary

Surgical robotic technology is now on the cusp of revolutionizing microsurgical capabilities. With the latest advancements in the field of RAMS, the armamentarium available to the plastic surgeons will be greatly expanded. The advantages are self evident. The use of RAMS technology during microsurgery will greatly improve the microsurgical outcome by providing surgeons with greater precision, elimination of hand tremors, increased range of motion and enhanced 3-D visualization. With the continued evolution of robotic surgical technology the robots are expected to become smaller, faster, lighter and dexterous with exponentially increased application in micro-vascular surgery.

The robots despite of technical advancements are never likely to replace the highly evolutionized human hand. The robots r ather than replacing the human hand will help to retain the benefits of the human hand along with its superlative optimization to achieve the goal of optimal precision and predictability. By combining the robotic technology with human skills, the RAMS system will allow the performance of more precise and more dexterous operations to the zenith. The present surgical training programmes must include some robotic training in their curriculum keeping in the mind its exploding potential and future use by the present and next generations of microsurgeons.

11. References

Brady, M & Paul R. (1984). Robotics Research: The First International Symposium, The intelligent connection of perception to action. *Artificial Intelligence*, 1984, MIT press.

Bushnell, P. (2001). Robotic Surgery: A New Role for Machines in Medicine; *Bon Secours Health System, Inc. TEWS- White Paper*; July 2001. Available from: http://www.bshsi.com/tews/docs/ROBOTIC%20SURGERY.pdf

Cubano, M; Poulose, BK; Talamini, MA et al. (1999). Long distance telementoring. A novel tool for laparoscopy aboard the USS Abraham Lincoln. *Surg Endosc* 1999; 13:673-8.

Cavusoglu, MC; Williams, W; Tintack, F; Satyr, SS. (2003). Robotics for telesurgery: Second generation Berkeley/UCSF laparoscopic telesurgical workstation and Looking towards the future applications. *Industrial Robot* 2003; 301: 22-9. Available from: http://www.emeraldinsight.com/Insight/View Content Servlet.

Camarillo, DB; Krummel, TM & Salisbury JK Jr. (2004). Robotic technology in surgery: past, present, and future. *Am J Surg* 2004; 188: Suppl: 2S-15S.

Dasgupta, P; Challacombe, BJ. (2005) . Telerobotic surgery. *Indian J Urol* 2005; 21:89-92

Edmonds, GO & Welch, RV. (1993). "Applying Robotics to HAZMAT". *Proceedings of the 4th National Technology Transfer Conference and Exposition*, In: *NASA Technology 2003* 1993; 2:279-87. Available from: http://trs-new.jpl.nasa.gov/dspace/bitstream/2014/35273/1/93-0854.pdf

Elble, RJ. (1996). Central Mechanisms of Tremor. *J Clin Neurophysiol* 1996; 13:133-44.

Howe, RD; Matsuoka, Y. (1999). "Robotics for Surgery." *Annual Review Biomedical Engineering* 1999, 01:213.

Hoznek, A; Zaki, SK; Samadi, B; Salomon, L; Lobontiu, A; Lang, P; et al. (2002). Robotic Assisted Kidney Transplantation: An Initial Experience. *J Urol* 2002; 167:1604-6.

Innovation-Robotic Microsurgery. (1997). Robotic Microsurgery to Make Difficult Procedures Easier; 1997. Available from: http://ipp.nasa.gov/innovation/Innovation52/robsurg.htm

Krapohl, BD; Siemionow, M & Zins, JE. (1999). [Applicability of the robot arm for microsurgical operations] [Article in German] *Handchir Mikrochir Plast Chir* 1999 Sep; 31(5):333-8.

Knight, CG; Lorincz, A; Cao, A; Gidell, K; Klein, MD; Langenburg, SE. (2005). Computer-assisted, robot-enhanced open microsurgery in an animal model. *J Laparoendosc Adv Surg Tech A* 2005 Apr; 15(2):182-5.

Katz, RD; Rosson, GD; Taylor, JA; Singh, NK. (2005). Robotics in microsurgery: use of a surgical robot to perform a free flap in a porcine model. *Microsurgery* 2005; 25(7):566-9.

Katz, RD; Taylor, JA; Rosson ,GD; Brown, PR; Singh, NK. (2006). Robotics in plastic and reconstructive surgery: use of a telemanipulator slave robot to perform micro vascular anastomoses. *J Reconstr Microsurg* 2006 Jan; 22(1):53-7.

Karamanoukian, RL; Finley, DS; Evans ,GR; Karamanoukian, HL.(2006). Feasibility of robotic-assisted micro vascular anastomoses in plastic surgery.*J Reconstr Microsurg* 2006 Aug; 22(6):429-31.

Karamanoukian, R; Bui, T; McConnell, MP; Evans, GRD; Karamanoukian H. (2006). Transfer of Training in Robotic-Assisted Micro vascular Surgery. *Annals of Plastic Surgery* 2006; 57(6):662-665.

Le, Roux; Peter, D; Das, H; Esquenazi, S; Kelly, J; Patrick, MD. (2001). Robotic assisted microsurgery: A feasibility study in the Rat. *Neurosurgery* 2001; 48:584-9.

Louw, DF; Fielding, T; McBeth, PB; Gregoris, D; Newhook P; Sutherland, GR.(2004). Surgical Robotics: A Review and Neurosurgical Prototype Development. *Neurosurgery* 2004; 54:523-37.

Marescaux J, Smith MK, Folscher D, Jamali F, Malassagne B, Leroy J. (2001) .Telerobotic Laparoscopic Cholecystectomy: Initial Clinical Experience With 25 Patients. *Ann Surg* 2001; 234:1-7.

Mohr FW, Falk V, Diegeler A, Autschbach R. (1999). Computer-enhanced coronary artery bypass surgery. *J Thorac Cardiovasc Surg* 1999; 117:1212-4.

Moran, ME. (2003). Robotic surgery: urologic implications. *J Endourol* 2003 Nov; 17(9):695-708.

Menon, M. (2003). Robotic radical retropubic prostatectomy. *BJU Int* 2003; 91:175-6.

Menon, M; Tewari, A; Peabody, JO, et al. (2004). Vattikuti Institute prostatectomy, a technique of robotic radical prostatectomy for management of localized carcinoma of the prostate: experience of over 1100 cases. *Urol Clin North Am* 2004; 31:701-717.

Morita, A; Sora, S; Mitsuishi, M; Warisawa, S; Suruman, K; Asai, D; Arata, J; Baba, S; Takahashi, H; Mochizuki, R; Kirino, T. (2005). Microsurgical robotic system for the deep surgical field: development of a prototype and feasibility studies in animal and cadaveric models. *J Neurosurg* 2005 Aug; 103(2):320-7.

Riviere, CN & Khosala, PK. (1997). Active hand-held instrument for error compensation in microsurgery. *Proceedings of Intelligent System and Manufacturing: Tech. Conf. on Microrobotics and minisystem fabrication*: Pittsburg; 1997. p. 86-95.

Riviere, CN; Radar, RS & Khosla, PK.(1997). Characteristics of hand motion of eye surgeons. *Proc. 19th Annual Conference of the IEEE Engineering in Medicine and Biology Society*: 1997. p. 1690-3.

Rosson, GD. Robotic-Assisted Microsurgery. (2005). *Reconst Microsurg Spring Summer* 2005; 16:17-8.

Robotic Surgery. (2005). Important Historic Robotic Companies and Systems. Available from:
http://biomed.brown.edu/Courses/BI108/BI108_2005_Groups/04/history.html

Schenker, PS; Das, H & Ohm, T. (1994). Development of a Master-Slave manipulator for Dexterity-Enhanced Microsurgery. *Telemanipulator & Telepresence Technologies*, SPIE Proc. 2351: Boston, MA; 1994.

Schenker, PS; Barlow, EC; Boswell, CD; Das, H; Lee, S; Ohm, TR et al. (1995). Development of a telemanipulator for dexterity enhanced microsurgery. *Proc 2nd Intl Symp Med Robot Comput Assist Surg* 1995. p. 81-8. Available from:
http://www.emeraldinsight.com/Insight/ViewContentServletEmeraldFullTextArticle/Articles/0490240212.html

Stephenson, ER; Sankholkar, S; Ducko, CT; Damiano, RJ. (1998). Robotically assisted microsurgery for endoscopic coronary artery bypass grafting. *Ann Thorac Surg* 1998; 66:1064-7.

Stephenson, ER; Sankholkar, S; Ducko, CT; Damiano, RJ. (1998). Successful endoscopic coronary artery bypass grafting: An acute large animal trial. *J Thorac Cardiovasc Surg* 1998; 116:1071-3.

Siemionow, M; Ozer, K; Siemionow, W; Lister, G. (2000). Robotic assistance in microsurgery. *J Reconstr Microsurg* 2000; 16:643-9.

Szymula, TP & Richter, V. (2001). Recenzie Endoscopy and Microsurgery, D. Pieptu, In the series "Update in Plastic Surgery. Manfred Fray (Ed) 2001, Spinger Wien New York. In *Romanian Journal of Hand and Reconstructive Microsurgery*: 2001. p. 1-2. Available from: http://www.rjhrm.ro/pdf/43.pdf

Schenker, PS; Das, H & Ohm, TR. (2001). A new robot for high dexterity microsurgery", in Ayache, N. (editors), Computer Vision, Virtual Reality and Robotics in Medicine. *Proceedings of 1995 Conference on Computer Vision,* Virtual Reality, Springer-Verlag: Berlin, Germany; 15-22.

Schaff TA. Robotic Surgery: The Future is Now Telerobotic Application. 2001. Available from: http://www.devicelink.com/mx/archive/01/03/0103mx024.html

Schiff, J; Li, PS & Goldstein, M. (2005). Robotic microsurgical vasovasostomy and vasoepididymostomy in Rats. *Int J Med Robot Comput* 1:122-6.

Taylor, RH; Mittelstadt, BD; Paul, HA; Hanson, W; Kazanzides, P. (1994). An image-directed robotics system for precise orthopaedic surgery. *IEEE Trans Robot Auto* 1994; 10:261-75

Turner, J Editor. (1997). Robotic Microsurgery to Make Difficult Procedures Easier. *Aerospace Technology Innovation*; 9th Ed: 1997. Available from: http://nctn.hq.nasa.gov/innovation/Innovation52/robsurg.htm

Tang, LW; D'Ancona, G; Bergsland, J; Kawaguchi, A; Karamanoukian, HL. (2001). Robotically assisted video enhanced endoscopic coronary artery bypass graft surgery. *Angiology* 2001; 52:99-102.

Zimmermann, M; Krishnan, R; Raabe, A; Seifert, V. (2002). Robot-assisted Navigated Neuroendoscopy. *Neurosurgery* 2002; 51:1446-52.

28

Prototypic force feedback instrument for minimally invasive robotic surgery

Ulrich Seibold, Bernhard Kuebler, and Gerd Hirzinger
Institute of Robotics and Mechatronics, DLR (German Aerospace Center)
Germany

1. Introduction

In recent years the success of the daVinci robotic surgery system (Intuitive Surgical Inc., Sunnyvale, CA, USA) has demonstrated the advantages of a telerobotic approach in minimally invasive surgery (MIS). The worldwide need and acceptance of robotic assistance systems for minimally invasive surgery can be seen with more than 600 sold systems worldwide[1]. Still haptic feedback, important to surgeons who generally rely on the sense of touch in assessing tissue properties, is missing. This is due to the lack of suitable instruments capable of measuring the manipulation forces inside the human body on one hand and the lack of haptic displays for conveying this force information in a comprehensible way to the surgeon on the other hand.

In this chapter we present a prototypic force feedback instrument as well as a surgeon workstation as part of a complete setup for minimally invasive robotic surgery (MIRS). The system serves as technology demonstrator showing the feasibility of integrating advanced manipulator technology, haptic feedback and (semi-) autonomous functionality in the context of MIRS. The system will be used to evaluate the impact and benefit of these technologies and hopefully help to improve the acceptance of advanced MIRS. A selection of surgical applications, notably suturing (anastomosis) of coronary vessels while following the motion of the beating heart (motion compensation), provide the requirements in terms of functionality and performance. In a first step, described in this chapter, components are built and the adherence to the required specifications is assured (objective performance measurement). In a future step the impact and benefit on the selected surgical tasks (subjective performance measurement) will be evaluated by defining relevant experiments and performance metrics. Over the course of the project emphasize is given to generic and modular concepts, as acceptance of MIRS technology will be improved by high usability and good integration into the clinical workflow.

After a short introduction into MIS and MIRS (Section 1.1 and 1.2) the DLR scenario is introduced in Section 2 followed by a selection of related research in Section 3. Main focus lies on an instrument and a surgeon workstation providing haptic feedback, which are presented in Section 4, together with initial results. The chapter is concluded with a critical review of the contributions (Section 5) and closes with an outlook about future research (Section 6).

---

[1] As of June 30, 2007. North America: 504, Europe: 108, rest of the world: 44 (Intuitive Surgical, 2007).

1.1 Minimally Invasive Surgery

Minimally invasive surgery is an often described and well established operation technique in the so called 1st world country's health care especially for standard procedures like cholecystectomies (gall bladder removals). We, therefore, content ourselves with a very brief description of this method.

In conventional MIS long, slender instruments providing only one functional degree of freedom (DoF), e. g. a grasper at their distal end, are used through small incisions into the patient's skin to access the intra-corporal operation field. For better access to abdominal organs the abdominal wall can be uplifted by insufflating gas (pneumoperitoneum, see Figure 1). The epidermis forms an effective barrier preventing direct view and manual access. Hence, dexterity is heavily restricted and hand eye coordination is disrupted due to the so called *chopstick-effect* (inversion of movement) and two missing DoF inside the patient caused by the invariant point of incision *(fulcrum point),* see Figures 1 and 2. Getting used to the handcraft of MIS, therefore, is very protracted and the falsified haptic and tactile feedback is considered to be a hinderance.

Advantages	Disadvantages
• reduced traumatisation • reduced loss of blood • reduced risk of wound infection • reduced postoperative pain • shorter hospital stays and rehabilitation time • faster social reintegration • cosmetically favorable results	• lost hand-eye coordination • constricted DoF in instrument handling • 2-D sight, falsification of color representation • significantly longer operating time • heavily diminished haptic/tactile feedback • complex reorientation after instrument changes • expensive and sophisticated equipment necessary • long learning curve, high training needs

Table 1. Summary of the most important reduced wound healing disorders advantages and disadvantages of MIS; note that almost all advantages affect the patient while almost all disadvantages affect the surgeon

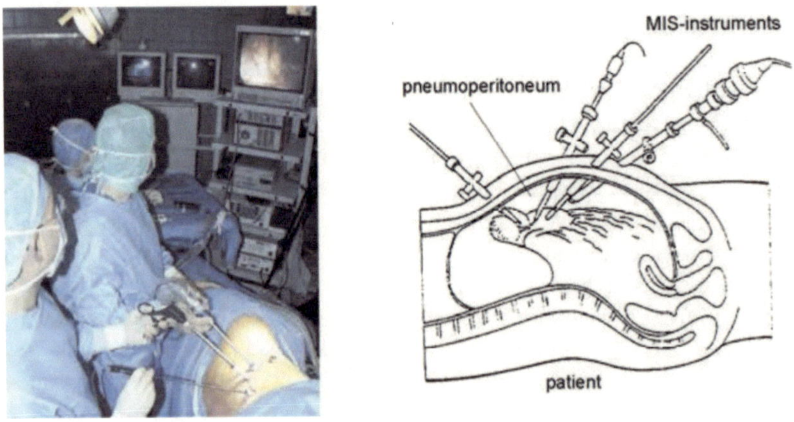

Figure 1. *Left:* Typical view in an operating room for MIS. In front: surgeons and patient; in the back: technical equipment with monitor. *Right:* Schematic diagram of instrument insertion in MIS (cholecystectomy)

Nevertheless, MIS provides fundamental advantages like drastically reduced surgical traumatisation with consecutively shortened time of convalescence and faster social reintegration. The objective is to treat patients with maximum care and, thereby, save costs due to shorter hospital stays and rehabilitation time.
It is evident that almost all advantages are in the interest of the patient while surgeons are burdened with most disadvantages of MIS. A summary of the most important advantages and disadvantages of MIS can be seen in Table 1.

1.2 Minimally Invasive Robotic Surgery

As stated above, the handcraft of conventional MIS is very protracted as instrument handling is counterintuitive to open surgery and additional DoF inside the patient are missing. Providing the surgeon with additional manual control elements to operate additional distal DoF was attempted (Tuebingen Scientific Medical, 2007; Frede et al., 2007; Inaki et al., 2007, also see Figure 5), but handling is even less intuitive than in conventional MIS.
Minimally invasive robotic surgery can overcome these drawbacks by using a teleoperated approach: the surgeon comfortably sits at a console controlling the surgical instruments guided by a patient sided surgical robot. Computational support allows for reestablishing hand-eye coordination, motion scaling, indexing (repositioning of the input devices to a comfortable working position while the instruments remain still) and even motion compensation (e. g. breathing motions).

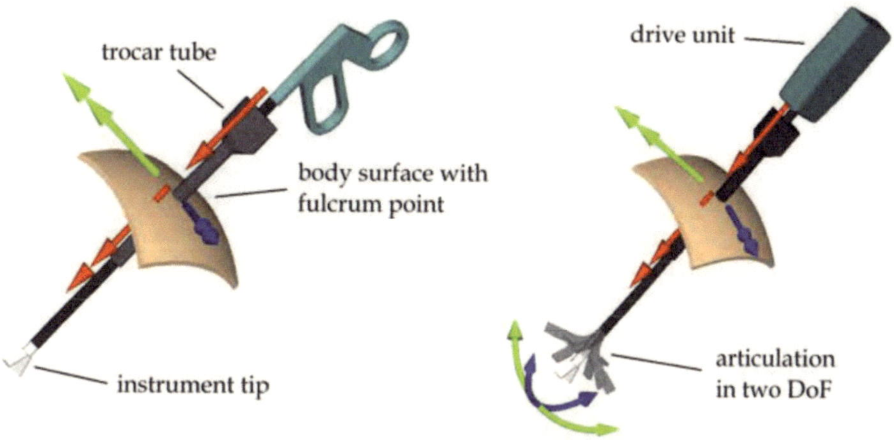

Figure 2. Schematic diagram of DoF in MIS. Rotational DoF indicated with a double arrowhead, translational DoF with a single one. *Left:* Diagram of the four available DoF in conventional minimally invasive surgery; the instruments are under constraint by the fulcrum point. *Right:* Diagram of two additional DoF at the distal end of the instrument. Intracorporal DoF are actuated from outside the patient

However, the entirely mechanically decoupled arrangement of surgeon and patient entails a total absence of haptic and tactile feedback, even more so than in conventional MIS. Visual judgement remains the only solution to get an impression of the forces applied to the environment. In fact, the deformation of tissue is patient dependent (Wagner et al., 2002) and even in the hands of experienced surgeons this is not sufficiently reliable and unsatisfying. Considering e. g. knot tying, it is impossible in this way to guarantee a reliable tightness of knots (Müller, 2004) because tension of a thread cannot be estimated only by inspecting it visually. Methods of resolution for this problem have been presented by Akinbiyi et al. (Kitagawa et al., 2004; Akinbiyi et al., 2006), but for high immersive surgical purposes this does not seem satisfying. Additionally the presented approaches do not consider gripping forces: Manipulating tissue without gripping force feedback holds the risk of unintentional damage to the tissue.

Advantages	Disadvantages
• reestablishment of hand-eye coordination • intuitive use, short learning curve • comfortable posture of user, indexing • minor fatigue, prolonged concentrated work • 3-D vision • tremor filtering • motion scaling	• high purchase cost • high maintenance cost • limited number of proven operation types • noteworthy setup time • cumbersome instrument change • longer operating time • usage only as a whole • no haptic/ tactile feedback • necessity of specially trained/educated back staff

Table 2. Summary of the most important advantages and disadvantages of MIRS

Looking at the presently only commercially available MIRS system (daVinci by Intuitive Surgical, Inc., Sunnyvale, CA, USA) a number of further drawbacks aside from the disadvantages related to the absence of haptic/tactile feedback have to be mentioned.

The still limited number of applications makes it difficult for small and mid-size clinics to have a fast and easy amortization of the considerable purchase and maintenance cost. Setup time of the system and intraoperative instrument changes are still cumbersome which extends the over all operation time even beyond conventional MIS. Obstructive for more universal usage is the fact, that the system can only be used as a whole; e. g. it is not possible to perform a conventional MIS procedure only with the aid of a daVinci camera guidance. The direct access for a surgeon to the patient with the daVinci-slave in position is largely obstructed. Table 2 shows the major advantages and disadvantages of minimally invasive robotic surgery as performed today.

2. The DLR Minimally Invasive Robotic Surgery Scenario

The DLR (German Aerospace Center) is currently developing an integrated environment for MIS. The system shown in Figure 3 is divided into a surgeon workstation and a patient-side manipulator setup.

The slave system consists of usually three surgical robots (Figure 3 bottom middle).

Two robots are carrying actuated and sensor integrated surgical instruments (Figure 3 bottom right) which provide additional DoF. The third is used as an automated robotic camera guidance system (Wei et al., 1997; Omote et al., 1999). The robotic arms are lightweight and dimensions are optimized for surgical applications, performing with the highest possible manipulability, dexterity, and accuracy in the important minimally invasive application areas of abdominal and cardiac surgery (Konietschke et al., 2003). Due to the chosen dimensions, this generic manipulator arm is also applicable for urological, gynaecological, orthopaedic, and otorhinolaryngological applications. The 7 DoF (kinematic redundancy) design allows for a more flexible operating room setup and facilitates collision avoidance with other manipulators or operating room equipment, as the elbow joint can be reoriented without altering the position and orientation of the robot's end effector.

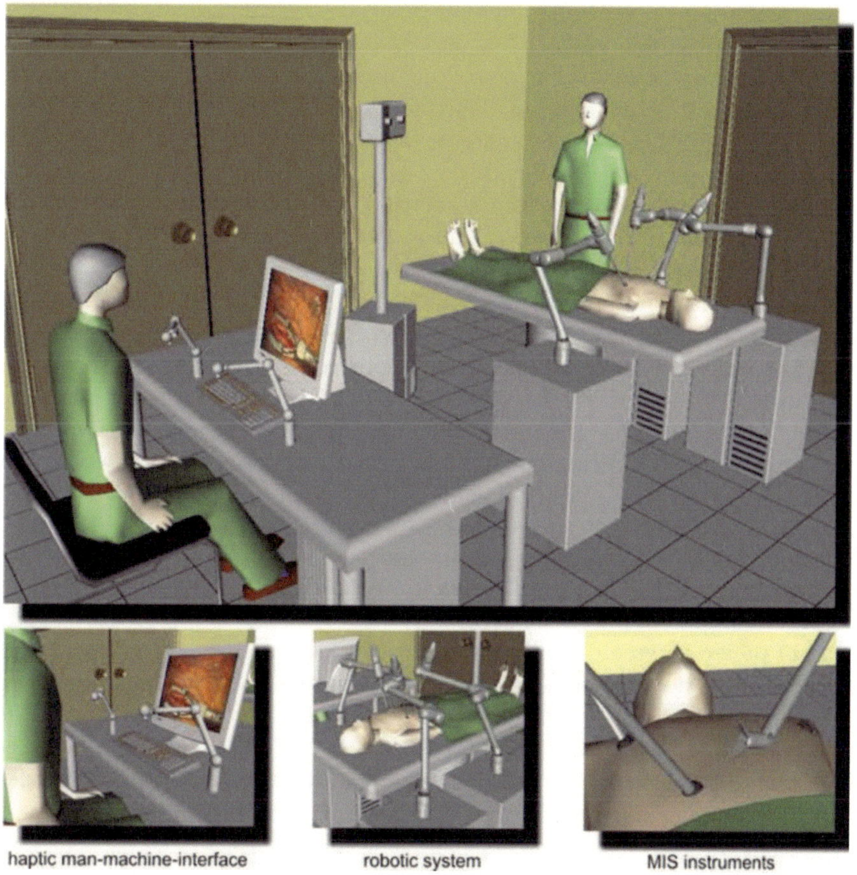

Figure 3. Main components of DLR MIRS system

The master console enables the surgeon to command the instruments and also provides a stereo image of the operation site. Haptic hand controllers not only register the surgeon's hand movements, but also display the intracorporal manipulation forces and torques, including gripping force (Figure 3 bottom left).

The DLR MIRS system will enable surgeons to perform new operation techniques requiring a high degree of manipulability like enteroanastomoses (Müller, 2004) or minimally invasive coronary artery bypass operations on the beating heart (Falk et al., 1999). It will also allow the realization of semi-autonomous functionality such as motion compensation of the beating heart (Ortmaier et al., 2003; Ortmaier, 2003; Nakamura, 2003). Furthermore, the system will include a self-guided robotic camera control system: when advised by the surgeon, the endoscope carrying surgical robot can follow the surgical instruments autonomously. All instruments are equipped with a color marker at the tip. Provided, the same color is not normally present at the operation site, the marker can be segmented from the video image with a high degree of robustness (Wei et al., 1997; Omote et al., 1999). Following the segmented positions a trajectory can be calculated which generates the target trajectory for the camera guidance robot. This application has been successfully clinically tested during laparoscopic cholecystectomies.

The MIRS system in development is completed by a preoperative planning and registration tool which allows optimal positioning of ports and robots for the intended operation. The access planning is performed prior to the procedure using the patient specific anatomical data obtained by a medical 3-D imaging modality preoperatively. In the OR, the position of the patient is registered with a 3-D laser scanner, so that the access data can be aligned to the actual patient location very precisely (Konietschke et al., 2004). Intraoperative repositioning of the robots as well as the necessity for placing additional ports intraoperatively can thus be avoided.

The need to perform routine long distance tele-operations is questionable, however, invoking external assistance or a remote expert opinion (teleconsultation) might be realized in the near future. The remote expert will be equipped with a console connected by broadband communication lines to the hospital where the operation takes place. This setup is also especially suited for new surgical training procedures where the remote expert trains the novice surgeon.

This chapter focuses on the development of actuated and sensor integrated forceps as well as on the surgeon input console and on sensory substitution approaches for providing haptic feedback. Details on the development of the surgical robot can be found in (Ortmaier et al., 2006; DLR - German Aerospace Center, Institute of Robotics and Mechatronics, 2007).

3. State of the Art

A selection of previous research will be introduced in this section. Improved dexterity and force feedback have shown beneficial effects (see Section 3.1, Section 3.2), however, studies on the effects of force feedback on task performance in laboratory settings are currently limited. Information on the effectiveness for the whole task of surgery does not exist at this point. Exploring the effects of improved dexterity and force feedback simultaneously while using telemanipulators was previously not possible since no setup was available combining intracorporeal degrees of freedom and force sensing capability.

Sensory substitution (auditory and visual instead of haptic feedback) has been shown to be a viable option of providing additional information on the tissue manipulation forces (see Section 3.5). However, the performance of sensory substitution has not yet been directly compared to haptic feedback. If proven effective, sensory substitution could not only be beneficial to the surgical task, but also lead to the development of cheaper surgeon input consoles. This potential is described in Section 4.4 in more detail.

3.1 The Impact of Dexterity on Surgical Performance

A comparison of laparoscopic skills performance between standard laparoscopic instruments and two surgical robotic systems was performed by Dakin et al. (Dakin & Gagner, 2003). In this study all 18 test subjects were skilled laparoscopic surgeons, although only two had prior exposure to telemanipulator systems. They were evaluated on the following tasks using conventional instruments, the daVinci, and Zeus (Computer Motion Inc., USA) robotic surgery system:

- 'Rope passing': A rope is incrementally passed in both directions using hand-to-hand technique.
- 'Bead drop': In this task beads with a diameter of 6 mm have to be placed on pegs.
- 'Peanut Task': Cotton balls have to be dropped in cylindrical beakers.
- 'Suturing' was evaluated on a piece of cloth supported by a foam block. Target sizes for the stitches are 1.0, 0.75, and 0.5 mm with distances of 5, 3, and 1 mm. Both knot tying and running stitches were evaluated.

The surgeon's work was evaluated for completion time as well as number of errors. None of the telemanipulator systems was faster than conventional technique, however, they seemed to allow slightly higher precision. The average number of errors, e. g. for running sutures using a particular suture material, was highest for manual technique, lowest for daVinci. In all the basic tasks, daVinci outperformed Zeus with regard to speed and showed some increased (although inconsistent) accuracy. It is likely that both the articulated EndoWrist® instruments and the presence of three-dimensional vision in the daVinci system contribute to its superior performance. Only the suturing task is representative for a real surgical task. The other tests, while investigating important task primitives (instrument positioning and grasping) are not sufficient to allow for the prediction of performance during a complex surgical task.

As in conventional laparoscopy, training has an important effect on the performance of the surgeons. The learning curve of six experts (more than 100 laparoscopic cholecystectomies, clinical experience in intracorporal knot tying) and seven novices (less than 50 cholecystectomies, no advanced laparoscopic experience) was evaluated by Hernandez (Hernandez et al., 2004). Using a daVinci surgical system and a small bowel anastomosis model, the study simulated a complex procedure that requires advanced planning and the use of a significant range of skills and entails a longer learning process. The use of a synthetic model makes the experiment reproducible, standardized and allows more objective comparisons. Shape, lumen, and strength of the anastomosis were evaluated as well as time, instrument path length, and the number of movements. No comparison to conventional MIS or manual techniques was included in the study.

Surprisingly, for the daVinci system, results after five training sessions did not significantly vary between novices and experts. The fact that eight out of thirteen subjects (two experts and 6 novices) reached a competent status after only five sessions could mean that the learning process in the daVinci system is shorter than it would be in conventional laparoscopic surgery. The likely conclusion is that the level of immersion and intuitive instrument handling provided by the daVinci system offers advantages for novice surgeons.

3.2 The Impact of Haptic Feedback on Surgical Performance

In conventional MIS there is little to no haptic feedback from the operation site. Friction generated within the instrument and between the instrument and the access port greatly exceeds manipulation forces at the operation site. Exerted forces cited in the literature range from 0.3 N for bypass grafting (Salle et al., 2004) to about 4 N normal and 50 N along the instrument shaft in cholecystectomy (Rosen, 2001). This unexpectedly large range is not sufficiently explained and will need to be investigated.

Surgeons are able, through experience, to interpret visual tissue deformation as a measure of external forces and thus compensate for the lack of haptic information. Unfortunately, tissue properties depend on the patient and may also vary with time (Wagner et al., 2002). The visual compensation can only be applied when handling soft elastic materials. It is not feasible with bone structures and suture materials due to their rigidity.

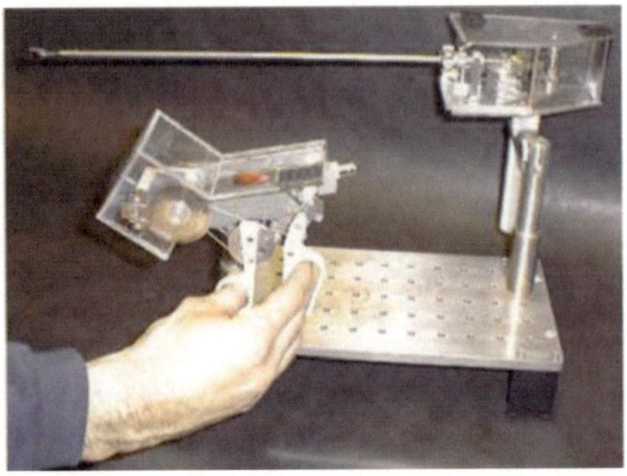

Figure 4. Force controlled gripper designed at the University of Washington (Rosen et al., 1999a)

An experimental sensor integrated gripping instrument was introduced by the BioRobotics Lab, University of Washington, USA (Rosen et al., 1999a). It consists of a conventional laparoscopic instrument which was separated into the gripper/shaft and handle portion (see Figure 4). Both, gripper and handle are actuated by servo drives and controlled in a bilateral force feedback scheme. Using this device several experiments were carried out evaluating the sensitivity and recognition rate while palpating tissue samples.

Test subjects were asked to palpate tissues of varying stiffness by hand, using a conventional laparoscopic grasper and using the sensor integrated instrument. Results were shown as mean square error (MSE) of recognition. As expected, the performance of the human hand defines the upper performance limit and the conventional instrument performed at the lower limit with the sensor integrated instrument performing at a level similar to a gloved hand. Subjective results also showed that the sensor integrated gripper significantly improved the rate of correctly recognized tissue samples. Accurately recognizing the stiffness of tissue will help surgeons to distinguish between different tissue types and assess the health of particular structures.

The role of force feedback in a blunt dissection task was evaluated by R. Wagner (Wagner et al., 2002). During this experiment participants operated on a model of an arterial structure surrounded by tissue. Hand controller and telemanipulator were PHANToM® (SensAble Technologies, Inc., Woburn, MA, USA) haptic hand controllers and forces in the instrument were recorded by a 6 DoF force torque sensor. Tissue was represented by material similar to children's play dough while arteries were represented by weatherstrip and caulking cord. The task was to dissect and expose the structure embedded in the tissue. Individual performance was measured by evaluating the applied force level, number of errors, as well as the rate and precision of the dissection. It was shown that force feedback reduced the magnitude of forces applied on the instrument tip. Higher forces were applied for longer durations when force feedback was not present. The number of errors, defined as punctures and scratches in the artery, was also reduced in the presence of force feedback. The rate of the dissection and the amount of tissue that was disturbed around the dissection area, however, were not significantly influenced by the presence of force feedback. It was hypothesized that at decreasing levels of force feedback the haptic information does not

constitute a physical constraint anymore but acts as supplemental information. A conscious response is required to take advantage of the available forces.
Participants of this study were novices. Experienced laparoscopic surgeons have developed perceptual and motor skills to deal with the constraints of MIS techniques. The influence of laparoscopic training on the benefit of force feedback needs to be investigated and a more realistic tissue model should be used.

3.3 Previous Instrument and Sensor Designs

The foremost example of articulated instruments for MIRS is the EndoWrist® by IntuitiveSurgical® as part of the daVinci robotic surgery system. The instrument design is highly integrated with a diameter of 8 mm, yet extremely rugged and provides two cable driven DoF in addition to the actuation of the functional end (forceps, scissors, and needle holders), thus providing full dexterity inside the body (Guthart & Salisbury, 2000; Intuitive Surgical, 2007). Recently IntuitiveSurgical® developed even smaller instruments with a diameter of 5 mm, featuring a cable driven spine kinematic for the 2 DoF actuation. However, both instruments are not sensor integrated and so do not allow the measurement of interaction forces and torques.
The Radius Surgical System by Tuebingen Scientific (Braun et al., 2004) closely resembles a conventional hand-held MIS instrument (see Figure 5). As major difference, the functional (distal) end consists of a 2 DoF (pitch-roll) joint, providing full manipulability at the gripper. These two additional degrees of freedom cannot be controlled by the scissor-handle used in conventional instruments. Therefore, an ergonomic handle providing additional functionality was incorporated in the design. The instrument closely resembles a conventional MIS instrument, therefore, providing straight forward integration in the clinical setting at comparably small cost. Surgeons experienced in MIS will adapt their skills readily to the Radius Surgical System. However, the disadvantages of the chop-stick effect and uncomfortable operating posture remains. In addition, demands on the surgeons manual dexterity are greatly increased, as 3 DoF have to be controlled in each hand.

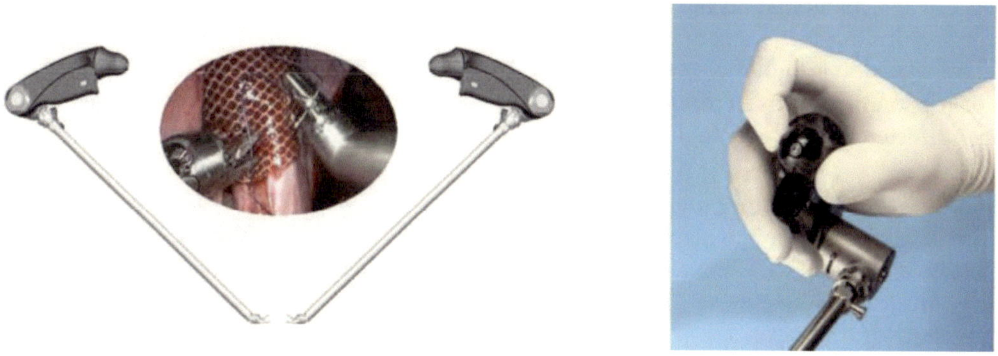

Figure 5. The Radius Surgical System, a novel manually articulated instrument for MIS with ergonomic handle design (Braun et al., 2004)

Full dexterity inside the patient as well as the decoupled determination of grasping force and interaction forces is deemed necessary for an appropriate immersion of the surgeon. Most systems comprising a force sensing modality only focus on one of these three requirements. At the Korean Advanced Institute of Science and Technology (KAIST) a

telepresence system for microsurgical tasks has been developed. As one of few systems it realizes six DoF force/torque reflection at the master console. Unfortunately, the instruments do not provide additional DoF inside the patient's body (Kwon et al., 1998).
Rosen et al. introduced a teleoperated gripper for MIS (see Figure 4), providing measurement and realistic feedback of endoscopic gripping forces (see Section 3.2). However, this system is limited to the measurement of gripping forces, and so interaction forces cannot be captured (Rosen et al., 1999b; MacFarlane et al., 1999).
Zemiti et al. introduced a force controlled laparoscopic surgical robot without distal force sensing. A standard force sensor was integrated into the trocar outside the patient. The measurement did not deteriorate by friction due to the double-walled design of the trocar (Zemiti et al., 2004). The placement of the sensor requires a very accurate gravity compensation of the results for every position of the Instrument. Additionally, the large distance between instrument tip and sensor entails a deterioration of the force/moment discernibility.
The sensor of the laparoscopic grasper developed by Tholey et al. is integrated in the gripper branches. Forces normal to the gripper branches as well as lateral and longitudinal forces inside the gripper can be registered. Unfortunately, the principle of measurement is not explained in detail but the assembly seems to be prototypic. The instrument has not yet been integrated into a robotic surgery system (Tholey et al., 2004).
Jan Peirs et al. have designed a 3-axis micro optical force sensor. Employing an optical measurement principle, the sensor is inert to electro-magnetic interference. The necessary force range was determined using strain gauges applied onto a needle driver. Future experiments with a laparoscopic system are planned (Peirs et al., 2004).
Several groups (Kitagawa, 2003; Mayer et al., 2004) have equipped daVinci instruments with strain gauges attached to the shaft, close to the joint. This placement does not require the electrical connection to be routed through the joint, which will prolong the life expectancy of the sensor. However, three sets of drive cables for the joint and the gripper are running through the sensor. Therefore, the sensor is subjected to the driving forces which greatly exceed the manipulation loads. The measurement range of the sensor must accommodate for the driving forces, thereby, greatly reducing the sensitivity to the manipulation loads. Compensation is highly difficult since all six cable forces at the sensor location, compensated for friction in the drive mechanism, are required. Additionally, manipulation forces have to be corrected for the joint angle.

3.4 Surgeon Work Station

The daVinci robotic surgery system by Intuitive Surgical® (Guthart & Salisbury, 2000; Intuitive Surgical, 2007) includes a surgeon console. The surgeon sits in a comfortable forward leaning posture at the main console, supported by arm and head rest. By placing the head on the visor, a 3-D image of the surgical field can be seen through a binocular viewer. The hands of the surgeon grasp the master controls, which are situated underneath the visor of the workstation. The placement of the vision system and the master controls convey the impression that the surgeon is looking down at the natural position of the hands and the user has an immersive view of the surgical field. In addition, a light barrier is integrated in the headrest which serves as safety feature. The input controls allow manipulation within a cube with 30 cm side length, however, do not provide realistic haptic feedback from the operation site.

Stand alone haptic feedback devices are available from various companies, including the PHANToM® as well as the delta.x and omega.x series (Force Dimension, Inc., Lausanne, Switzerland). None of the above are currently available with 7 active force feedback DoF. Force Dimension has recently added an active grasping DoF and 3 passive (wrist) rotations to the original omega.3, creating the omega.7. An extension to the PHANToM® including a collocated, semitransparent display is available by Reachin Technologies (Inc., Stockholm, Sweden). However, the restricted workspaces of all devices require some indexing or clutch function in order to provide the full range of motion required for various surgical procedures (e. g. exploration of the abdominal cavity or harvesting of the Arteria mammaria). Therefore, a collocated semitransparent display is not usable as the collocation of video image and hand position cannot be guaranteed.

3.5 Haptic Feedback and Sensory Substitution

A comparison of the effectiveness of visual and haptic feedback in a laparoscopic grasping procedure was done by Tholey (Tholey et al., 2003). For visual feedback, the participant is shown an isometric view of the grasper and tissue sample (n.b. This description of visual feedback refers only to providing a video feed of the test sample and is not identical to visual augmentation described by Kitagawa below). No grasping force is measured in this setting. This experiment is equivalent to a surgeon observing the visible deformation of manipulated tissue, estimating the strain through experience and assumptions of the tissue properties. Next, for the haptic feedback, the motor torque required to grasp the tissue was recorded and interpreted as a measure for tissue stiffness. In Tholey's experiment, the participants only saw the deformation on the screen or felt the opposing force provided by a PHANToM®, while the gripper was closed autonomously to identical angles for every experiment. Several trials were conducted to test the effect of using only the video feed, only force, as well simultaneous video feed as force feedback on rating the stiffness of three samples. The rate of correctly characterizing tissue stiffness was highest for direct exploration by hand, followed by simultaneous video feed and force feedback. The video feed alone produced the lowest rate of success.

The effect of sensory substitution on suture manipulation forces for surgical teleoperation was investigated by Kitagawa (Kitagawa, 2003). Suture forces during knot tying were compared for direct manipulation, conventional MIS technique, and using a telemanipulator setup. The coefficient of variance (CV) between optimal and actually applied suture forces was measured. The results indicate that the manual instrument ties provide a CV that is more similar to the hand ties than do the robot ties. The hand tie had the lowest CV of all methods, meaning suture forces were consistently applied close to their optimum level. Use of a telemanipulator setup mitigated the difference in skill levels between novice and expert participants. The knot tying procedure using the telemanipulator setup was repeated, providing either only the video image (no feedback) or a visual representation of forces (bargraph or gauge: augmented visual feedback) or an audible tone when the force reached the optimal value (auditory feedback). The provision of any kind of feedback showed significantly improved results. Direct haptic feedback was not provided in this experiment, therefore, a comparison between haptic feedback and sensory substitution feedback was not performed.

Aside from a technical report by Computer Motion, Inc., that only mentioned the possibility of using visual feedback for manipulation forces, no other relevant studies on sensory substitution in MIS were found.

4. Description of the Setup

As shown in Figure 3 and described in Section 2 the surgical instrument shown in Figure 6 is carried by the DLR KineMedic® (Ortmaier et al., 2006; DLR - German Aerospace Center, Institute of Robotics and Mechatronics, 2007) surgical manipulator arm for MIRS applications. The robot is mechanically, electrically, and electronically interconnected to the propulsion unit of the instrument (proximal part, see Section 4.1). At the distal end of the instrument two actuated DoF, a force/torque sensor, and the functional end (e. g. gripper) are located (see Section 4.2 and 4.3). The instrument shaft passes through the hollow axis of the last rotational joint of the KineMedic®, so that the instrument can be rotated around its longitudinal axis. With the two additional DoF at the distal end of the instrument full dexterity inside the patient is possible as well as a basic ability to reach behind intracorporal structures. Due to the kinematically redundant design of the KineMedic®, its posture can be altered intraoperatively without changing position and orientation of the instrument. Thereby, collisions of robot arms with each other, the patient or other OR equipment can be avoided.

4.1 Instrument: Propulsion unit

The instrument is located at the TCP of the KineMedic®, therefore, light and compact design especially of the propulsion unit is important not to influence dynamics and performance of the KineMedic® in a negative way. Thus, it is possible to move robot and instrument with the relatively high acceleration necessary to follow the movements of the beating heart.

The propulsion unit provides actuation for the distal joints and gripper, signal conditioning for the force/torque sensor, and contains additional sensors to determine the absolute position of the drive cables. Since the conventional way of sterilization in a hospital is autoclavation and the distal end is in direct patient contact, the instrument has to withstand the according conditions[2]. Therefore, all thermo instable components are placed in the proximal propulsion unit. The distal end (with patient contact) can be detached and autoclaved. The decoupling mechanism allows for relatively simple handling, connectable by technically untrained staff under operation room conditions. The mechanism separates the drive train at the output of the propulsion unit, hence, it is mandatory for satisfactory position control that it is entirely free of backlash and play even after several coupling/decoupling cycles.

4.2 Instrument: Distal Force Torque Sensor

To obtain realistic force information a sensor is preferably placed close to the instrument tip, minimizing the errors due to friction between the instrument and the trocar. The sensor should be decoupled from the drive mechanism to prevent the influence of driving forces, backlash, and friction on the sensor's performance (Seibold & Hirzinger, 2003). A placement between the gripper and joint was selected, as the sensor is only subjected to the gripper actuation force at this location. It is not influenced by the joint actuation forces as in placements proximal to the joint. The gripper actuation force is measured for the calculation of the gripping force, so the force/torque sensor (FTS) output can be compensated for simultaneously. However, the electrical connections to the sensor have to be routed through the joint, requiring highly flexible, isolated, multi-strand wires. This location requires the

[2] Hypertensive water steam at up to 156° C and up to 2 bar positive pressure for at least 25 min.

sensor to be of roughly cylindrical shape with a preferably central hollow section to accommodate for the gripper drive cable and mechanics.
A Stewart Platform based FTS was chosen for its high stiffness, adaptable properties, annular shape, and scalability. Furthermore, only longitudinal force transducers are required, which facilitates the future application of force transducers other than resistive strain gauges. Analysis and properties of Stewart Platform transducers were presented previously by Sorli et al. (Sorli & Pastorelli, 1995) who outlined a set of variables (R, L, a, β, γ, shown in Figure 7 left) sufficiently describing the geometry and, thus, the properties of the sensor. The characteristic matrix $\mathbf{A} \in \mathbb{R}^{(6\times 6)}$ describing the transformation of link forces to externally applied loads

$$[F_x, F_y, F_z, M_x, M_y, M_z]^T = \mathbf{A} \cdot [F_1, F_2, F_3, F_4, F_5, F_6]^T \tag{1}$$

is calculated using the method described by Sorli:

$$\begin{bmatrix} F_x \\ F_y \\ F_z \\ M_x \\ M_y \\ M_z \end{bmatrix} = \begin{bmatrix} -2n & 2n & \sqrt{3}m+n & \sqrt{3}m-n & -\sqrt{3}m+n & -\sqrt{3}m-n \\ -2m & -2m & m-\sqrt{3}n & m+\sqrt{3}n & m+\sqrt{3}n & m-\sqrt{3}n \\ -2q & -2q & -2q & -2q & -2q & -2q \\ 2aq & 2aq & -aq & -aq & -aq & -aq \\ 0 & 0 & aq\sqrt{3} & aq\sqrt{3} & -aq\sqrt{3} & -aq\sqrt{3} \\ -2an & 2an & -2an & 2an & -2an & 2an \end{bmatrix} \cdot \begin{bmatrix} F_1 \\ F_2 \\ F_3 \\ F_4 \\ F_5 \\ F_6 \end{bmatrix} \tag{2}$$

with

$$m = \cos(\alpha)\cos(\beta)$$
$$n = \cos(\alpha)\sin(\beta)$$
$$q = \sin(\alpha)$$

To find a sensor geometry that is well conditioned and optimized for the force range expected in a surgical application, the following search method is used. The radius of the base R and the link length L (see Figure 7 left) are determined by the space available in the instrument. For all geometrically valid combinations (non-intersecting links), the parameters R, L, a, β, γ, are used to calculate **A**. Various sets of maximally expected external loads $[F_x, F_y, F_z, M_x, M_y, M_z]^T$ are selected. These sets must contain at least one load in each of the 6 principal directions.
Every member of the external load set is pre-multiplied by $\mathbf{A}^{-1}$, yielding the corresponding set of internal leg forces $\mathbf{J} = [F_1, F_2, F_3, F_4, F_5, F_6]^T$. The conditioning number of the internal leg force set (denoted in Figure 8) is a measure of the isotropy of the sensor structure with respect to the external load set. This, however, is not an isotropy in the classical definition as the external loads in the principal directions need not be equal.
For the load set $F_{x,y,z}$ = 10 N, $M_{x,y}$ = 150 Nmm, M_z = 100 Nmm the following parameters were selected as optimal sensor geometry: R = 4.2 mm, L = 3.9 mm, a = 65°, β = 90°, γ = 36°, yielding a conditioning number of 6.3 and a joint separation of i = 1.1 mm.
For a sensor of less than 10 mm diameter, ball or universal joints normally used in Stewart Platforms are not suitable due to their high complexity of manufacturing and assembly. These are replaced by flexural joints creating a monolithic sensor structure as shown in Figure 7 right (Seibold, 2002). Given appropriate design of flexural hinges and leg cross-

section, the results of an FEM analysis are in very good agreement with the prediction by the ideal analytical model (Seibold & Hirzinger, 2003; Lobontiu, 2002).

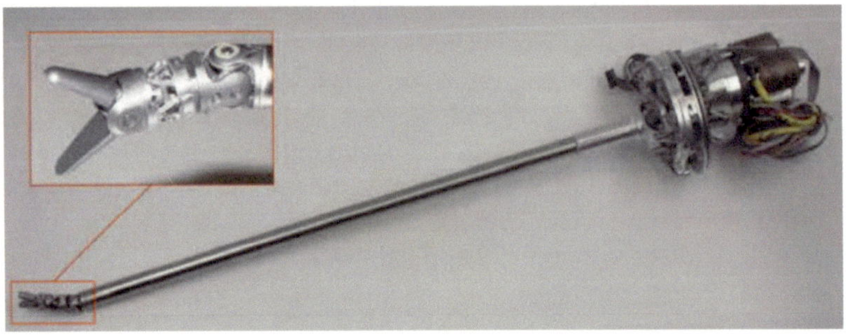

Figure 6. General view of the DLR MIRS instrument and detailed view of its distal end

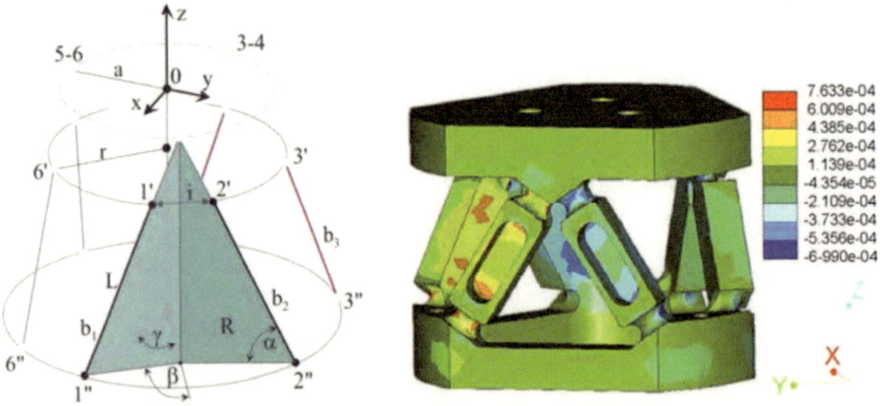

Figure 7. *Left:* Geometrical parameters of Stewart Platform: Base radius R and platform radius r. *Right:* Average strain on force/torque sensor for load $F_y = 30$ N

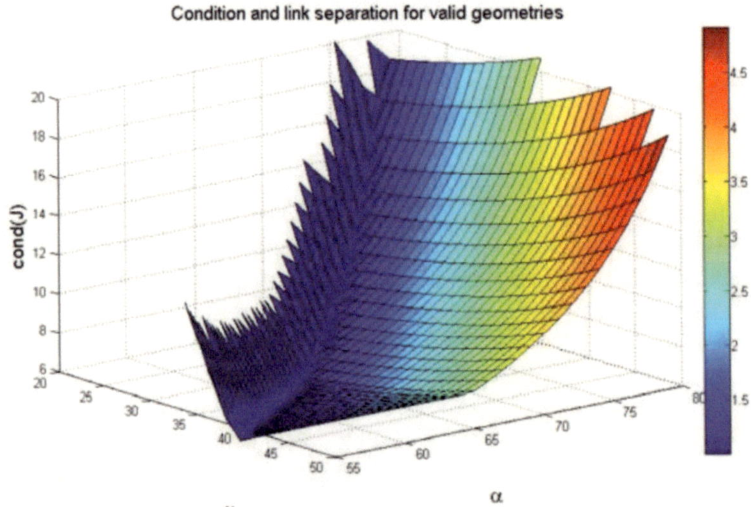

Figure 8. Condition number of internal forces. Colors denote leg separation i at the platform in mm

After fabrication and assembly of the strain gauges, the sensor is calibrated using a set of known weights applied in the six principal directions. The sensor is subjected to at least one complete loading/unloading cycle to determine the amount of hysteresis. Results of the calibration for one sensor are shown in Figure 9, with output values for all six load directions being shown in each graph. Output values for the load direction corresponding to the applied external load show an approximately linear unity response, whereas, outputs for all other load directions are expected to remain zero.
An earlier version of the sensor was mounted to the tip of an experimental surgical knife (see Figure 10) and dissection tasks similar to the experiments conducted by Wagner et al. were performed using this setup (Wagner et al., 2002). While the dissection was on average performed 50% faster by conventional MIS, the damage to the simulated arteries was 20% lower when using a telemanipulator with force feedback. For detailed discussion of the results see (Deml et al., 2005).
Due to a Quarter-Wheatstone-Bridge configuration and subsequently necessary high amplification the force signal contained 3 bit of noise after 12 bit digitization and was sensible to temperature changes. Especially the F_z component was susceptible to large temperature drift due to self heating of the strain gauges. Since this resistive heating affects all gauges equally, the increase in resistance is recorded as apparent force in z-direction. In newer versions the strain gauge configuration was, therefore, changed to a Half-Bridge configuration in order to increase the usable sensor signal and decrease the effects of self heating, effectively decreasing noise, and drift.

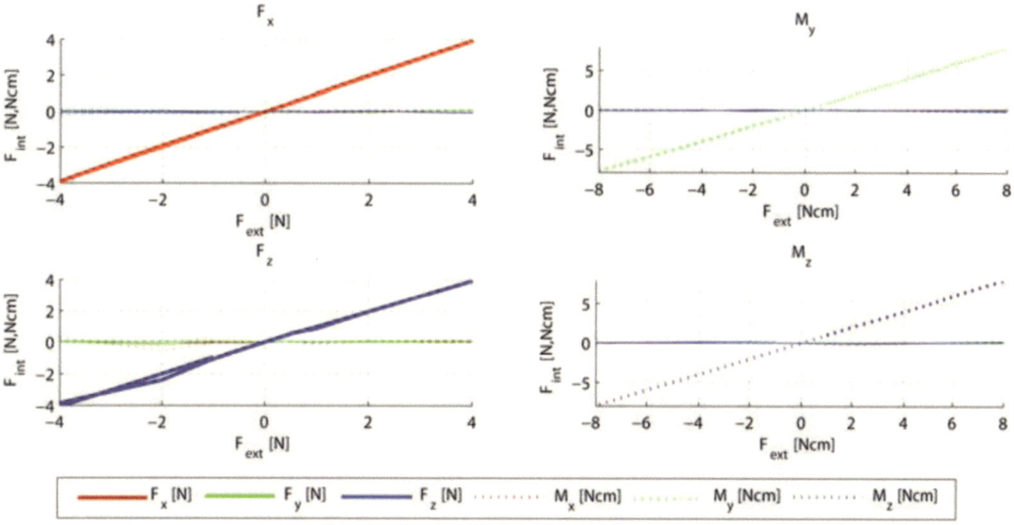

Figure 9. Response of the FTS to externally applied loads

4.3 Instrument: 2 DoF Wrist

The length of the distal joint assembly is restricted during surgery by manipulability considerations, as well as the distance between skin and operation site. For abdominal procedures this distance can be increased by insufflation, but due to the rigidity of the ribcage this is not an option for heart procedures. The joint and gripper mechanics should,

therefore, be kept as short as possible, this is even more important as the sensor increases the length of the distal assembly.
The articulated joint shown in Figure 11 closely resembles a universal joint with intersecting axes, actuated by steel cables. The drive cables in the joint run tangent to the joint pulleys at all times, therefore, the lengths of both cable loops remain constant for every joint position. The middle of each cable loop is fixed at the distal part of the joint, while the proximal ends are connected crosswise at the actuators. With this particular layout only two rotary drives are needed in the propulsion unit to fully actuate the joint, yielding linear transmission characteristics. Driving only one actuator results in a tilting motion of the instrument tip at 45° angle to the principal axes of the joint:

$$\begin{aligned}\theta_8 &= \frac{r_M}{2r_a}(\beta - \alpha),\\ \theta_9 &= \frac{r_M}{2r_a}(\beta + \alpha)\end{aligned} \tag{3}$$

with r_M: radius of motor pulley, r_a: radius of joint pulley (3 mm), α, β: actuator positions and θ_8, θ_9: joint angles. To guarantee zero backlash, the cables are prestressed with the maximum expected driving force.

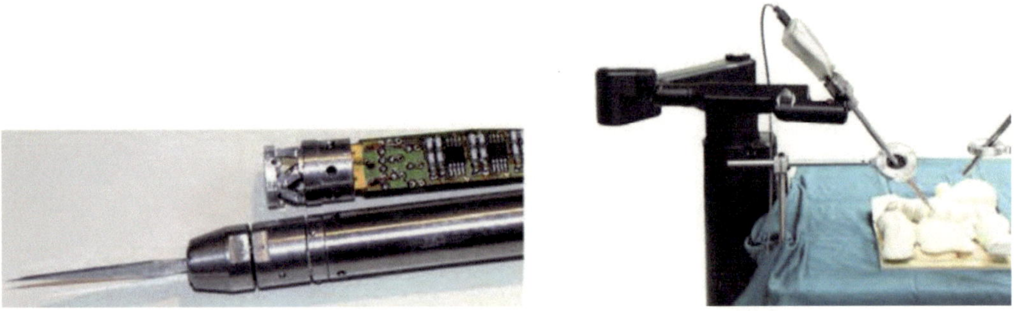

Figure 10. Application of the sensor in an experimental surgical knife, attached to a Zeus manipulator

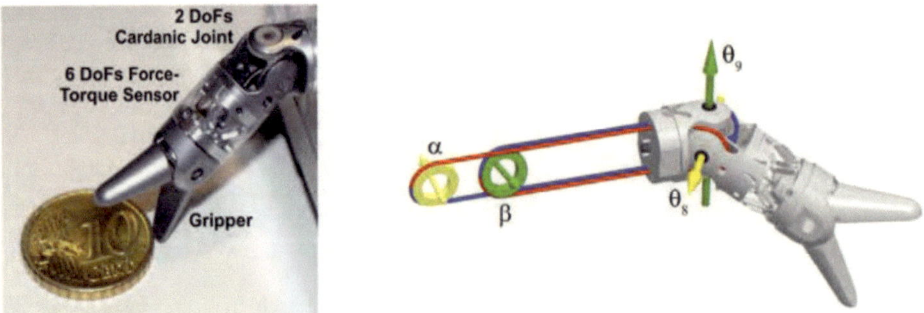

Figure 11. Prototype of instrument tip and layout of the drive cables

4.4 Haptic Workstation

To accomplish surgical procedures, the surgeon has to control the instruments, the endoscope, and additional surgical functions (e. g. electrocoagulation, irrigation, suction). The user interface of the daVinci system by Intuitive Surgical® is a good example for ergonomics and usability. However, as proprietary system and integral part of the daVinci setup it cannot be used in experimental MIRS systems. A surgeon input console for MIRS commonly includes a (stereo) display and two hand controllers to command the surgical manipulators with up to 7 DoF. Most hand controllers consist of articulated mechanical arms with four to six active and/or passive joints. The position of the surgeon's hands is measured by encoders in every joint. In order to provide a smooth, backlash-free motion these arms consist of a mechanically complicated setup including precisely machined parts and bearings. The console, integrating two arms and a display, is expensive and tends to take up significant space in the operating room. To provide full active force feedback, motors have to be integrated for every joint of the hand controller in addition to the encoders.

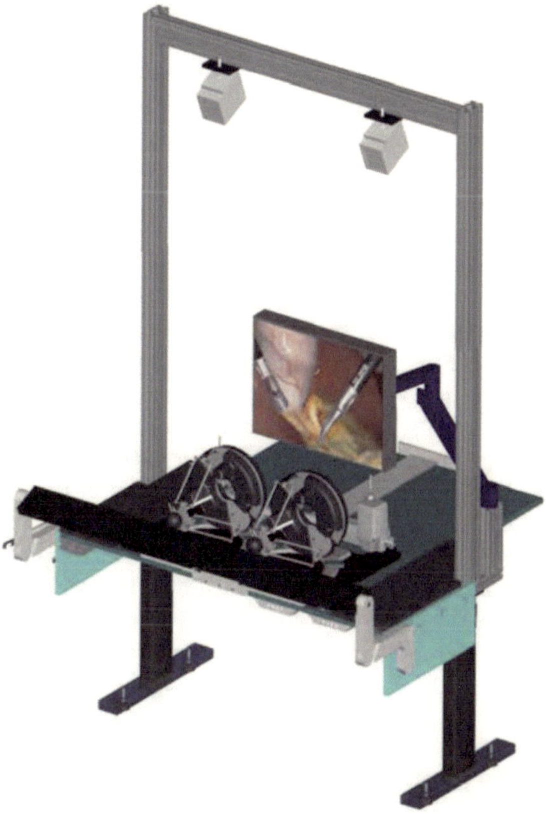

Figure 12. CAD depiction of the proprietary developed telesurgical workstation (master console)

The DLR MIRS workstation will provide intuitive manipulation of up to three instruments, including indexing functions to enlarge the available workspace. Important aspects of this concept are 3-D visualization without the use of shutter glasses or head up displays, haptic feedback, as well as comfortable and strain-free working environment from the 5th percentile female to 95th percentile male. Also, a compact design of the workstation is desired to minimize the spatial requirements in the OR, reduce separation between the surgeon and the surgical team, allowing direct visual contact to the anaesthesia area and to ease transportation.

At the current point of the project it is important to provide a generic and open setup, conducive to experimentation with a range of different input and feedback strategies, rather than a finished product.

As haptic input devices commercially available omega.7 devices by ForceDimension are chosen for their reasonable size, sufficient resolution, and high stiffness. The omega.7 device only provides force feedback in 4 DoF (3 translations and gripper). At this point, however, no device capable of satisfying all requirements exists. To enhance the precision for intricate tasks, the robotic workstation will provide the possibility of force and motion scaling, generally between 1 : 1 and 1 : 10. The devices are mounted on the workstation facing the surgeon frontally. This way the workspace of the haptic input devices best matches the required workspace for various surgical procedures (Schechner, 2007), however, the handles need to be angled outward to allow for a more natural hand position.

Unlike open surgeries, in MIS the surgeon has no direct visual access to the operation site. Conventionally, an assistant guides the camera, however, this is a strenuous task and requires practice and good collaboration. To compensate for this drawback and to allow for efficient working it is necessary to provide a fast camera control to the surgeon, which can be operated simultaneously to surgical task. As surgeons have emphasized in conversations, the ability to switch between camera positions, such as detail and overview or memory positions, is desired. Since different camera guidance modalities are to be evaluated, camera control is provided with foot pedals, but autonomous camera guidance can also be used (Wei et al., 1997). An auto-stereoscopic LCD display, including eye tracking to adjust for the position of the user, was chosen to provide 3-D visualization.

Comfortable working postures for surgeons of different height require many sections of the workstation to be adjustable. Before determining appropriate ranges, a fixed point of reference was chosen. In airplanes and for microscopic applications the eyes are chosen as fixed point to ensure the best viewing conditions. In cars, generally the fixed point is determined by the position of the foot pedals. For the workstation design, the option of choosing the eyes as fixed point is not reasonable as the view is not determined by a windshield as in cars or airplanes. To the contrary, it is relatively easy to adjust the display according to the posture of the user. The floor is chosen as fixed point, because this allows resting the feet on the ground and also moving the chair with the feet. Furthermore, the surgeon can easily change the position between standing and sitting. Table 3 shows the appropriate adjustment ranges based on ergonomics data.

An armrest is added to the workstation to minimize the load on the shoulder neck area and to allow a strain-free working for the surgeon. The armrest has to be adjustable relatively to the haptic devices in height and depth allowing for support of elbow, forearm, or hand. Fail-safe operation of the workstation is of paramount importance. To prevent unintentional operation of the instruments, a pressure sensitive switch is integrated in the armrest to disable movement and force feedback when contact between the surgeon's hands and the armrest is lost.

The generic and open concept of the Surgeon Console described in this section allows for comprehensive experiments, in order to determine the respective impact and benefit of these technologies.

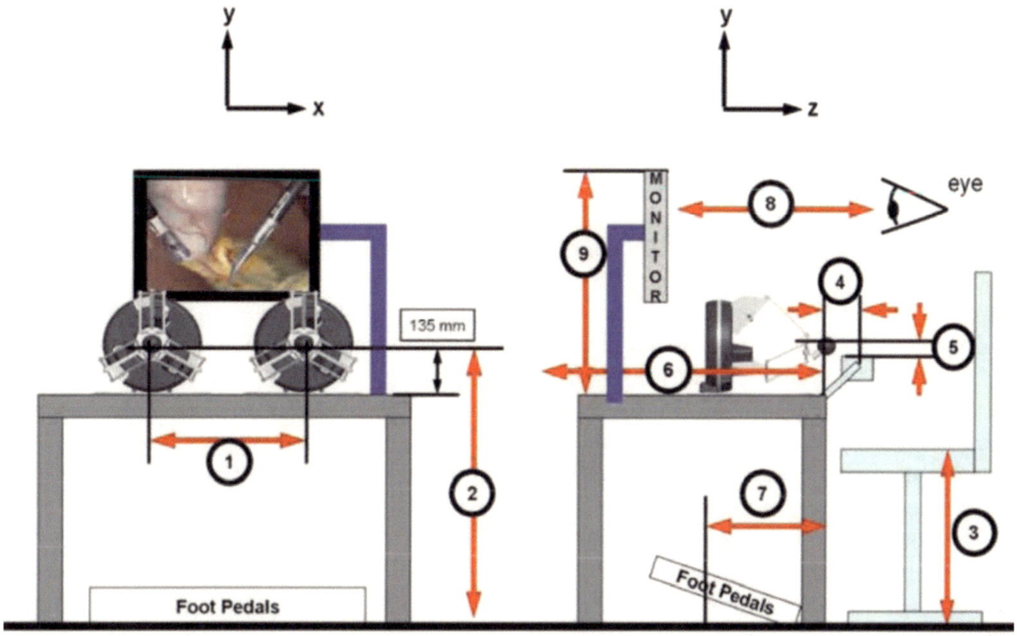

Figure 13. Range of adjustability for the haptic workstation (Schechner, 2007)

Description according to Figure 13	Adjustment range
1. haptic devices relative to each other (x)	300 *mm* to 600 *mm*
2. height of the work center (y)	600 *mm* to 1250 *mm*
3. height of the chair (y)	375 *mm* to 490 *mm*
height of the standing stool (y)	700 *mm* to 850 *mm*
4. distance between armrest and device (z)	60 *mm* to 510 *mm*
5. distance between armrest and device (y)	−50 *mm* to 50 *mm*
6. haptic device/optical tracking position (z)	0 *mm* to 600 *mm*
7. distance between foot pedals and table edge (z)	250 *mm* to 350 *mm*
8. distance eye - monitor (z)	500 *mm* to 700 *mm*
9. distance monitor - table (y)	575 *mm* to 665 *mm*

Table 3. Adjustment ranges of the workstation (Schechner, 2007)

5. Contributions

In Section 1, three main goals for this project were stated:

1. Demonstrating the feasibility of integrating a force/torque sensor inside an articulated instrument for MIRS.
2. Evaluating the impact and benefit of providing haptic feedback during MIRS.
3. Improving the acceptance of this advanced technology by providing a generic and modular setup applicable to a large number of procedures.

Although the entire system is targeted for minimally invasive as well as for open procedures, minimally invasive cardiac bypass grafting on the beating heart was selected as exemplary application due to the high demands on dynamics, accuracy, and workspace of the manipulator. Two requirements in particular apply to the presented instrument. As determined in infeeding tests of surgical needles into cadaveric tissue, intracorporal suturing requires gripping forces of ~10 N to securely hold a needle and several Newton to securely tie a suture. Furthermore, motion compensation on the beating heart necessitates an actuation frequency of ~3.5 Hz to follow the motion of the heart surface according to previous research (Ortmaier, 2003). Preliminary experiments showed that specifications could be met with a compact, light weight instrument, consisting of a self contained propulsion unit with integrated motion control and sensor conditioning electronics. An articulated 2 DoF wrist joint and 7 DoF force/torque sensor could be placed inside the distal end of a 10 mm diameter shaft, thereby, achieving the first goal. With the presented instruments not only pure *kinaesthetic* feedback can be achieved, also *tactile* impressions, like rigidification of tissue, can be recognized to some degree: taking tissue between the gripper jaws gives a comparably good impression of rigidity. Surfaces with inconsistent properties can be explored by drawing the tip over the surface with constant contact force; depth of impression will give at least an idea of tissue elasticity. By moving the instrument tip along a surface even coarse textures (surface roughness) can be felt. However, the tactile impressions are not comparable to the sensitivity and resolution of the human skin.

The second goal, assessing the impact and benefit of haptic feedback during surgery, requires the entire system (surgical manipulators, instruments, surgeon workstation, vision system, control hardware) to be assembled and integrated. Only then meaningful experiments can be conducted, comparing the performance of surgeons without haptic feedback and with various forms of feedback at an identical setup. Evaluating the performance of a MIRS force feedback system in an engineering fashion is difficult, since subjective perception (e. g. usability, immersion, user-friendliness) which is not always measurable objectively, plays an important role. Indirect measures like applied forces or time required to complete a defined task can be consulted. With previous hardware a preliminary user study was performed, comparing the dissection of an artery from surrounding tissue using tissue models. It was shown that the surgeon can benefit from high quality haptic feedback. Applied forces were reduced and the procedure was performed more cautiously (Deml et al., 2005), which on the other hand resulted in increased task completion time. It was also shown that high levels of haptic feedback are distracting, whereas low levels provide a more subtle guidance. The hardware is since being improved, and more studies based on tasks required for the proposed application of coronary surgery will need to be performed. Experiments might include tasks comparable to Section 3.1 but also more complex tasks like banding a hollow organ (e. g. a vessel) or performing a suture. The observation of simplified and standardized tasks will lead to better understanding of the whole system performance and future requirements. Additionally, subsequent motion analysis and the recognition of target oriented movements as well as auxiliary motions can be performed. A performance metric has to be found accounting for e.g. the tradeoff between task completion time and error rate. Assembly of the new system is currently in progress.

The third goal can be seen as overall design guide for the system development. Initially, the system will be used for research. It is, therefore, important to ensure modularity so that components can be tested separately, as well as providing generic components that can easily be adapted to the task at hand. This design guide has the added benefit of allowing the system to be used in a number of configurations. Examples include different numbers and arrangements of manipulators, working without MIS instruments for some neurological

or orthopedic procedures, or employing the system just as autonomous endoscope carrier. The system can also be used as a virtual reality trainer displaying previously recorded procedures to novice surgeons and providing means for learning assessment and quality assurance. This large spectrum of possible applications will help with improved capacity utilization in the OR and, therefore, a better cost benefit ratio. Ensuring the steam sterilizability of all components with direct patient contact falls into the same category, as it allows following the normal clinical workflow.
For the three goals - creating a technology demonstrator, evaluating its impact/benefit, and improving its acceptance - either solutions or research approaches could be demonstrated.

6. Future Research/Outlook

The DLR surgical instruments currently allow for one functional DoF which can take shape as gripper, scissors, or clip applicator. The instrument diameter of 10 mm is in a usual MIS range, but for further improved patient protection as well as for higher manipulability and dexterity in small body cavities, it is desired to further reduce the instrument diameter. Additional functionality like laser application, monopolar electrosurgery in combination with argon plasma coagulation (APC), or ultrasound dissection are standardized methods in surgery which have to be supported. Especially the integration of electrosurgery necessitates the cautery current carrying parts to be insulated from highly sensitive sensor elements, the drive unit with control electronics, and of course tangible parts.
Concerning the everyday use of common surgical robots, instrument changes require a significant portion of the operation time. Reintroducing a new instrument into the body should, for safety reasons, still be guided by an assistant. However, remembering the last instrument position, removing, and switching the instrument could be automated. This would reduce reorientation time and prevent unintended tissue damage during the relocation process.
The presented system is at this point designed as modular research platform rather than for a clinical environment. Therefore, some aspects which are important in a production system (suitability for series production, life-time analysis, etc.) will have to be addressed with the input from experienced industrial partners. Sterilizability was considered, for components with direct patient contact even steam sterilizability, however, in many cases mostly in material selection and not fully in geometrical arrangement. Consequently, a significant amount of work is left in those areas, as well as in refining the "touch and feel" of the system for maximum immersion, necessitating the cooperation with surgeons, industry, and industrial psychologists.

7. References

Akinbiyi, T.; Reiley, C.E.; Saha, S.; Burschka, D.; Hasser, C.J.; Yuh, D.D. & Okamura, A.M. (2006). Dynamic augmented reality for sensory substitution in robot-assisted surgical systems, in: *Proceedings of the 28th IEEE EMBS Annual International Conference*, pp. 567-570, New York City, NY, USA

Braun, M.; Schurr, M.; Hausam, V. & Buess, G. (2004). Erweiterte Freiheitsgrade mechanischer Manipulatoren für die minimalinvasive Chirurgie, in: *Biomedizinische Technik*, vol. 49, pp. 126-127

Dakin, G. & Gagner, M. (2003). Comparison of laparoscopic skills performance between standard instruments and two surgical robotic systems, *Surgical Endoscopy,* vol. 17:pp. 574-579

Demi, B.; Ortmaier, T. & Seibold, U. (2005). The touch and feel in minimally invasive surgery, in: *HAVE 2005 IEEE International Workshop on Haptic Audio Visual Environments and their Applications. Ottawa, Ontario, Canada.,* pp. 33-38

DLR - German Aerospace Center, Institute of Robotics and Mechatronics (2007). KineMedic Homepage, Web-site, URL http://www.dlr.de/rm-neu/desktopdefault.aspx/tabid-3 82 8 /

Falk, V.; Diegeler, A.; Walther, T.; Löscher, N.; Vogel, B.; Ulmann, C.; Rauch, T. & Mohr, F.W. (1999). Endoscopic coronary artery bypass grafting on the beating heart using a computer enhanced telemanipulation system, *Heart Surgery Forum,* vol. 2:pp. 199-205

Frede, T.; Hammadya, A.; Klein, J.; Teber, D.; Inaki, N.; Waseda, M.; Buess, G. & Rassweiler, J. (2007). The radius surgical system - a new device for complex minimally invasive procedures in urology?, *European Urology,* vol. 51:pp. 1015-1022

Guthart, G. & Salisbury, J. (2000). The intuitive telesurgery system: Overview and application, in: *Procedings of the IEEE International Conference on Robotics and Automation (ICRA),* vol. 1, pp. 618-621, San Francisco, CA, USA, ISBN 0-7803-5886-4

Hernandez, J.; Barm, S.; Munz, Y.; Moorthy, K.; Datta, V.; Martin, S.; Dosis, A.; Bello, F.; Darzi, A. & Rockall, T. (2004). Qualitative and quantitative analysis of the learning curve of a simulated surgical task on the daVinci system, *Surgical Endoscopy,* vol. 18:pp. 372-378

Inaki, N.; Waseda, M.; Schurr, M.; Braun, M. & Buess, G. (2007). Experimental results of mesh fixation by a manual manipulator in a laparoscopic inguinal hernia repair model, *Surgical Endoscopy,* vol. 21(2):pp. 197-201

Intuitive Surgical, Inc. (2007). Company profile of Intuitive Surgical, Inc., Sunnyvale, CA, USA, Website, URL http://www.intuitivesurgical.com

Kitagawa, M.; Dokko, D.; Okamura, A.M.; Bethea, B.T. & Yuh, D.D. (2004). Effect of sensory substitution on suture manipulation forces for surgical teleoperation, in: *Annual Medicine Meets Virtual Reality Conference (MMVR),* Newport Beach, CA, USA, submitted

Kitagawa, M. (2003). *Indirect Feedback of Haptic Information for Robot-Assisted Telemanipulation,* Master's thesis, Johns Hopkins University

Konietschke, R.; Ortmaier, T.; Weiss, H.; Engelke, R. & Hirzinger, G. (2003). Force propagation models in laparoscopic tools and trainers, in: *2nd Conference of the German Society of Computer and Robotic Assisted Surgery (CURAC),* Nürnberg, Germany

Konietschke, R.; Ortmaier, T.; Weiss, H.; Hirzinger, G. & Engelke, R. (2004). Manipulability and accuracy measures for a medical robot in minimally invasive surgery, in: *9th International Symposium on Advances in Robot Kinematics*

Kwon, D.S.; Woo, K.Y.; Song, S.K.; Kim, W.S. & Cho, H.S. (1998). Microsurgical telerobot system, in: *Proceedings of the IEEE/RSJ International Conference on Intelligent Robots and Systems (IROS),* pp. 945-950

Lobontiu, N. (2002). *Compliant Mechanisms: Design of Flexure Hinges,* CRC Press Inc., ISBN-10: 0849313678, ISBN-13: 978-0849313677

MacFarlane, M.; Rosen, J.; Hannaford, B.; Pellegrini, C. & Sinanan, M. (1999). Force-feedback grasper helps restore sense of touch in minimally invasive surgery, *Journal of Gastrointestinal Surgery,* vol. 3(3):pp. 278-285

Mayer, H.; Nagy, I.; Knoll, A.; Schirmbeck, E. & Bauernschmitt, R. (2004). Upgrading instruments for robotic surgery, in: *Australasian Conference on Robotics & Automation*

Müller, J. (2004). Charite, Klinik für Allgemein-, Visceral-, Gefäß- und Thoraxchirurgie, Campus Mitte, from discussion, Berlin, Germany

Nakamura, Y. (2003). Virtual stillness and small size robot system that occupies less space in OR, in: *Proceedings of the IEEE International Conference on Robotics and Automation (ICRA), Workshop Recent Advances in Medical Robotics,* Taipei, Taiwan

Omote, K.; Feussner, H.; Ungeheuer, A.; Arbter, K.; Wei, G.Q.; Siewert, J.R. & Hirzinger, G. (1999). Self-guided robotic camera control for laparoscopic surgery compared with human camera control, *The American Journal of Surgery,* vol. 117:pp. 321-324

Ortmaier, T.; Weiss, H. & Hirzinger, G. (2003). Minimally invasive robotic surgery: Foundations and perspectives, in: *Proceedings of the IEEE International Conference on Robotics and Automation (ICRA), Workshop on Recent Advances in Medical Robotics,* Taipei, Taiwan

Ortmaier, T.; Weiss, H.; Hagn, U.; Grebenstein, M.; Nickl, M.; Albu-Schäffer, A.; Ott, C.; Jörg, S.; Konietschke, R.; Le-Tien, L. & Hirzinger, G. (2006). A hands-on-robot for accurate placement of pedicle screws, in: *Proceedings of the IEEE International Conference on Robotics and Automation (ICRA),* Orlando, Florida, USA

Ortmaier, T. (2003). *Motion Compensation in Minimally Invasive Robotic Surgery,* VDI Verlag, PhD Thesis

Peirs, J.; Clijnen, J.; Reynaerts, D.; Brussel, H.V.; Herijgers, P.; Corteville, B. & Boone, S. (2004). A micro optical force sensor for force feedback during minimally invasive robotic surgery, *Sensors and Actuators A,* vol. 115:pp. 447-455

Rosen, J. (2001). Human machine interfaces in minimally invasive surgery, in: *Medicine Meets Virtual Reality (MMVR), Workshop on Simulating Minimally Invasive Surgical Procedures in Virtual Environments*

Rosen, J.; Hannaford, B.; MacFarlane, M. & Sinanan, M. (1999a). Force controlled and teleoperated endoscopic grasper for minimally invasive surgery - experimental performance evaluation, IEEE *Transactions on Biomedical Engineering,* vol. 46(10)

Rosen, J.; MacFarlane, M.; Richards, C.; Hannaford, B. & Sinanan, M. (1999b). Surgeon-tool force/torque signatures - evaluation of surgical skills in minimally invasive surgery, in: *Annual Medicine Meets Virtual Reality Conference (MMVR),* vol. 7

Salle, D.; Bidaud, P. & Morel, G. (2004). Optimal design of high dexterity modular MIS instrument for coronary artery bypass grafting, in: *Procedings of the IEEE International Conference on Robotics and Automation (ICRA),* vol. 2, pp. 1276-1281, ISSN: 1050-4729, ISBN: 0-7803-8232-3

Schechner, V. (2007). *Concept and Ergonomics of a Bi-Manual Haptic Workstation for Minimally Invasive Robotic Surgery,* Master's thesis, Lehrstuhl für Ergonomie, Technische Universität München, Munich, Germany

Seibold, U. (2002). Monolithic Force-Torque Sensor (Kraft-Moment-Sensor), German Patent 102 17 018.5

Seibold, U. & Hirzinger, G. (2003). A 6-axis force/torque sensor design for haptic feedback in minimally invasive robotic surgery, in: *MICRO.tec - 2nd VDE World Microtechnologies Congress*, pp. 239-244

Sorli, M. & Pastorelli, S. (1995). Six-axis reticulated structure force/torque sensor with adaptable performances, *Mechatronics*, vol. 5(6):pp. 585-601

Tendick, F. & Cenk Cavusoglu, M. (1997). Human-Machine Interfaces for Minimally Invasive Surgery, Proceedings of the 19th Annual International Conference of the IEEE Engineering in Medicine and Biology Society, pp. 2771-2776, Chicago, IL, USA

Tholey, G.; Desai, J.P. & Castellanos, A.E. (2003). Evaluating the role of vision and force feedback in minimally invasive surgery: New automated laparoscopic grasper and a case study, in: *Proceeding of the Medical Image Computing and Computer-Assisted Intervention (MICCAI)*

Tholey, G.; Pillarisetti, A.; Green, W. & Desai, J.P. (2004). *Design, Development, and Testing of an Automated Laparoscopic Grasper with 3-D Force Measurement Capability*, vol. 3078, Springer Berlin / Heidelberg

Tuebingen Scientific Medical, G. (2007). Homepage of Tuebingen Scientific Medical, Inc., Tuebingen, Germany, Website, URL http://www.tuebingen-scientific.de

Wagner, C.; Stylopoulos, N. & Howe, R. (2002). The role of force feedback in surgery: Analysis of blunt dissection, in: *Proceedings of the 10th Symposium on Haptic Interfaces for Virtual Environment and Teleoperator Systems (HAPTICS)*, pp. 68-74, ISBN: 0-7695-1489-8

Wei, G.; Arbter, K. & Hirzinger, G. (1997). Real-time visual servoing for laparoscopic surgery, IEEE *Engineering in Medicine and Biology*, vol. 16(1)

Zemiti, N.; Ortmaier, T.; Vitrani, M. & Morel, G. (2004). A force controlled laparoscopic surgical robot without distal force sensing, in: *Proceedings of the International Symposium on Experimental Robotics (ISER)*

29

"RoboLase": Internet-accessible robotic laser scissors and laser tweezers microscope systems

Linda Z. Shi[1], Michael W. Berns[1, 2, 3] and Elliot Botvinick[2, 3]
[1]*Department of Bioengineering, University of California, San Diego,*
[2]*Beckman Laser Institute, University of California, Irvine,*
[3]*Deparment of Biomedical Engineering, University of California, Irvine*
USA[1]

1. Introduction

The advent of the internet has opened the door to remote computing, remote file sharing and remote instrumentation control. We have taken advantage of these capabilities to: (1) satisfy our need for 24-hour access to the laser-microscope, and (2) facilitate collaboration and networking with investigators from other locations around the world. The remote operation of microscope systems has been demonstrated for electron microscopes (Chumbley, et al., 2002, Hadida-Hassan, et al., 1999, Takaoka, et al., 2000, Yamada, et al., 2003), for light microscope evaluation of fixed samples (Kaplan et al., 2002, Molnar, et al., 2003), and for laser scanning confocal microscopy (Youngblom, et al. 2001). Though there has been significant progress in developing real-time microscopy and radiological image sharing over the internet, this has not been extended to the domain of real-time interventional manipulation of live cells, tissues, and organelles (Botvinick & Berns, 2005).
Technology is revolutionizing the biomedical field with the latest development of automatic image processing algorithms and real-time robotic devices in the study of scale of microns and even nanometers. Automated image processing algorithms have been successfully applied to tracking neurons (Cohen, et al., 1994, He, et al., 2003), Caenorhabditis elegans (Bao, et al., 2006), and sperm cells (Shi, et al., 2006a & 2006b, Nascimento, et al., 2006), identifying Sphacelaria algae (Yeom & Javida, 2006) and soil bacteria (Bloem, et al., 1995), and live embryos (Brodland & Veldhuis, 1998). Robotic telemicroscopy has been developed for general applications (Lin, et al., 2003, Botvinick & Berns, 2005) and is currently being applied to pathology (Szymas, et al., 2001, Della Mea, et al., 2000, Burgess et al., 2002) and microsurgery (Knight, et al., 2005, Kuang, et al., 2005).
Lasers are useful tools for micromanipulation of biological specimens (Prasad, 2003). With the addition of tightly focused laser beams, microscopes have been turned into elaborate tools that not only allow detailed observation of a specimen but also the capture, displacement, and microdissection of biological samples in vitro with astonishing ease and

[1] All three authors contributed equally to this work

accuracy (Conia, et al., 1997). Some commercial optical trapping and scissors systems are available, such as The LaserTweezers® Workstation and The LaserScissors® Workstation from Cell Robotics Inc, and PALM MicroLaser Systems from P.A.L.M. Microlaser Technologies. A review of this field is published in Methods in Cell Biology (Berns & Greulich, 2007)

We have developed a system with remote operational capabilities using several different standard microscope platforms that have evolved from a multi-parametric laser microscope described over two decades ago (Berns, et al., 1981). At that time, however, there was neither the computing power nor the internet of today, two of the key technologies that are combined with current opto-electronic microscopic systems. One goal of the "systems-integrated" microscope (RoboLase) is to develop a platform that can be accessed by collaborators via the internet. The system has been used to image, ablate, and/or trap cells and their organelles by remote-control. In the laser ablation mode (laser scissors), all the electronic components, such as the microscope, cameras, laser power and ablation coordinates, are controlled by the local host computer but can be operated by remote collaborators. Delicate microsurgery on cell organelles, such as individual microtubules, spindle fibers, chromosomes and centrioles can be performed to study each organelle's role in cell function. In addition, localized DNA damage inside the cell nucleus can be patterned to study DNA repair mechanisms. In the laser trapping (laser tweezers) mode, phase contrast images of swimming sperm are digitized to the computer at a video rate (30 frame per second) or higher (up to 90 frames per second). The custom trapping algorithm places a region of interest (ROI) centered about a sperm in response to a mouse click by a remote collaborator. All subsequent real-time tracking and trapping of the sperm are performed automatically to study relationships between sperm swimming force and swimming speed. With this system we have studied the effects of laser trap duration and power on sperm motility and are integrating real-time measurements of sperm energetics assessed by fluorescent molecules (Nascimento, et al., 2006).

2. Robotic Laser Scissors Microscope System

2.1 Microscope

The robotic laser microscope is comprised of a motorized inverted microscope stand, external optics to direct the ablation laser into the microscope, a CCD digital camera, and a hardware-software suite for the control of laser power and firing position, mechanical shutters in the laser path, the specimen stage, and microscope stand focus and illumination.

The major brands of research microscopes have all developed motorized versions of their inverted microscopes. Our system utilizes a Zeiss Axiovert 200M (Zeiss, Thornwood, NY) with motorized objective turret, reflector turret (for fluorescent filter cubes), condenser turret, halogen lamp shuttering with intensity control, mercury arc lamp shuttering, camera port selection, objective focus, and parfocality switching between objective lenses. The microscope also has a motorized optovar turret to increase the system magnification by 1.6X or 2.5X. For laser ablation experiments, a 63X, phase III, NA1.4 oil immersion microscope objective is used. The microscope stand has a built in computer which uses a controller area network (CAN) to communicate with motors and encoders within the microscope stand. The CAN can receive commands through a serial interface typically attached to a computer running an image acquisition/microscope control program. Rather than using the software provided with the microscope manufacture which we found to be cumbersome and slow,

we have developed custom control software capable of communicating with the CAN as described below.
Features of the motorized microscope that are especially relevant to remote operation of a laser microscope are the shift-free reflector turret, microscope light path selection, illumination control and objective focus. The shift-free reflector turret allows the user to repeatedly switch between any of 5 fluorescent filter cubes in the turret without a detectable pixel shift in the image. This is of great importance when performing resolution-limited targeting for laser ablation as it ensures that the laser will always focus at the expected pixel location. Likewise, the Axiovert microscope can switch from camera port to laser ablation port and back to camera port with no detectable pixel shifts when initiating an ablation sequence.
Specimens are mounted in an X-Y stepper stage (Ludl Electronic Products Hawthorne, NY) controlled with a PXI-7344 stepper motor controller (National Instruments, Austin, TX) and an MID-7604 power drive (National Instruments). The motion board is mounted in a PXI chassis (National Instruments), which is connected to the host computer through two MXI4 boards (one in the PXI chassis, the other in the host computer) through the MXI-3 fiber-optic cable (National Instruments). Motorized objective focus control is achieved through the CAN by Zeiss' Harmonic Drive DC motor providing 25nm steps with 10 mm travel for precise focus control over multiple objectives' working distances. To achieve stable temperature control for specimens imaged by an oil-immersion objective lens both the specimen and the objective lens are heated. Specimens in 35 mm Petri dishes are heated with a stage heater (heater: DH-35; controller: TC-324B; Warner Instruments Corporation, Hamden, CT) while the objective is heated with a collar-type objective heater (OBJSTD with controller, Bioptechs, inc., Butler, PA).

2.2 External laser optics and hardware

Optics outside the microscope stand guide the ablation laser into the microscope and supplies RoboLase system with automated laser power control, laser shuttering, and laser positioning (Figure 1). The laser ablation light source is a diode-pumped Vanguard with a second harmonic generator (SHG) providing TEM_{00} mode 532 nm laser light linearly polarized with 100:1 purity, 76 MHz repetition rate, 12 ps pulse duration and 2W average power(Spectra-Physics, Mountain View, CA). The unattenuated laser power is far in excess of the threshold for resolution-limited subcellular laser ablation (Botvinick, et al., 2004) and left unattenuated is well above the plasma threshold causing catastrophic damage to cells in the vicinity of the laser. We built a beam attenuator from dual linear polarizers. The laser beam polarization purity is considerably increased from 100:1 through the first glan linear polarizer (CLPA-12.0-425-675, CVI Laser, LLC, Albuquerque, NM) with a 5 x 10^5 extinction ratio rotated for maximum transmission (95%). Laser power is controlled by rotating an identical glan linear polarizer placed in series to the first and mounted in a motorized rotational mount driven by an open loop 2-phase stepper motor with 0.05° accuracy (PR50PP, Newport Corp, New Port, CA). The stepper motor rotates the polarizer from its vertical orientation with maximum transmission (95%) to its horizontal orientation with minimum transmission well below the damage threshold of biological samples. The stepper motor is controlled via the motion board in the PXI chassis. Light exiting the second polarizer is partially reflected by a laser-line beam sampler with dual antireflection-coated surfaces. The sampled beam is measured by a photodiode (2032 photo receiver, NewFocus,

San Jose, CA) and converted to a voltage. A calibrated photometer (1825-C, Newport Corp) is used to determine the relationship between the photodiode voltage and average laser power in the main beam. A mechanical shutter (Vincent Associates, Rochester, NY) with a 3ms duty cycle gates the main laser beam to provide 'short' bursts of pulses to the microscope (Botvinick & Berns, 2005).

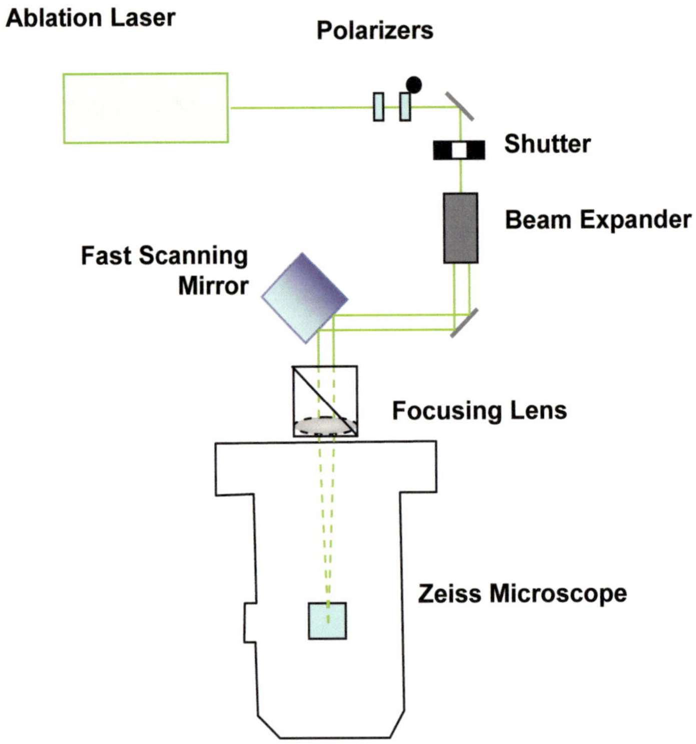

Figure 1. External laser light path of robotic laser scissors microscope system

The laser beam is then expanded using an adjustable-beam expander (2-8X, 633/780/803nm correction, Rodenstock, Germany) and lowered to a height just above the optical table by two additional mirrors. Telecentric beam steering is achieved by placing a dual-axis fast scanning mirror (Newport Corp) at an image plane conjugate to the back focal plane of the microscope objective. This image plane is formed by a 250 mm biconvex lens positioned with its front focal plane at the image plane of the microscope Keller-Berns camera port (We refer to the entry port underside the microscope as the Keller-Berns port as opposed to the Keller-port because the first Zeiss microscope with this port was built by Zeiss following the design requirements of Berns for the construction of the LAMP CATS microscope in the early 1990's (see Berns, et al., 1998). In order to access the Keller-Berns port, the microscope is raised 70 mm above the table via custom machined metal alloy posts to leave room for a 45° mirror which vertically redirects incident laser light running parallel to the table through the Keller-Berns port. Once inside the microscope stand, the laser light passes through the tube lens and one of the five fluorescent filter cubes of the reflector turret before entering the back of the objective lens. The reflector turret can be set up either with one filter slot blank, or since the turret is automated, the system can position a fluorescent filter cube into place with appropriate laser transmission characteristics. All external mirrors in the ablation laser light path are virtually loss-less dielectric mirrors optimized for 45° reflections of 532nm S-polarized light (Y2-1025-45-S, CVI Laser LLC). It is important to note that the selection of the laser for RoboLase system was based upon our desire to produce cellular damage using multiphoton processes of the picosecond green second harmonic wavelength. We have built several other RoboLase systems using other short-pulsed lasers, such as the femtosecond Titanium sapphire laser at 800 nm (see Botvinick, et al., 2005, Wakida et al, 2006 and Gomez-Godinez, 2007).

2.3 Cameras

A high quantum efficiency digital camera is used to capture transmitted and fluorescent images. RoboLase implements a Hamamatsu Orca-AG deep-cooled 1344 x 1024 pixel, 12-bit digital CCD camera with digital (fire wire) output (Hamamatsu Photonics, K.K., Hamamatsu, Japan). The ORCA can read out sub regions of the chip for increased frame rates, bin pixels for increased signal-to-noise, and adjust gain and exposure time to trade off between signal-to-noise characteristics and arc lamp exposure times. RoboLase uses Hamamatsu's Video Capture Library for LabVIEW (ver 1.0) communicate with the ORCA camera controller through its DCAMAPI driver.

2.4 Software

The control software is programmed in the LabVIEW 8.2 (National Instruments) language and is responsible for control of the microscope, cameras and external light paths. The control software also manages image and measurement file storage. It communicates with the user through the graphic user interface or the 'front panel' in LabVIEW. The front panel receives user input and displays images and measurements. The control software interprets commands sent by the user into appropriate hardware calls and returns the results of that action to the front panel and/or computer's hard drive. Emphasis was placed on the design of the front panel, such that it would be easy to learn while providing the features needed to search for a cell of interest and then to perform cellular manipulation on that cell.

Figure 2 shows an image of the front panel of Robolase. The upper-left panel/tab contains laser parameter controls. This panel contains: 1) the Turn-on-Laser button to control the emission of the ablation laser inside the laser cavity, 2) the LaserShut button to control the laser's internal shutter, 3) the % Power slider to select a percent of maximum laser ablation power (100% percent corresponding to 3.5 mW at the focal spot after the objective), 4) the Scissors-Filter-Cube selector to choose the filter cube turret position during ablation, 5) two fire buttons, Cut ROI and Fire at (0,0), to fire the laser either at user-drawn positions or the center of the field respectively.

Once either fire button is pressed, the control software calls the microscope CAN to select the Keller-Berns port and the appropriate filter cube. The control software then continuously queries the CAN to ensure the completion of both actions before opening the mechanical shutter in the laser path for a pre-defined laser burst time. Beam steering is sufficiently faster than the camera port and filter turrets such that a quarry of its position prior to opening the shutter in unnecessary.

The center panel on the left of the front panel of Robolase in Figure 2 contains 5 tabs: 1) The 'Stage Ctl' tab contains left/right and up/down rockers to move the microscope stage with position feedback. A similar pair of rockers moves the microscope objective for focus control. The 'Click and Move' control is a novel control designed to minimize exposure of the cells to the arc lamp light during stage movements. The user simply chooses the crosshairs tool from the toolbar to the left of the image and clicks on an object of interest in the image. The program then calculates that pixel's displacement from the field center and moves the stage to center the object. 2) The 'Coor List' tab allows the user to store the current position in a list or to return to any stored coordinate. It also allows the user to load an old list of coordinates, to clear the current list, or to save the current list to the hard drive. 3) The 'Cut ROI' tab contains controls for beam steering and for laser ablation through a series of z-coordinates. The user can select a shape tool (dot, line, rectangle, irregular shapes) from the tool bar and draw one or more shapes on the image. The region of interest (ROI) of that shape can be caved by firing single macropulse (one opening of the mechanical shutter which will pass multiple individual laser pulses). Since the laser causes near diffraction limited ablation (Botvinick, et al., 2004), the program calculates the number of macropulses necessary to fill in the shape based on the pixel dimensions of the shape and the pixel extent of a single diffraction-limited ablation. 4) The 'Camera Ctl' tab contains controls for camera gain, digitization offset, exposure time and binning. It also contains an area-of-interest control to only transfer image data from an area of interest defined with the rectangle tool in the image display. 5) The 'Microscope Ctl' tab contains controls for the microscope stand to select the objective, filter cube, condenser filter, optovar, and image port.

The lower panel on the left of Robolase front panel in Figure 2 contains image acquisition controls. The 'Image Acquisition' tab contains controls for exposing single images (Expose), continuous acquisition (Focus), image save and image printing. The user can select the filter cube for fluorescence image acquisition, whether to open the arc lamp during the exposure. The 'Root Directory' control specifies the top directory for file saving using our automated file naming system, and an indicator displaying the full path and name of the last saved image. The file path and name are designed to prevent accidental overwriting of data during successive operations of the program coding the file name with the current time. The 'Time Series' tab contains controls for acquiring a time series of images. The time series uses setting from the 'Image Acquisition' tab and contains controls for the number of images and the duration between images as well as an indicator of the last image saved in the time series.

The lower panel on the right of Robolase front panel in Figure 2 displays the last acquired image plus the slider to control/indicate the brightness of the halogen lamp. The upper panel on the right contains a message box and the image histogram. The message box displays important messages, such as error notifications or equipment status, and draws user attention by pulsing the large green digital LED to the left of the message box when a new message arrives. The gray box controls the image display lookup table for mapping 12-bit images to the 8-bit display. This control uses four modes of look-up table: 1) Full-dynamic, in which the range of non-zero intensities are divided into 256 equally spaced bins, 2) 90%-dynamic, in which the dynamic range containing the middle 90% of the cumulated histogram of the image is divided into 256 equally spaced bins, 3) Given-range, in which the range of grayscale values specified by the 'Maximum Value' and 'Minimum Value' slider controls are equally divided into 256 bins, and 4) Down-shift, in which the grayscale values are shifted to the right in 8-bit increments as specified by a control. An image histogram displays the pixel intensity histogram of the last acquired image to aid in the selection of an appropriate lookup table.

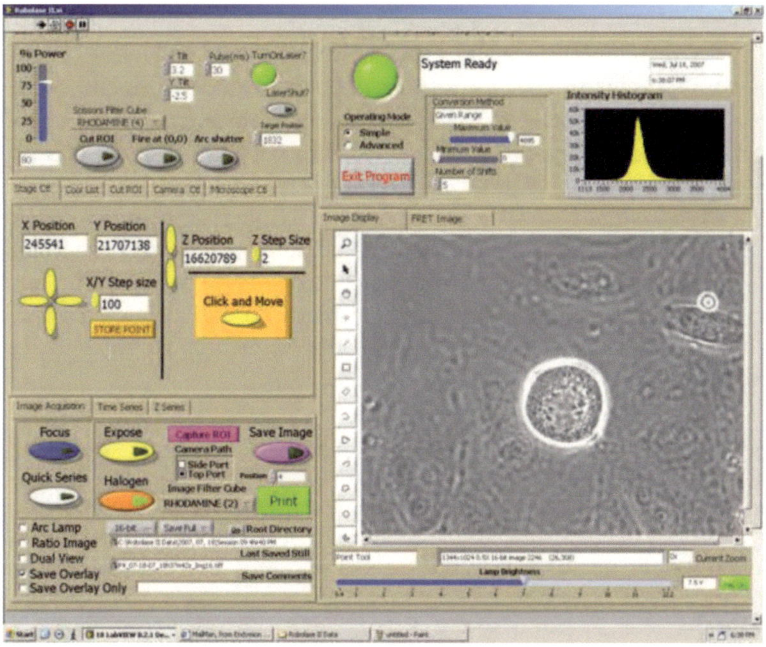

Figure 2. Front panel of robotic laser ablation microscope system

2.5 Internet-based laser ablation control

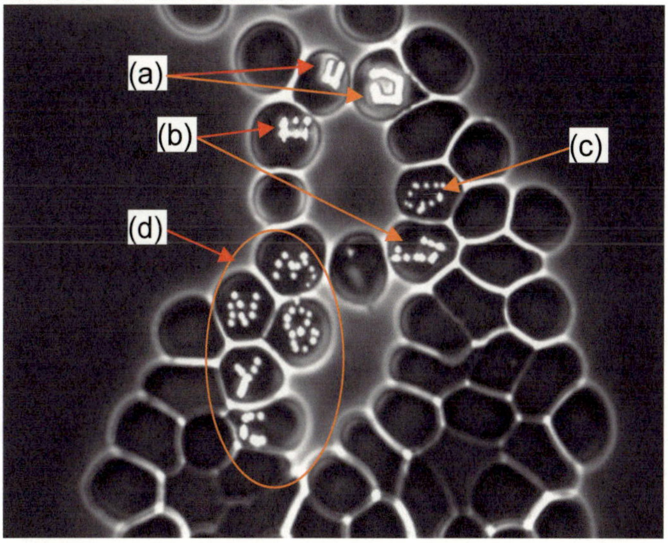

Figure 3. Irregular shape laser cuts on red blood cells on robotic laser scissors microscope system via internet. The irregular shapes were cut out with the ablation distance smaller than the actual ablation radius (3μm) at high laser power as shown in (a). The discrete ablation spots can be clearly seen with bigger ablation distance at high laser power in (b) and at low laser power in (c). The patterns (MB and NYC) is laser-etched in 4(d) (Shi, et al., 2006c, © 2006 IEEE)

The robotic laser ablation microscope system at University of California, San Diego/Irvine can be operated via the internet using most internet accessible devices, including laptops and desktop computers. The experiment testing irregular shape cutting through the internet was conducted from New York City using the www.logmein.com web server as shown in Figure 3. Red blood cells were deposited on a microscope cover glass, allowed to air-dry, and mounted in a cell culture chambers (rose chamber, Shi, 2006a). The collaborator in New York City logged in to RoboLase system and drew multiple shapes on the captured image at San Diego. That collaborator also modified the ablation power and the ablation distance between the two ablation spots in the front panel of RoboLase as shown in Figure 3 (higher laser power and bigger ablation distance was used in (a), higher laser power and smaller ablation distance in (b), lower laser power and bigger ablation distance in (c), patterns of alphabet letters of MB and NYC were laser-etched in (d)).

3. Robotic Laser Tweezers Microscope System

The robotic laser tweezers microscope system can be designed in the robotic laser scissors microscope system similar to that discusses in Botvinick & Berns 2005 (the trapping laser was directed behind the microscope in the arc lamp illumination light path to merge the two light paths). The robotic laser tweezers microscope system may be designed and built as a stand-alone system as described in Shi, 2006c. Real-time automatic tracking and trapping of sperm (RATTS) is discussed in this paper as an example of RoboLase system.

3.1 Hardware and optical design of RATTS

A single point gradient trap was generated using a Nd:YVO_4 continuous wave 1064nm wavelength laser (Model BL-106C, Spectra Physics) coupled into a Zeiss Axiovert S100 microscope and a 40x, phase III, NA 1.3 oil immersion objective. The optical design is shown in Figure 4. Laser light is reflected off two dielectric mirrors to orient the beam parallel to the table and along the optical axis of the microscope. The beam is expanded by two lenses (plano-concave lens, f = -25.5mm at λ = 1064nm, and plano-convex lens, f = 76.2mm at λ = 1064 nm) in order to fill the objective's back aperture. A third lens (biconvex lens, f = 200mm) focuses the beam onto the side port of the dual video adaptor to ensure the beam is collimated at the objective's back aperture. The dual video adaptor contains a filter cube with a dichroic mirror that allows laser light entering the side port to be transmitted to the microscope while reflecting visible light to the camera attached to the top port for imaging. A low pass filter (D535/40M, Chroma Technology Corp., Rockingham, VT) is placed in the filter cube to block back reflections of IR laser light while allowing visible light to pass. The laser trap remains stationary near the center of the field of view. In order to trap a sperm the microscope stage is moved to bring the sperm to the laser trap location. The laser trap location is determined prior to each experiment by trapping 10μm-diameter polystyrene beads suspended in water within a 35 mm diameter glass bottom Petri dish. The trap depth within the sample is kept to approximately 5 μm (approximately one sperm head diameter) above the cover glass. This ensures that the trap geometry is not sensitive to spherical aberrations from the surrounding media (Nascimento, et al., 2006). Laser power in the specimen plane is attenuated by rotating a polarizer (**CVI Laser LLC**) that is mounted in a stepper-motor-driven rotating mount (PR50PP, Newport Corp). The mount is controlled by a custom program that allows the experimenter to set the power decay rate (rotation rate of polarizer) and record laser power at the moment a sperm escapes the trap. The specimen is imaged by a CCD camera (XC - 75, Sony, Sony, Japan operating at 30 frames per second or Cohu, Model 7800, San Diego, CA, operating up to 90 frames per second), coupled to a variable zoom lens system (0.33 - 1.6 X magnification) to demagnify the field of view. For video rate RATTS operation, analog output (RS-170 format) from the Sony CCD is distributed to a TV monitor, a Camcorder (DCR-PC101, Sony, Japan) for recording, and the image acquisition board PXI-1409 (National Instruments) through a video distribution amplifier (IN3218HR,Extron Electronics, Anaheim, CA). For cases to acquire the sperm swimming images in higher frame rate, the digital output (RS-422 format) from the Cohu camera is connected to the 16-bit digital image acquisition board PCI-1422 (National Instrument) for image display and streaming. Note that only one camera is used at a time in RATTS.

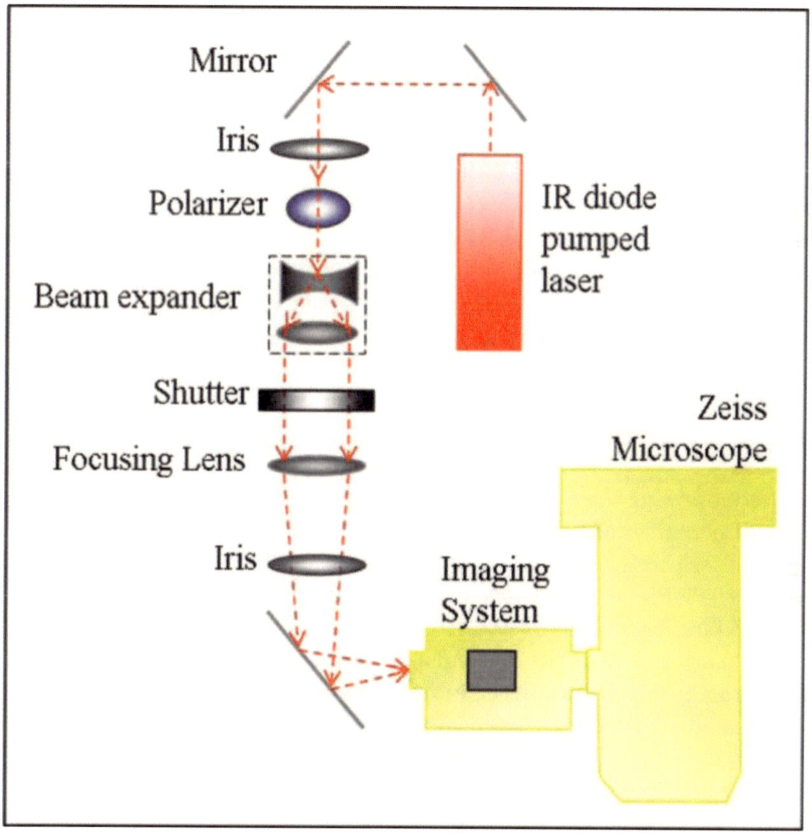

Figure 4. External laser light paths of robotic laser trapping microscope system

3.2 Software design of RATTS

RATTS is custom coded in the LabView 8.2 language (National Instruments) to process streaming images, calculate sperm trajectories, and drive the motion hardware (Shi, et al, 2006b). RATTS implements the image segmentation and sperm tracking algorithm (SSTA) in real time (Shi et al., 2006a). Images are digitized by the image acquisition board and transferred into a continuous buffer from which they are retrieved for image analysis and displayed in the front panel as shown in Figure 5. The bright dots in the image window are living sperm in a rose chamber. The command tab allows the user to define different features in the experiment:

1. AutoStop: if checked, RATTS will track a sperm for pre-defined duration. If not checked, RATTS will track the sperm until the user press StopTracking or StropProgram button.
2. RealTime: if checked, the live images of sperm swimming are acquired and displayed on the front panel. If it is not checked, RATTS will load the saved image based on the directory in SSTA tab.
3. Decay: if checked, laser power is decayed after a sperm is trapped. Parameters are entered for maximum (or constant) laser power, rate of power decay, and if appropriate, duration of the trap in the Decay tab. If Decay is not checked, the laser power is held constant (0-420 mW at focal spot after the objective) for a fixed duration in the trapping phase of the experiment.

During real-time experiments, image analysis detects when a tracked sperm has reached a defined rectangular boundary near the extremity of the field of view. RATTS moves the microscope stage to position the sperm centroid at the center of the field of view. If Chase is checked (in command tab, Figure 5), the sperm centroid position is extrapolated using a multi-thresholding method to predict the sperm's position beyond the most recent image in order to compensate for swimming during the stage movement. Swimming parameters are calculated and saved in a continuously updated data file. Since new images arrive at 30 (or up to 90) frames per second, it is necessary to restrain net computation and data writing time to less than 33 ms (or less for the higher frame rates) in order to capture and process each image. RATTS is coded to use the most recent frame in the buffer. Sperm were recorded and tracked for extended durations to demonstrate variability in swimming parameters and variation in the swimming speed as a function of track length and track time.

The automated trapping mode of RATTS replaces our manual protocol as previously described (Nacimental, et al., 2006). User input is limited to setting parameters prior to an experiment and selecting, via the computer mouse, a sperm for analysis within the continuously updated image display. During the experiment, the user selects a sperm to be analyzed by clicking on its image with the arrow curser on the front panel of RATTS in Figure 5. The curser coordinate is registered, passed to the tracking algorithm and computation proceeds with no further intervention. Once the specified number of frames has been processed, the stage is moved to place the sperm under the laser trap and the shutter is opened.

During the trapping phase of the experiment, RATTS implements an escape detection subroutine to detect the presence of a sperm in the laser trap and to respond if the sperm escapes the trap. The subroutine monitors a small square pixel region (representing approximately 10 μm per side) centered about the laser trap. Using SSTA algorithms (Shi, et al., 2006a), the subroutine segments the image within this region and uses size threshold to detect the presence or absence of a sperm. A sperm must remain in the trap for a continuous 15 frames or the subroutine declares a failed trapping attempt.

During constant-power trapping experiments, the escape detection subroutine is used to ensure that, the sperm was successfully trapped, and second that it does not escape the trap during the trapping phase of an experiment. If the sperm is not initially trapped, RATTS will use the SSTA algorithm to again find the sperm and continue tracking it for a user-defined number of frames after which a new trapping attempt is made. RATTS will repeat this either until the sperm is trapped, or for a user-defined number of attempts. If a sperm escapes before the trap duration is completed, the algorithm will continue to track that sperm and attempt to re-trap it.

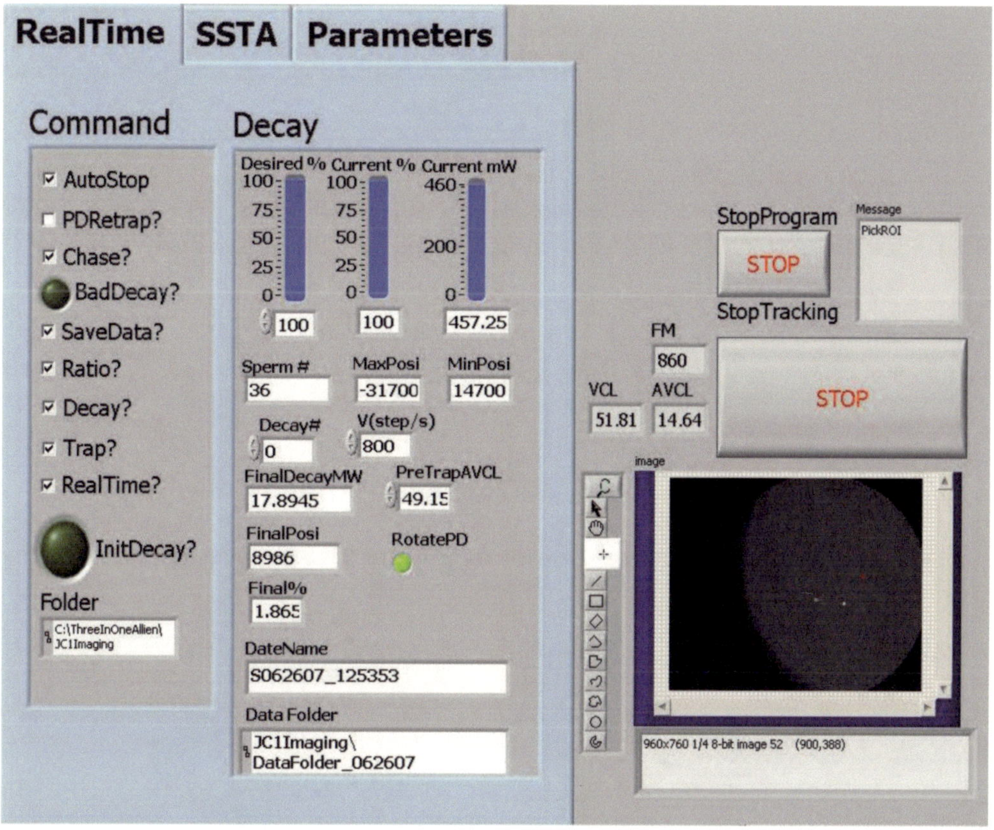

Figure 5. Front panel of RATTS system

In power decay experiments, the escape detection subroutine is used to ensure that a sperm is stably trapped. The laser power used to first trap a sperm is a user-defined percentage of maximum power (or maximum transmission through the polarizer). Once a sperm is stably trapped, RATTS automatically decays the laser power by rotating the polarizer until the sperm is capable of swimming away from the trap. Once the escape is detected, the polarizer position (and thus laser power) is written to hard disk and the polarizer is automatically rotated back to its starting position. A running file is updated at video rate or higher to record real-time swimming parameters including frame-by-frame centroid coordinates, position, and escape power. Figure 6 shows a flow diagram of the RATTS algorithm for power decay experiments.

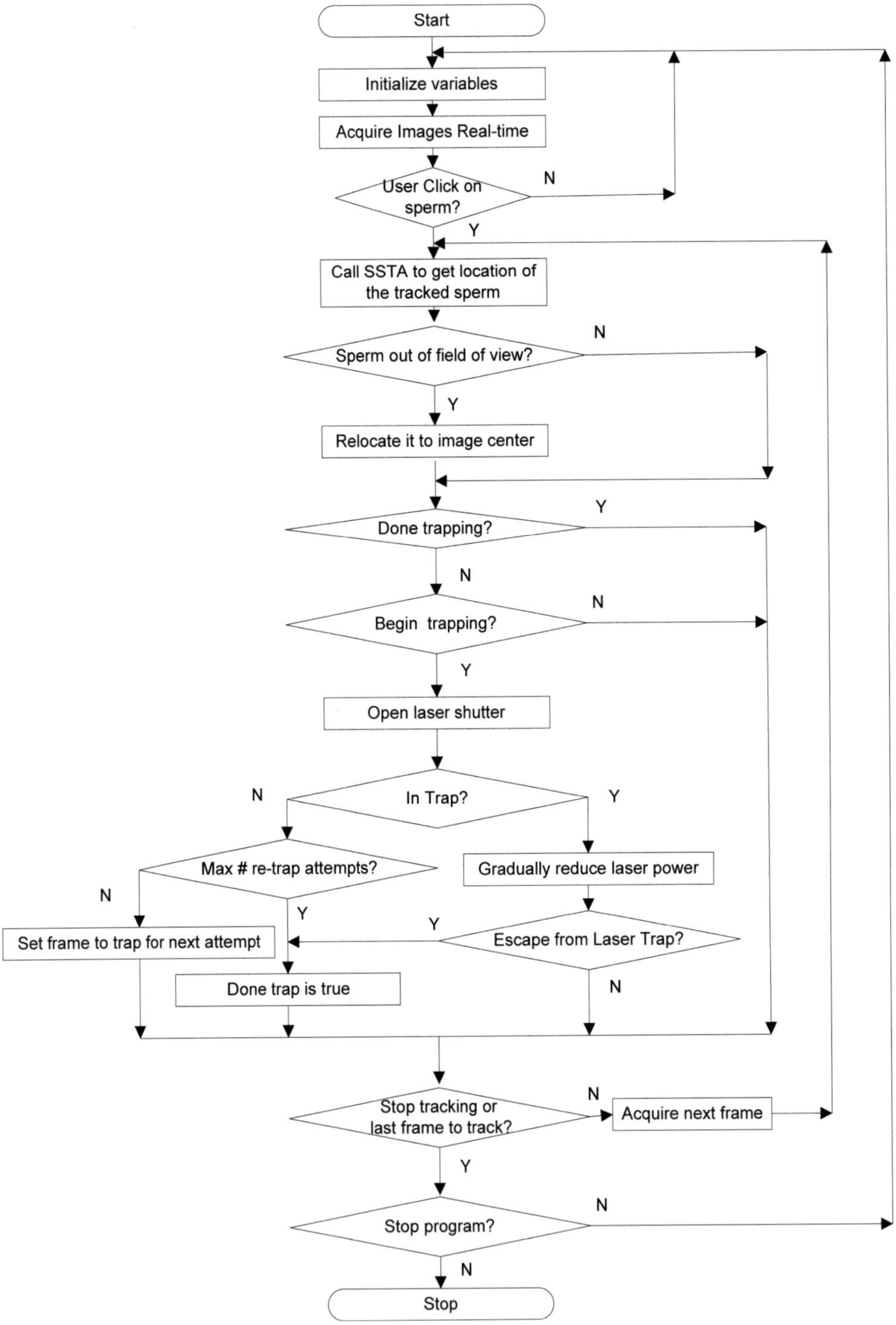

Figure 6. Flowchart of RATTS in power decay mode using the robotic laser tweezers microscope system (Shi, et al., 2006b)

4. Biological Experiments using Robolase Systems

The robotic laser scissors microscope system has been used to perform nano-surgery on both single microtubules as well as microtubule spindles in living cells (Botvinick & Berns, 2004, Wakida, et al., 2006, Conia, et al., 1997, Baker, et al., 2006, Shi, et al., 2006c). As Figure 7 demonstrates, a diffraction limited spot within a single fluorescent microtubule (transfected with a cyan fusion protein)in a live rat kangaroo kidney epithelial cell (Ptk2) can be ablated and the post-irradiation depolymerization can be observed in subsequent images . The single microtubule (Figure 7(a)) was positioned under the laser ablation crosshairs as shown in Figure 7(b). By pressing the "Fire at (0,0)" button (Figure 2), a 20ms macropulse (Botvinick, et al. 2004) was delivered to the microtubule. Figure 7(c-f) showed the microtubule depolymerizing at 1 s (Figure 7(c)), 5 s (Figure 7(d)), 10 s (Figure 7(e)), and 15 s (Figure 7(f)) post ablation.

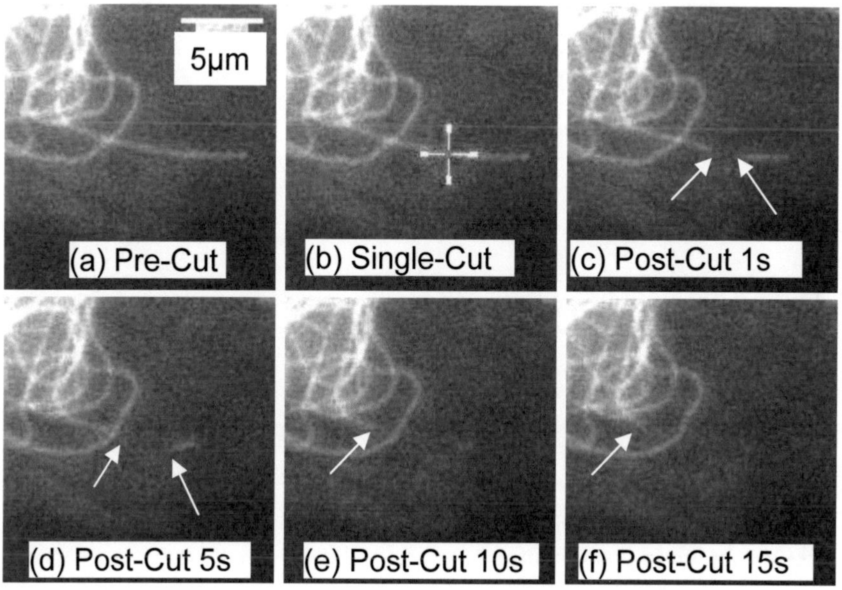

Figure 7. Effects on single microtubule of PTK2 cells using robotic laser scissors system. (a) Fluorescent image before laser exposure. (b) Crosshairs depict exact location of laser focal point during laser exposure. (c-f) Images captured immediately after laser exposure show a loss of fluorescence in the targeted region. (Shi, et al., 2006c, © 2006 IEEE, images courtesy of Nicole Wakida, University of California, Irvine)

Experiments using the robotic laser scissors microscope system have also shown that ablation across both mitotic half spindles (severing microtubule connections between the spindle pole and chromosome at the metaphase plate) immediately after anaphase-onset results in either the prevention or delay of cytokinesis. The machinery by which chromosomes move from the metaphase plate to the poles appeared to be unaffected in cells of the rat kangaroo line (PTK2) stably transfected by ECFP-tubulin (Figure 8). Anaphase onset can be observed in either phase contrast (Figure 8(a)) or fluorescence (Figure 8(b)) microscopy. The experimenter draws two rectangular regions of interest (Figure 8(c, d)) each of which are scanned by the ablation laser. Figure 8(e) shown a fluorescent image acquired 90 seconds after ablation demonstrating recovery of the mitotic spindle. The chromosomes still underwent pole-ward anaphase movements via spindle contraction as shown in the phase contrast (Figure 8(f)) and fluorescence (Figure 8(g)), but cytokinesis did not occur after several hours as shown in Figure 8(h).

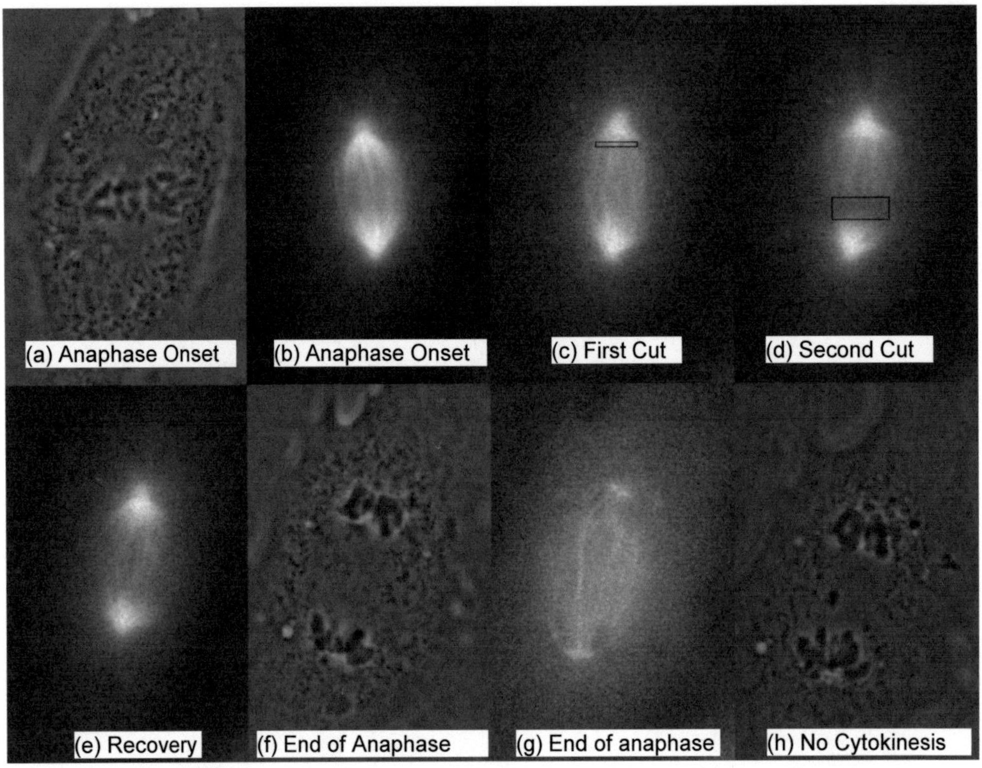

Figure 8. Anaphase spindle cutting of PTK2 cells using robotic laser scissors system. (a) Anaphase onset shown in phase contrast image. (b) Fluorescence image of anaphase onset. (c) Fluorescent image after the first cut. (d) Fluorescent image after the second cut. (e) Fluorescent image during recovery. (f) Phase contrast image at end of anaphase. (g) Fluorescent image at end of anaphase. (h) No cytokinesis after several hours (Shi, et al., 2006c, © 2006 IEEE, images courtesy of Norman Baker, University of California, San Diego)

The robotic laser tweezers microscope system has been used to study the sperm motility and swimming force (RATTS). RATTS can track and trap fast moving sperm in real-time (Figure 9). The continuous tracking mode can track single sperm over long durations. The longest duration we achieved was 11260 frames (6.25 min) for a dog sperm; its swimming trajectory is shown in Figure 9(a) (Note that the average survival time after the dog sperm is loaded to the microscope is about 20 min). The swimming trajectory of the sperm appears to be a relatively straight line when viewed in a stationary field of view as shown in the rectangle box (lower right corner) in Figure 9(a). The curvilinear velocity (VCL) in Figure 9(a) is 52 μm/s. Figure 9(b) shows an example of a single sperm tracked for 3 seconds, trapped it for 10 seconds (at 350 mW at focal spot), released, and tracked again for 3 seconds. The sperm changed swimming direction after laser trapping.

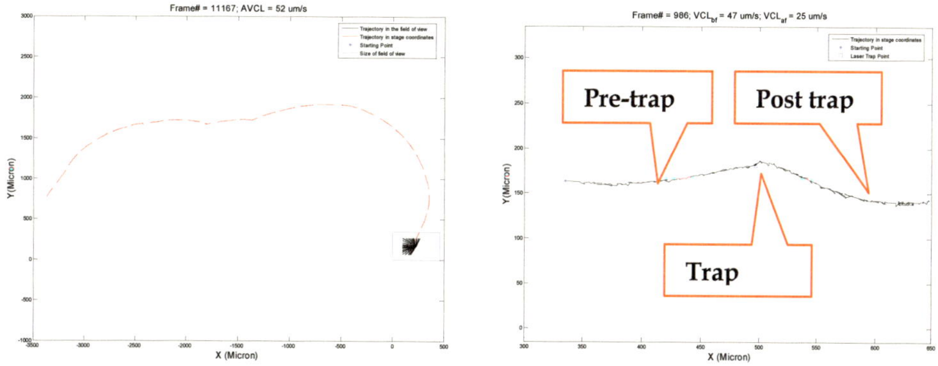

(a) (b)

Figure 9. Sperm trajectories using laser tweezers system. (a) Continuing tracking of single sperm for 6.25 min (b) Track and trap single sperm (Shi, et al., 2006b)

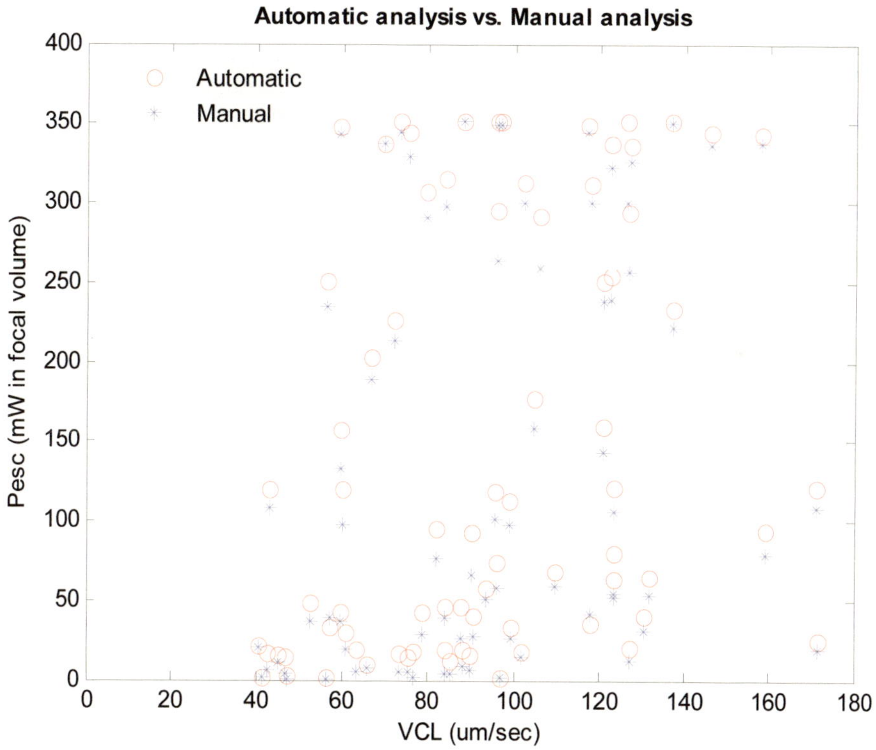

Figure 10. Escape power assessed manually and automatically. The scatter plot shows escape power determined by RATTS (◦) and by user mouse click (*) as a function of curvilinear swimming speed (VCL). Delay time is defined as the RATTS measurement minus the manual measurement. Delay times between RATTS and manual detection of escape had a mean and standard deviations of [0.46, 0.4] seconds with delays as long as 3

seconds. Scatter plots (not shown) of error against either VCL or the RATTS measurement show no non-linear relationship. Linear regression of errors as a function of VCL yields [slope = 0.06, $R^2 = 0.04$, $p = 0.1$], which casts doubt on a non-random relationship. Linear regression of errors against the RATTS measurement yields [slope = 0.02, $R^2 = 0.05$, $p < 0.05$], which indicates a very weak relationship, if any, with poor predictive power. Thus manual measurements cannot be corrected retrospectively (Shi, et al., 2006b)

To compare escape power measurements assessed manually or by RATTS, a subroutine was written to record the polarizer orientation when escape is register by the user (register as a mouse click) and by RATTS. The power decay continues until both RATTS and the user respond. Latency in the human response result in negatively biased laser power measurements since the polarizer continues to rotate until the mouse is clicked. Figure 10 shows escape laser power of each individual sperm measured manually (*) and by RATTS (◦). Manual measurements were less than or equal to those of RATTS 95% of the time. Delay times between RATTS and manual detection of escape had a mean and standard deviations of [0.46, 0.4] seconds with delays as long as 3 seconds (Shi, et al, 2006b).

The RATTS system can also be accessed through the internet (Logmein.com server) as showed in Figure11. Collaborators from the University of Queensland, Brisbane, Australia accessed RATTS. Dog sperm were loaded into a rose chamber and onto the Robolase at University of California, San Diego. Images of the sperm swimming were seen in Australia through the internet. One of the collaborators in Australia clicked on a swimming sperm "of-choice" (Figure 11(a)) to initialize the RATTS to track the sperm for the next 5 seconds. The sperm was then relocated to the laser trap position and held under the trap (410 mW at focal spot) for 10 seconds (Figure 11(b)).

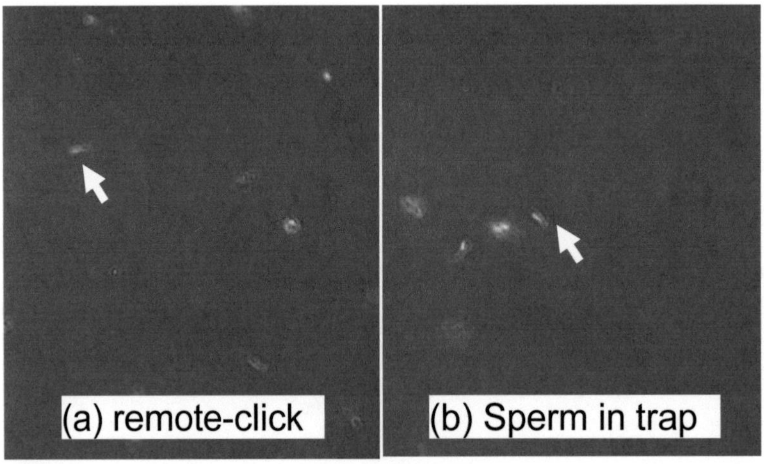

Figure 11. Remote-control of RATTS. (a) Collaborator from Australia clicked on a selected swimming dog sperm on the image screen in Australia which then activated RATTS in the UCSD lab. (b) The same sperm in (a) was held in the laser trap after tracking it for 5 seconds. It was trapped for 10 seconds (Shi, et al., 2006c, © 2006 IEEE)

5. Conclusion and future work

In this paper, the structure and features of the robotic laser scissors and laser tweezers microscope systems are presented. The Robolase systems are shown to be accessible through the internet using the Logmein program, making it feasible to perform biological experiments with remote collaborators. Future developments may involve the creation of separate log-in software for simultaneous use by more than two users/collaborators as well as the use of dedicated fiber-optic lines between different locations.

The robotic laser scissors microscope system can be used to ablate a single microtubule and to study the subsequent depolymerization. Ablating of both mitotic half spindles immediately after anaphase-onset was shown to prevent or delay cytokinesis while preserving chromosome pole-ward movement. We demonstrated that the robotic laser tweezers microscope system can be used to study sperm motility by integrating real-time measurements of swimming parameters and laser tweezers assessment of swimming force. To facilitate remote operation of experiments, the user is allowed to select from different types of sperm analysis experiments: continuous tracking experiments to measure motility within a population, track and trap experiments at constant power to determine affects on sperm motility, and track and trap experiments with decaying laser power to study the relationship between sperm motility and sperm swimming force.

The RoboLase systems are now being used in a variety of other biological experiments, including the molecular mechanism of DNA repair. Since the laser ablation can generate patterned DNA damage in defined areas of the nucleus at defined points in the cell cycle (Lisby & Rothstein, 2004), it is becoming a very powerful tool to study DNA repair mechanisms (Gomez-Godinez, et al., 2006). The studies involve studying the molecular mechanisms underlying the activation of checkpoints and the control of the progression through the cell cycle following laser-induced DNA damage (results not shown). Note that different pulse energies and irradiances will produce different damage modalities, and likely recruit different repair molecules. The Robolase project is pursuing this in multiple Robolase systems with nano, pico, and femto second lasers, as well as cw UV lasers (Chen, et al., 2005, Wakida, et al., 2006, Gomez-Godinez, et al., 2006, Baker, et al., 2006).

6. Acknowledgements

This work was supported by grants of the United States Air Force (AFOSR # F9620-00-1-0371) and of the National Institute of Health (NIH RR 14892). Dr. Botvinick would like to thank the Arnold and Mabel Beckman Foundation's Beckman Fellow's program for supporting his research. We would like to give special thanks to David Little and George Wu, for helping develop the code of RoboLase, Jaclyn Nascimento and Charilie Chandsawangbhuwana for their contribution of RATTS, Norman Baker for the mitotic study (Figure 8), and Nicole Wakida for the microtubule study (Figure 7). We also thank Halina Rubensztein-Dunlop and her laboratory at the University of Queensland Australia for participating as "remote" users in the on-line proof of concept experiments.

7 References

Baker, N. M., Botvinick, E. L., Shi, L. Z., Wu, G. & Berns, M. B. (2006). Mitotic spindle studied using laser scissors, *SPIE Optics & Photonics conference*, San Diego, August 2006, 6326.

Bao, Z., Murray, J. I., Boyle, T., Ooi, S. L., Sandel, M. J. & Waterston, R. H. (2006). Automated cell lineage tracing in Caenorhabditis elegans. *Proc Natl Acad Sci*, U S A., February 2006, Vol. 103(8), pp. 2707–2712

Berns, M. W. & Greulich, K. O (2007). *Laser Manipulation of cells and tissues. In Methods in Cell Biology*. Academic Press Inc. ISBN-13: 978-0-12-370648-5, San Diego, CA, USA.

Berns, M. W., Tadir, Y., Liang, H. & Tromberg, B. (1998) *Laser scissors and tweezers. In: Methods in Cell Biology*. M. P. Sheetz (ed.). Academic Press, Inc, San Diego, CA, Vol. 55, pp. 71-97.

Berns, M. W., Botvinick, E. L., Liaw, L., Sun, C-H. & Shah, J. (2005). Micromanipulation of chromosomes and the mitotic spindle using laser microsurgery (laser scissors) and laser-induced optical forces (laser tweezers), *Cell biology: a laboratory handbook*. Burlington, MA: Elsevier Press

Bloem, J., Veninga, M. & Shepherd, J. (1995). Fully Automatic Determination of Soil Bacterium Numbers, Cell Volumes, and Frequencies of Dividing Cells by Confocal Laser Scanning Microscopy and Image Analysis. *Appl Environ Microbiol*. Vol. 61(3), pp. 926-936

Brodland, G. W. & Veldhuis, J. H. (1998). Three-dimensional reconstruction of live embryos using robotic macroscope images. *IEEE Trans Biomed Eng*. Vol. 45(9), pp. 1173-1181

Botvinick, E. L. & Berns, M. W. (2005). Internet-based robotic laser scissors and tweezers microscopy, *Microsc Res Tech*. Vol. 68(2), pp. 65-74

Botvinick, E.L., Venugopalan, V., Shah, J.V., Liaw, L.H., Berns, M,W.(2004). Controlled ablation of microtubules using a picosecond laser.*Biophys J*. Vol. 87(6), pp. 4203-12

Burgess, J. R., Sandberg, G. D., Myers, C. P., Bigott, T. R. & Greenspan, R. B. (2002). Use of robotic telepathology for frozen-section diagnosis: a retrospective trial of a telepathology system for intraoperative consultation, *Mod Pathol*. Vol. 15(11), pp. 1197-1204

Chen, B. P.C., Chan, D. W., Kobayashi, J., Burma, S., Asaithamby, A., Yano, K., Botvinick, E. F., Qin, J. & Chen, D. J. (2005). Cell cycle dependence of DNA-PK phosphorylation in response to DNA double strand breaks. *J. Biological Chemistry*, Vol: 280, pp. 14709-15

Chumbley L.S., Cassucio G., Kritikos D., Lentz H., Mannes C. & Mehta K. (2002). Development of a web-based SEM specifically for K-12 education. *Microsc Res Tech*, Vol. 56(6), pp.454-461

Cohen, A. R., Roysam, B. & Turner, J. N. (1994). Automated tracing and volume measurements of neurons from 3-D confocal fluorescence microscopy data. *J Microsc*. Vol. 173(2), pp. 103-14

Conia, J., Edwards, B. S. & Voelkel, S. (1997). The micro-robotic laboratory: optical trapping and scissing for the biologist, *J. Clin Lab Anal*., Vol. 11(1), pp. 28-38

Della Mea, V., Cataldi, P., Pertoldi, B. & Beltrami, C. A. (2000). Combining dynamic and static robotic telepathology: a report on 184 consecutive cases of frozen sections, histology and cytology, *Anal Cell Pathol.* Vol. 20(1), pp. 33-39

Gomez-Godinez, V., Wakida, N. M., Dvornikov, A. S., Yokomori, K. & Berns, M.W. (2007). Recruitment of DNA damage recognition and repair pathway proteins following near-IR femtosecond laser irradiation of cells. *J Biomed Opt.* Vol. 12(2), 020505

Hadida-Hassan M., Young S. J., Peltier S. T., Wong M., Lamont S. & Ellisman M. H. (1999). Web-based telemicroscopy. *J Struct Biol.* Vol. 125(2-3), pp. 235-245

He, W., Hamilton, T. A., Cohen, A. R., Holmes, T. J., Pace, C., Szarowski, D. H., Turner, J. N. & Roysam, B. (2003). Automated Three-Dimensional Tracing of Neurons in Confocal and Brightfield Images. *Microsc Microanal.* Vol. 9(4), pp. 296-310

Kaplan K. J., Burgess J. R., Sandberg G. D., Myers C. P., Bigott T. R. & Greenspan R. B. (2002). Use of robotic telepathology for frozen-section diagnosis: a retrospective trial of a telepathology system for intraoperative consultation. *Mod Pathol.* Vol. 15(11), pp. 1197-1204.

Knight, C. G., Lorincz, A., Cao, A., Gidell, K., Klein, M. D. & Langenburg, S. E. (2005). Computer-assisted, robot-enhanced open microsurgery in an animal model, *J Laparoendosc Adv Surg Tech A.* Vol. 15(2), pp. 182-185

Kuang, W., Shin, P. R., Oder, M. & Thomas Jr. A. J. (2005) Robotic-assisted vasovasostomy: a two-layer technique in an animal model. *Urology.* Vol. 65(4), pp.811-814

Lin, W., Wilder, J., Grossman, S. & Foran, D. J. (2003). A network-reactive model for distributed telemicroscopy. *J Telemed Telecare.* Vol. 9(2), pp. 78-83

Lisby, M. & Rothstein R. (2004). DNA damage checkpoint and repair centers, Current opinion in Cell Bio., Vol. 16, pp. 328-334.

Parkin S., Knöner G., Singer W., Nieminen T. A., Heckenberg N. R., Rubinsztein-Dunlop H. (2007). Optical torque on microscopic objects. *Methods Cell Biol.* Vol. 82, pp. 525-61

Prasad, P. N., (2003). *Introduction to biophotonics*, John Wiley & Sons, Inc., Hoboken, New Jersey

Molnar B., Berczi L., Diczhazy C., Tagscherer A., Varga S. V., Szende B. & Tulassay Z. (2003). Digital slide and virtual microscopy based routine and telepathology evaluation of routine gastrointestinal biopsy specimens. *J Clin Pathol*, Vol. 56(6), pp.433-438

Nascimento, J. M., Botvinick, E. L., Shi, L. Z., Durrant, B. & Berns, M. W. (2006). Analysis of sperm motility using optical tweezers. *J. Biomed Opt.*, Vol. 11(4), 044001

Shi, L. Z., Nascimento, J. M., Berns, M. W. & Botvinick, E. L. (2006). Computer-based tracking of single sperm. *J. Biomed Opt*, Vol. 11(5), 054009

Shi, L. Z., Nascimento, J. M., Chandsawangbhuwana, C., Berns, M. W. & Botvinick, E. L. (2006). Real-time Automated Tracking and Trapping System (RATTS) for Sperm. *Microsc Res Tech.* Vol. 69(11), pp. 894-902

Shi, L. Z., Nascimento, Wakida, N., Dvornikov, A., Baker, N., Botvinick, E. L. & Berns, M. W. (2006). "RoboLase", A robotic laser scissors and laser tweezers microscope. *40th Asilomar Conference on Signals, Systems, and Computers*, pp. 173-177, Asilomar, CA, Oct. 2006, IEEE Processing.

Szymas, J., Wolf, G., Papierz, W., Jarosz, B. & Weinstein, R. S. (2001). Online Internet-based robotic telepathology in the diagnosis of neuro-oncology cases: a teleneuropathology feasibility study. *Hum Pathol.* Vol. 32(12), pp. 1304-1308

Takaoka A., Yoshida K., Mori H., Hayashi S., Young S. J. & Ellisman M. H. (2000). International telemicroscopy with a 3 MV ultrahigh voltage electron microscope. *Ultramicroscopy,* Vol. 83(1-2), pp. 93-101

Wakida, N. M., Lee, C. S., Botvinick, E. L., Shi, L. Z., Dvornikov, A. & Berns, M. W. (2006). Laser Nanosurgery of Single Microtubules Reveals Time and Location Dependent Depolymerization Rates. *J. Biomed Opt,* Vol. 12(2)

Yamada A., Hirahara O., Tsuchida T., Sugano N., Date M. (2003). A practical method for the remote control of the scanning electron microscope. *J Electron Microsc.* Vol. 52(2), pp. 101-109.

Yeom, S., Javidi, B. (2006). Automatic identification of biological microorganisms using three-dimensional complex morphology. *J Biomed Opt.* Vol. 11(2), 024017

Youngblom J. H., Youngblom J. J., Wilkinson J. (2001). TelePresence Confocal Laser Scanning Microscopy. *Microsc Microanal,* Vol. 7(3), pp.241-248

30

Robot Attack on Vascular Surgery

Petr Štádler
Na Homolce Hospital, Department of Vascular Surgery and Department of Cardiovascular Surgery, Charles University, First Medical Faculty and General Teaching Hospital, Prague Czech Republic

1. Introduction

Over the past few years, technological developments in global medicine have given rise to a whole series of new surgical techniques, particularly in minimally invasive surgery (Dion et al., 1996). Few people can now imagine general surgery or gynaecology without laparoscopic techniques, although this was not initially the case. Laparoscopic interventions reduce patient trauma, lower treatment and recovery times and, finally, also reduce overall treatment costs. Major developments in laparoscopic surgery in the 1990s have had an impact on vascular surgery. Minimally invasive approaches used in general surgery have gradually become a novel technique used in vascular surgery. Laparoscopy was introduced into vascular surgery much later than other areas and was approached with far greater apprehension, as well as with limited interest, by a number of renowned vascular surgeons, who were censorious of it from the very beginning (Dion et al., 1998). The main reasons for this lack of interest in laparoscopic vascular surgery were the difficulties associated with suturing of the vascular anastomosis, the long clamping times and complications in accessing the aorta and pelvic arteries, which are located low down next to the spine. On an imaginary scale of difficulty, vascular laparoscopic techniques would score extremely high, vascular surgeons in general have very little experience of laparoscopy and the learning curve is a long one. These are probably the main reasons preventing the further expansion of vascular laparoscopy, although there are centres in both Europe and the United States that are actively using vascular laparoscopic methods. Total laparoscopic aortoiliac surgery can be performed on patients with occlusive diseases and aneurysms.
Robotics, which began to appear in 2000, is a state-of-the-art surgical technology (Marescaux et al., 2001). The Department of Vascular Surgery at Prague's Na Homolce Hospital has been performing laparoscopic reconstructions since 2003 and these have been robot-assisted since the end of 2005. Under the direction of Dr. Petr Štádler, the robotic vascular team has not only created its own modified transperitoneal approach for these interventions, but has catapulted Czech robotic vascular surgery to the forefront of this modality worldwide. (Fig. 1. Robotic master console).

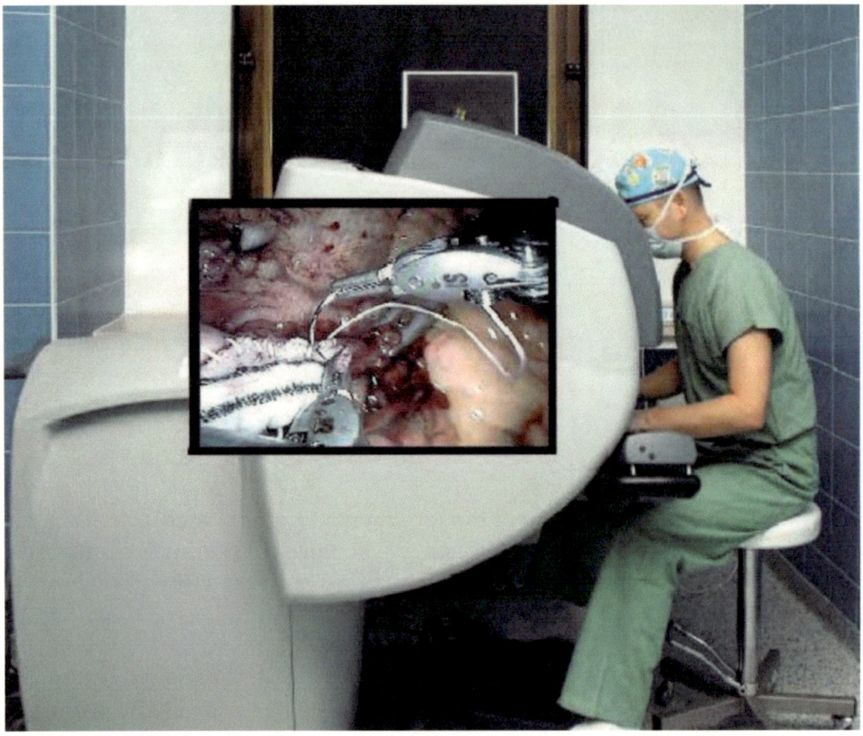

Figure 1. Robotic master console

2. Robotic Surgery and Medical Simulation

Robotic surgery and medical simulation have much in common: both use a mechanized interface that provides feedback from the patient to the health care professional, or physician, both use monitors to visualize the performance of the procedure, and both use computer software applications through which the physician interacts. Both technologies are experiencing rapid adoption and are viewed as modalities that allow physicians to perform increasingly complex minimally invasive procedures while enhancing patient safety.

The growing experience of physicians with medical simulation and robotic surgery brings new benefits (O'Toole et al., 1999). The increasing success and use of robotics will lead to a growth in the need for trained physicians with the appropriate licence to provide patients with complex medical services. The role played by simulation in the certification of these professionals also forms an important part of medical training programmes. Many professional medical societies and training programmes use this type of technology to assess the ability of health care professionals during the certification procedure.

2.1 Robotic Surgery

Robotic surgery can be characterized as an operation that uses a computer-controlled robotic system. The advantage of this technique is that it does not require direct contact between the patient and surgeon, while also significantly enhancing the precision of the surgery by eliminating tremor from the surgeon's hands and providing perfect 3D visualization. It is also now possible to perform surgical interventions in places that would be hard to access using classical surgical or laparoscopic techniques. This means that this type of operation can significantly enhance patient safety (Talamini et al., 2003).

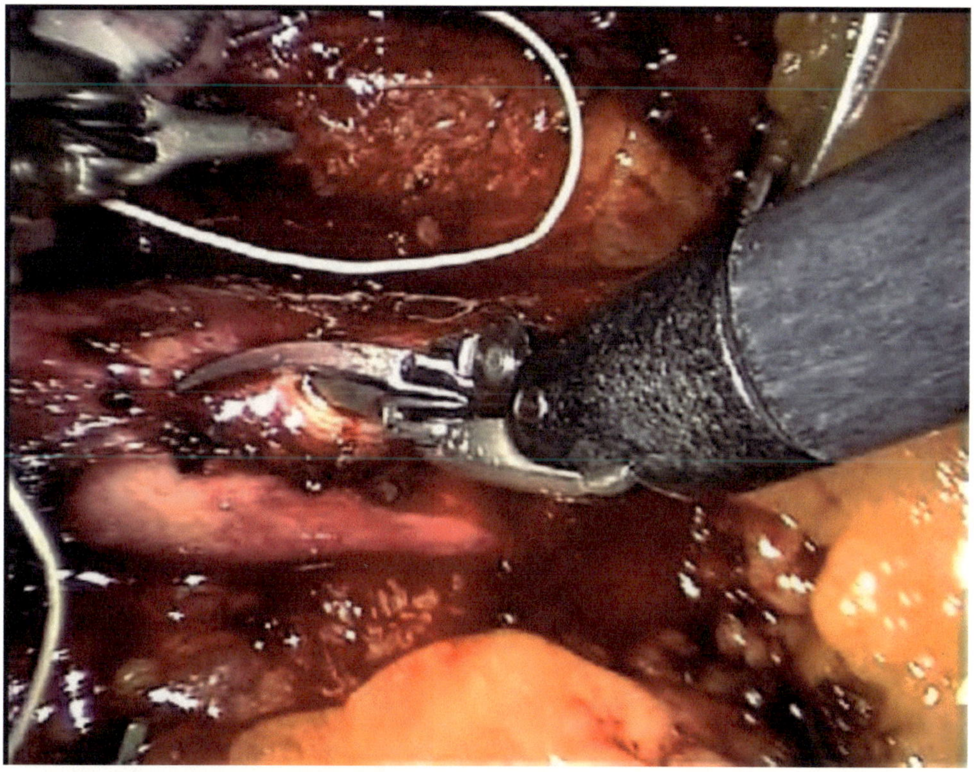

Figure 2. Robotic scissors - aortotomy

2.2 The da Vinci Robotic System

The da Vinci surgical robot is a system with multiple arms and composed of three principal parts. The first is the patient-side cart, which can have three or even four arms. The second part is the instrument tower and the third the surgeon's console, from which the arms and instruments are operated and where the 3D visualization provides the surgeon with a perfect view of the operative field in the patient's body. Other surgical team members can follow the procedure on television screens located in the operating theatre itself. A powerful computer is an essential part of the system.

Unlike laparoscopic instruments, which do not have flexible ends, robotic instruments copy the movements of the human hand (using the Endo-Wrist® technology) and are easy to manipulate, even in more inaccessible areas. The computer adjusts all movements in order to enhance the safety and precision of the surgical instruments in the patient's body. This, together with the elimination of tremor from the surgeon's hands, significantly reduces the risks associated with surgery (Nio et al., 2005).

The da Vinci robot was originally developed by NASA for the American army to use on aircraft carriers or during space flights, enabling surgeons to perform remote interventions from base. The civilian version of the robot has been available for use by physicians since 2000.

This is not a classical robot in the narrower sense of the word, as the procedure is performed by a surgeon who uses the technology to enhance his/her surgical skills. The robot cannot perform the intervention itself and simply translates the movements of the surgeon's hands.
Robot-assisted surgery has raised laparoscopic surgery to a higher level of quality and, given the almost perfect movements of the instruments, the system inflicts less damage on the surrounding tissues. The successful use of robotics in surgery depends on an understanding of all the technical functions of the robotic equipment, sufficient experience of classical laparoscopy and teamwork. No less important is the improved orientation of the surgeon in the operative field, with the new opportunities afforded by the robotic visualization and instrument flexibility. (Fig. 2. Robotic scissors - aortotomy).
In the USA and the western states of the European Union, a highly efficient training course has been developed for robotic surgical teams, which is required as part of the delivery package for robotic surgery centres.
The first level prioritises the understanding of all the technical functions of the equipment, coordination and teamwork, and preparing patients for the procedure, while the second stage focuses on the surgeon's orientation in the operating field using the new options offered by robotic visualization and the mobility of the equipment. During the third stage, which is seen as building additional endoscopic skills, the surgeon is shown clinically tested procedures that are robotically assisted in his/her area of specialization.

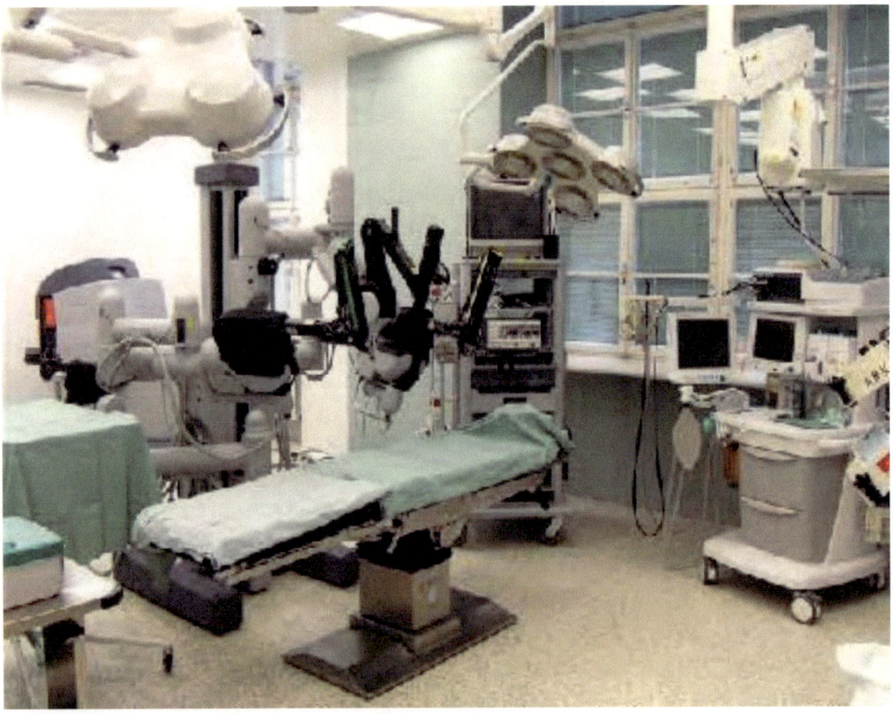

Figure 3. Robotic Surgery Centre

2.3 The Multidisciplinary Robotic Surgery Centre

Robotic surgery today is developing into a multidisciplinary modality used by surgical departments that deal with the soft tissue structures in the abdominal or thoracic cavities. It also uses all the advantages of minimally invasive methods. It is specifically used for general abdominal surgery, gynaecology, urology, oncosurgery, thoracic surgery, vascular surgery and cardiac surgery. (Fig. 3. Robotic surgery centrum).

Robotic surgery centres are generally established as a separate multidisciplinary operating theatre, shared among the individual specialists to perform field-specific procedures. Over time, a number of these multidisciplinary centres have become characterized by dominant specialities led by individuals who have achieved exceptional outcomes in robotic surgery, often becoming single-disciplinary specialized robotic units, which may often require a separate robotic system to be established in the same health care facility. This leads to a concentration of highly specialized care and an increase in the number of procedures from a wider catchment area. The final outcome of this process is a dramatic rise in the quality of care, as a correlation of the number of interventions performed.

2.4 The Introduction of Robotics into Vascular Surgery

The introduction of robotics has led to a fundamental turning point for laparoscopic vascular surgery, which has always entailed relatively difficult manipulation with instruments and required a long time to construct the anastomosis, leading to long aortal clamping times. The robotic system removes these fundamental disadvantages of laparoscopy and opens up the possibility of expanding robot-assisted laparoscopic surgery in this area (Wisselink et al., 2002).

At the present time, the Department of Vascular Surgery at Na Homolce Hospital performs a range of vascular reconstructions of the pelvic arteries and abdominal aorta. This has ranked the hospital alongside a small number of centres worldwide, these can be counted on the fingers of one hand, where robotic-assisted vascular reconstructions are routinely performed. Our physicians are planning future expansion of the "range" of these procedures to include other types of vascular reconstructions (Štádler et al., 2006,b).

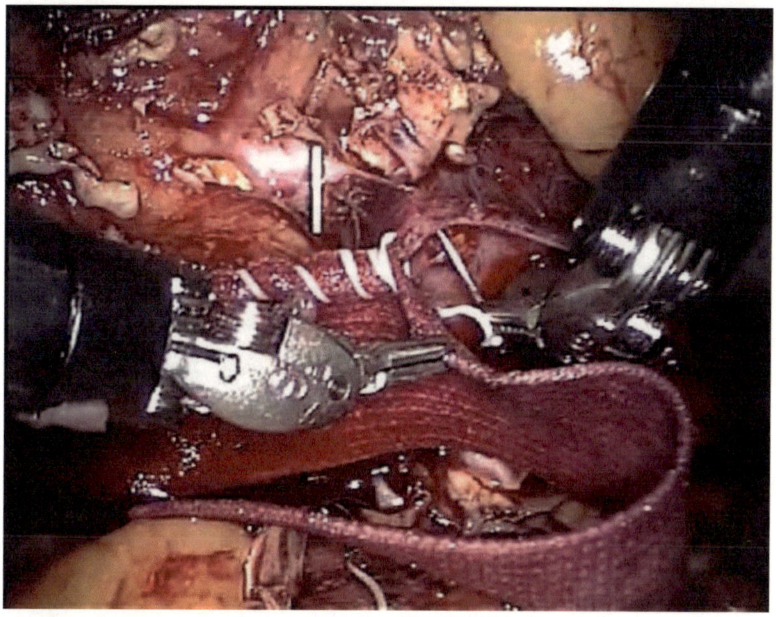

Figure 4. Aortoiliac prosthetic patch

Thanks to the early introduction of robotic surgery in the Czech Republic and the progressive nature of the robotic team, the opportunity has arisen, with the support of the manufacturer, to create another training centre for central and eastern European states in the Czech Republic. We should not fail to mention the international recognition achieved by the vascular robotic team at Prague's Na Homolce Hospital, a team that, through its perseverance and excellent medical outcomes, is training new teams in countries such as the USA, the country that originated robotic surgery. As an example, the first robotic-assisted abdominal aortal reconstruction was performed in the first week of February 2007 by a team of surgeons from the Baptist Memorial University Hospital in Memphis in the American state of Tennessee, under the direction of Dr. Petr Štádler from Na Homolce Hospital in Prague.

3. Robotic Surgery in the Czech Republic

November 2005 saw the beginning of an era of robot-assisted minimally invasive surgery in the Czech Republic. The first facilities to decide to install a Centre of Robotic Surgery with the da Vinci robotic system have now taken a wide lead. They are lecturing on their successes both at home and abroad, attend courses abroad not only as trainees but now also as trainers, even in the da Vinci robotic system's country of origin. These centres are negotiating with professional associations, health insurance companies and political representatives and are creating the environment for those who are now deciding to introduce robotic surgery.

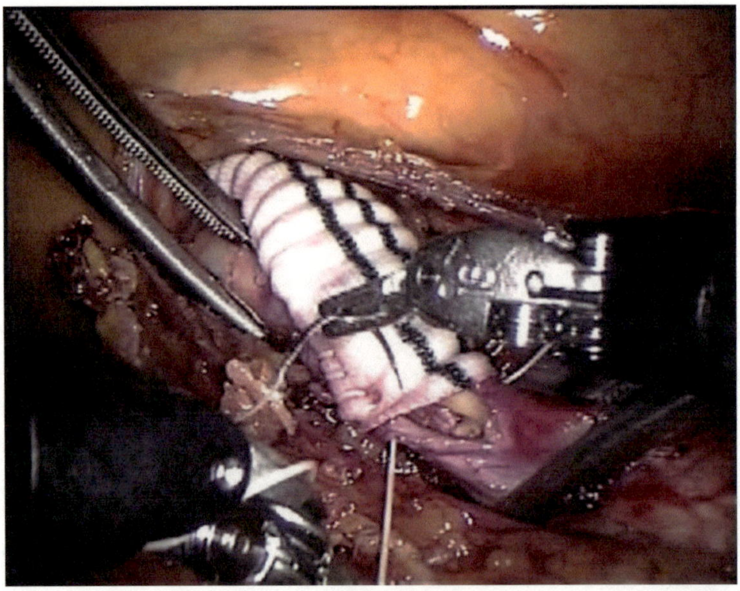

Figure 5. Central anastomosis of a right iliofemoral bypass

3.1 Robotic Vascular Surgery in Na Homolce Hospital, Prague

The da Vinci 1200 robotic system has been used in Na Homolce Hospital, Prague for a range of surgical disciplines since November 2005. The hospital's robotic vascular surgery achievements rank it among the world-class institutions performing these procedures and,

in terms of their number and outcomes, would be at the top of an imaginary ladder of globally renowned centres. Some of these procedures have been performed for the first time ever with robotic assistance (an operation on an isolated common pelvic arterial aneurysm or the reconstruction of the abdominal aorta by prosthetic patch). (Fig. 4. Aortoiliac prosthetic patch). The fact that the experience of the Homolka vascular robotic team is accepted, not only by Czech centres, but that there is also great interest in its work from abroad, is evidenced by the number of international lectures and publications they produce.
To date, over 70 robotic-assisted arterial reconstructions have been performed in the aorto-iliac area and a total of over 120 general laparoscopic vascular procedures (including robot-assisted). Experience of laparoscopic vascular surgery is seen as a prerequisite for performing robot-assisted vascular operations.
The robotic vascular surgery team in Prague's Na Homolce Hospital, led by Dr. Petr Štádler, has developed surgical procedures for aorto- and ilio- femoral bypasses, endarterectomies of the abdominal aorta and resection and replacement of abdominal aortal aneurysms, which are now performed as standard practice. (Fig. 5. Central anastomosis of an right iliofemoral bypass, Fig. 6. Aortoiliac thromboendarterectomy, Fig. 7. Distal anastomosis of AAA). The physicians have been able to find optimal locations for ports to facilitate the use of the robotic system in vascular surgery. The basis for robotic vascular reconstruction is the modified transperitoneal approach, a description of which was published in Europe and in the USA.

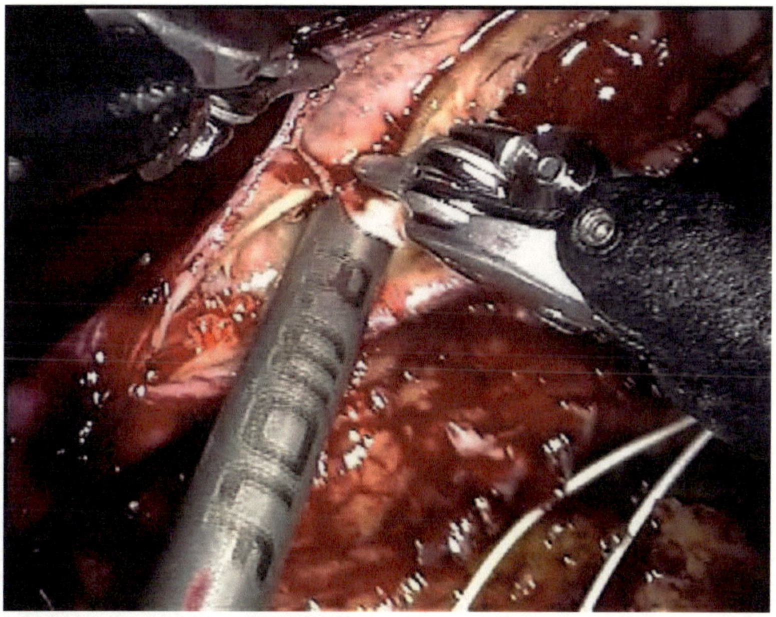

Figure 6. Aortoiliac thromboendarterectomy

3.2 A Modified Technique of Transperitoneal Direct Approach

This modified procedure is offered to all robot-assisted patients. The da Vinci robotic system is positioned for use on the patient's right side. The patient is placed on his or her right side at a 30-45° angle, in a mild Trendelenburg position (10° to 15°), with the left arm lying along the length of the body. Trocar positioning is slightly different from conventional laparoscopy because of the volume of the articulating robotic arms. The pneumoperitoneum

is secured via a minor left subcostal incision with an abdominal pressure of 12 mm Hg. An 12-mm trocar for the robotic arm is introduced. The next three 12-mm trocars are inserted below the costal margin for the laparoscopic instruments during the first part of operation and for the robotic arms, for the assistant´s port and the robotic camera in the second part. Two 12-mm ports are inserted on the midline for the central and distal aortic or pelvic clamp. (Fig. 8. Position of trocars). Dissections of the aorta and iliac arteries are performed laparoscopically. The retroperitoneum is opened on the left side of the aorta from its bifurcation to the left renal vein alongside the left gonadal vein. The posterior peritoneum with preaortic fat and ganglia is liberated as necessary up to the right aortic wall and stitched up to the parietal peritoneum (Štádler et al., 2006,a). Thus, mobilization of the entire descending colon is not required. (Fig. 9. Fixed posterior peritoneum - perioperative view)
The subrenal aorta and both common iliac arteries are exposed, and the inferior mesenteric artery is usually temporarily clipped except for abdominal aortic aneurysm (AAA) resection. In patients who have had an AAA, the inferior mesenteric artery is interrupted and visible lumbar arteries are clipped. After the aneurysmal sac is opened, the robotic technique is used to internally control the remaining lumbar arteries with free 4-0 shortened polytetrafluoroethylene stitches. Tunnelling is performed from one or two groins under the direct view of the laparoscopic video camera using a long DeBakey aortic vascular clamp. A conventional knitted Dacron vascular prosthesis (Albograft, Sorin Biomedica Cardio, SpA, Saluggia, Italy), with attached shortened 3-0 or 4-0 Gore-Tex suture (W. L. Gore & Associates, Flagstaff, Ariz) is inserted into the abdomen through an 12-mm trocar. The robotic system is used to construct the central anastomosis (twice for both anastomoses in the case of tube grafts), to perform a thromboendarterectomy, and mostly for posterior peritoneal suturing. The role of the assistant at the patient's side is limited to exposure, assisting in the dissection, haemostasis, and maintaining traction on the running sutures performed by the robot.

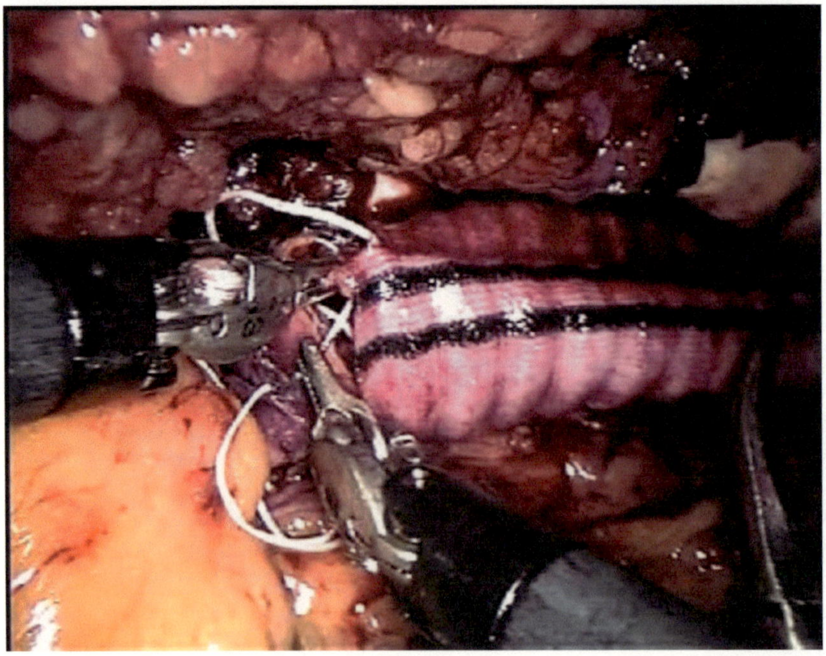

Figure 7. Distal anastomosis of AAA

3.3 Advantages and Disadvantages of the Robot-Assisted Vascular Procedure

From a practical point of view, the greatest advantage of the robot-assisted procedure has proved to be the speed of construction of the vascular anastomosis. This has helped to eliminate the largest disadvantage of laparoscopic vascular reconstruction - lengthy clamping time. Reducing the time needed to construct the anastomosis also shortens the period of ischaemia temporary of the lower limbs while the aortal clamps are being placed. This represents a significant reduction in the level of stress placed on the heart and muscular reperfusion and leads to better post-operative results, including morbidity and mortality. These times are now comparable to those of standard vascular surgery, and provide all the advantages of minimally invasive surgical techniques. Patients mainly benefit through shorter hospitalization periods and an early return to their normal activities and working life, which, in most cases, is not significantly restricted. Another important factor is the excellent cosmetic result. A further advantage of this method is that it can also be used with obese patients, where standard interventions are technically demanding and often involve problems with the healing of wounds after laparoscopy. The main disadvantage is still the high price, not only of the robotic system, but also of the individual instruments, which have a pre-determined life expectancy, and in the case of vascular surgery, the need to combine robotic and standard laparoscopy.

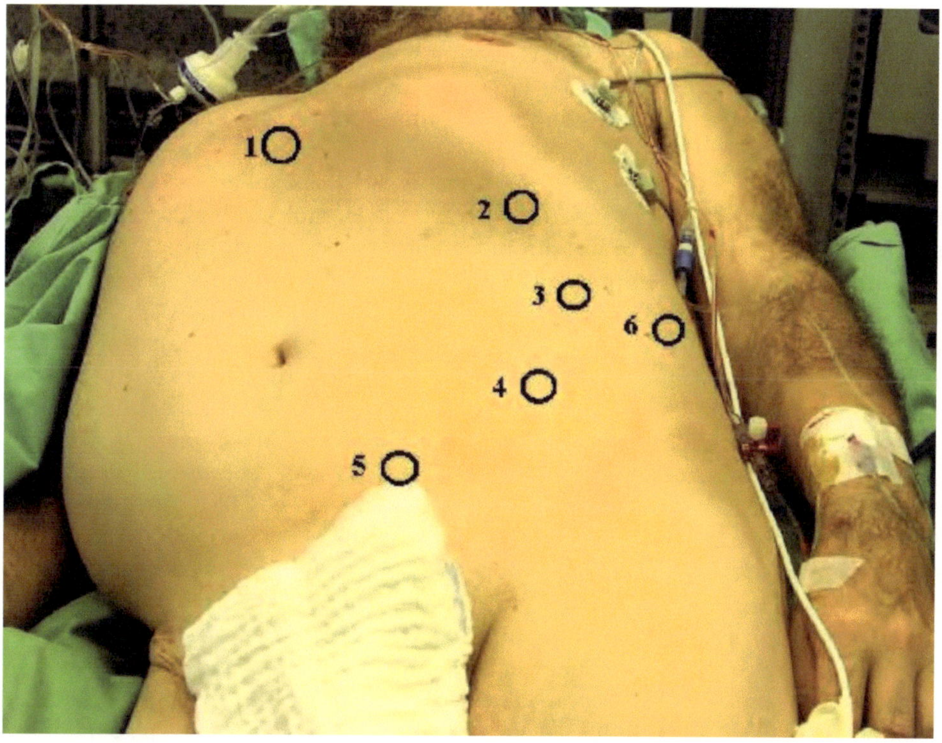

Figure 8. Position of trocars (1, central clamp; 2, and 4, robotic arms; 3, robotic camera; 5, distal clamp; 6, assistant´s port)

When this method was being introduced, particularly at the beginning, mostly younger patients, with no associated disorders, were being indicated. Alongside the increasing experience of the team, the circle of suitable candidates for robotic-assisted procedures is constantly being widened. However, operations on the abdominal aorta are generally extremely traumatic for patients and are associated with a high level of risk, particularly for polymorbid patients with more serious forms of ischaemic heart disease and failing renal and respiratory functions. Patients suffering from acute forms of obstructive pulmonary disease are not suitable for either laparoscopic or robot-assisted procedures, given the need for a capnoperitoneum. A contraindication for capnoperitoneum automatically entails a contraindication for laparoscopic-robotic vascular procedures. On the other hand, physicians from Prague had a successful experience with two patients with severe left ventricular dysfunction after myocardial infarction (25 and 29%). They performed robot-assisted procedures with low pressure pneumoperitoneum (8-10 mm Hg).

Neither may patients be indicated for these interventions after major intra-abdominal operations with numerous peritoneal accretions, but adhesions after previous laparotomy may sometimes help to create a clear working field. Obesity is no longer a major contraindication.

3.4 Results of our own Robot-Assisted Vascular Procedures

Robot-assisted vascular surgery can be of value in overcoming the long learning curve for laparoscopic suturing of vascular anastomoses. In the reported total laparoscopic procedures by Štádler team, the mean operating time was 259 minutes (range, 150 to 420 minutes), and the clamping time was 69 minutes (range, 35 to 150). When compared with our robot-assisted vascular procedures, the times for laparoscopic procedures and aortoiliac cross-clamping were longer.

From November 2005 to June 2007, 70 robot-assisted aortoiliac reconstructions were performed at the Department of Vascular Surgery, Na Homolce Hospital in Prague, Czech Republic. They included 3 aortoiliac thromboendarterectomies with prosthetic patch, and 12 iliofemoral, 28 aortounifemoral, and 20 aortobifemoral bypasses. Six patients were treated for AAA and one for common iliac artery aneurysm (CIAA). Among these patients, there were 56 men and 14 women, with a mean age of 61 years (range, 38 to 78 years). Mortality in the cohort mentioned above was 0%. In three cases (4.3%) conversion to mini or full laparotomies was required and two patients (2.8%) experienced nonlethal post-operative complications. The duplex scans demonstrated 100% graft patency.

Conversion to mini-laparotomy occurred in one patient, because difficulties were encountered with the Endo Gia stapler during the exclusion of CIAA after completion of the robotic anastomosis. The second conversion to a full laparotomy was required on the first postoperative day because of a haemoperitoneum, caused by bleeding from a clipped lumbar artery. The third conversion to mini-laparotomy was caused by prolonged bleeding from lumbar arteries after robotic creation of a central anastomosis of an aortic tube graft. The first converted patient had postoperative fever and methicillin-resistant Staphylococcus aureus (MRSA) was detected from the central venous catheter and haemoculture. In this case antibiotics were applied over the six weeks. One patient had an incisional hernia in the port nine months after the first operation, which was treated under local anaesthesia.

Median operating time was 238 minutes (range, 150 to 360 minutes), with a median clamp time of 52 minutes (range, 25 to 120 minutes). Median anastomosis time was 27 minutes (range, 12 to 60 minutes). Median blood loss was 420 mL (range, 50 to 1500 mL), median intensive care unit (ICU) stay was 1.7 days (range, 1 to 5 days), median ventilator support was 6 hours (0 to 48 hours), and median hospital stay was 5.2 days (range, 4 to 10 days). Nearly all patients began a liquid diet 1 day after surgery and a solid diet after 2.5 days.

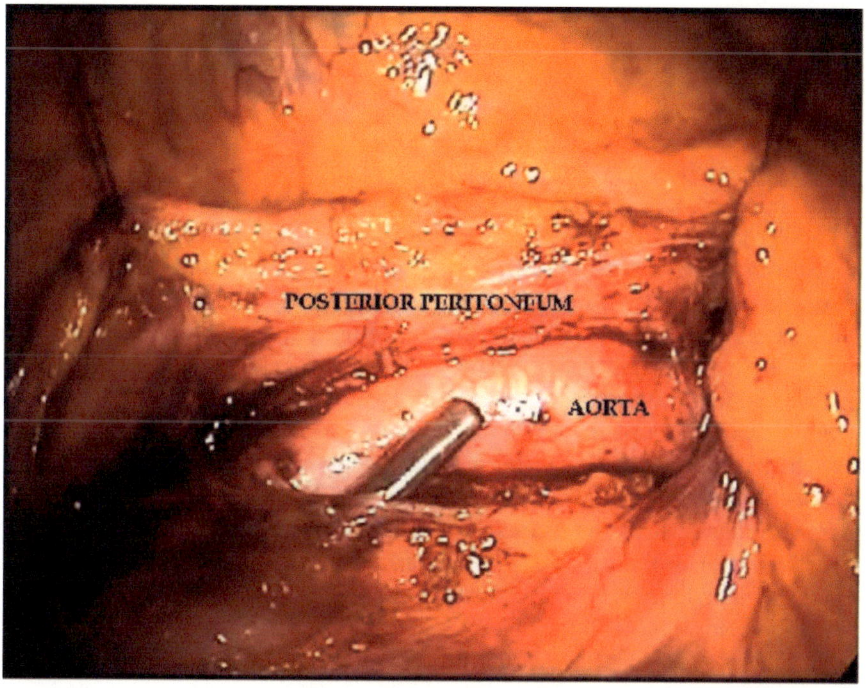

Figure 9. Fixed posterior peritoneum - perioperative view

4. The Future of Robotic Vascular Surgery

Robot-assisted surgery was first introduced in cardiac surgery. Although the da Vinci system has been used by a variety of disciplines for laparoscopic procedures, including cholecystectomies, mitral valve repairs, radical prostatectomies, reversal of tubal ligations, and many gastrointestinal surgeries, nephrectomies, and kidney transplantations, the use of robots in vascular surgery is still relatively unique.

In the view of Dr. Petr Štádler, robot-assisted vascular procedures represent a modality that has a great future. Major benefits can be expected from their introduction into hybrid procedures, primarily on the abdominal and thoracic aorta. In robotic vascular surgery, Na Homolce Hospital in Prague is ranked among the world-class centres that are intensively involved in cutting-edge technology in the field of vascular surgery. The patients are the first to profit from these minimally invasive procedures. On the other hand, it is obviously necessary to underline the economic cost of this new technology and the need for accurate indications. The number of robotic systems established throughout the world must also be calculated in order to ensure that they are used to maximum effect. We hope that in the future robotic procedures will be less financially burdensome and that, given the funds saved in post-operative care and the low numbers of demanding complications requiring treatment, these new methods will prove to be economically profitable.

Because robot-assisted aortoiliac procedures have to be combined with conventional laparoscopic surgery, previous experience of conventional laparoscopic vascular surgery is very important. By combining robotic technology with surgical skills, the da Vinci Surgical System can allow the performance of more precise and more types of minimally invasive procedures in vascular surgery.

5. References

Dion, Y. M.; Gracia, C. R. & Demalsy, J. C. (1996). Laparoscopic aortic surgery. *Journal of vascular surgery,* Vol. 23, No. 3, (539), ISNN 0741-5214.

Dion, Y. M.; Gracia, C. R.; Estakhri, M.; Demalsy, J. C.; Douville, Y.; Piccinini, E. et al. (1998). Totally laparoscopic aortobifemoral bypass: A review of 10 patients. *Surgical laparoscopy & endoscopy,* Vol. 8, No. 3, (165–170), ISSN 1051-7200.

Marescaux, J.; Smith, M. K.; Folscher, D. et al. (2001). Telerobotic laparoscopic cholecystectomy: Initial clinical experience with 25 patients. *Annals of surgery,* Vol. 234, No. 1, (1–7), ISSN 0003-4932.

Nio, D.; Diks, J.; Linsen, M. A. M.; Cuesta, M. A.; Gracia, C.; Rauwerda, J. A. & Wisselink, W. (2005). Robot-assisted laparoscopic aortobifemoral bypass for aortoiliac occlusive disease: Early clinical experience. *European journal of vascular and endovascular surgery,* Vol. 29, No. 6, (586-590), ISNN 1078-5884.

O'Toole, R. V.; Playter, R. R.; Krummel, T. M.; Blank, W. C.; Cornelius, N. H.; Roberts, W. R.; Bell, W. J. & Raibert, M. (1999). Measuring and developing suturing technique with a virtual reality surgical simulator. *Journal of the American College of Surgeons,* Vol. 189, No. 1, (114-127), ISSN 1072-7515.

Štádler, P.; Šebesta, P.; Vitásek, P.; Matouš, P. & El Samman. K. (2006, a). A modified technique of transperitoneal direct approach for totally laparoscopic aortoiliac surgery. *European journal of vascular and endovascular surgery,* Vol. 32, No. 5, (266-269), ISNN 1078-5884.

Štádler, P.; Matouš, P.; Vitásek, P. & Špaček M. (2006, b). Robot-assisted aortoiliac reconstruction: A review of 30 cases. *Journal of vascular surgery,* Vol. 44, No. 5, (915-919), ISNN 0741-5214.

Talamini, M. A.; Chapman, S.; Horgan, S. et al. (2003). A prospective analysis of 211 robotic-assisted surgical procedures. *Surgical endoscopy,* Vol. 17, No. 10, (1521–1524), ISSN 0930-2794.

Wisselink, W.; Cuesta, M. A.; Gracia, C. & Rauwerda JA. (2002). Robot-assisted laparoscopic aortobifemoral bypass for aortoiliac occlusive disease: A report of two cases. *Journal of vascular surgery,* Vol., 36, No. 5, (1079-1082), ISNN 0741-5214.

31

Mechanical error analysis of compact forceps manipulator for laparoscopic surgery

[1]Takashi Suzuki, [2]Yoichi Katayama, [3]Etsuko Kobayashi and [3]Ichiro Sakuma
[1]Advanced Biomedical Engineering and Science, Tokyo Women's Medical University,
[2]Graduate School of Frontier Sciences, The University of Tokyo,
[3]Graduate School of Engineering, The University of Tokyo
Japan

1. Introduction

Laparoscopic surgery, sometimes called "keyhole surgery", is one of minimally invasive surgical techniques. All procedures are completed inside abdominal cavity through 3-4 small holes on the abdomen using rigid thin videoscope and long-handled surgical instruments such as clamp, scissors, and scalpel. This patient-friendly technique has a lot of merits compared with conventional laparotomy; less pain, shorter hospital stay, and lower medical costs. It is, however, a difficult procedure. As the linear-shape forceps are bound at the incision hole, symmetrical motion is required around the fulcrum. Surgeons have only four Degrees of Freedom (DOF); two DOFs are for the orientation of forceps, and the other two for axial rotation and longitudinal translation of forceps (Fig. 1), so that laparoscopic surgery needs highly-skilled surgeons with enough experiences.

As one of engineering solutions responding to these clinical issues, surgical manipulators are developed and some of them, such as da Vinci® Surgical System, are clinically applied. These manipulators are aiming to enhance surgeons' ability and dexterity, not for automatic robot surgery. While great contribution to high-quality surgical procedure using three-dimensional view and dexterous robotic hands, one of the drawbacks of surgical manipulators is their size. Conventional operating theatre is too small to install the robotic surgery system. Thus, space-saving, miniaturized manipulator is required.

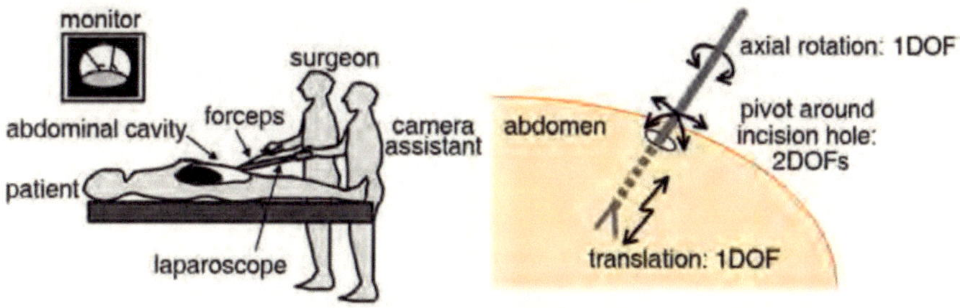

Figure 1. Laparoscopic surgery; surgeon manipulates forceps watching video from laparoscope controlled by camera assistant (left). Limitation of degrees of freedom (rotation, translation, and pivot) is one of causes that make laparoscopic surgery difficult for surgeon (right)

We have developed a compact forceps manipulator using "friction wheel mechanism" (FWM) and "gimbals mechanism" (Suzuki, et al., 2002) and evaluated it (Suzuki, et al., 2005). In this paper, we 1) introduce the mechanism of the manipulator and 2) describe the mathematical analysis of the mechanical error and correction factor based on mechanism of manipulator and the measured error.

2. Method

2.1 Mechanical configuration

In laparoscopic surgery, at least four DOFs are required for forceps motion: axial rotation and longitudinal translation of the forceps, and pivot motion around the incision hole on the abdomen (Fig. 1). We realize only four DOFs because redundancy may disturb the miniaturization and simplification of mechanism; those are important factors for clinical application and commercialization. The compact forceps manipulator we have developed consists of two mechanical subcomponents; Friction Wheel Mechanism (FWM) and Gimbals mechanism. The FWM provides axial rotation and longitudinal translation of forceps using friction drive mechanism. Gimbals mechanism realizes pivot motion of forceps. The prototype is shown in Fig. 2. Dimensions of manipulator are 80×150×320 mm^3 and weight is 1.7 kg.

2.2 Friction wheel mechanism

Friction wheel mechanism consists of a couple of friction wheel that has three tilted driving rollers and outer case (Fig. 3).

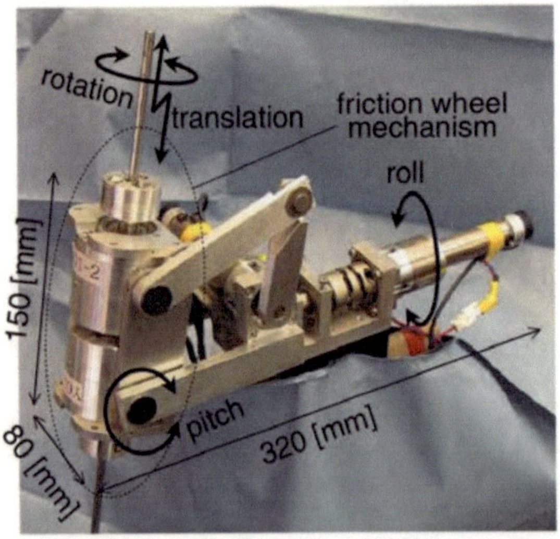

Figure 2. Prototype of compact forceps manipulator; friction wheel mechanism provides rotation and translation of forceps, gimbals mechanism realizes pivot motion (roll, pitch)

Three rollers are radially-located in the case with 120-degree gap, and the forceps shaft is inserted among those rollers. When the outer case is rotated, the rollers travel on the surface of forceps spirally. The shaft is relatively driven by the driving rollers using friction force between rollers and surface of forceps in spiral trajectory. We adopted hollow-shaft ultrasonic actuators with optical encoder (rated torque 50mNm, custom order, Fukoku, Japan) because of various advantages of ultrasonic motor; compact size and light weight for miniaturization, high holding torque, clean environment for future clinical application, and suitable for hollow-shaft configuration. We use a couple of friction wheels with opposite tilting angle. They provide symmetrical spiral motions like right-handed and left-handed screws, and they are combined to generate rotation and translation (Fig. 4).

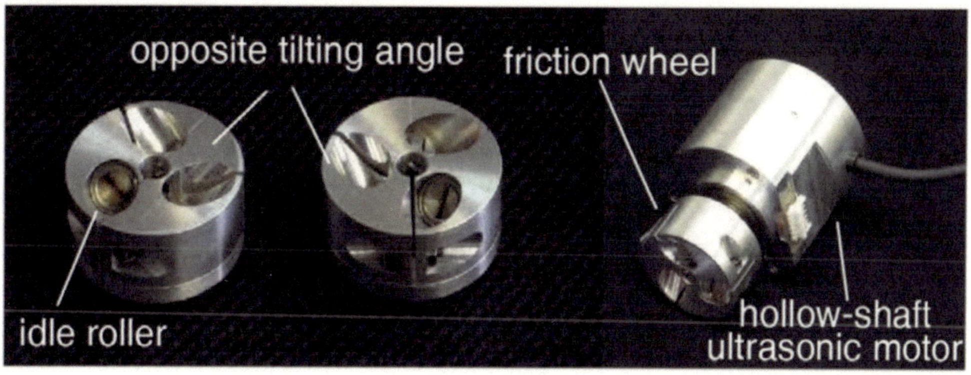

Figure 3. A couple of friction wheel; Each friction wheel has three tilted driving rollers with opposite tilting angle (left). Hollow-shaft ultrasonic motor is adopted for actuation (right)

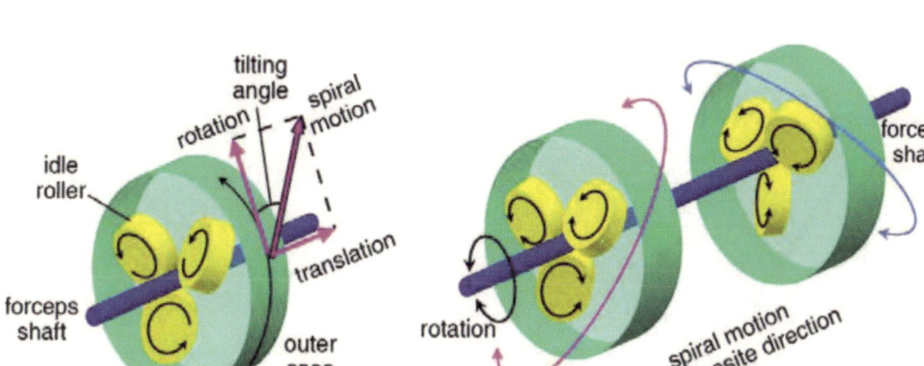

Figure 4. Friction wheel mechanism; friction wheel travels spirally around the forceps shaft (left). Opposite tilting angle generates two different spiral shapes like right-handed and left-handed screws (right)

For the axial rotation of forceps shaft, two friction wheels are rotated in the same direction. In that case, driving rollers and shaft does not have relative speed, so that spiral motions are not generated and forceps shaft rotates at the same speed of friction wheel. For the longitudinal translation, two friction wheels are rotated in the opposite direction. In this case, spiral motions are generated. The rotational components of spiral motion are cancelled mutually and remaining translation drives the forceps (Fig. 5).

The mechanism to generate translation can be shown using mathematical expression (Fig. 6).

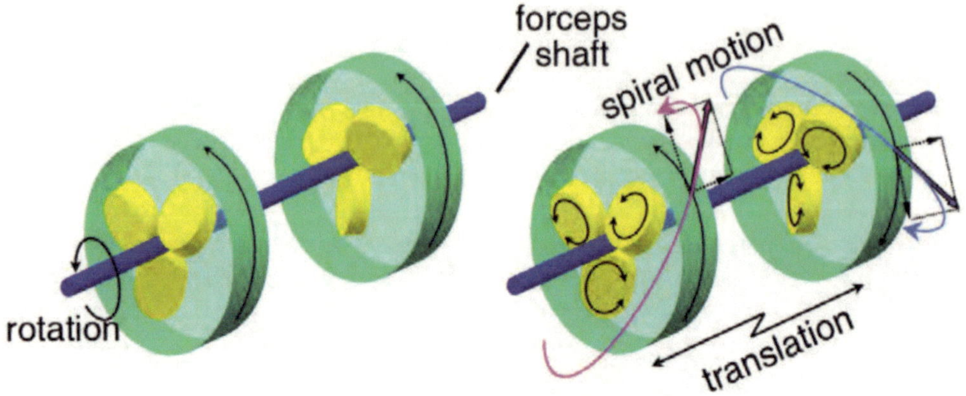

Figure 5. Driving principle of friction wheel mechanism: Rotational motion is generated by rotating both motors in the same direction (left). When each motor is driven in the opposite direction, rotational motions are cancelled mutually and remaining translational motion drives forceps in the longitudinal direction (right)

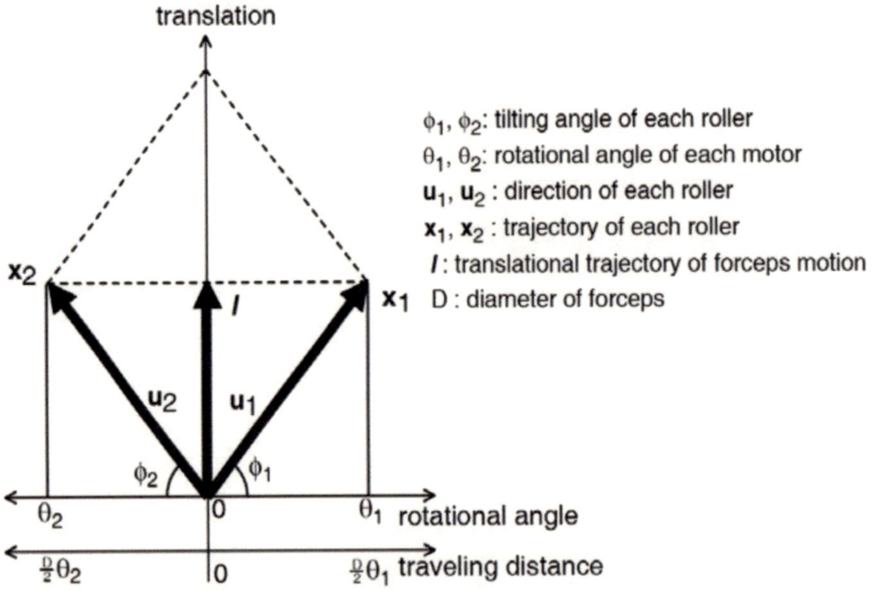

Figure 6. Translational motion can be shown by expanding the surface of forceps to a plane

Here, each roller has tilting angle of ϕ_1 and ϕ_2. When outer cases are rotated by θ_1 and θ_2, trajectory of each roller is as follows;

$$\begin{cases} x_1 = \frac{D}{2}\theta_1 u_1 = \frac{1}{2}\begin{bmatrix} D\theta_1 \\ D\theta_1 \tan(\phi_1) \end{bmatrix} \\ x_2 = \frac{D}{2}\theta_2 u_2 = \frac{1}{2}\begin{bmatrix} D\theta_2 \\ D\theta_2 \tan(\phi_2) \end{bmatrix} \end{cases} \quad (1)$$

As the traveling distance is written as the average of two friction wheels, translation can be express using rotational angle of each motor (θ_1 and θ_2) and tilting angle (ϕ_1 and ϕ_2);

$$
\begin{aligned}
l &= \frac{x_1 - x_2}{2} \\
&= \begin{bmatrix} \frac{D}{4}(\theta_1 - \theta_2) \\ \frac{D}{4}(\theta_1 \tan(\phi_1) + \theta_2 \tan(\phi_2)) \end{bmatrix} \\
&= \begin{bmatrix} \frac{D}{4}(\theta_1 - \theta_2) \\ \frac{D}{4}(\theta_1 + \theta_2)\tan(\frac{\pi}{6}) \end{bmatrix} & \left(\phi_1 = \phi_2 = \frac{\pi}{6}\right) \\
&= \begin{bmatrix} 0 \\ \frac{D}{2}\theta \tan(\frac{\pi}{6}) \end{bmatrix} & \left(\theta_1 = \theta_2 = \theta\right) \qquad (2)
\end{aligned}
$$

Here, we used 30 deg ($\pi/6$ rad) for tilting angle of rollers and θ for rotational angle of each motor. As shown in eq. (2), the translational distance is controlled by the rotational angle of actuator like a ball screw.

This mechanism is proposed by Vollenweider for surgery simulator (Vollenweider, et al, 1998). Ikuta, et al. also adopted the similar mechanism for axial rotation and longitudinal translation of colonoscope in the virtual endoscope training system (Ikuta, et al., 1998). To the best of authors' knowledge, this is the first prototype that uses this kind of rotation and translation mechanism not for simulator but for real manipulator.

2.3 Gimbals mechanism

Gimbals mechanism has two mutually-perpendicular intersectional rotational axes and realizes pivoting motion of forceps with wide working range around the trocar port. The simple kinematics eases numerical control.

A concern about the location of rotational centre of the mechanism should be discussed. Many studies have proposed the necessity of the remote centre of motion (RCM) mechanism to realize pivot motion with no mechanical part at the trocar port; such as R-guide (Mitsuishi, et al., 2003) and parallel-linkage mechanism (Taylor, et al., 1995, Madhani, et al., 1998, and Kobayashi, et al., 2002). As gimbals mechanism has its rotational centre inside it, not at the incision hole, the rotational centre is located above trocar port and forceps pulls abdominal wall accompanying its pivot motion. As we reported in the past publication (Suzuki, et al., 2002), the result of preliminary in-vivo experiment using pig showed no problem; such as expansion of incision hole and bleeding. We conclude that gimbals mechanism will not damage the abdominal wall because abdominal muscle got relaxed under anaesthesia and incision hole follows the motion of forceps, although the required torque increased to pull the abdominal wall according to the pivot motion of forceps and actuators should be carefully selected. We adopted DC servomotor (ENC-185801, CITIZEN CHIBA PRECISION Co., LTD) to control each rotational axis.

3. Evaluation

3.1 Separation between translation and rotation

One of advantages of FWM is that it realizes rotation and translation with one miniaturized mechanism. For appropriate rotation and translation, we need two conditions; one is the shape of each spiral and the other is rotational speed of each motor. In other words, the lead length of each spiral motion generated by friction wheel should be the same, and rotational speed of each motor should be the same. This is because rotational component of spiral motion must be the same to be cancelled mutually. Our former studies, however, showed that the friction wheel mechanism provided rotational error in translation. We measured the rotational error when 90 mm translation, equivalent to 1800 deg rotation of actuator, was input. The rotating angle of each actuator was controlled using pulse signal from rotary encoders mounted on the motor. The rotating angle of forceps shaft was measured using digital microscope (VH-7000C, Keyence, Japan) with 0.5 deg resolution. The result of error evaluation is shown in Table. 1 (Suzuki, et al., 2005). Measured error was large compared to the required specification we set for this manipulator.

input	error factor	required spec.	average +/- S.D.
translation (90 mm, 1800 deg)	rotation	less than1 deg	14.5 +/- 3.0 deg

Table 1. Rotational error of friction wheel mechanism in translational input

3.2 Error analysis based on mechanical error

For the error correction, we analyze the cause of rotational error in translational motion. As mentioned above, the error motion is caused by different spiral shape generated by each friction roller and/or different rotating angle of each actuator. As we control the actuators using rotary encoders, we can omit the possibility of different rotating angle. Thus, the cause of unstable motion is mismatch of lead length between each friction roller. Lead length error is caused by tilting angle error of the friction rollers. The angle error is determined by the machining error in prototyping process.

We discussed the cause of rotational error in translation and its correction method based on the mechanism of friction wheel. Error analysis is shown here using Fig. 7.

Rotational error is shown as follows;

$$\Delta\theta = \frac{1}{2}(\hat{\theta}_1 - \hat{\theta}_2) \tag{3}$$

Because the forceps shaft is rigid, the translational distance generated by each roller is the same, and sum of rotational angle are the same between each roller.

$$\begin{cases} \hat{\theta}_1 \tan(\phi + \Delta\phi_1) & = & \hat{\theta}_2 \tan(\phi + \Delta\phi_2) \\ \hat{\theta}_1 + \hat{\theta}_2 & = & \theta_1 + \theta_2 \end{cases} \tag{4}$$

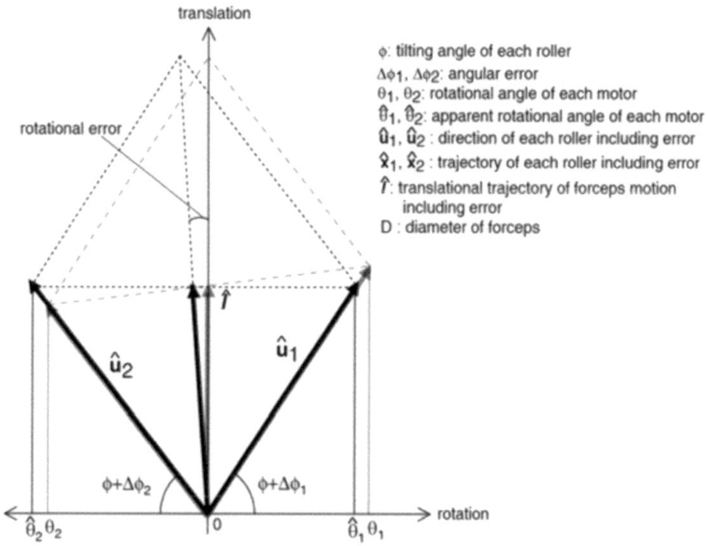

Figure 7. Error analysis of rotational error in translational motion

When these simultaneous equations (4) are solved for $\hat{\theta}_1$ and $\hat{\theta}_2$, they are shown as follows;

$$\begin{cases} \hat{\theta}_1 = \dfrac{\tan(\phi+\Delta\phi_2)}{\tan(\phi+\Delta\phi_1)+\tan(\phi+\Delta\phi_2)}(\theta_1+\theta_2) \\ \hat{\theta}_2 = \dfrac{\tan(\phi+\Delta\phi_1)}{\tan(\phi+\Delta\phi_1)+\tan(\phi+\Delta\phi_2)}(\theta_1+\theta_2) \end{cases} \tag{5}$$

Consequently, Δθ (eq. (3)) is shown using eq.(5).

$$\begin{aligned} \Delta\theta &= \frac{1}{2}(\hat{\theta}_1-\hat{\theta}_2) \\ &= -\frac{1}{2}\frac{\tan(\phi+\Delta\phi_1)-\tan(\phi+\Delta\phi_2)}{\tan(\phi+\Delta\phi_1)+\tan(\phi+\Delta\phi_2)}(\theta_1+\theta_2) \end{aligned} \tag{6}$$

This means that the rotational error is proportional to the sum of input rotating angle (θ_1, θ_2), and that the coefficient is determined using only mechanical error of tilting angle ($\Delta\phi_1$ and $\Delta\phi_2$), thus the error could be compensated using correction factor. On the assumption that rotational error of Δθ is observed when angle of θ_0 is input to generate translation, the correction factor is analyzed. As the condition, we have following equations. Equation (7) means the translational distance is expressed in two ways. The first equation in eq.(8) means input angle for each driving roller is the same in the case of translational input, and other equations are geometrically trivial.

$$\hat{\theta}_1\tan(\phi+\Delta\phi_1)=\frac{1}{2}\left(\theta_1\tan(\phi+\Delta\phi_1)+\theta_2\tan(\phi+\Delta\phi_2)\right) \tag{7}$$

$$\begin{cases} \theta_1 = \theta_2 & = & \theta_0 \\ \tan(\phi + \Delta\phi_1) & = & \dfrac{\hat{l}}{\hat{\theta}_1} \\ \tan(\phi + \Delta\phi_2) & = & \dfrac{\hat{l}}{\hat{\theta}_2} \end{cases} \tag{8}$$

When equations (8) are assigned to eq.(6) and (7), $\hat{\theta}_1/\theta_0$ and $\hat{\theta}_2/\theta_0$ are shown as eq.(9).

$$\begin{cases} \dfrac{\hat{\theta}_1}{\theta_0} = \dfrac{-2k+1+\sqrt{4k^2+1}}{2} \\ \dfrac{\hat{\theta}_2}{\theta_0} = \dfrac{2k+1+\sqrt{4k^2+1}}{2} \\ \left(k = \Delta\theta/\theta_0\right) \end{cases} \Rightarrow \begin{cases} \dfrac{\hat{\theta}_1}{\theta_0} = 1-k \\ \dfrac{\hat{\theta}_2}{\theta_0} = 1+k \\ (k \ll 1) \end{cases} \tag{9}$$

As they are the error coefficient of driving rollers, the inverse of those coefficients are the correction factor C_1 and C_2 (eq.(10)).

$$\begin{cases} C_1 = \dfrac{\theta_0}{\hat{\theta}_1} = \dfrac{1}{1-k} = 1+k \\ C_2 = \dfrac{\theta_0}{\hat{\theta}_2} = \dfrac{1}{1+k} = 1-k \\ \qquad (k \ll 1) \end{cases} \tag{10}$$

Consequently, the correction factor can be expressed using k that is determined by input angle ($\Delta\theta$) and measured error angle (θ_0).

3.3 Re-evaluation of separation after compensation

We measured rotational error again. In this measurement, we applied the correction factor k by assigning 1800 deg to θ_0 and 14.5 deg to $\Delta\theta$. Result is shown in Table 2 comparing the result of the case without correction factor. The rotational error was reduced more than 90 % by the error correction factor (Suzuki, et al., 2005).

input	error factor	correction factor	average +/- S.D (deg)
translation (90 mm, 1800 deg)	rotation	without	14.5 +/- 3.0
		with	1.0 +/- 1.0

Table 2. Rotational error of friction wheel mechanism in translational input with/without correction factor

4. Discussion

For realization of stable forceps manipulation using friction wheel mechanism, we analyzed the mechanical configuration of manipulator and proposed a correcting factor based on the input rotating angle and measured rotational error, so that the error was reduced by 90%. When the 90 mm translation is input, the error was approximately 1.0 deg. In laparoscopic surgery, innermost target is sometimes located 300 mm from incision hole. In that case, the rotational error will increase up to approximately 3.0 deg. As it does not meet the required specification of 1deg accuracy, we have to find other causes of unstable motion.

One of possible causes is the variation of correction factor. We calculated the correction factor as a constant value from limited number of sets of measured error and input rotating angle. The error correction factor may change depending on the surface condition of forceps shaft, so we need to change correction factor dynamically. Another cause is slip between friction rollers and forceps shaft. In the current prototype, the forceps position is calculated from encoder value and controlled in semi-closed feedback loop. We do not consider position error caused by slight slip or its accompanying accumulated error.

These issues could be solved by closed feedback control loop using direct sensing of forceps position. As implementation methods, we can use three dimensional optical position sensor and/or texture recognition system like optical mouse.

5. Conclusion

In this study, we introduce a compact forceps manipulator with four DOFs for laparoscopic surgery. It consists of two mechanical parts; friction wheel mechanism and gimbals mechanism. Friction wheel mechanism is space-saving and realizes two degrees of freedom of rotation and translation using a couple of friction wheel. Gimbals mechanism realizes wide working range and easy control. One of the drawbacks of FWM, rotational motion error in translational input, was shown and analyzed mathematically based on the mechanical configuration of manipulator. Rotational error was reduced more than 90 % by the error correction factor calculated from the mathematical analysis of mechanical configuration.

In the future works, we will work to modify mechanical configuration based on the results of this study and improve control method from semi-closed feedback control using rotary encoders to closed feedback control using direct position sensing method, such as three-dimensional optical position sensor. As another future work, we will integrate this forceps manipulator with robotized forceps, such as laser coagulator forceps with CCD camera (Suzuki, et al., 2004).

6. Acknowledgement

This work is partly supported by following grants;

-"Research for the Future Program (JSPS-RFTF 99I00904)" funded by Japan Society for the Promotion of Science

-Electro-Mechanic Technology Advancing Foundation

-"Research and Development of the Compact Surgical Robot System for Future Medical Care" funded by New Energy and Industrial Technology Development Organization (NEDO)

-"Research on medical devices for analyzing, supporting and substituting the function of human body" funded by Ministry of Health, Labour and Welfare
-JPSP(#18680041).

7. References

Ikuta, K. et al (1998). Virtual Endoscope System with Force Sensation. In :*Proceedings of the first international conference on medical image computing and computer-assisted intervention - MICCAI98, Lecture Note in Computer Science* 1496, pp.293-304, ISBN:3-540-65136-5, Cambridge, MA, USA, October, 1998, Springer.

Kobayashi, Y. et al (2002). Small Occupancy Robotic Mechanisms for Endoscopic Surgery. In : *Proceedings of the 5th international conference on medical image computing and computer assisted intervention* (MICCAI2002), *Part 1, Lecture Note in Computer Science* 2488, ISBN:3-540-44225-1, Tokyo, Japan, September, 2002, Springer.

Madhani, A. et al (1998). The Black Falcon: a teleoperated surgical instrument for minimally invasive surgery. In : *Proceedings of IEEE/RSJ international conference on intelligent robots and systems - IROS1998, vol.2,* pp.936-944, Victoria, BC, Canada, 1998, October, IEEE.

Mitsuishi, M. et al (2003). Development of a remote minimally-invasive surgical system with operational environment transmission capability. In :*Proceedings of the 2003 IEEE international conference on robotics and automation - ICRA2003,* pp. 2663-2670, Taipei, Taiwan, September, 2003, IEEE.

Suzuki, T. et al (2002). A new compact robot for manipulation forceps using friction wheel and gimbals mechanism. In : *Proceedings of the 16th international congress and exhibition computer-assisted radiology and surgery - CARS2002,* pp.314-319, ISBN:3-540-43655-3, Paris, France, 2002, June, Springer.

Suzuki, T. et al (2004). Development of a robotic laser surgical tool with an integrated video endoscope. In :*Proceedings of the 7th international conference on medical image computing and computer assisted intervention*–MICCAI2004, *Part II, Lecture Note in Computer Science* 3217, pp.25-32, ISBN:3-540-22977-9, Saint-Malo, France, September, 2004, Springer.

Suzuki, T. et al (2005). Compact forceps manipulator using friction wheel mechanism and gimbals mechanism for laparoscopic surgery. In :*Proceedings of the 8th international conference on medical image computing and computer assisted intervention–MICCAI2005, Part II, Lecture Note in Computer Science 3750,* pp.81-88, ISBN:978-3-540-29326-2, Palm Springs, CA, USA, October, 2005, Springer.

Taylor, RH. et al (1995). A telerobotic assistant for laparoscopic surgery. *IEEE Engineering in Medicine and Biology Magazine,* vol.14, no.9, May/Jun 1995, pp.279-288, ISSN:0739-5175.

Vollenweider, M. et al (1998). Surgery simulator with force feedback. In :*Proceedings of the 4th international conference on motion and vibration control - MOVIC98,* Zurich, Switzerland, 1998.

32

Dental Patient Robot

Hideaki Takanobu
Dept of Mechanical Systems Engineering, Kogakuin University, Tokyo
Japan

1. Introduction

Conventional robotics research in medicine is usually related to supporting surgical procedures and doctor's questions to patients during interviews [1]. However, there are not many examples on the development of patient robots for supporting clinical training of medical staff such as doctors and nurses. It is commonplace to use static models for therapeutic training in medicine. However, training based on the use of such models is inadequate due to differences between the models and actual patients [2]. Thus there are high expectations in the development of animated patient robots for use in medical training. Further, the development of simulators is being widely pursued in the field of dental therapy training but there are few examples of research on robots. The author has been developing patient robots for dental therapy training.

2. Practice in Dentistry

2.1 Dental school education

Recent dental school graduates of Japanese universities are said to lack clinical skills and experience in treating patients. The main reason is attributed to inadequate clinical training. Currently, so-called 'phantoms' (Fig. 1) consisting of a simple functional cephalic region and an arrangement of teeth are used for clinical training but these models are considerably different than actual patients. Until recently, clinical training was carried out on consenting volunteer patients. However, recent changes in ethical issues related to environmental studies, medicine and dentistry have made such clinical training difficult. Thus the potential danger of declining clinical skills is a problem in dental therapy training. Dental therapy skills often depend on the competence and ability of clinicians and it is necessary for them to have extensive experience using methods and models that accurately reflect actual treatment procedures and conditions.

2.2 Operating conditions

To become a dentist, it is necessary to graduate from dental school by passing a national examination in Japan. This examination is based on multiple choice (mark-sheet) questions. This method is used to reduce the possibility of unfair examinations that may result if tests were based on interviews and monitoring clinical ability. However, as described above, it can be said that in spite of the well known lack of skills of dental students, universities are still producing graduates based on knowledge instead of hands on, clinical ability. It is known that there are many accidents in the first few years after graduating from dental school.

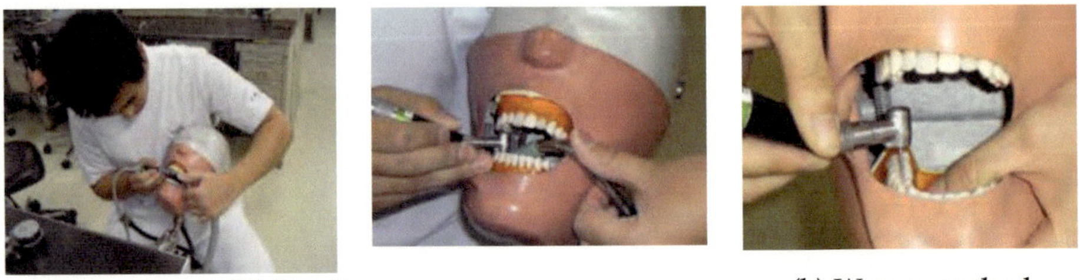

(a) Practice scenery (b) Wrong method

Figure 1. Phantom for practical training

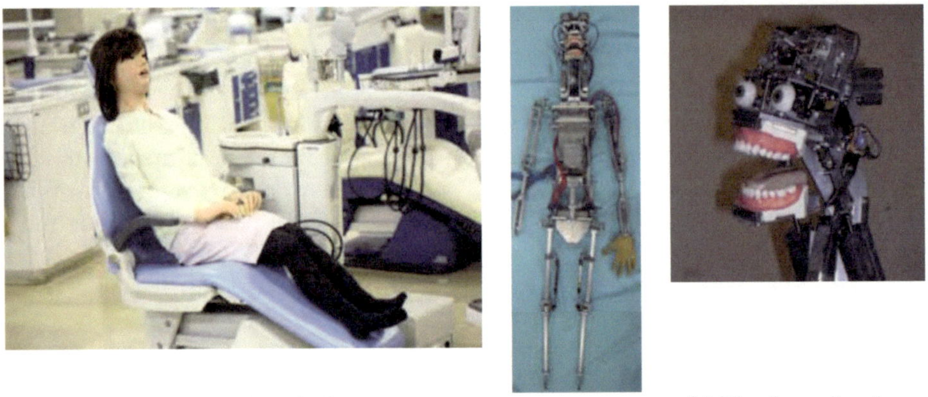

(a) Whole view (b) Head mechanism

Figure 2. Patient Robot

3. Specification of robot

3.1 External structure

The patient robot has a height of 165cm. The skeleton is made of metal and FRP is used for the skull (Fig. 2). The teeth in the conventional model used for direct therapy training, can be polished and can be easily replaced. The artificial outer skin is made from a special vinyl chloride based gum reproducing the form and sensation of actual skin. The robot has a total of 36 degrees of freedom (DOF), with patient movements being achieved by low pressure compressed air from an air cylinder as in Table 1. The other joints are passive components (Fig. 3). Further, by implementing almost human-like joints, it is possible to install the robot in an actual dental therapy unit[3][4].

3.2 Actuation system

An air cylinder is used in the drive sections. The main pressure is set at 0.7[MPa] and differential pressure to 0.35[MPa]. Further, blinking of the eyes and tongue movement are achieved by a diaphragm with a simple structure. Due to the high density of mechanical parts housed in the cephalic region, a wire is attached internally to the tongue which has 3-DOF, and the tongue is moved by pulling on the wire using a diaphragm attached to the body of the robot.

3.3 Control system

The patient robot is controlled by electro pneumatic regulators and electromagnetic valves using an air cylinder. Since it is possible to control the electro pneumatic regulator by minute changes in pressure, feedback from a PC enables fine movement of the neck and mouth. An electromagnetic valve is used for simple ON-OFF movements such as arms and eye lids. Feedback control is achieved by setting a potentiometer in parts where electro pneumatic regulators are used (Fig. 4).

3.4 Interface

The patient robot is controlled using a PC (Fig. 5). Position control of the patient robot's mouth and neck is achieved using voice recognition software that reacts to the trainee's instructions as in Fig. 6. Further, the supervising doctor can manipulate the interface to produce movements due to coughing and reactions to pain to which trainees as expected to respond. After the robot exhibits sudden movements, a five level point rating is displayed above the interface and the supervisor can grade the trainee's response in real time. A record of the type and timing of sudden movements and their evaluation is stored as a table. This table can be used in conjunction with video footage of training sessions by trainees to check their performance.

3.5 Image recoginition

The patient's eye is simulated by a small camera embedded into the patient robot's right eye. The camera has been successfully used to recognize and track trainees and instruments used during treatment. Imaging recognition is achieved using the RGB colors of video images where the color of the trainee's hair is electronically recognized and the robot's line of sight shown to the trainee (Fig. 7). By this procedure, it is possible to carry out therapy under conditions where the trainee is being watched by the patient.

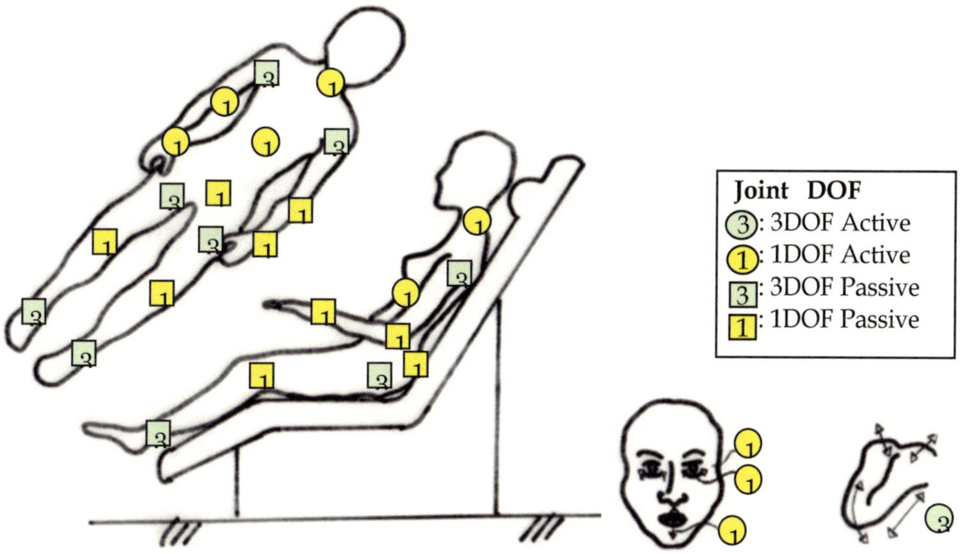

Figure 3. DOF of Patient Robot

Number	Item	DOF	Motion
1	Eyeball	1 (Active)	Right and Left
2	Eyelid	1 (Active)	Open and Close
3	Jaw	1 (Active)	Open and Close
4	Tongue	3 (Active)	Protrusion and Retraction
			Tip Up and Down
			Expansion
5	Throat	1 (Active)	Open and Close
6	Neck (Head)	3 (Active)	Nod
			Rotation
			Tilt
7	Chest	1 (Active)	Breath
8	Shoulder	3×2 (Passive)	
9	Right Elbow	1 (Active)	Bend and Stretch
10	Right Wrist	1 (Active)	Up and Down
11	Left Elbow	1 (Passive)	
12	Left Wrist	1 (Passive)	
13	Waist	1 (Passive)	
14	Hip Point	3×2 (Passive)	
15	Knee	1×2 (Passive)	
16	Ankle	3×2 (Passive)	

Table 1. DOF configurations of patient robot

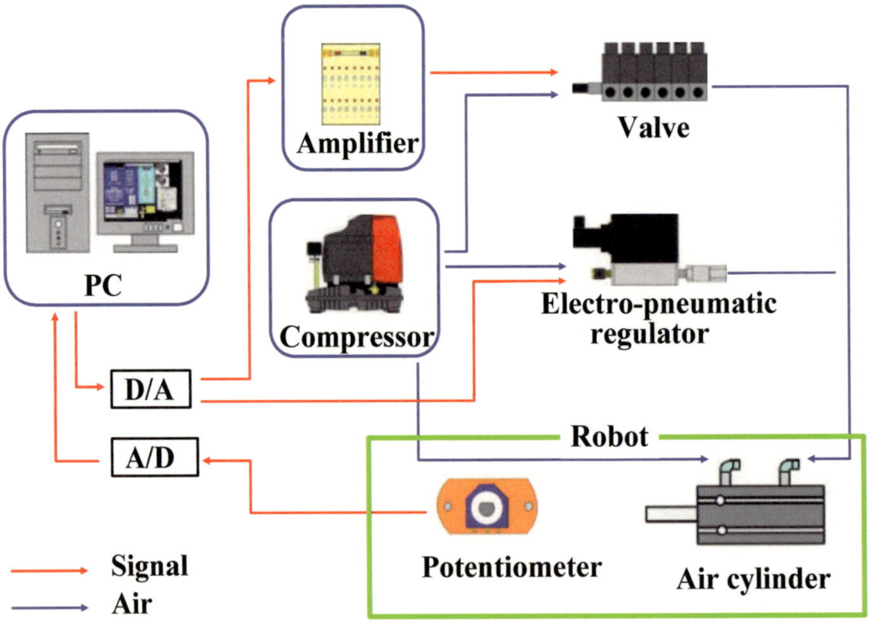

Figure 4. Control System

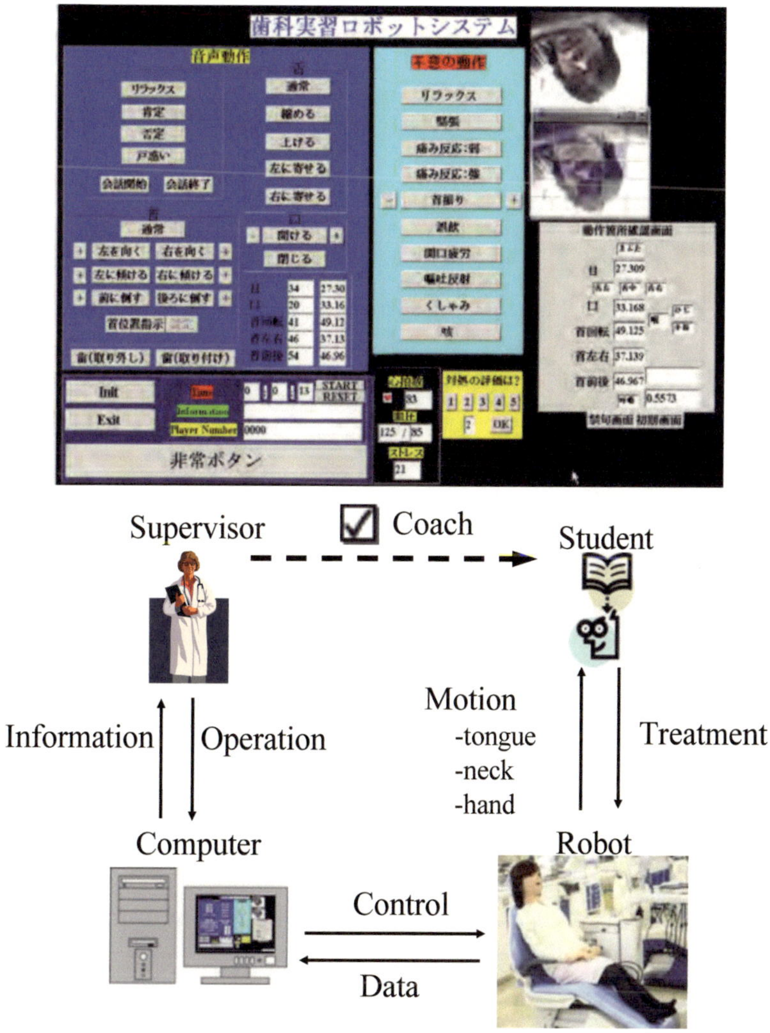

Figure 5. Interface and Total System

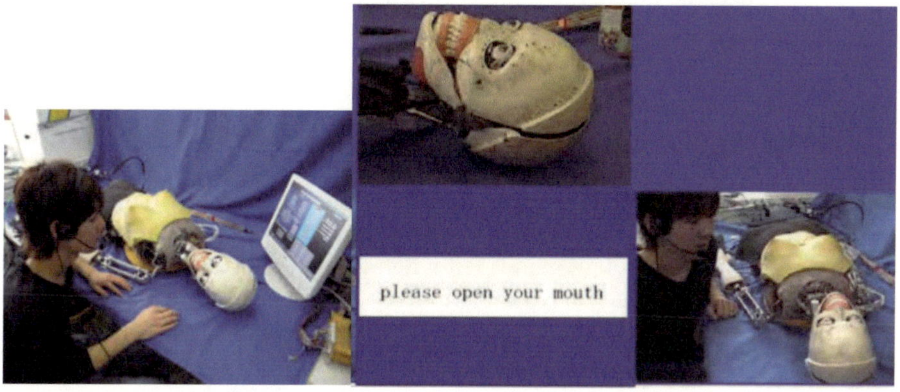

Figure 6. Voice recognition

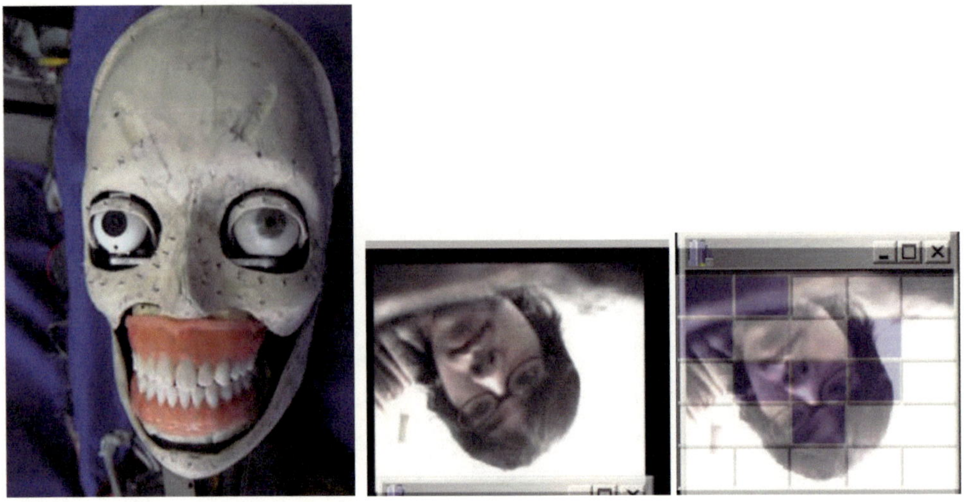

Figure 7. Target tacking by camera

Also, the voice recognition software is useful for creating more realistic conditions to simulate actual conversation with patients during training [4]. Further, we also reproduced the psychologically induced backward movement of the head when endodontic instruments appear in the patient's line of sight. This was made possible by attaching a vinyl tape of a color not found in the treatment room.

4. Oral Cavity

4.1 Structure of the teeth

Starting from the outer surface, human teeth consist of enamel, dentine and pulp (Fig. 9). Enamel is the hardest outer surface of teeth. It is colorless and semi-transparent with a hardness equivalent to a Moha hardness of 6-7, which is comparable to that of quartz. Further, the thickness of teeth depends on their type, with molar teeth being typically 1.1~1.3[mm]. Dentine is covered with cement and produces the shape of teeth with the pulp inside. Further, dental tubules are 2~3[μm] diameters pipes, and are slightly harder than bones but have elasticity and are flexible. The pulp fills the pulp cavity at the center of teeth and serves to produce dentine and supply it nutrition; repair the dentine; protect it against bacterial infection; and transmit sensory perception.

4.2 Drilling teeth

Drilling enamel does not produce pain but pain does arise when the air turbine reaches the pulp. The body's tissue fluids circulate inside the dental tubule and intersect with the tooth pulp. During drilling, fluctuations arise in the tissue fluid of the pulp tubule which stimulate nerve ends and ultimately leads to the sensation of pain. The pain due to tooth decay is the same. The sensation of pain is felt when cold and hot substances are consumed, where tissue fluids in the tubules move and stimulate nerve ends due to temperature related expansion and contraction of fluids in the tubules. That is, pain is felt when the dentine is drilled and the level of pain increases for prolonged drilling due to heat generated by friction. Further, acute pain is felt if drilling is continued into the pulp.

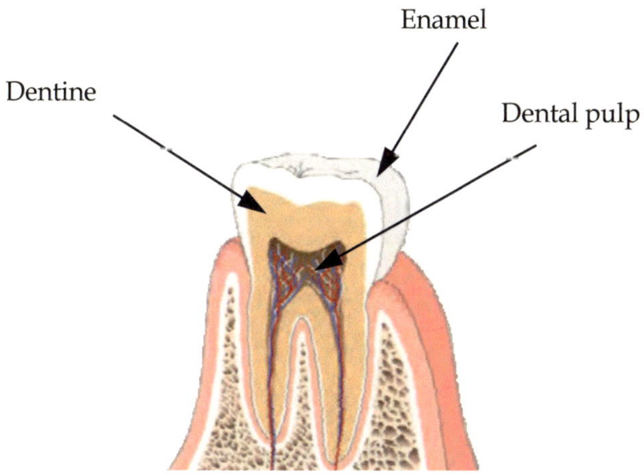

Figure 8. Tooth model [6]

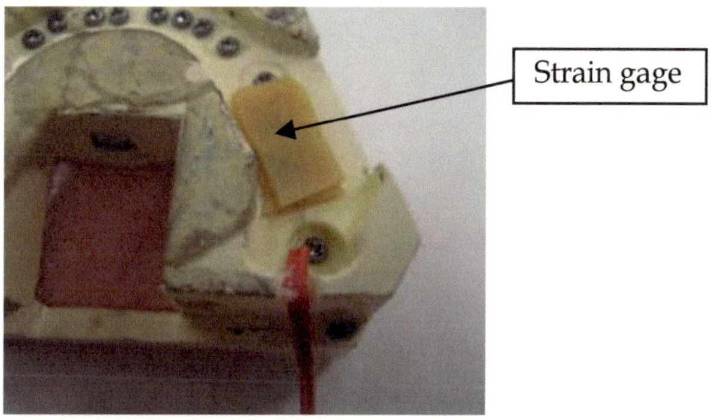

Figure 9. Installation of tooth sensor (bottom view)

4.3 Force sensor for drilling and grinding of teeth

Force sensing is achieved by monitoring the load of drilling during surgery by a sensor embedded in one of the 2nd molar teeth on the left side. The sensor consists of a strain gauge sandwiched in gum, which is attached to the teeth arrangement model (Fig. 9). In this way, when the spring is compressed under the action of a load, a screw is pushed and the strain gauge sandwiched in the gum is bent (Fig. 10). During this procedure, the voltage of the strain gauge is recorded which is a measure of the load acting on the tooth.

4.4 Effusion of bleeding

For dental students and trainees, the effusion of blood is one of several unexpected situations. Thus, in order to train students to react calmly to unexpected bleeding during surgery, the patient robot is designed to reproduce the effusion of blood. The main locations for bleeding in the oral cavity are regions inside of both cheeks and areas ranging from the surface to below the tongue.

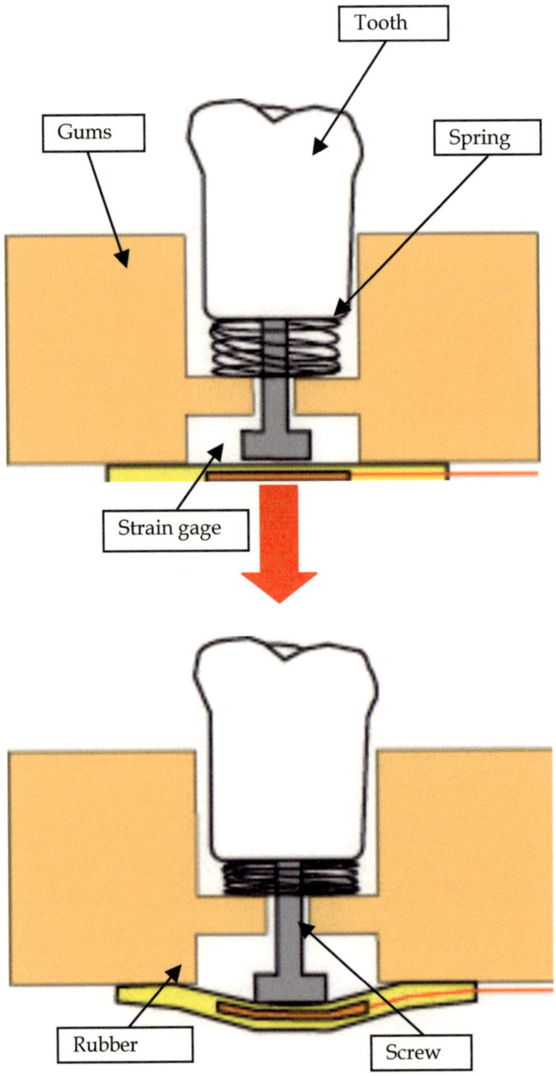

Figure 10. Mechanism of tooth sensor

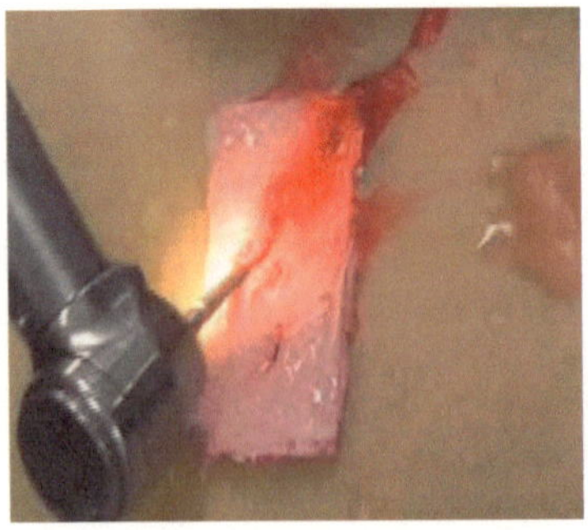

Figure 10. Bleeding results

The main reason for bleeding in these regions is due to accidental contact of the air turbine with the cheeks or tongue during surgery of the 2nd molar, when patients are prone to move their tongue. For these reasons, the patient robot is also designed so that bleeding results under the above conditions from both cheeks and the tongue regions as described. This is implemented as a three layered structure, consisting of red pigmentation sandwiched between two silicone resin plates. This structure is only a mere 0.4[mm] thick, and suitable for fitting into the oral cavity.

4.5 Saliva

The ease of performing dental surgery is affected by the amount of saliva. In particular, it is desirable that the surface of teeth be dry when inserting fillings. If the volume of saliva is large then the moist surface hinders adhesion of the fillings. Thus we have fitted a saliva mechanism to the patient robot. Since 2/3 of saliva secretion is exuded from the parotid gland, the saliva is produced from the parotid gland of the patient robot. The tube from an externally connected air pump is placed into a water tank, an air pump is used to push into the tube which flows out at the location of the parotid gland inside the oral cavity. The saliva flow volume for a patient at rest is 0.3 [ml/min]. External stimulation results in this volume increasing to between 1.0~1.7[ml/min]. The patient robot is able to produce 7.7 [ml/min], which reproduces the saliva flow patients undergoing surgical procedures.

4.6 Uvula

This robot have a uvula sensor that simulates human vomiting reflex. As in Fig. 11, a touch sensor was installed in the oral cavity. The robot vomits when something touches it. In the training situation, supervisor clicks the vomiting button to evaluate the trainee's reaction for the robot's vomiting.

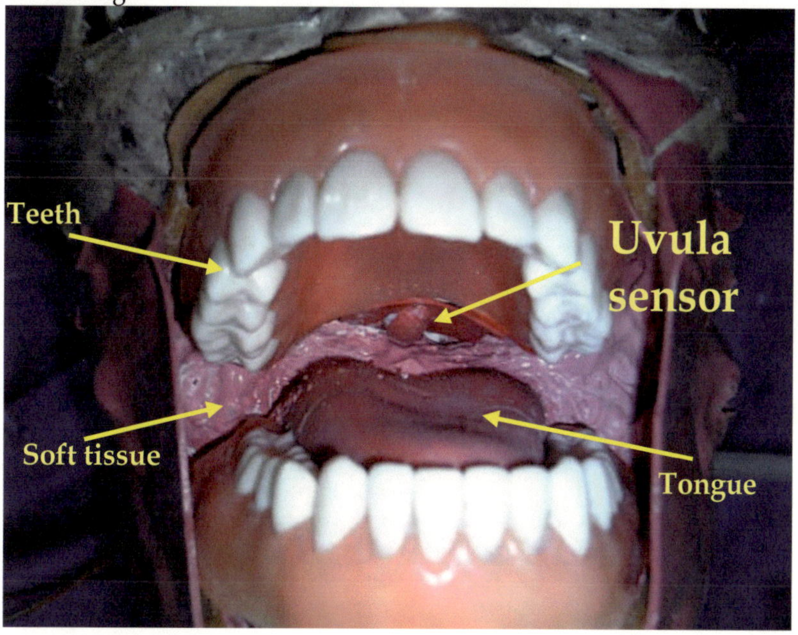

Figure 11. Uvula sensor

5. Experiment

5.1 Method

The performance of the patient robot was evaluated by 32 members of Showa University (two clinical interns, 29 students in the 5th year who had completed basic clinical training using phantom heads; and one veteran doctor). The experiments were conducted using the functions available at the present time and involved cavity preparation and drilling of the 2nd molar on the left side of the jaw, that is, drilling of back molars. The experiments were conducted in groups consisting of a trainee and two assistants. The supervisor evaluated the performance of the students by giving instructions to the patient robot via the interface of the PC (Fig. 12). The view from the camera embedded in the patient robot is shown in Fig. 13.

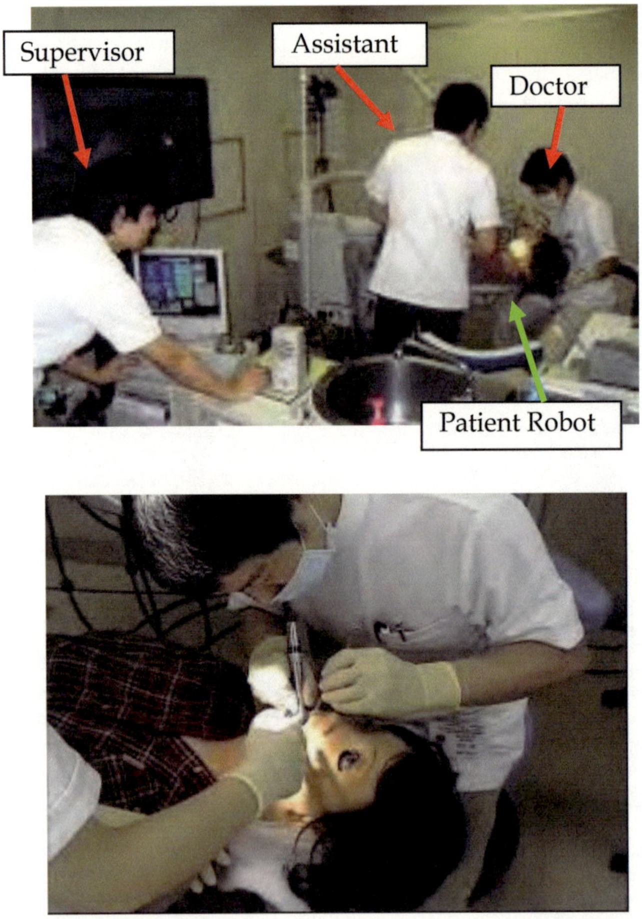

Figure 12. Practice scenery that uses Patient Robot

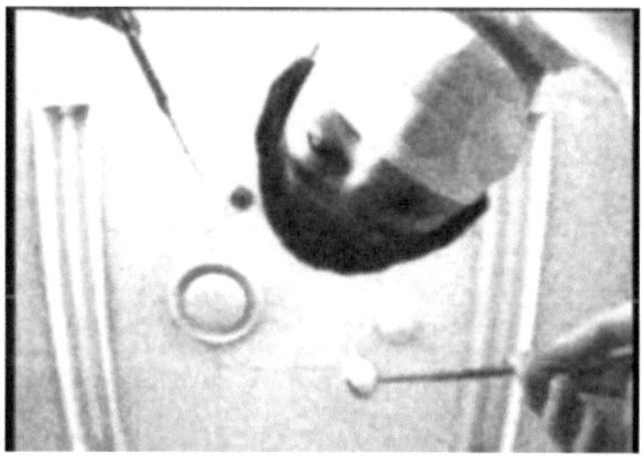

Figure 13 View from camera of Patient Robot

5.2 Experimental results

Fig. 14 shows a selection of the results of a questionnaire following the training.

Which components of the robot were well reproduced?

- Movement of the eyes, mouth and head and hardness of the lips.
- Unexpected movements (neck, vomiting, sudden closure of the jaw)
- Respiration, the act of swallowing, raising of hand
- The slow closure of the mouth during treatment

What components of the robot were not well reproduced?

- The opening of the mouth was too small and the tongue movement insufficient.
- The lips and buccal mucous membrane were too tight. The angle of the mouth too rigid.
- The pharynx was too deep inside the oral cavity
- Respiration movement was too large

What are the effective features of the patient robot?

- Reproduction of the movement as found in actual patients during surgery was instructive for learning about the difficulties of treatment.
- Treatment was difficult due to hard lips. Unexpected movements were realistic.
- Different to conventional machines thus enabling interactive learning.
- Voice recognition enabled students to respond individually.
- The importance of talking became apparent.
- A certain degree of tension was generated during training.

What aspects were ineffective?

- Cavity formation would become difficult to understand if the robot were to be used from the beginning.
- The lips and jaw angle were rigid.
- I do not think that patients move in the same way as the robot.
- The timing of the mouth closing was a little different from reality.
- There were occasions when there was not a response to the actions of the trainee.
- I did not understand the reasons for certain reactions during treatments.

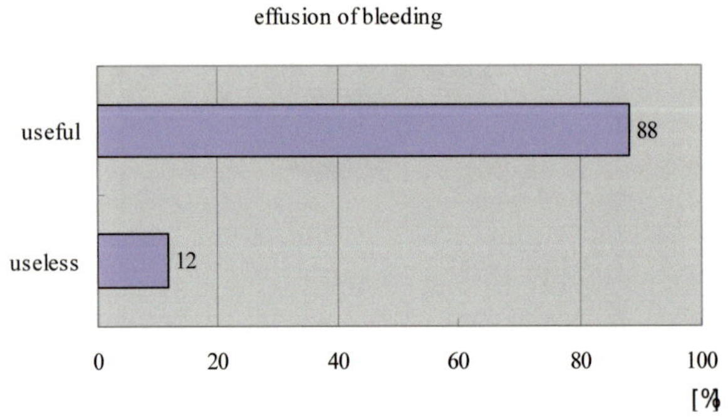
effusion of bleeding
useful
88
useless
12
0
20
40
60
80
100
[%]

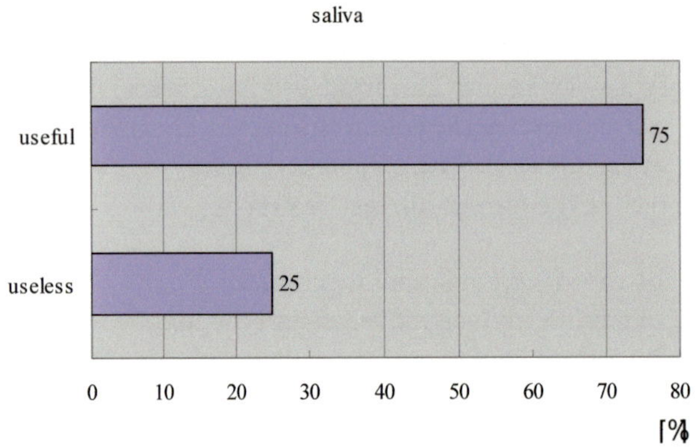
saliva
useful
75
useless
25
0
10
20
30
40
50
60
70
80
[%]

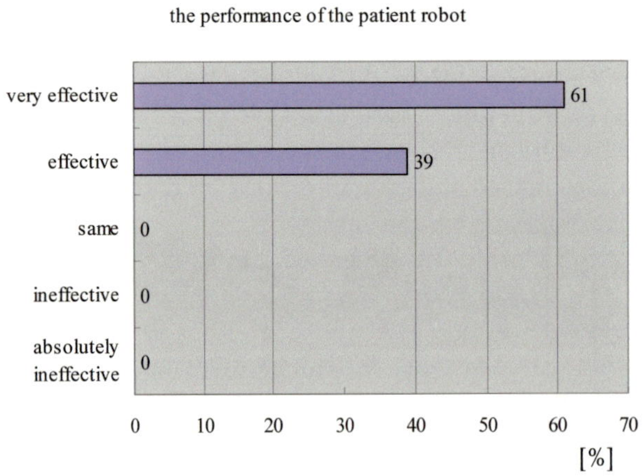
the performance of the patient robot
very effective
61
effective
39
same
0
ineffective
0
absolutely ineffective
0
0
10
20
30
40
50
60
70
[%]

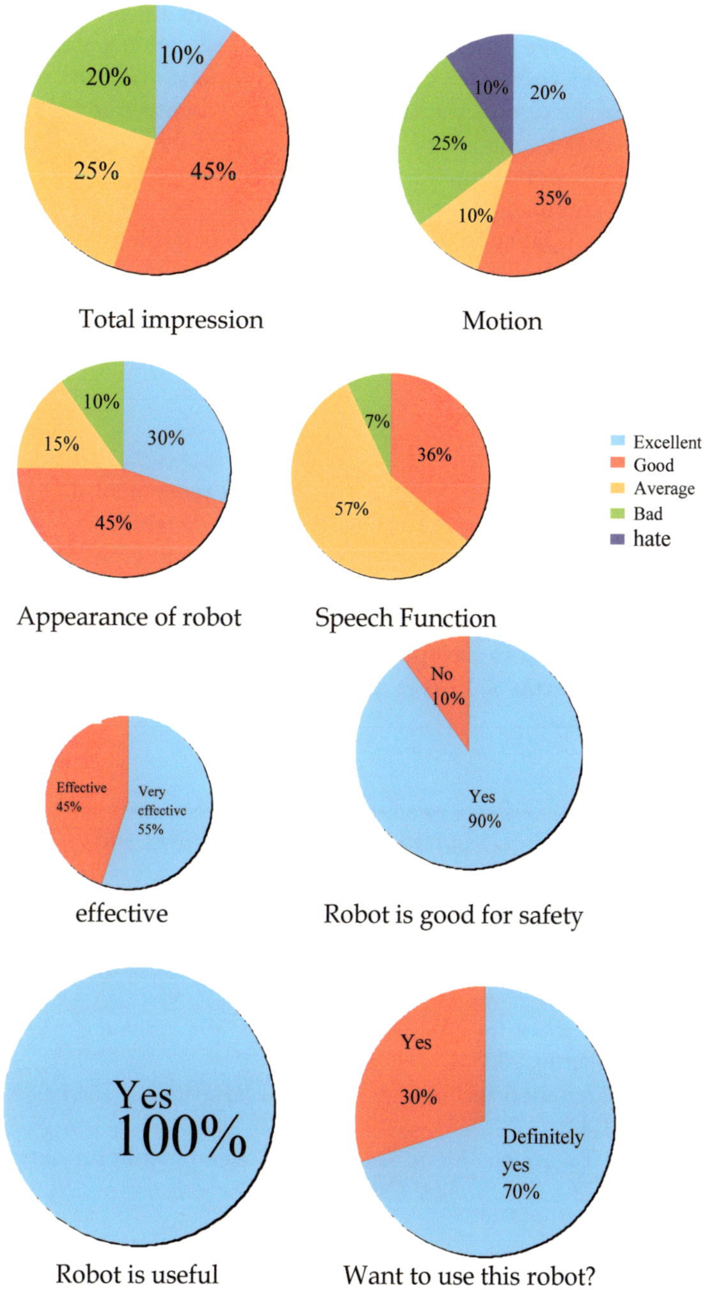

Figure 13. Result of questionnaire

Regarding comments about the ineffectiveness of reactions during treatment, I think that improving the performance of the sensors will resolve these problems. Also, I have consulted with dentists and been told that the rigidity of the mouth is acceptable as designed and hence this issue is not a problem. The major differences of opinion between the clinical residents and students were the volume of the mouth opening and stiffness of the lips. Clinical residents have actual experience of treating patients and are familiar with the rigidity of the lips and volume of the mouth opening and used the robot as in usual procedures. However, in the case of students who have not operated on actual patients yet, there were many instances of comments about the rigidity of the lips, volume of the mouth opening and signs of forcibly opening the mouth.

This is because the phantom usually used by dental students for training, has a larger sized mouth opening than actual patients and thus they find it difficult to carry out procedures using actual sized models. Also, since students performed surgery by looking only into the oral cavity, they did not notice the patient robot raising its hand in response to pain. This cannot be reproduced using a training phantom and is another useful feature of the patient robot.

6. Conclusions and future works

A patient robot with an oral cavity mimicking unexpected movement due to vomiting and pain and functions to induce bleeding and saliva flow was developed and used for clinical training. Trainee students and clinical residents were asked to complete a questionnaire about the patient robot. The results showed the patient robot to be effective as a means of training students to respond to unexpected movements during surgical procedures.

In the future, the author intend to incorporate additional sensors such as those used in the oral cavity, to enhance reactions to due pain so that clinical students could train by themselves without supervision.

7. Aknowlegement

This is a joint research with Prof. Koutaro Maki of Showa Univ., and Associate Prof. Kenji Suzuki and Prof. Hirofumi Miura of Kogakuin Univ. The author expresses great thanks for their and all staff's support on developing this robot.

8. References

Taro Gotoh etc: Analogue robot for medical training, *The 8th Annual Conference The Virtual Reality Society of Japan*, 2003 [1]

Buchanan JA: Use of simulation technology in dental education *J Dent Educ.* 2001 Nov. ; 65(11) * 1225-31. [2]

Akihisa Okino, Hideaki Takanobu, Atsuo Takanishi: Development of a jaw robot for study and education. *The 15th Annual Conference of The Robotics Society of Japan*, pp.707-708, 1997 [3]

Hideaki Takanobu, Akihisa Okino, Atsuo Takanishi, Mutsumi Madokoro, Yoshikazu Miyazaki, Koutarou Maki: Dental Patient Robot, *IROS2006*, pp. 1273-1278, 2006. [4]

Hideyuki Yanagiya, Hideaki Takanobu, Kenji Suzuki, Hirofumi Miura, Atsuo Takanishi, Mutumi Madokoro, Koutaro Maki: Dental Patient Robot, *The 45th Annual Conference of research reports of a student member* , pp.191-192 , 2006.[5]

Structure of the teeth, http://www.yic.ac/kenkou/kouzou.html [6]

33

Neuro- and Fascial Anatomy in the Male Pelvis for Robotic Radical Prostatectomy

Atsushi Takenaka[1], Ashutosh K. Tewari[2] and Masato Fujisawa[1]
[1]*Division of Urology, Kobe University Graduate School of Medicine*
[2]*Department of Urology, Weill Medical College of Cornell University, New York*
[1]*Japan,* [2]*USA*

1. Introduction

Prostate cancer is the most commonly diagnosed cancer and the second leading cause of cancer-related deaths in men in the US [Parker et al., 1997]. In the Prostate Specific Antigen (PSA) era, minimally invasive and nerve-sparing radical surgery for prostate cancer, e.g., conventional and robot-associated laparoscopic prostatectomy, is widely performed throughout the country.

Robotic prostatectomy started in 2000 [Menon et al., 2004], and it is estimated that 33,500 cases were performed during 2006. Robotic prostatectomy is increasing rapidly, and is becoming an important option for the management of localized prostate cancer. The da Vinci Robot® (Intuitive Surgical, Sunnyvale California) with its magnified 3-D vision and multi-jointed instruments facilitated the performance of radical prostatectomy with consideration of the pelvic anatomy (Figure 1). It is possible to view almost all pelvic anatomic structures during robotic prostatectomy. This enables the surgeon, in theory, to perform the operation with respect to anatomic findings using the multi-jointed instruments, compared with conventional for laparoscopic radical prostatectomy.

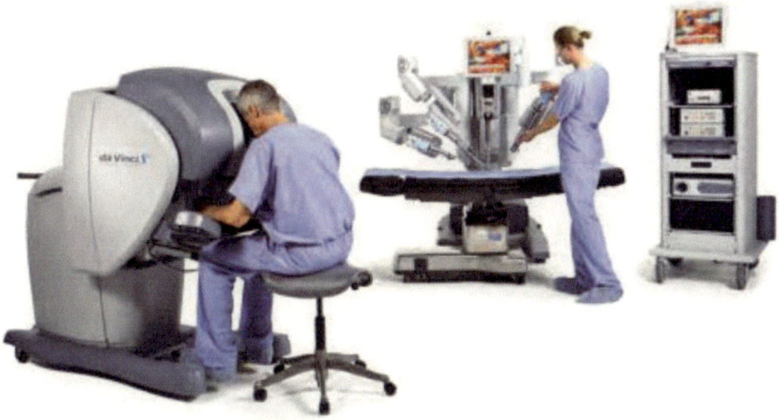

Figure 1. da Vinci system®. It consists of a surgeon's console, a patient-side cart with three or four interactive robotic arms, a high-performance *InSite*® Vision System and proprietary *EndoWrist*® Instruments

Although mapping for nerve-sparing during radical retropubic prostatectomy was laid down by the pioneering contributions [Walsh et al., 1982], there is some need reemphasize these anatomic principles in the robotic prostatectomy era.
Therefore, we felt the need to revisit these anatomic foundations in order to understand the macroscopic and microscopic findings and tailor them to the robotic approach. In the present paper, we review the pelvic neuro- and fascial anatomy with respect to robotic prostatectomy and demonstrate the procedures and critical points of nerve-sparing robotic radical prostatectomy based on novel anatomic concepts.

2.Materials and Methods

Anatomy of the autonomic nerves, ganglion cells and fasciae around the prostate, e.g., endopelvic fascia, Denonvilliers' fascia, was elucidated using 40 donated fresh cadavers and 60 donated fixed cadavers. The former were frozen at less than 12 to 36 hours after death and stored at -20C until dissection mainly for macroanatomic study. The latter were used for histologic study. The age at death was over 60 years for all cadavers. Robotic prostatectomy video tapes from 205 patients treated by one of the authors (A. K. T.) between January 2005 and December 2005 were reviewed step by step to understand the procedures anatomically. We used the Cornell Institute technique described previously [Tewari et al., 2005].

3. Neuroanatomy

3.1 Tri-zonal concept

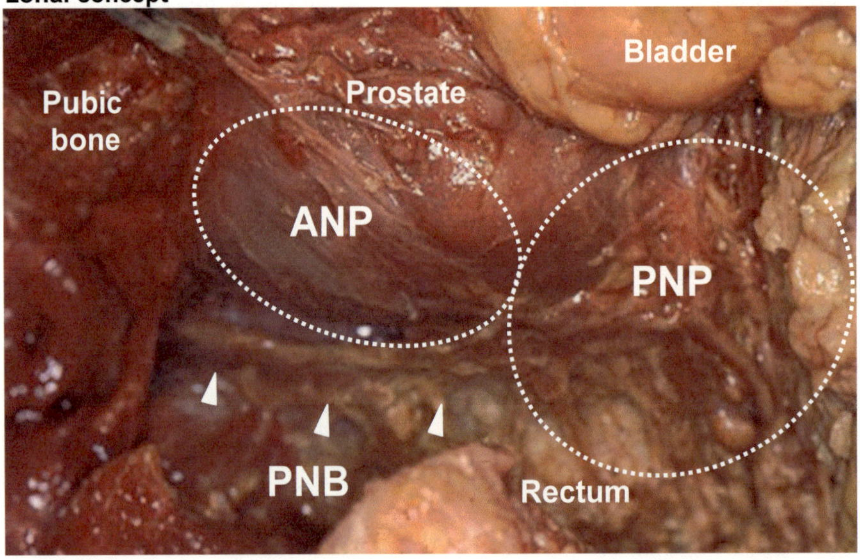

Figure 2. Tri-zonal concept of autonomic neural architecture around the prostate, proximal neurovascular plate (PNP), predominant neurovascular bundles (PNB, arrowhead), and accessory neural pathways (ANP)

In the classical concept, the neuroanatomy for nerve-sparing radical prostatectomy has been described in a limited area, i.e., only the posterolateral aspect of the prostate and the seminal vesicle [Lepor et al., 1985]. Many urologists have conceived of the preserved neural

3.1.1 Proximal neurovascular plate (PNP, Figure 3)

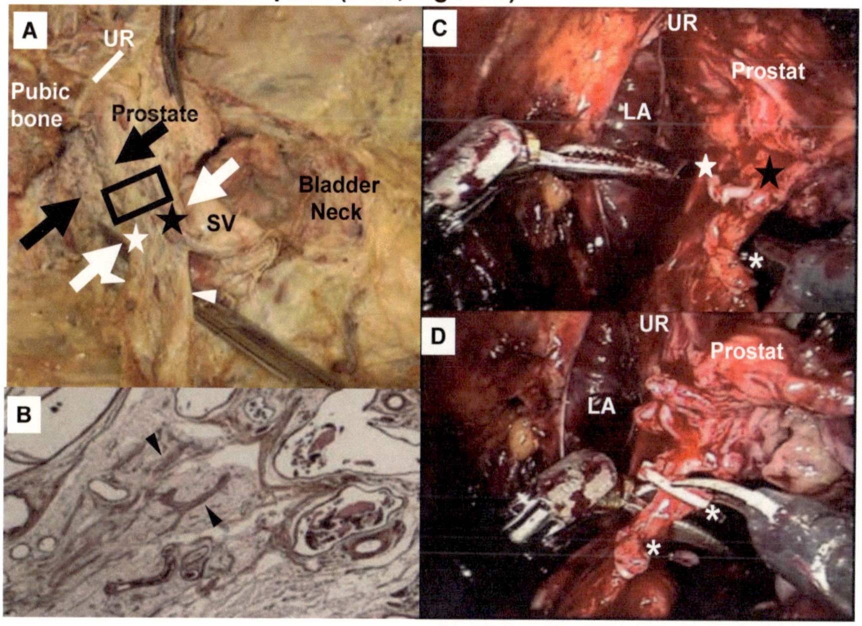

Figure 3. Control of vascular pedicle. Panel A is cadaveric dissection showing the relationship between seminal vesicle (SV) and proximal neurovascular plate (PNP, white arowhead) according to the procedure of robotic prostatectomy. Bladder neck transaction is performed, and the prostate is lifted up by the forceps. PNP is intermingled with vascular pedicle (black star) of the prostate. Black arrow, PNB; white arrow, intermingled structure of vascular and neural (white star) component. Panel B is histologic study stained by hematoxylin and eosin in small square in Panel A. Black arrowhead, ganglion cells. Panel C and D are the surgical procedure. Viewing these structure laterally, we should estimate where is the approximate border between neural (white star) and vessel component (black star), although they are actually intermingled. We have already cut a part of the vessels using a clip (asterisk). Panel D shows we insert the tip of the left hand instrument into the border, ligate the residual vessels using clip, and are cutting sharply. UR, urethra; LA, levator ani

The PNP is an integrating center for the processing and relay of neural signals. This plate is located lateral to the bladder neck, the seminal vesicles and branches of the inferior vesical vessels and is thick in the center near the seminal vesicles. Specifically, depending on variations in anatomy and prostate size, the PNP is located 5-10 mm (average 5 mm) lateral to the seminal vesicles, and within 4-15 mm (average 6 mm) of the bladder neck, within 2-7 mm (average 5 mm) of the endopelvic fascia.

The PNP extends posterolaterally to the base of the prostate, and distally continues as the classical neurovascular bundle while a few branches travel through the fascial and capsular tissue of the prostate as accessory pathways.

3.1.2 Predominant neurovascular bundles (PNB, Figure 4)

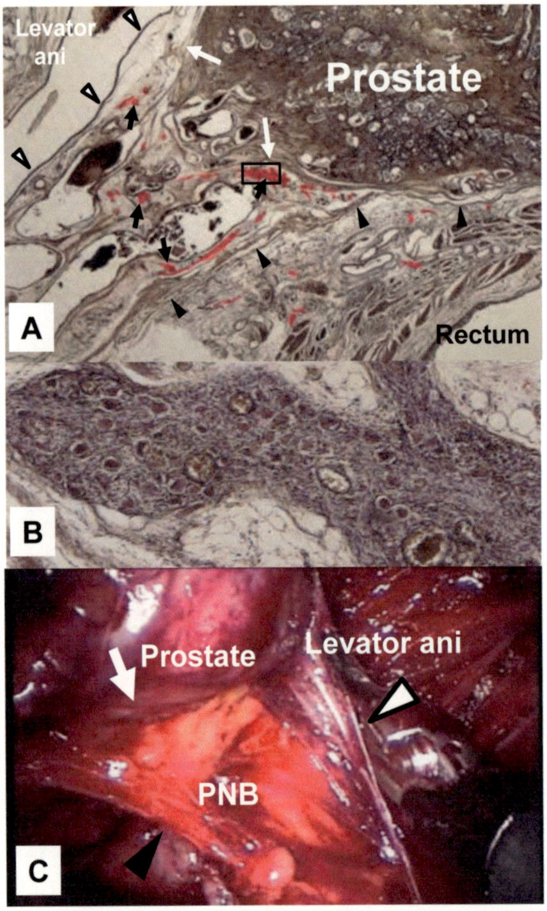

Figure 4. Release of predominant neurovascular bundles (PNB). Panel A is horizontal section of the posterolateral prostate. Ganglion cells (black arrow) in PNB are along or attaching to the posterolateral aspect of the prostate capsule (white arrow). Ganglion cells exist in the triangle of the prostate capsule, lateral pelvic fascia (white arrowhead), and Denonvillier's fascia (black arrowhead). Red, neural component. Panel B is a magnification of small square in Panel A. Hematoxylin and eosin stain. Panel C is the surgical procedure. We should imagine PNB as a triangle, which is seen in Panel A.

This corresponds to the classical bundle, however, it carries the neural impulses not only to the cavernous tissue, but also urethral sphincter and to the end of the levator ani muscle. The PNB is enclosed within the layers of levator fascia and / or lateral pelvic fascia and is located at the posterolateral aspect of the prostate. The course varies from the base to the prostatic apex.

The PNB occupies a groove between the prostate and rectum, is thickest at the base and has a highly variable course and architecture near the apex. Our anatomic study [Takenaka et al., 2004] showed the cavernous nerve candidate continued to the PNB through the distal part of the PNP. The fibers from HGN are more ventral and from PSN are more dorsal at the base of the prostate.

3.1.3 Accessory distal neural pathways (ANP, Figure 5)

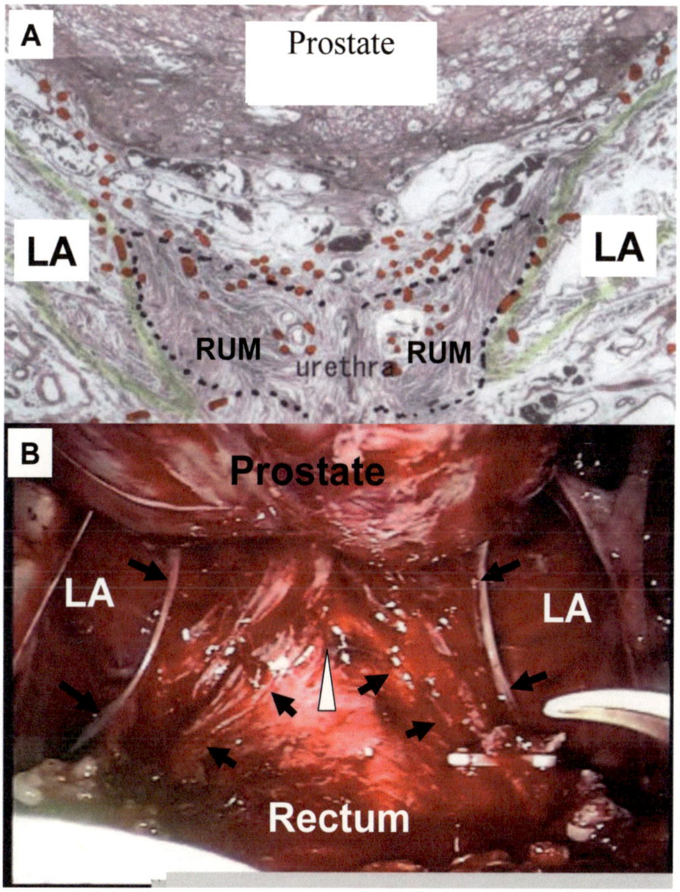

Figure 5. Apical transaction. Panel A is a frontal section through the apex of the prostate. Many nerve fibers exist behind the apex of the prostate between bilateral levator ani (LA). Some of them penetrate the rectourethral muscle (RUM) encircled by dots. Hematoxylin and eosin staining. Panel B is the surgical procedure. We can see the many nerve fibers behind the apex of the prostate during robotic prostatectomy. Bilateral PNB (black arrow) overlapped behind the apex, and formed posterior plexus (white arrowhead)

There have been discussions about putative accessory pathways besides PNB around the prostate [Lunacek et al, 2005, Menon et al, 2005]. These are usually described within the layers of the levator fascia and / or lateral pelvic fascia, on the anterolateral and posterior aspect of the prostate, which may serve as additional conduits for neural impulses.
Additional accessory branches occasionally formed an apical plexus on the posterolateral aspect of the prostatic apex and urethra incorporating fibers from both the PNB. This distal plexus was observed in 35% of cases, penetrating the recto-urethral muscle. This could potentially act as a neural pathway for not only cavernous tissue but also the urethral sphincter. It could also serve as a safety mechanism to provide backup neural crosstalk between the two sides.

3.2 Distribution of autonomic ganglion cells

To our knowledge, we were the first to report the distribution of autonomic ganglion cells (GCs) in the male pelvis [Takenaka et al, 2005a]. Pelvic autonomic GCs exist not only in macroanatomic nerve components but also along the viscera. In nerve-sparing prostatectomy, major components for preservation include sparing the nerve bundles only. GCs have received little consideration in this strategy. Since GCs cannot repair themselves, special consideration should be given to these structures during nerve-sparing surgery.
We examined the distribution of ganglion cells in detail, according to the robotic procedure (Table 1).

Specimen	M1	M2	M3	M4	M5	M6	M7	average
PNP	1113	332	250	-	534	411	575	535.8±307.7
PNB	698	230	448	66	908	96	500	420.9±313.3
ANP								
• Bladder, posterior	172	48	44	0	10	162	567	143.3±199.1
• B / P junction	78	280	135	53	50	232	211	148.4±93.2
• SV, posterior	163	25	78	-	212	45	273	132.7±99.2
• Prostate, posterior	155	101	0	65	230	15	535	157.3±184.7
• Prostate, anterior	0	0	10	-	3	0	0	2.2±4.0
• Prostate, apex	15	0	10	109	177	104	387	114.6±136.8
Other site								
• HGN	604	945	276	-	248	-	825	579.6±314.8
• PSN	1262	396	223	84	853	285	765	552.6±420.9
• Sacral ganglion	1566	687	-	249	1092	849	1884	1054.5±596.2
• levator ani	0	0	-	16	0	3	0	3.2±6.4

Table 1. Pelvic ganglion cell numbers and distribution in male hemipelvis using semiserial sections at 1-mm intervals

At 1-mm interval sections, we could detect many GCs in the PNP (250 to 1113 cells) and the PNB (66 to 908 cells). In the PNP, we recognized an intermingled structure comprised of GCs and a vascular component (Figure 3B). GCs were distributed widely throughout the PNB, especially laterally or posteriorly (Figure 4A, 4B). In particular, these ganglion cells were attached to the prostatic capsule or even embedded within the capsule. In the ANP, some ganglion cells existed in the bladder/prostate junction, the posterior aspect of the seminal vesicle, and posterior aspect of the prostate, however they didn't touch the plane by our nerve-sparing robotic technique. However, almost all nerve fibers and GCs converged at the apex. Some cavernous nerve candidates penetrated the recto-urethral muscle, which filled the space between the bilateral levator ani muscle behind the urethra.

As shown above, intersubject differences were evident at all sites. Significant variations were noted in the posterior aspect and near the apex of the prostate. There were almost no ganglion cells in the anterior aspect of the prostate and levator ani muscle.

3.3 Robotic Technique based on the neuroanatomy

With respect to the distribution of GCs along the prostate, we revaluated each step of the nerve-sparing robotic technique at our institution. Although all steps of surgery should be performed skillfully, we note the most critical procedures neuroanatomically, control of the pedicle, release of the PNB and the apical transaction. These are extremely important steps in the preservation of the GCs, because there are several GCs along the plane of dissection.

3.3.1 Control of the vascular pedicle

This is one of the most critical procedures, because neural fibers and GCs were intermingled with the vascular component in the distal end of the PNP. Furthermore, the issue becomes even more complex when we must preserve the ANP, which is present in the anterolateral aspect of the prostate. We avoided electrocautery and bulldog clamp during this phase of surgery. First, the assistant lifted the prostate ventrally and laterally in the direction contralateral to treatment. Viewing the PNP from the proximal and lateral side, we dissected the vessels in smaller packets using the EndoWrist forceps (Intuitive Surgical, CA, USA), to identify vessels entering the prostate and control these athermally using small clips (Figure 3C, 3D). The key was to stay close to the prostate, where the vessels and neural components gradually separated. This meticulous separation is necessary, because there is no clear border between the vessels and neural component. Dissection becomes further complicated due to the competing goal of avoiding the cancer containing prostatic capsule. It is crucial to remain right on the surface of prostatic fascia to avoid inadvertent entry to a deeper plane, which might compromise cancer control, especially if there is pathological capsular penetration.

3.3.2 Release of PNB

Once the prostate is freed from the vascular pedicle, it becomes more mobile with the support of the assistant. The prostate can be rotated to expose a potentially avascular triangle that is bounded posteriorly by the Denonvilliers' fascia, laterally by the levator fascia / lateral pelvic fascia, and medially by the prostatic capsule. Once this triangle leaves the prostate, the dissection appears very elegant and usually can be performed by gently pushing the prostate. We must avoid traction injury of the PNB by excessive pulling and blunt dissection (Figure 4C).

If patients have a small (5%) focus of less than Gleason 7 prostate cancer, we may choose to preserve the anterior ANP, i.e., using the Veil technique by Menon's group. To the contrary, we developed dissection planes within the fatty tissue of the PNB (incremental nerve sparing) and therefore stayed away from the capsule in cases where there was high risk of extra capsular extension.

3.3.3 Apical transaction

This is also one of the most critical steps, because almost all nerve fibers and GCs converge to the apex circumferentially. The assistant pulls the prostate ventrally again, and we push down the rectal wall gently using the left instrument. We performed sharp meticulous dissection not only at the PNB but also at the posterior aspect of the apex. It was very important to dissect the neural component together with the recto-urethral muscle (Figure 5C).

After complete apical separation from the PNB and posterior plexus, we stitched the dorsal vein complex at the apex with a small needle. After viewing the apex from various aspects and determining the shape of the apex, we cut the dorsal vein complex and anterior wall of the urethra. Finally, the posterior wall of the urethra is sharply cut, while avoiding the PNB and posterior plexus injury.

Of patients who were pre-operatively potent (SHIM score > 22) and who had nerve sparing surgery, 80% were able to have an erection firm enough to have an intercourse, or were actively having sexual intercourse, at 1 year of follow-up [Tewari et al., in press].

4. Fascial anatomy

Although the fascia or the membrane covering a structure is a very important landmark for separation of a structure, it might sometimes be anatomically tiny or thin. Therefore, there are some descrepancies between the actual anatomic construction and the pre-operative surgical planning. Because it is sometimes very difficult to demonstrate the fascial structure on micro- and macroanatomic study, the fascial anatomy occasionally might differ and might be understood arbitrarily or practically. In this section, we describe the anatomy of the endopelvic fascia (EPF) and Denonvilliers' fascia (DVF) which are extremely useful structures for improving the oncological and functional outcomes in robotic prostatectomy.

4.1 Endopelvic fascia

EPF is thought to refer to the fascia in the transitional area between the pelvic wall and pelvic viscera. However, the fascial anatomy near the prostate is not accepted anatomically, i.e., the existence and implications of the fascia of the levator ani (FLA) are not considered. The FLA is folded back at the anterior or lateral aspect of the prostate behind the EPF. The overlap of the EPF and the foldback resemble a condensed white collar, i.e., the fascial tendinous arch of the pelvis [Takenaka et al, 2005b]. In other words, the fascial tendinous arch of the pelvis is not the anatomic ligament structure. The lowest part connected to the pubo-prostatic ligament (Figure 6). When the prostate was small, the fascial tendinous arch connected to the anterior aspect of the prostate and the pubo-prostatic ligament is clearly seen to be connected to the bladder. We identify this as the pubo-vesical ligament. In large prostate cases, the location of the fascial tendinous arch is sometimes lateral, and pubo-vesical ligament was unclear. When the thin EPF was incised within the fascial tendinous arch of the pelvis, the collar and the levator ani could be separated laterally. This collar distally attached to the under surface of pubic symphysis to form pubo-prostatic ligaments. The EPF, FLA, and pubo-prostatic ligaments formed a sheet covering the pelvic floor. The shape of the collar was variable, depending on the prostate shape, volume, and pelvic shape. Pubo-prostatic ligaments were very close to the dorsal vein complex, however, we could separate this structure in fresh cadavers.

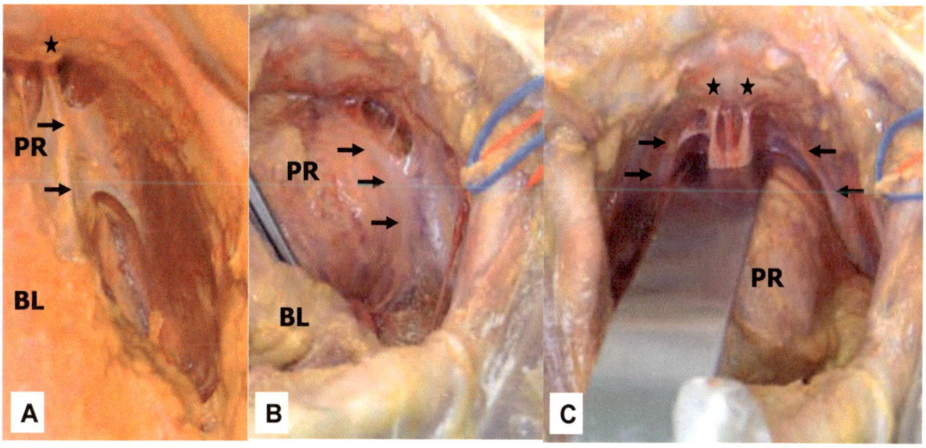

Figure 6. The various shape of the endopelvic fascia and the pubo-prostatic ligaments (star) in the fresh cadavers. The prostate in Panel A is very small. We can easily understand the fascial tendious arch of the pelvis (arrow) connects to the pubic symphysis to form the pubo-prostatic (-vesical, in this case) ligament. In Panel B, large prostate case, the endopelvic fascia is incised along the arrows, the condensed collar, i.e., the fascial tendious arch of the pelvis (arrow) and the levator ani could be separated laterally (Panel C). PR, prostate; BL, bladder

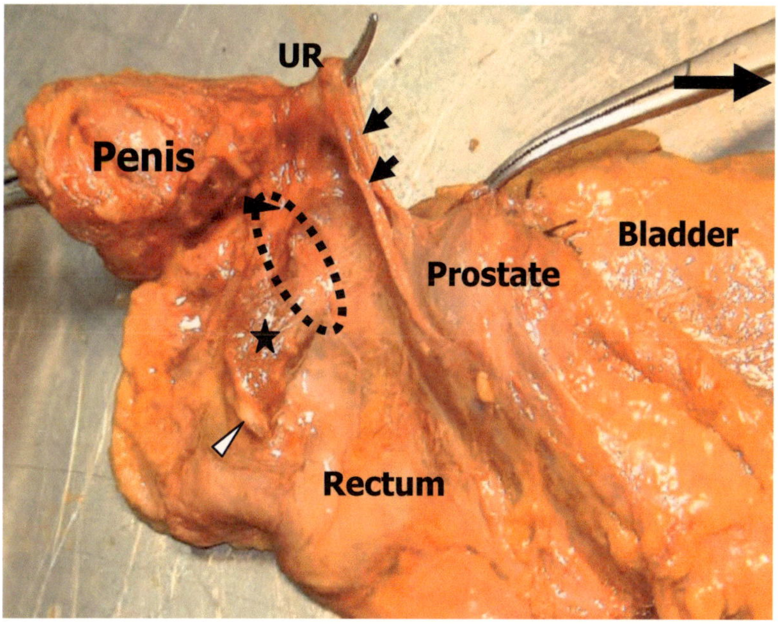

Figure 7. The rhabdosphincter, the urethra, and the pupo-perinealis muscle in the fresh cadaver. The urethra is cut at the apex of the prostate, and the forceps is inserted into the urethra retrogradely. The pubo-perinealis muscle (star) and pubo-prostatic ligaments (white arrowhead) are separated from the pubic symphysis and droop over the rectum. The rhabdosphincter is Ω shape, and the dorsal fibers coursed to the pubo-perinealis muscle and the apex of the prostate (black arrowhead and black arrow, respectively). The puboperinealis muscle terminated at the perineal body (encircled by dots). UR, urethra

The pubo-perinealis muscle was attached behind the insertion of the pubo-prostatic ligament (Figure 7). It was anteromedial to the levator ani [Myers et al., 2000] and formed a hammock around the urethra. That is to say, the pubo-prostatic ligament and the fascial tendinous arch together formed a pubo-prostatic collar on the pelvic floor. The pubo-perinealis muscle, which formed the inner layer of the levator ani muscle and connected to the urethral sphincter, attached to the back of the pubo-prostatic ligament. These three structures surrounded and supported the periurethral area, horizontally, sagittally, and frontally, as a complex.

4.2 Robotic approach to the EPF

4.2.1 Preservation of pubo-prostatic collar

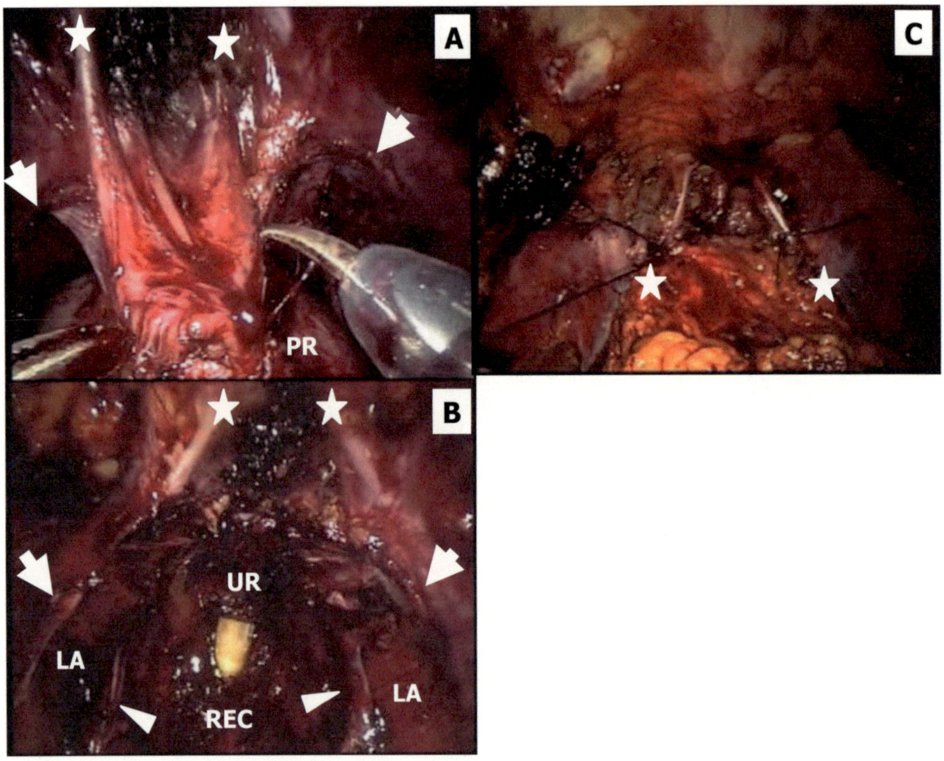

Figure 8. Panel A: After the separation of the fascial tendious arch of the pelvis, the dorsal vein complex is cut proximal to the pubo-prostatic ligaments (closed star). Arrow, the fascial tendious arch of the pelvis; PR, prostate; Panel B: The preserved fascial tendious arch of the pelvis (arrow) and the pubo-prostatic ligaments (closed star) form a plate of the pubo-prostatic collar. LA, levator ani; REC, rectum; UR, urethra; white arrowhead, preserved nerve plate; Panel C: The accomplishment of the pubp-perineoplasty. The open star shows the position of the most proximal tie

The EPF was incised just medial to the fascial tendious arch. However, at this time we stopped the incision short of the pubo-prostatic ligament in order to avoid excessive separation around the apex [Takenaka et al, 2007a]. Because the antegrade approach is performed in robotic prostatectomy, dissection of the dorsal vein complex and apex should be the final step. After the dorsal vein stitch at the middle of the prostate, bladder neck transaction, seminal vesicle dissection, separation of the prostate and rectum, control of the vascular pedicle, and release of the predominant neurovascular bundles were performed. We separated the apex carefully from the pubo-prostatic collar complex. First, we cut the dorsal vein complex proximal to the pubo-prostatic ligaments (Figure 8A). Cautery is used at the ventral part of the dorsal vein complex, but is not used at the dorsal part in any case. Second, after viewing the apex from various aspects and determining the shape of the apex, it was completely but minimally separated from the rhabdosphincter and pubo-perinealis muscle. Finally, the urethra is sharply cut. Pubo-prostatic ligaments and the fascial tendinous arch were preserved in all cases (Figure 8B).

4.2.2 Pubo-perineoplasty

A running vesico-urethral suture is made using a tied suture of 9-inch dyed and 9-inch undyed 3-0 Biosin with a small needle (CV-23) as described previously [Menon et al., 2004]. After finishing the anastomosis, it was suspended to the collar of residual tissues using three 3-0 sutures on each side (Figure 8C). The technique is easy and requires only 5 minutes to complete. This modification helped in the early return of continence. The continence rate was 29% in the first week, 62% at 6 weeks, 88% at 12 weeks, and 95% in 16 weeks after catheter removal [Tewari et al., 2007].

4.3 Denonvilliers' fascia

In 1863, Charles Denonvilliers first described a thin layer structure separating the rectum from the bladder, seminal vesicles, and prostate. This structure has become important for urologic and colorectal surgeons, because it is an important landmark indicating a pathway between urogenital and digestive organs [Ophoven et al, 1997].

However, there is no consensus on usage of the term "Denonvilliers' fascia" during urologic and colorectal surgeries. The first reason for the confusion is that we were not able to obtain a panoramic view of the rectogenital septum. The second reason is that the clinical anatomy is quite different from histology. Consequently, surgeons might use the term "Denonvilliers' fascia" conceptually.

During robotic prostatectomy, we can directly and antegradely observe a magnified view behind the prostate. The aim of the present study is to elucidate the clinical anatomy of the Denonvilliers' fascia.

In all cases of robotic prostatectomy, we identified a membranous structure attached to the posterior aspect of the prostate near the base of the seminal vesicle or slightly distal of the base. After cutting this membrane, we encountered a mesh-like structure behind the posterior aspect of the prostate. Histologically, there existed the disorderly loose connective tissue between Douglas' cul-de-sac and the rectourethral muscle, which could correspond to the mesh-like structure in Robotics. In addtion, there was the tight and thick membrane including smooth muscle fibers between cul-de-sac and posterior aspect of the prostate near the base of the seminal vesicle (Figure 9). There isn't two-layer structure in histology, either [Takenaka et al, 2007b].

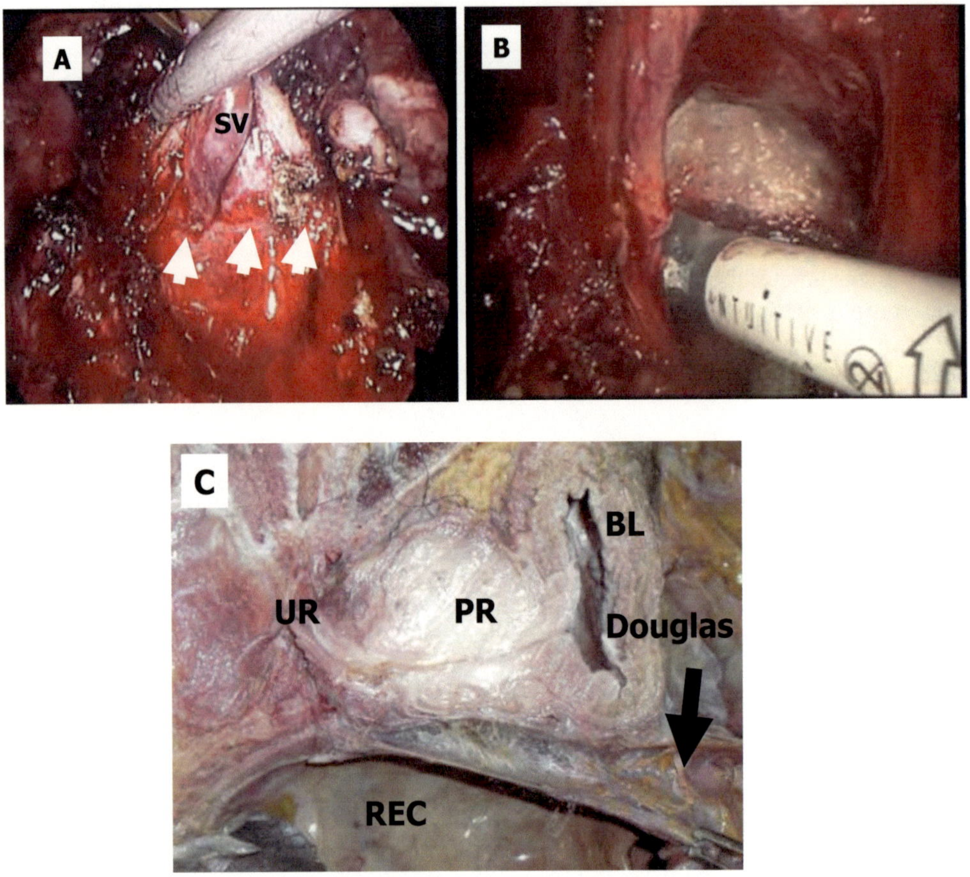

Figure 9. Panel A, After the seminal vesicle (SV) was lifted up, the arrows indicated the line where the thick membrane from the the cul-de-sac attaches. Panel B, After cutting the thick membrane, we can see the mesh-like connective tissue and the anterior surface of the rectum. Panel C, Mid-sagittal section of fresh cadaver illustrates the mesh-like connective tissue between the prostate (PR) and the rectum (REC). UR; urethra, BL; bladder, Douglas; Douglas pouch

4.4 Surgical approach to the DVF

As described above, after cutting the thick membrane between the cul-de-sac and posterior aspect of the prostate near the base of the seminal vesicle, we can easily find the flexible way to the apex, because there is a mesh-like structure, which is not a two-layered structure. Due to the angle of the anterior rectal wall and Endowrist™, we easily reach the rectal wall. To avoid rectal injury, and to preserve the neural components around the apex of the prostate, we must turn the tip of the Endowrist™ to the ventral side. If there is an advanced cancer at the border of the posterior aspect of the prostate, we can keep the dissection plane adjacent to the rectal wall.

5. Conclusion

These tri-zonal and ganglion cell concepts may be beneficial to new surgeons undertaking nerve-sparing robotic radical prostatectomy. An anatomic approach to the EPF might lead to improvement of the functional outcomes. Anatomically, there was no two-layer structure of the Denonvilliers' fascia. It is important to delineate the difference between embryologic concept, surgical anatomy, and histologic findings in order to avoid misunderstanding of the term "Denonvilliers' fascia.

6. References

Costello, A. J.; Brooks, M. & Cole, O. J. (2004). Anatomical studies of the neurovascular bundle and cavernosal nerves. *BJU Int*, 94, 1071-1076.

Lepor, H.; Gregerman, M.; Crosby, R.; Mostofi, F. K. & Walsh, P. C. (1985). Precise localization of the autonomic nerves from the pelvic plexus to the corpora cavernosa: a detailed anatomical study of the adult male pelvis. *J Urol*, 133, 207-212.

Lunacek, A.; Schwentner, C.; Fritsch, H., Bartsch, G. & Strasser, H. (2005). Anatomical radical retropubic prostatectomy: 'curtain dissection' of the neurobascular bundle. *BJU Int*, 95, 1226-1231.

Menon, M.; Tewari, A.; Peabody, J. O.; Shrivastava, A.; Kaul, S.; Bhandari, A. & Hemal, A. K. (2004). Vattikuti Institute prostatectomy, a technique of robotic radical prostatectomy for management of localized carcinoma of the prostate: experience of over 1100 cases. *Urol Clin N Am*, 31, 701-717

Menon, M.; Kaul, S.; Bhandari, A.; Shrivastava,; Tewari, A. & Hemal, A. (2005). Potency following robotic radical prostatectomy: a questionnaire based analysis of outcomes after conventional nerve sparing and prostatic fascia sparing techniques. *J Urol*, 174, 2291-2296.

Myers, R. P.; Cahill, D. R.; Kay, P. A.; Camp, J. J. Devine, R. M.; King, B. F. & Engen, D. E. (2000). Puboperineales: muscular boundaries of the male urogenital hiatus in 3D from magnetic resonance imaging. *J Urol*, 164, 1412-1415.

Ophoven, A. & Roth, S. (1997). The anatomy and embryological origins of the fascia of Denonvilliers: a medico-historical debate. *J Urol*, 157, 3-9.

Parker, S. L.; Tong, T.,;Bolden, S. & Wingo, P. A.(1997). Cancer statistics, 1997. *CA Cancer J Clin*, 47, 5-27.

Takenaka, A.; Murakami, G.; Soga, H.; Han, S. H.; Arai, Y. & Fujisawa, M. (2004). Anatomical analysis of the neurovascular bundle supplying penile cavernous tissue to ensure a reliable nerve graft after radical prostatectomy. *J Urol*, 172, 1032-1035.

Takenaka, A.; Kawada, M.; Murakami, G.; Hisasue, S; Tsukamoto, T. & Fujisawa, M. (2005a). Interindividual variation in distribution of extramural ganglion cells in the male pelves: a semi-quantitative and immunohistochemical study concerning nerve-sparing pelvic surgery. *Eur Urol*, 48, 46-52.

Takenaka, A.; Hara, R.; Soga, H. Murakami, G. & Fujisawa M. (2005b). A novel technique for approaching the endopelvic fascia in retropubic radical prostatectomy, based on an anatomical study of fixed and fresh cadavers. *BJU Int*, 95, 766-77.

Takenaka, A.; Tewari, A.; Leung, R. A.; Bigelow, K.; El-Tabey, N.; Murakami, G. & Fujisawa, M. (2007a). Preservation of the puboprostatic collar and puboperineoplasty for early recovery of urinary continence after robotic prostatectomy: anatomic basis and preliminary outcomes. *Eur Urol*, 51, 433-440.

Takenaka. A.; Soga, H.; Tewari A.;, Leung, R.; Miyake, H.; Tanaka, K. & Fujisawa, M. (2007b). Does Denonvilliers' fascia consist of anterior and posterior layers?: An anatomic study of cadaveric dissections and robotic prostatectomy findings. *Urology*, 20 (suppl. 3A), 233.

Tewari, A.; El-Hakim, A.; Horninger, W.; Peschel, R.; Coll, D. & Bartsch, G. (2005). Nerve-sparing during robotic radical prostatectomy: use of computer modeling and anatomic data to establish critical steps and maneuvers.*Curr Urol Rep*, 6, 126-128.

Tewari, A.; Takenaka, A.; Mtui, E.; Horninger, W.; Peschel, R. & Bartsch, G. (2006). The proximal neurovascular plate (PNP) and the tri-zonal neural architecture around the prostate gland -importance in Athermal Robotic Technique (ART) of Nerve Sparing Prostatectomy. BJU Int, 98, 314-323.

Tewari, A.; Bigelow, K.; Rao, S.; Takenaka, A.; El-Tabi, N.; Te, A. & Vaughan, E. D. (2007). Anatomic restoration technique of continence mechanism and preservation of puboprostatic collar: a novel modification to achieve early urinary continence in men undergoing robotic prostatectomy. *Urology*, 69, 726-731.

Tewari, A.; Ramanathan, R. & Takenaka, A. (in press). Anatomical foundations for nerve preservation during prostatectomy -trizonal concept and athermal robotic technique. *Contemp Urol.*

Walsh, P. C. & Donker, P. J. (1982). Inpotence following radical prostatectomy: Insight into etiology and prevention. *J Urol*, 128, 492-497

Robotic assistance in microvascular surgery

M.G.W. van den Heuvel and R.R.W.J. van der Hulst
Department of Plastic, Reconstructive and Hand Surgery, University Hospital Maastricht
The Netherlands

1. Introduction

The introduction of minimally invasive surgery in the early 1990s has rapidly changed the performance of surgical procedures in a wide range of surgical specialities. Postoperative pain, discomfort and morbidity are caused by trauma created by trying to gain access to the area of surgery, rather than by the surgical procedure itself. Through the application of minimally invasive surgery, several advantages are offered to the patient. Decreased post-operative pain, shorter hospitalisation, a more rapid return to work, improved cosmetics and reduced risk of wound infection and other post-operative complications are achieved by the performance of laparoscopy [1-5].

However, laparoscopic surgery also has it's limitations. The most important disadvantage is that only a two-dimensional image of the operating field can be provided, with a decreased depth perception as a result. Through experience, processing of monocular cues can be learned and depth perception improved. The adaptation of monocular cues, however, is a learning process through which performance times are significantly improved [6]. These adaptations are accounted for the increased mental fatigue and strain found with two-dimensional imaging. Other important limitations of laparoscopy are the limited manoeuvrability of effecter instruments, small working spaces, fixed angles at the trocar level to place sutures and the loss of direct contact with organs causing insufficient tactile information [1, 3, 6, 7]. Furthermore, the surgeon's tremor is amplified by the long instruments, which causes the use of laparoscopy in microsurgery to be problematic. Through all these limitations, a steep learning curve exists for the performance of laparoscopy [8].

Nowadays, minimally invasive surgery is widely applied in general surgery, gynaecology, urology and thoracic surgery. There is only little use of it in the divisions of plastic surgery, cardiothoracic surgery and vascular interventional surgery. Despite the technical advantages, laparoscopy is more difficult to be performed and more skills are required from a surgeon than with the performance of traditional surgery. The use of laparoscopy is especially problematic in microsurgery. A solution to all these problems can be provided by robotic surgery. Research has shown that robotic surgery is superior to traditional laparoscopy [8, 9]. By the participants of this study it was felt that robotic surgery was easier to learn than traditional laparoscopy. However, application of robotic surgery for the purpose of performing microsurgery is only in the first stage of development. This is unfortunate, while utilisation of robots in microsurgery offers the possibility to work really precise. An area where that feature is really important is the performance of microvascular surgery. Up to now, there has been only little experience with robotic surgery in this area.

2. Why use robots?

Surgery is a technology driven profession. The development of robotic surgery was originally started for the possibility of tele-surgery. Surgical tele-manipulation is performing an operation through communication technology and robotics without being physically present at the operating table. This offers great possibilities for performing surgery on patients that are inaccessible. Inaccessibility could be due to several reasons: 1) unavailability of a surgeon (a surgeon in one hospital with particular expertise can assist a colleague in another institution or country), 2) the patient being in a hazardous environment (e.g. in case of a battlefield or a nuclear accident), 3) the patient presents a danger to the surgical team (radioactive contamination or contagious infection) or 4) the surgical team is a danger to the patient (e.g. an immunodeficient patient). The first operation where the surgeon was virtually present was performed in France by Professor Marescaux, where the surgical console was present in New York City and was connected to the three arms of the Zeus system in France [2]. This type of procedures would not have been possible without the advent of high-speed broadband internet technology to rapidly deliver the surgical commands from the console to the robot arms.

Today, robotic surgery is widely utilized in different medical professions, e.g. general surgery, gynaecology, urology, thoracic surgery and neurosurgery. The use of robotic surgery is mainly twofold. It is widely used for endoscopic procedures to perform minimally invasive surgery (MIS), while another area of utilization is the use of robots in microsurgery because robots offer the possibility to work really precise. The role of automation is to standardize a procedure. Surgical robots can reduce variations in patient outcome among surgeons and for an individual surgeon.

The use of robotic assistance has enabled humans to transcend their limitations by information gathering and sensing or by improved delivery on a microscale basis or in difficultly accessible areas [3]. Surgeons are allowed to perform tasks that currently require more than one person, dexterity is increased, a three-dimensional image is provided and the possibility to operate in very confined spaces is offered. A master-slave manipulator allows performance of superhuman tasks that would not be possible without computer enhancement [3]. These manipulators also regulate filtration of tremor and downscaling of robotic movements through removing all high-frequency oscillating motions and reducing all large movements into microscopic movements at the instrument tips. The only disadvantage of master-slave manipulators is that they make a system mechanically and electrically complicated from the perspectives of safety and maintenance [3].

3. Robotic systems

First-generation surgical robots consisted mainly of robotic arms that assisted the primary surgeon by holding and positioning instruments. Nowadays, surgical robots are the primary surgeon's hands through a digital interface. Currently, two surgical telemanipulators are capable of performing remote telerobotic surgery: the da Vinci Robotic Surgical System (Intuitive Surgical, Mountain View, California, USA) and the Zeus Robotic Surgical System (Computer Motion, Goleta, California, USA). Surgical developed the da Vinci system at the urging of the Pentagon, in order to be able to perform remote operations without surgeons being at the front line or at sea [10]. With both systems, the surgeon is sitting at a console, the instruments appear right in front of his eyes and the controllers are in the same eye-

hand-target axis as found in open surgery, giving the impression that the instruments are an extension of the surgeon's hands [1].
Although there are many resemblances, there are also some technical differences between the two systems. With the da Vinci, surgeons are provided with a true 3D image obtained through binocular vision: different images are presented to each eye from a dual light source and dual cameras [2]. The 3D image on the Zeus system is achieved by viewing alternating 2D images on a monitor wearing special glasses. Manipulation systems are also different between the two systems. The da Vinci instruments are manipulated through friction-free devices held between forefinger and thumb, whilst Zeus instruments are manipulated by moving a ball-like hand interface. Both systems articulate at a "wrist" and offer seven degrees of freedom motion for the instruments. The master-slave can reduce tremor and downscale movements by 5:1 for the da Vinci and by 10:1 for the Zeus system. The advantage of the Zeus system is that, on the contrary of the da Vinci, it has three separate arms that provide the robot with a greater flexibility [2].
Both systems provide high visual magnification, movement scaling and tremor filtration, allowing for precise tissue dissection [11]. However, limitations in the current robotic systems are the lack of tactile feedback and potential interference between robotic arms [11]. A study of Sung and Gill showed that robotic laparoscopic procedures can be performed effectively using either the da Vinci or the Zeus system [11]. In this study, however, the learning curve and operating times were shorter and execution of the technical movements appeared inherently more intuitive for the da Vinci system [11].

4. Use of robotics in vascular surgery

Cardiac surgeons were the first to accept the application of robotic assistance in their surgery. Since robotic assisted technology became available, it has been successfully applied for aortic anastomoses in animal models. Surgical correction of aortic disease used to require a large incision in the abdomen and shifting of the abdominal viscera [12]. Through the use of robotic surgery the procedure has become minimally invasive, resulting in less post-operative pain and complications and improved cosmetics. Furthermore, robotic technology provides the vascular surgeon with the accuracy demanded to perform the delicate tissue handling necessary for aortic procedures.
From 1998 to 2000 Martinez et al. gained experience in using robotic surgery for performing aortic grafts in animal models [12]. In february 2001, Wisselink and collegues completed the first human aortic reconstruction using the Zeus system [12]. The procedure was performed in two patients. Since then, similar robotic surgery has been performed on many patients more. Research has confirmed the advantages of robotic use for aortic reconstruction. Kolvenbach and co-workers compared robotic versus manual aortic anastomosis times and found that times were shorter in the robotic group [12]. In addition, Stadler et al. found that the da Vinci robotic system facilitated the creation of the aortic anastomosis and shortened aortic clamp time in comparison to laparoscopic techniques [10].
Robotic surgery appears to be of most benefit in the area of microsurgery, while it can manipulate in a small space and finer and more controlled movements can be made without tremor. The use of robotics in microvascular surgery is the most recent area of development. And although not much experience has been gathered in this area, it holds great promises for the future...

5. Current experience in robotic microvascular surgery

Robot-assisted microvascular surgery was first introduced in cardiac surgery. Endoscopic instruments lacked the necessary degrees of angulation required and were insufficiently long to achieve a precise microvacular anastomosis in the chest [13]. In order for these problems to be solved, robotic surgery was introduced. In june 1998 Loulmet and colleagues performed the first clinical, totally endoscopic, computer-enhanced arrested heart coronary artery bypass in Paris [13]. A study performed on porcine hearts showed that a vascular anastomosis is easier performed by three-dimentional visualisation combined with robotic assistance than manually [13]. In 2000, the performance of arrested heart coronary artery bypass surgery was repeated with the Zeus system by Reichenspurner and his team in Munich [13]. The first report of coronary revascularization on a beating heart was in 2001 [2]. Using both the Zeus and the da Vinci System, over 2000 coronary bypass procedures were performed by the first half of 2002 [1]. From 2002 to 2004 robotic assisted TECAB surgery was performed on 98 patients divided over 12 centres [14].This study demonstrated that it is safe and efficient to perform this operation in patients by robotic means.

Except for the use of robotics in cardiac surgery, robots are still rarely used in microvascular surgery. Especially the area of reconstructive microsurgery demands optimal visualization, technical skill, precise surgical manipulations and minimization of tremor. All these demands are well sufficed by robotic surgery. Experienced microsurgeons operate at an accuracy of 50 μm; robotic assistance refines this accuracy by a factor of 10, to 5 μm [4]. Although high free-flap success rates are achieved by microsurgeons, the loss of a free flap is a dramatic event for the patient. Mostly, a compromised free flap is the result of a technical error. The frequency of these technical errors may be reduced by the use of robotic surgery. Several studies on this subject are already performed.

Already in 2000 the Robot Assisted MicroSurgery (RAMS) was used to perform vascular anastomoses of the rat femoral artery, both in vitro and in vivo. The RAMS system proved to be applicable in microsurgery, with the advantages of greater precision and more rapid manipulation compared to the surgeon [15]. Remarkable was that macro movements take more time accomplished by the robot than by the surgeon, while micro maneuvers are performed equally fast or even more rapid by the RAMS system than by the surgeon. Thus, when a surgical procedure approaches the micro level, the time difference between the surgeon and the robotic system is equilibrated.

In 2001 Le Roux and colleagues also used the RAMS system (NASA's Jet Propulsion Laboratory, Pasadena, CA and MicroDexterity Systems Inc., Memphis, TN) to anastomose carotid arteries in rats [16]. All vessels were patent and the error rate was similar to that of conventional techniques. However, using the RAMS system was associated with a significant increase in operating time, particularly due to an increase in time required for needle positioning and knot tying [16]. This increase in operative time may reflect a learning curve. The RAMS system improved the performance of medical students and engineers doing the same task and that of plastic residents carrying out a variety of microsurgical procedures [16].

Karamanoukian et al. used the Computer Motion Zeus Robotic Surgical System to anastomose 1-mm arterial vessels harvested from explanted pig hearts. They concluded that the Zeus robotic technology had certain advantages over the conventional human assistant, with the major advantage being the ability of scaling down the surgeon's movements to a microscopic level [17]. Another experiment of their group showed an important conclusion.

It proved that robotically assisted microanastomoses can be mastered equally well by surgical trainees and fully trained vascular surgeons [18]. Prior experience with open microsurgical procedures does not facilitate use of the robotic system. This conclusion may have important consequences for the future of microsurgery. Nowadays, only few surgeons share the experience to perform microsurgery. However, when robotic assistance would be used, microsurgery can be performed equally well by all surgeons and residents. This way, microsurgery can be applied amply in the medical world. Furthermore, anastomosis times were significantly longer using the robot compared to traditional freehand technique for the residents as well as for the fully trained surgeons.

In addition, research on performing end-to-end anastomoses in rat femoral arteries with Zeus showed that the Zeus system is effective at performing complex, open, microsurgery tasks in vivo, although there was no measurable benefit from robot-enhanced surgery [19]. A remarkable degree of tremor filtration was observed by the surgeon in the robot-enhanced cases as well as the feeling of exerting a greater precision when placing sutures. Anastomoses done by hand were significantly faster than those done with Zeus. This, however, could be a result of the large instruments available for Zeus. While they are three to five times larger than microsurgical instruments, it is more difficult to perform microsurgery with them [19]. This could also have contributed to the outcome of another experiment where vascular anastomoses were performed using the Zeus system on prosthetic conduits in a laparoscopic training box [20]. Although vascular anastomoses could be made with equal quality compared to manual procedures, robotic assistance resulted in significant longer suture and knot tying time, more failings during the procedures and more actions needed to perform the procedure. These problems may decrease when working with robotic instruments that are suitable for microsurgery.

In 2005 the first experimental microvascular surgery was performed in a pig using the da Vinci Surgical system. The robot was used to perform vessel adventitiectomy and microanastomoses. In performing a free flap the robotic assistance offered numerous advantages: elimination of tremor, scalable movements, fully articulating instruments with six degrees of spatial freedom and a dynamic three-dimensional visualization system. Despite the advantages, drawbacks were also present, with the absence of true microsurgical instruments being the most important one [21]. Preparation of the robot, including draping and positioning the arms, was performed in 27 minutes. The time to perform the microsurgical procedures (adventiectomy, arterial and venous anastomosis) took 44 minutes.

Recently, our department has gathered the first clinical experience in reconstructive robotic microvascular surgery when we performed a microvascular anastomosis in a muscle sparing free TRAM-flap. Using the da Vinci Surgical System (Intuitive Surgical, Inc, Sunnyvale, US) the arterial adventectomy and anastomosis was performed using 9/0 nylon sutures. The time to perform this anastomosis was about 40 minutes, which is significantly longer than the standard technique (around 20 minutes). To put a sterile draping around the robot took 20 minutes, but did not increase operating time while it was performed during dissection of the flap. Conclusions from this experiment are that the advantages of robotic surgery were not yet translated into a clear advantage, e.g. decreased operating time, however that can be achieved with more experience [22]. Again, the increase in operating time is partially due to the fact that this robot is not suited for the performance of microvascular surgery.

In 2006 a group of plastic and cardiothoracic surgeons used the Aesop robotic arm (Computer Motion Inc, Santa Barbara, CA, USA) to harvest internal mammary vessels for breast reconstruction in 20 patients [23]. The vessels were brought out through a passage in the second intercostal space. However, there is no need for such a complex procedure, while removing cartilage from the third or fourth rib provides a vessel long enough to perform an anastomosis. Their study also revealed a high incidence of complications. Although the study of Boyd et al. did not show convincing advantages, it should be further investigated whether there could be a role for robotic surgery in harvesting internal mammary vessels in breast reconstruction.

6. Advantages of robotic assistance in microvascular surgery

Normally, the full potential of microsurgery is limited by the manual dexterity of the individual surgeon. The physical and intellectual possibilities of surgeons differ. On top of that, the microscope magnifies and exaggerates all movements while it limits visual field and depth. Microsurgery requires that the surgeon spends long hours in a relatively fixed posture, which can be really tiring and can adversely affect the surgeon's technical performance. Finally, the microsurgical instruments act as extensions of the surgeon's hands and magnify physiological tremor [16]. In order to perform microsurgery optimal visualisation, technical skills, precise surgical manipulations and minimalization of tremor are important. These aspects are better sufficed by a robot than a surgeon. Advantages obtained by use of robotic assistance are a three-dimensional view, greater three-dimensional precision, better access to difficult areas, a larger range of motion, down scaling of movements to tissue level, tempering of incorrect movements or tremor, consistent reproducibility of movements and improved ergonomics [4, 6, 16-20, 24-26]. Furthermore, robots are not subjected to fear, stress or fatigue. Through all these advantages robotic surgery can potentially diminish tissue damage.
Prasad et al. compared the accuracy of robotic assistance without motion scaling to robotic assistance with the addition of motion scaling in a trial. There was a significant improvement in accuracy of 20-30 % for the groups with motion scaling [4]. This indicates that motion scaling is mainly responsible for the improvement in accuracy when using robotic assistance. A smaller role in accuracy seems to be assigned to tremor filtration [4]. Motion scaling also has the possibility to reduce operating time and to equalize the performance of the dominant and non-dominant hand [4].
Three-dimensional vision offers the advantage of improved depth perception and accuracy. A study showed that novice and advanced surgeons performing anastomotic drills with the da Vinci robot, were both 65 % faster and more accurate when working in three dimensions than in two [8]. Prior robotic experience was not necessary to benefit from 3D viewing [8]. Another study using the da Vinci robotic system showed that drill performance times were significantly reduced by using 3-dimensional vision when compared to 2-dimensional vision [6]. Error rates were also significantly improved by using 3-dimentional vision. The subjective impression of surgeons experienced in working with 2D and 3D view was that in performing anastomoses on a pig heart 3D-visualization improved coordination between the right and left instrument [25]. This facilitated handling of the needle. Especially transfer of the needle from one instrument to the other was easier, which reduced the forces applied to the needle and suture.

Research has shown that no transfer of training exists in performing microvascular anastomoses with robotic assistance for it requires totally different skills. This implies that when robots are developed for performing microvascular anastomoses, this procedure can also be carried out in peripheral hospitals instead of only in microsurgical centres, which is the case nowadays. This will be an extreme booster for the application and development of microvascular surgery.

The development of robotic systems to assist surgeons in performing microsurgery is a growing field of research. Robotic surgery holds promises for an evolutionary future. Expectations are that with more experience microvascular anastomoses can be performed more rapidly and with greater precision when using robotic assistance.

7. Problems concerning robotic microvascular surgery

Robots provide excellent opportunities for the future of microvascular surgery. However, at this point of time no robots have been adjusted for performing microvascular surgery. The current robots exhibit some problems. First of all there is no software designed for handling blood vessels, restricting the robot's range of motion and performing microvascular anastomoses. Furthermore, robots cannot operate with true microsurgical instruments what makes it difficult to manipulate the blood vessels effectively. In addition, their needle holders are too large to place a microsurgical suture [19, 21]. Another possible point of improvement is the creation of the anastomosis. Sutures need to be performed by multiple persons, while the use of small metal clips (nitinol clips) can decrease anastomosis time [27]. This possibility should be further examined in the near future.

The most discussed problem is the lack of haptic feedback [3, 15, 24]. Surgeons have to rely on visual cues to estimate the forces that they exert on the tissue. This is often a cause of broken sutures and torn delicate tissues, resulting in prolonged operative times and possible injury to the patient [24]. On the other hand, there are also surgeons that do not experience the lack of haptic feedback as an important issue. According to them, traditional microsurgery does not rely on haptic feedback, as before a microsurgeon can feel the small forces when a needle tears through a 1-mm vessel, the surgeon should see the vessel being stretched. This is found to be similar when using the robot [21]. Research has indeed shown that the lack of haptic feedback is partially compensated by visually observing deformation of the tissue [24]. Several studies have been done investigating the effect of haptic feedback. From all these studies it was concluded that haptic/ force feedback lowered suture tension and the amount of tension applied was significantly more consistent than without feedback [24, 28]. The force magnitudes applied with any force-feedback method more closely approximate the manual suture tension than forces applied without feedback [28]. Forces achieved with sensory -substitution modes did not vary significantly from the manual forces achieved with hand ties [28]. The consistency of these robot-assisted ties is equivalent or superior to those attained with hand ties [28]. Conclusively, sensory feedback improves the consistency of robotically applied forces [28]. Furthermore, research has shown that visual feedback systems were not as effective as vibrotactile feedback systems [28].

A huge drawback is the cost of a robot: it ranges from $ 750,000 to $ 1 million [11, 15, 21]. And also the maintenance costs should be considered. On top of that, the application of robotic surgery requires specially trained personnel and a dedicated surgical team. However, in the long run, these costs can be covered through the advantages of robotic surgery, e.g. by working more efficient more patients can be operated on in a shorter period

of time and with less assistance, and hospitalization will be shortened because of the decreased complication rate.
Some ethical issues have been raised concerning the use of robotic surgery. It is questioned who takes responsibility for harm caused by robotic surgery and when it is ethically appropriate for robots to be used? These questions can only be answered satisfactionally when experience in robotic surgery has been gathered.
However, the advantages of minimally invasive surgery justify the development of robotic surgery. Reducing robotic drawbacks should expand the use of robotic surgery. Thorough research needs to be performed in order to optimalize the use of robotic systems in surgery. For that to happen, a less conservative surgical community and an adapting industry are needed.

8. Does a learning curve exist in robotic surgery?

Many studies have demonstrated that there is a learning curve for robotic-assisted surgery [4]. Although a learning curve exists, it can be methodically overcome [1, 26]. The role of the mentor is critical in the process to overcome the challenges and flatten the learning curve [26]. Research has shown that educational experience of the fellow revealed improved operative times [26]. Mean robotic setup time, mean total robotic operative time and mean total operative time were all significantly improved when more experience was gathered [26].
In a study where surgeons performed a synthetic small bowel anastomosis in a closed box simulator, performance significantly increased between the first and the last task and also operative time was significantly reduced [1]. The number of movements also significantly reduced between the first and the last task and appeared to be a useful tool to measure performance [1]. A research performed on patients executing coronary bypass surgery on the beating heart indicated that there is a significant moderately steep learning curve, which is mitigated by further experience [29]. In CABG anastomoses on the beating heart, there existed a learning curve during the first 18 to 20 patients [29]. From the first to the last quintile there was a significant 40 % decrease in operating time [29]. Another study in which anastomoses were performed with the Zeus system showed that in the early cases, the surgeon broke sutures and bent the needles frequently [19]. After this learning period, these were both rare events.
Another remarkable finding was done. No significant difference in performance or time was measured between experienced and nonexperienced surgeons performing synthetic small bowel anastomoses [1, 9]. In another study where surgeons performed an anastomosis on a pig heart using the Zeus telemanipulator system, novice and experienced surgeons showed quite similar learning curves and anastomosis times [25]. This indicates that there is no transfer of traditional microsurgical skills to robotic microsurgical skills.
From all these studies it can be concluded that a learning curve indeed exists for the performance of robotic surgery. However, it is demonstrated from different studies that the learning curve for robotic-assisted surgery is actually shorter compared to that of traditional laparoscopic surgery [9, 18]. In combination with all the other advantages that robotic surgery holds over laparoscopic surgery, it can be concluded that the use of robotic assistance in microvascular surgery in time will definitely be worth wile.

9. Future expectations

Because robotic surgery offers great possibilities for the future of microvascular surgery, more and more surgeons and technicians will gather their strengths to improve the current technology and create robots that are perfectly suited to assist surgeons in the performance of microvascular surgery. Developments will probably focus on designing robots specialized in open procedures, creating software for the handling of blood vessels and performing microvascular anastomoses, adjusting needle holders to safely place microsurgical sutures and developing a haptic feedback system for the surgeon. These developments may have important impact on the future of supermicrosurgery, which is defined as anastomosis of blood vessels 0.5-0.8 mm in diameter [30, 31].

It is expected that robots will be designed that are specialized in microvascular surgery. This brings surgeons the opportunity to perform microvascular anastomoses more precisely and more successfully. With more experience microvascular anastomoses are expected to be performed more rapidly than in the conventional way. Because no transfer of training exists, microvascular surgery can also be performed in small hospitals, which will be an extreme booster for the application and development of microvascular surgery.

Robotic technology has the potential to mutinously increase patient safety in surgery in the next decades. Further clinical trials are needed to explore the clinical potential of robot-assisted microvascular procedures.

10. References

Hernandez, J.D., et al., Qualitative and quantitative analysis of the learning curve of a simulated surgical task on the da Vinci system. *Surg Endosc,* 2004. 18(3): p. 372-8. [1]

Deeba, S., et al., Cardiac robotics: a review and St. Mary's experience. *Int J Med Robot,* 2006. 2(1): p. 16-20. [2]

Furukawa T, M.Y., Ozawa S, Wakabayashi G, Kitajima M, The revolution of computer-aided surgery -- the dawn of robotic surgery. *Min Invas Ther & Allied Technol,* 2001. 10(6): p. 283-288. [3]

Prasad, S.M., et al., Surgical robotics: impact of motion scaling on task performance. *J Am Coll Surg,* 2004. 199(6): p. 863-8. [4]

Stephenson, E.R., Jr., et al., Computer-assisted endoscopic coronary artery bypass anastomoses: a chronic animal study. *Ann Thorac Surg,* 1999. 68(3): p. 838-43. [5]

Byrn, J.C., et al., Three-dimensional imaging improves surgical performance for both novice and experienced operators using the da Vinci Robot System. *Am J Surg,* 2007. 193(4): p. 519-22. [6]

Yohannes, P., et al., Comparison of robotic versus laparoscopic skills: is there a difference in the learning curve? *Urology,* 2002. 60(1): p. 39-45; discussion 45. [7]

Badani, K.K., et al., Comparison of two-dimensional and three-dimensional suturing: is there a difference in a robotic surgery setting? *J Endourol,* 2005. 19(10): p. 1212-5. [8]

Sarle, R., et al., Surgical robotics and laparoscopic training drills. *J Endourol,* 2004. 18(1): p. 63-6; discussion 66-7. [9]

Stadler, P., et al., Robot-assisted aortoiliac reconstruction: A review of 30 cases. *J Vasc Surg,* 2006. 44(5): p. 915-9. [10]

Sung, G.T. and I.S. Gill, Robotic laparoscopic surgery: a comparison of the DA Vinci and Zeus systems. *Urology,* 2001. 58(6): p. 893-8. [11]

Martinez, B.D. and C.S. Wiegand, Robotics in vascular surgery. *Am J Surg*, 2004. 188(4A Suppl): p. 57S-62S. [12]

Boyd, W.D., et al., A comparison of robot-assisted versus manually constructed endoscopic coronary anastomosis. *Ann Thorac Surg*, 2000. 70(3): p. 839-42; discussion 842-3. [13]

Argenziano, M., et al., Results of the prospective multicenter trial of robotically assisted totally endoscopic coronary artery bypass grafting. *Ann Thorac Surg*, 2006. 81(5): p. 1666-74; discussion 1674-5. [14]

Siemionow, M., et al., Robotic assistance in microsurgery. *J Reconstr Microsurg*, 2000. 16(8): p. 643-9. [15]

Le Roux, P.D., et al., Robot-assisted microsurgery: a feasibility study in the rat. *Neurosurgery*, 2001. 48(3): p. 584-9. [16]

Karamanoukian, R.L., et al., Feasibility of robotic-assisted microvascular anastomoses in plastic surgery. *J Reconstr Microsurg*, 2006. 22(6): p. 429-31. [17]

Karamanoukian, R.L., et al., Transfer of training in robotic-assisted microvascular surgery. *Ann Plast Surg*, 2006. 57(6): p. 662-5. [18]

Knight, C.G., et al., Computer-assisted, robot-enhanced open microsurgery in an animal model. *J Laparoendosc Adv Surg Tech A*, 2005. 15(2): p. 182-5. [19]

Nio, D., et al., The efficacy of robot-assisted versus conventional laparoscopic vascular anastomoses in an experimental model. *Eur J Vasc Endovasc Surg*, 2004. 27(3): p. 283-6. [20]

Katz, R.D., et al., Robotics in microsurgery: use of a surgical robot to perform a free flap in a pig. *Microsurgery*, 2005. 25(7): p. 566-9. [21]

van der Hulst, R., J. Sawor, and N. Bouvy, Microvascular anastomosis: is there a role for robotic surgery? *J Plast Reconstr Aesthet Surg*, 2007. 60(1): p. 101-2. [22]

Boyd, B., et al., Robotic harvest of internal mammary vessels in breast reconstruction. *J Reconstr Microsurg*, 2006. 22(4): p. 261-6. [23]

Bethea, B.T., et al., Application of haptic feedback to robotic surgery. *J Laparoendosc Adv Surg Tech A*, 2004. 14(3): p. 191-5. [24]

Gulbins, H., et al., 3D-visualization improves the dry-lab coronary anastomoses using the Zeus robotic system. *Heart Surg Forum*, 1999. 2(4): p. 318-24; discussion 324-5. [25]

Ali, M.R., J. Rasmussen, and B. Bhaskerrao, Teaching robotic surgery: a stepwise approach. *Surg Endosc*, 2006. [26]

Hamman, B.L. and C.H. White, Interrupted distal anastomosis: the interrupted "porcupine" technique. *Ann Thorac Surg*, 2004. 78(2): p. 722-4. [27]

Kitagawa, M., et al., Effect of sensory substitution on suture-manipulation forces for robotic surgical systems. *J Thorac Cardiovasc Surg*, 2005. 129(1): p. 151-8.[28]

Novick, R.J., et al., Analysis of the learning curve in telerobotic, beating heart coronary artery bypass grafting: a 90 patient experience. *Ann Thorac Surg*, 2003. 76(3): p. 749-53. [29]

Kim, J.S., et al., The replantation of an amputated tongue by supermicrosurgery. *J Plast Reconstr Aesthet Surg*, 2007. [30]

Schoeller, T., et al., Modified free paraumbilical perforator flap: the next logical step in breast reconstruction. *Plast Reconstr Surg*, 2003. 111(3): p. 1093-8; discussion 1099-1101. [31]

35

Cooperative robotic system to support surgical interventions

Raúl A. Castillo Cruces, H. Christian Schneider and Jürgen Wahrburg
University of Siegen, Center for Sensor Systems (ZESS)
Germany

1. Introduction

Currently computer assisted surgery is dominated by use of navigation systems. These systems track the position of surgical instruments by the use of a 3D digitizing system and insert a corresponding symbol in the pre-operative image on the computer screen. First originating from applications in neurosurgery, Ear-Nose-Throat (ENT) and spinal surgery, such systems have found wide acceptance in most bone-related surgical interventions. However, surgical instruments are still guided manually. Unintentional deviations caused, for example, by hand tremor, slipping or inhomogeneous bone structure can occur.

Robotic systems for computer assisted surgery have gained a lot of interest and are investigated by several research groups, but they are rarely found in clinical practice. The concept of commercial systems like Robodoc (Kazanzides, 1999) and CASPAR (Grueneis, 1999), which have been introduced for milling the stem cavity in total hip replacement surgery, has turned out to be not convincing. Many of those have been removed from the OR. There are other robotic solutions for surgery, including tele-manipulator systems like the daVinci system from Intuitive Surgical Inc., and robots for endoscope guidance in abdominal surgery, like the AESOP system (developed by Computer Motion, Inc.) or the EndoAssist from Armstrong Healthcare (Davies, 2000). However, the operational mode of these systems is not based on computer assisted pre-operative planning and intra-operative registration, and they will not be discussed in this paper.

The interaction between surgeon and robotic system is a very important issue when thinking about its introduction within surgical interventions. Autonomous systems have lost acceptance in the surgical community because the surgeon wants to be in charge of the operation instead of acting only as an observer. In such scenario, the human experience, intuition, capability of react in front of unexpected situations is lost. An alternative solution is to provide a cooperative system where benefits of both can be derived. Some work has been done in relation to haptic interface for direct cooperation between surgeon and robot. Robotic systems like the JHU Steady Hand Robot from the Johns Hopkins University (Bettini, 2004) and the Hands-On Robot, also known as Acrobot (Davies, 2004), use active constraints to limit the motion of the robot within predefined regions.

This paper discusses the concept of a cooperative robotic system to support medical interventions in several surgical disciplines. A modular structure facilitates the adaptation of a common basic hardware platform to specific applications by adding associated software modules as well as appropriate robot mounted surgical tools. Our approach represents a versatile surgical assistance system which is based on the combination of an optical navigation system, a robotic arm, and a haptic interface based on a force-torque-sensor mounted at the robot's wrist. Compared to manual instrument guidance in pure navigation, the integrated system offers significant additional advantages by guaranteeing precise positioning and guidance of surgical instruments according to pre-operative planning. Moreover, the system offers an intuitive interaction between surgeon and robot; where the surgeon has complete control over the operation by grabbing the tool mounted on the robot's wrist and moving it with his own hands. The issue of mishandling is avoided with the introduction of virtual constraints based on the pre-operative planning. In this way, regions outside the operating zone can be avoided or the surgeon can virtually guide the tool along a certain path. Any intent to move the robot along a forbidden direction will be rejected. The virtual constraints are defined in relation to the patient thanks to the information provided by the 3D digitizing system.

2. Concept of a navigated robotic system for universal surgical application

2.1 Combination of Navigation and Robotics

Although navigation solves the basic problem of providing the surgeon with information for the exact localization of his instrument in the anatomic structure of the patient, there are two important issues which can be significantly improved by adding a robotic component to the navigation system. First, mechatronic supported instrument guidance eliminates the need for the surgeon to constantly move his attention from the operating area to the computer screen where he has to monitor the instrument position. This means he can concentrate fully on the operating area. Second, no unintentional deviations caused, for example, by hand tremor or slipping can occur.

Our patented approach, using robotic systems in surgery, is based on the integration of a navigation system and robotic arm into one system that appears as a single unit, combining the specific advantages of each of the two components. Patient registration is performed by using only the navigation system, while the robotic arm positions and guides the surgical instruments during the intervention.

Instead of designing specific robotic systems which are exclusively tailored to certain applications, our approach adapts the design philosophy of existing commercial navigation systems. A common hardware platform is used for all applications, i.e. a robotic system which fulfils basic requirements, such as easy setup, sufficiently large working space, high safety standards, etc. Adaptation to various surgical procedures is carried out by adding procedure specific software modules and specific tool systems to be mounted at the wrist of the robotic arm. Fig. 1 shows the different components of the navigated robotic system.

A control computer system is used to synchronize the operation of the robotic arm and the optical 3D digitizing system. An important integration aspect is the alignment of the various coordinate frames that are assigned to all relevant system parts and structures, including the base frame of the digitizing system and the base frame of the robotic arm, the surgical instruments and the patient structure to be operated on. The actual position and orientation of the frames can be measured by fixing small rigid bodies (DRB = dynamic reference base elements) to them which can be localized by the stationary cameras of the 3D digitizing system. Part of our research is dedicated to determining homogeneous transformation matrices which establish mathematical relations between the various frames.

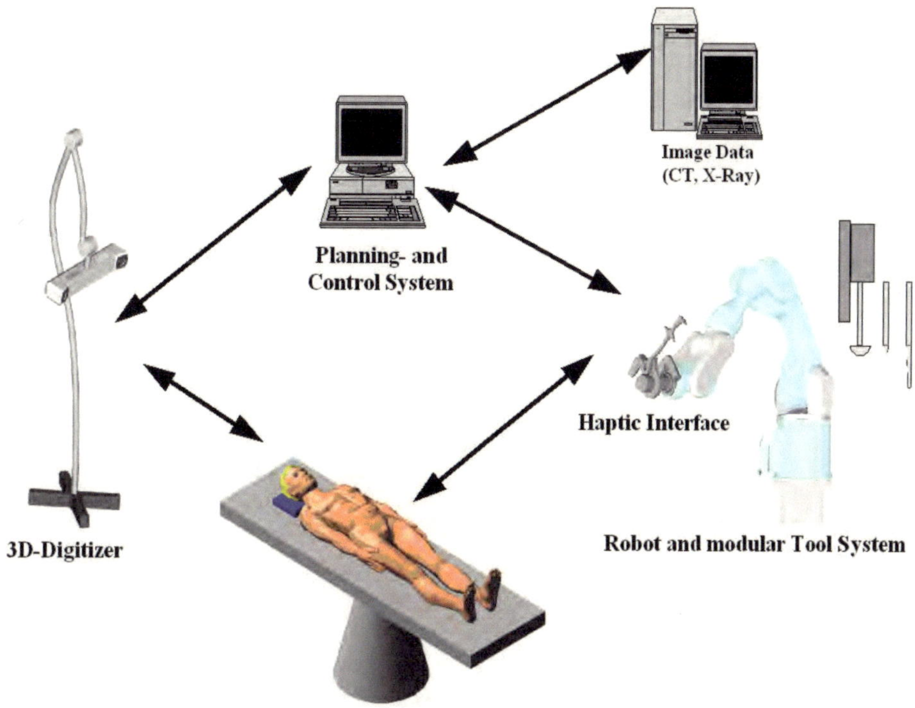

Figure 1. Components of the navigated robotic system for surgical assistance

For example, a setup procedure is carried out during system initialization to align the coordinate systems of the robotic arm and the digitizing system. Once the corresponding transformation matrix, transforming the position of the arm into the coordinates of the navigation system, has been determined, all arm movements can also be specified with reference to the coordinate system of the digitizing system. The robotic arm may then be regarded as a mechatronic unit of the navigation system for automatic positioning and guiding of surgical instruments. Furthermore, the DRB element mounted at the wrist of the arm also provides redundant measurement of the surgical tool position by two completely independent systems: a) the digitizing system detecting the DRB element, and b) the in-built encoders of the arm joints. This is an important feature to meet the high safety requirements applicable to surgical robotics.

A special feature of the robotic arm is its ability to automatically track potential movements of the patient in real time, eliminating the need for rigid fixation of the anatomic structure that is to be operated upon. In the first step, a DRB element of the navigation system is attached to the bony structure by a suitable fixation mechanism and the patient anatomy is registered using common procedures of the navigation system. If any patient movements are detected during the surgical intervention, a control computer generates corresponding motion commands which move the mechatronic arm to follow the patient, thus keeping the surgical instrument always in the pre-planned position and orientation related to the patient anatomy.

2.2 Cooperative interaction

The robotic arm is equipped with a haptic interface based on a force-torque-sensor mounted at its wrist. This feature facilitates manual-driven motion of the arm, back and forth on the working area. The surgeon easily guides the arm by grabbing a handle, and by pulling it in the desired position. This means the arm is seamlessly integrated into the operating procedure because there is no need to use any input-device like a mouse, a touch screen or a keyboard. The real-time patient-tracking mode of the arm can only be activated when the surgical tool has reached a predefined small working space around the operating area. During the intervention the surgeon can stop the tracking mode at any time to manually move the arm back and then pull it to the operating area again. It will automatically resume tracking exactly at the position before the interruption occurred.

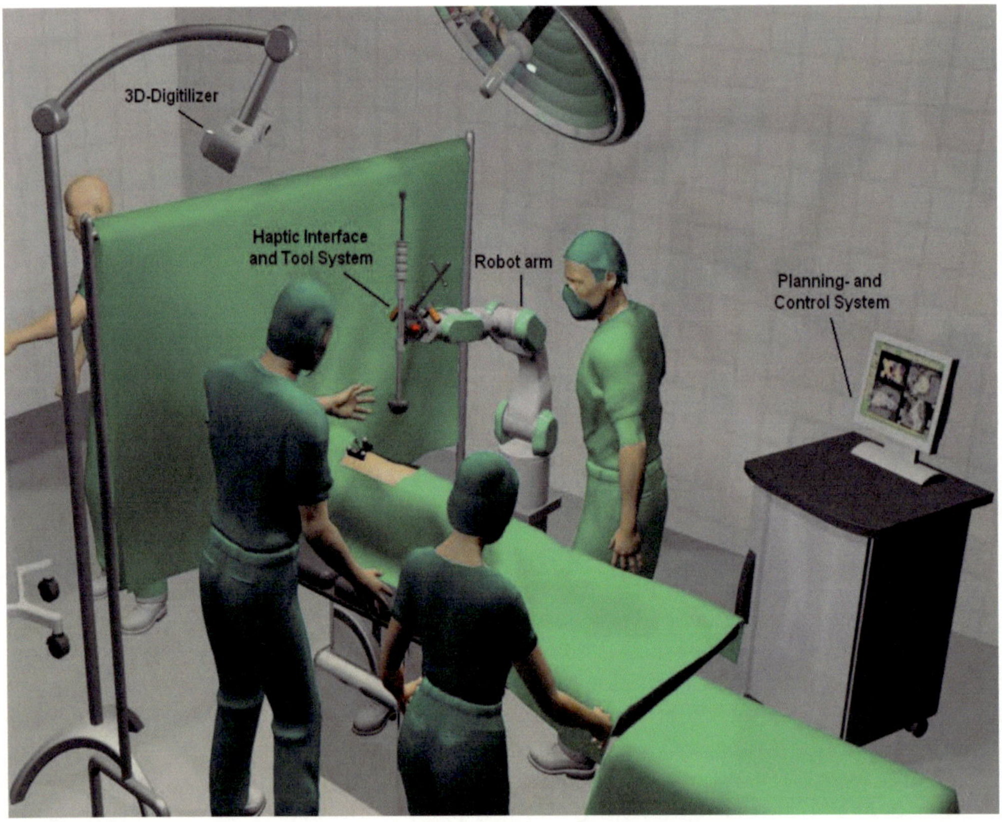

Figure 2. Example of surgical intervention scenario

Figure 2 illustrates the setup of the system for a surgical intervention in the OR. Notice that the surgeon has freedom to move the robot at any time; however, safety measurements are applied in order to avoid any danger to non-specified regions. Therefore, any movement commanded by the surgeon is virtually constrained, which means the system can only move along allowed directions defined in relation to the patient. The constraints can vary depending of the proximity to the patient, where the stiffness and allowed degrees of freedom are switched to achieve different effects. For instance, at first a simple linear movement on the operating normal direction with high stiffness is applied in order to get out of the critical area nearby the patient in a safety way. After a certain distance, the virtual constraint is shifted to an inverted conic form giving the possibility to locate the robot out of the way not to obstruct any other activity of the surgeon. On the same way, once the robot is pulled back to the working area, the virtual constraints procure that the final operating position and orientation are achieved (Marayong et al., 2003).

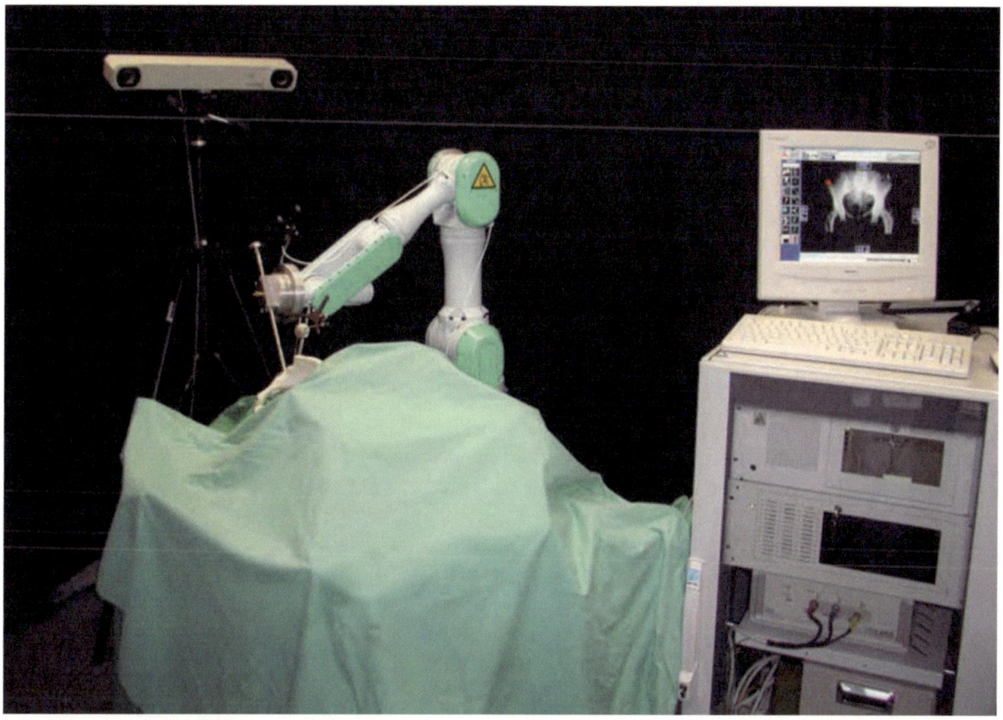

Figure 3. Prototype of the navigated robotic system

3. Setup of a prototype system

3.1 System components

A prototype of the navigated surgical assistance system has been set up in our laboratory. It consists of an optical 3D "Polaris" localizer from NDI Inc., a light weight (35 kg) robotic arm from Mitsubishi Heavy Industries, Ltd. and a mini45 force-torque-senor from ATI Industrial Automations. Fig. 3 shows a photo of the whole system. This hardware is embedded into the development of our "modiCAS" system (modular interactive Computer Assisted Surgery), which comprises hard- and software-modules to facilitate the use of CAS techniques at different levels, starting form pure pre-operative planning, intra-operative registration, up to mechatronic-supported interventions. It is possible to upgrade the system to a higher level by adding further modules, while maintaining a common user interface and retaining the experience already gained. A modular surgical tool system can be mounted to the wrist of the arm. In combination with appropriate software modules, it tailors the systems to various surgical applications.

3.2 Software architecture

The modiCAS framework is developed to maintain modularity as the backbone of its software architecture, making distinctions between fundamental functionalities of the system and application-oriented tasks. The latter makes use of the former to satisfy its specific requirements. Such distribution allows the flexibility to adapt the system to fulfil the demands of different surgical procedures.

On the one hand, the fundamental functionalities are implemented in an embedded target computer that runs a real-time operating system. This guarantees deterministic behaviour of the time critical tasks. On the other hand, a second computer (the Host) runs Microsoft Windows to implement the graphical user interface (GUI) as well as the application-oriented tasks. Both computers are connected by a fast Ethernet link.

The Host computer communicates with the Target using a Command-Based architecture, which provides access in the form of commands, to all functionalities available at the Target. Fig. 4 illustrates the organization of this architecture. The command interface looks like a simple library of functions that can be called on by the Host. Plausibility is checked by the Target each time a command is requested before it can be executed.

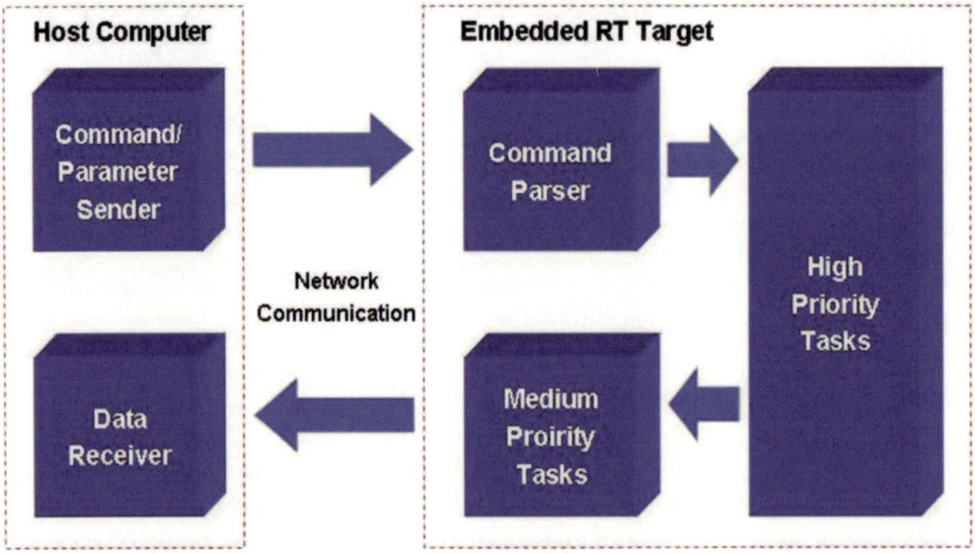

Figure 4. Command-based architecture

4. Application in various surgical procedures

In comparison to conventional navigation systems which are still based on pure manual instrument handling, precise instrument guidance by navigated mechatronic assistance systems offers significant additional advantages. Those include:
the use of novel minimal invasive operating techniques

- application of new surgical instruments (such as medical laser systems or micro tools which cannot be used in manual surgery)
- high certainty in the execution of pre-operative plan even under difficult circumstances (minimizing the risk of cost intensive post-operative treatment)
- the possibility to reduce the assistant staff numbers in the operating theatre

This will lead to patient benefits, better support of the surgeon and improved cost/benefit ratios.

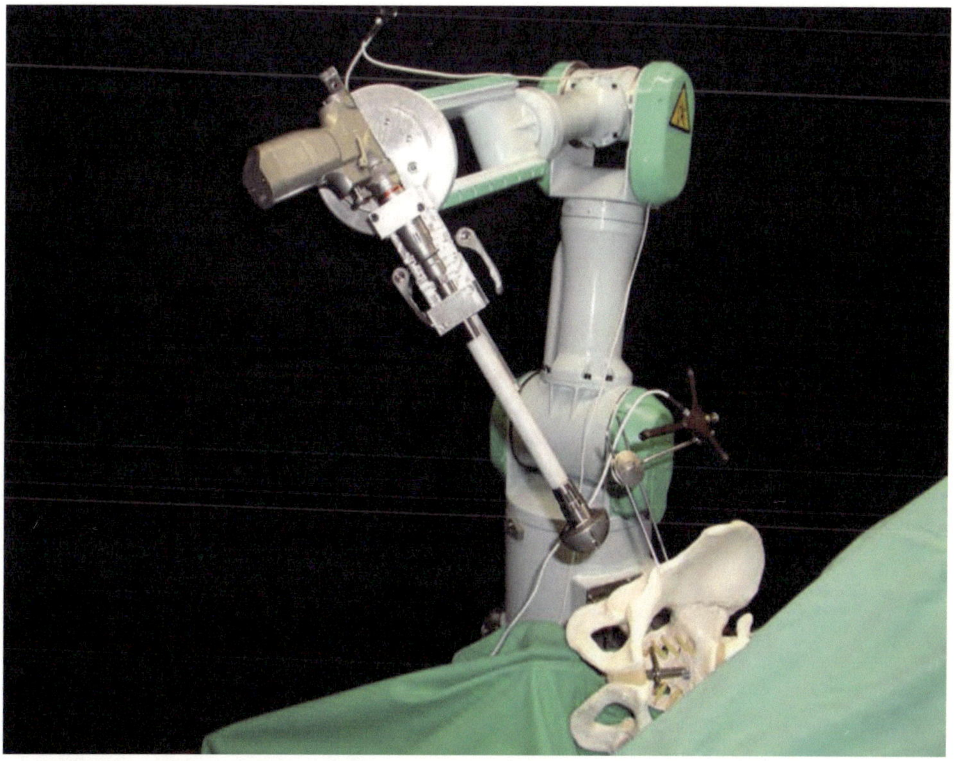

Figure 5. Preparation for the cup implant in total hip replacement surgery

1. Orthopaedic surgery: The first clinical application of the robotic assistance system has been carried out in total hip replacement surgery. It has been world's first robotic system to support the implantation of the acetabular cup, which has been facilitated by using its unique patient tracking capability (Kerschbaumer et al, 2003). A specific tool system for mechatronic-based preparation of the bony bed and mechatronic-supported placement of the cup implant has been developed. It is based on the design of conventional components (reamers, surgical drives, etc), see Fig. 5. The tools are fixed

on a one-degree-of-freedom linear slider mounted at the wrist of the robot. The operation of the surgical tool itself is still manually controlled by the surgeon. In this way he keeps control over the operation, while he can be certain that the tool maintains its correct orientation and that there are no unintentional deviations caused by inhomogeneous bone structure. Furthermore the system prevents the surgeon from reaming too deep into the acetabulum.

2. ENT surgery: The application under investigation is Functional Endoscopic Sinus Surgery, a standard minimal invasive procedure in ENT. In conventional operating technique the surgeon requires one hand to guide the endoscope and can use only one instrument with the other hand. Single-handed operating can become extremely frustrating during delicate manoeuvres. It is therefore a significant improvement if the robotic assistance system can be configured to partly guide the endoscope but fully controlled by the surgeon. It therefore facilitates safer and more comfortable two-handed operating. In haptic mode, the wrist of the arm can be manually positioned close to the desired operating zone above the patient's head. Then either cooperative or teleoperative moves the endoscope to the pre-operatively planned intranasal location, taking the meatus nasi externus as a relative pivot point and respecting pre-operatively defined safety regions. The virtual constraints assure that the correct direction is maintained and prevent the endoscope from reaching dangerous internal regions in the patient.

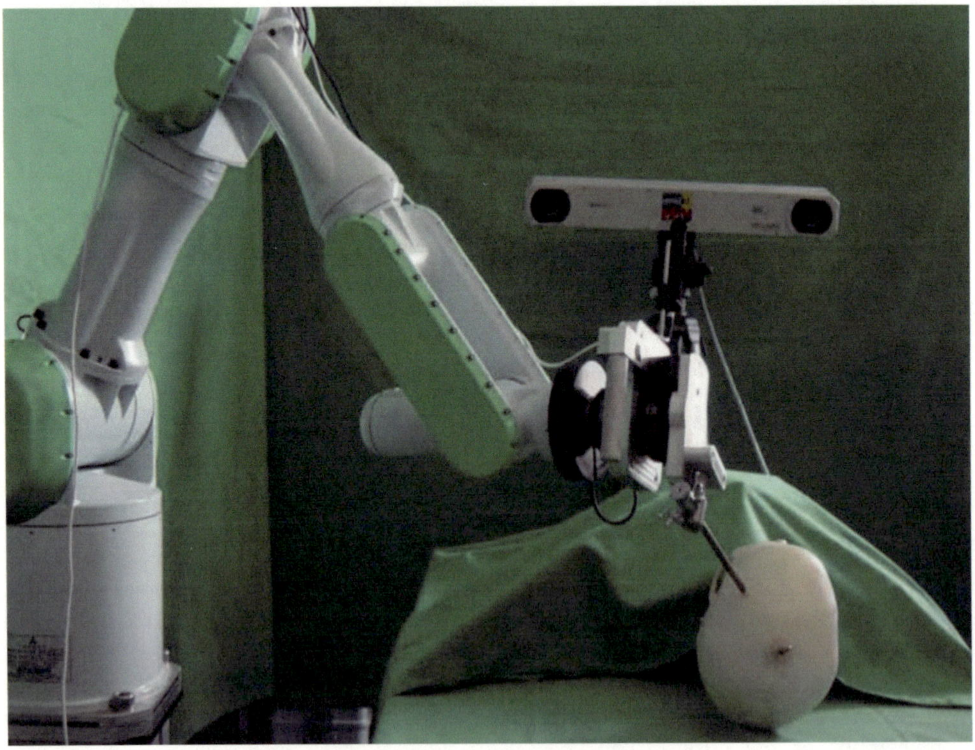

Figure 6. Endoscope guidance for neurosurgical applications

3. Neurosurgery: Intracranial endoscopic approaches require high accuracy to reach the target point. The free-hand approach, combined with neuronavigation, is usually used for a precise access to small ventricles or cysts. To improve the accuracy and to provide a stable holding system, the navigated robotic system will be used for guiding the endoscope. Once the burr hole has been made and the dura has been incised, the endoscope is inserted by the robotic arm along the planned trajectory to the target point. It can be moved by the arm under teleoperative control while the surgeon is looking at the monitor screen or directly, in a cooperative fashion, using the haptic interface. At the end of the intervention, the endoscope is retrieved manually exactly along the trajectory as it has been inserted. Fig. 6 illustrates the laboratory setup.

5. Conclusion

The interactive robotic assistance system can be considered as an intelligent instrument that supports surgeons to achieve more precise and reproducible surgery. It combines the advantages of navigation and mechatronics by using the navigation system for registration and position measurement, and the robotic arm for precise positioning and guidance of the surgical instruments. The integrated haptic interface offers a seamless incorporation of the robotic system in surgical intervention. The surgeon maintains full control over the operation procedure. Moreover, safety measurements are introduced, using the concept of virtual constraints, in order to avoid any mishandling due to excessive manipulability freedom. For instance, by defining forbidden regions that the robot is not allowed to enter, or guiding the tool along a desired direction through direct cooperation between surgeon and robot.

A command-based architecture is used for the software development to provide a solid foundation for a flexible and scalable framework. This is divided by hardware in two main parts: The embedded target with a pool of modules for the different functionalities, and the Host, which use these modules together with the GUI to build the different applications. The modular system design facilitates its adaptability to a variety of surgical applications. In particular, in cooperation with clinical and scientific partners, we will further investigate the robotic-guided application of new surgical instruments (e.g. laser systems, micro tools, radiation devices) which cannot be used in manual surgery, in order to demonstrate their benefits in surgical treatment.

6. References

Bettini, A., Marayong, P., Lang, S., Okamura, A. M., Hager, G. D., (2004). Vision-Assisted Control for Manipulation Using Virtual Fixtures, *IEEE Transactions on Robotics*, Vol. 20, No. 6, December 2004.

Davies, B. (2000) A review of robotics in surgery, *Proceedings of the I MECH E Part H Journal of Engineering in Medicine*, Vol. 214, No. 1, pp. 129-140, January 2000.

Davies, B. L. , Harris, S. J., Rodriguez y Baena, F., et al., (2004). Hands-On Robotic surgery: Is This the Future?, Medical Imaging and Augmented Reality, In: *Proceedings 2nd Int. Workshop*, Guang-Zhong Yang, Tianzi Jiang (Eds.), 27-37, Springer, ISBN 3-540-22877-2, Beijing, China.

Grueneis, C., Richter, R., et al., (1999). Clinical introduction of the CASPAR system: problems and initial results, *4th International Symposium of Computer Assited Orthopaedic Surgery, CAOS'99*, Davos, 17-19 March 1999, Switzerland.

Kazanzides, P., (1999). Robot Assisted Surgery: The ROBODOC Experience, *Proceedings 30th International Symposium on Robotics*, pp. 281-286, Tokyo, 1999, Japan.

Kerschbaumer, F., Künzler, S., Wahrburg, J. (2003). Minimally Invasive Total Hip Replacement - Application of Intraoperative Navigation and Robotics, In: *Navigation and Robotics in Total Joint and Spine Surgery*, J.B.Stiehl, W.Konermann, R. Haaker (Eds.), pp 145-150, Springer, Heidelberg/New York.

Marayong, P., Li, M., Okamura, A. M., Hager, G. D., (2003). Spatial Motion Contraints : Theory and Demonstrations for Robot Guidance Using Virtual Fixtures, *Proceedings of the IEEE International Conference on Robotics and Automation*, pp 14-19, September 2003, Taipei, Taiwan.

36

Robotics in General Surgery

James Wall, MD, Venita Chandra, MD and Thomas Krummel, MD
Stanford University Department of Surgery, Stanford, California
USA

1. Introduction

General Surgery has seen an evolution over the last several decades toward minimally invasive approaches to procedures that were classically performed though large open incisions. The former assumption in the surgical world that "a big surgery requires a big incision" is no longer true. The benefit of significant reductions in the size of incisions is clear to surgeons who appreciate fewer wound complications and to the educated public who value less post-operative pain and rapid return to normal activities. As incisions and access ports become smaller and fewer, the tools to enable complex tasks through these ports are being developed. Robotics is one of the primary tools being incorporated into the surgical environment. The term robot comes from the Czech word *robota* for "compulsory labor"[1].

While many modern definitions of 'robot' include a component of automation, such a component has yet to be significantly integrated into General Surgery machines. Thus, for the purpose of this chapter, a surgical robot is defined as a machine that performs various complex surgical tasks in a master-slave configuration.

Surgical robots offer many advantages in the area of minimally invasive General Surgery and have made significant contributions to the field in the last twenty years. Robotics was first introduced to the General Surgery operating room in the form of surgeon controlled robotic arms for laparoscopic camera manipulation. More recently, robotic surgical systems that allow the surgeon to operate from a remote console have been introduced. Significant challenges remain for the field including the cost-effectiveness, safety, training, and adoption. However, the benefits of robotics in the operating room are becoming clear and further development will see the maturation of a field with significant promise to improve patient care.

2. The Surgeon Assistant

The first surgical robot was approved by the FDA in 1994 for use in General Surgery. The Aesop® (Automatic Endoscopic System for Optimal Position, Computer Motion Inc., Goleta CA) is a system designed to assist the surgeon in the era of laparoscopy by taking control of the laparoscopic camera[2, 3]. The system is composed of an articulated, electromechanical arm mounted to the operating room table. The arm provides 7 degrees of freedom (7-DOF) that is completely controlled by the surgeon via foot control, hand control, or voice recognition[4]. Aesop® was designed to reduce the need for an assistant to operate the camera during laparoscopic procedures and was subsequently found to have benefits in reducing smudging, fogging, inadvertent movements and overall operative time[5, 6]. The EndoAssist (Prosurgics, High Wycombe, England) is another FDA approved laparoscopic camera control system that relies on a head mounted sensor. The system is a stand alone cart with an electro-mechanical robotic arm that is activated by a foot pedal, and moves according to the desired viewing direction of the surgeon (Figure 1). The system can be quickly learned and offers similar benefits to the Aesop® [7]. The EndoAssist and Aesop® systems were found to be equally effective in task performance in a study by Wagner and colleagues[8] while Nebot and colleagues[9] found the EndoAssist guidance more efficient than the voice commanded Aesop®. Both studies, however, noted some drawback to the size of the EndoAssist and its separation from the operating table.

3. The Teleoperator Era

Since their introduction in 1994, robotic applications in General Surgery have evolved from simple surgical assist devices, to more sophisticated systems capable of enhancing surgical performance. The primary class of robots used in General Surgery today, are "master-slave" machines, where the robot mimics the movement of the surgeon. In these units the "master" control console, from which the surgeon operates, is physically separated from the "slave" unit, composed of the robotic arms performing the surgery. As a result of this separation, these systems are also referred to as teleoperators or telemanipulators.

While the foundation of teleoperator surgical systems can be traced back to the United States National Aeronautics and Space Administration (NASA) in the 1970s, their major development was funded by DARPA (Defense Advanced Research Project Administration) as a potential military tool for remote surgical care of the injured soldier. Two main teleoperator surgical robots were developed from the research; the da Vinci® Surgical System (Intuitive Surgical, Inc., Sunnyvale, CA) described in detail below and the Zeus® system (Computer Motion, Goleta, CA). Intuitive Surgery and Computer Motion merged in 2003, resulting in a single FDA approved robotic platform on the market today that carries the name da Vinci®.

3.1 The da Vinci ® Platform

The da Vinci® surgical system (Figure 2), which obtained FDA approval in September 2001, has two main components: the surgeon's console and a patient's side cart. The surgeon's console houses the sophisticated visual display system, surgeon's control handles, and the user interface panels. The patient side cart is the actual robotic device, and electro-mechanical arms that move in response to the surgeon's motions at the console.

The surgeon console (Figure 3) consists of a workstation, which can be located up to 10 meters away from the operating table, from which the operator controls a video endoscope and two to three robotic arms. The surgeon is seated at the workstation and places his or her head inside a viewing space. The console contains the surgeon controls which act as high resolution input devices that read the position, orientation, and grip commands from the surgeon's finger tips. The surgeon's motions are relayed from the console to the robotic arms, which, in turn, manipulate the instruments (i.e. needle drivers, forceps, scissors) and the endoscope. The surgeon's console also holds commands for special enhancement functions such as motion scaling and tremor reduction.

The da Vinci® surgical system utilizes a sophisticated optic display. High-resolution images of the operative site are projected to the surgeon through a dual-lens, three-chip digital camera

system. Each camera transmits to different medical grade cathode ray tube (CRT) monitors located inside the console, which display a separate image to each eye. These are fused in the surgeon's brain, to create a three-dimensional image. In addition, the images are anatomically aligned with the position of the surgeon's hands, creating the feeling of being immersed into the surgical field—where the surgeons feels as if their hands are virtually inside the patient's body.
The da Vinci® robotic arms are attached to a patient-side cart (Figure 4) that contains the 2 to 3 arms that control the operative instruments as well as a center arm that controls the video endoscope. The cart is mobile allowing its position to be adapted to the specific operation being performed. Once locked in place and engaged within the patient, however, the cart cannot be re-positioned without entirely disengaging the system. The standard array of 8 mm da Vinci® instruments are outfitted with an EndoWrist® technology (Figure 5) with bidirectional articulation that provides 7-DOF. All instruments respond to the movement of the control handles with "wrist-like" movements that mimic the human hand. A variety of instrument tips are available including forceps, needle drivers, and scalpels, as well as both monopolar and bipolar electrocautery devices (Figure 6).

4. Advantages of Telerobotic Surgical Systems

Robotic surgery was introduced into clinical practice in the late 1990s, after conventional laparoscopic surgery had already made a significant impact on modern surgical practice. The primary advantages of the robotic surgical systems stem from their ability to address many of the limitations of conventional minimally invasive techniques. Modern laparoscopic instruments challenge the surgeon to perform manipulations with rigid shafted instruments through access ports. Undesirable effects of the current approach include counter intuitive movement at the instrument tip (fulcrum effect), reduced degrees of freedom, and the optical limitations of a 2-dimensional view through a single lens.
Telerobotic surgical systems enhance dexterity in several ways. Internal software filters out the natural tremor of a surgeon's hand, which can become particularly evident under high magnification and problematic when attempting fine maneuvers in very small fields[10]. In addition, the system can scale movements such that large movements of the control handles can be transformed into smaller movements inside the patient[10-12]. Lastly, the "wristed" 7-DOF instruments significantly enhance dexterity as compared with the 5-DOF of standard laparoscopic instruments. Robotic instruments permit a larger range of motion and rotation, similar to the natural range of articulation of the human wrist. This increased dexterity may be particularly advantageous during complex operations in limited spaces that require fine dissection and intracorporeal suturing.
During conventional minimal access surgery, instruments pivot around the fulcrum of the insertion point, thus movement in the surgical field is always opposite to the direction of motion of the surgeon's hand. In the robotic surgical systems electronic separation of the instrument tips from the handles eliminates the effects of instrument length, minimizes the fulcrum effect, and restores a more intuitive non-reversed instrument control[13].
The sophisticated vision system of the da Vinci® described above, is another significant advantage of robotic technology, adding a measure of safety and surgical control beyond what is available with traditional laparoscopy. The three dimensional display improves depth perception, and the ability to magnify images by a factor of ten allows extremely sensitive and accurate surgical manipulation. The alignment of the visual axis with the surgeon's hands in the console further enhances hand-eye coordination.

Lastly, teleoperator systems feature ergonomically designed workstations designed to minimize physical strain and fatigue associated with long minimally invasive procedures[14-16]. This may prove to become a particularly significant issue as the field of bariatric surgery expands, due to the high levels of surgeon fatigue seen when operating on the larger size and thicker body walls of bariatric patients.

5. Disadvantages of Telerobotic Surgical Systems

While robotic surgical systems have successfully provided several key advantages over standard minimal access surgery, there are a number of limitations that have prevented this technology from reaching its full potential. Foremost among these is the loss of force feedback (haptics). While such feedback is reduced in standard minimal access surgery, compared to open surgery, it is further reduced with the robotic interface. The operating surgeon must therefore rely on visual cues such as tissue compression and blanching, and suture stretch (e.g. knot deformation), to determine the tensile strength of tissue and sutures[17, 18].

Another significant limitation of robotic technology is the extremely high initial cost of purchasing a robot (~$1,200,000) as well as the relatively high recurring costs of the instruments (~$2500 per 10 usage disposable instrument) and maintenance (~$100,000 per year)[19]. A strong argument for the cost-effectiveness of robotic surgery has yet to be made with recent studies comparing robotic procedures with conventional operations revealing that the absolute cost for robotic operations is significantly higher[20].

Lastly, the robotic systems are large and bulky and have complex, time-consuming setups, requiring additional specialized training for the entire operating room team. This translates into robotic procedure times that are predictably longer when compared to conventional laparoscopic approaches, at least until the surgical team becomes facile with the use of the new technology. Even with an experienced team, setup times have been reported to require an additional 10 to 35 minutes at the beginning of each robot-assisted case[21]. Undoubtedly, many of these issues will be remedied in the next generation of equipment as the technology continues to improve. Table 1 summarizes the advantages and disadvantages of robot-assisted surgery in comparison to conventional minimal access surgery.

6. Current Applications of Robotics in General Surgery

To date, the majority of published clinical experience using robotic technology has consisted primarily of retrospective case reports and case series. Robotic surgical systems have been used in many different surgical disciplines including Urology, Cardiac Surgery, Gynecology, General Surgery and Pediatric Surgery. Despite the important role General Surgery has played in advancing minimally invasive surgical techniques, General Surgeons have been relatively slow to pick up on robotics in comparison to other surgical specialists particularly Urologists. Nonetheless, telerobotic surgical techniques have been applied to a rapidly growing list of General Surgery procedures (Table 2). Highlights of selected procedures are discussed below.

6.1 Cholecystectomy

The introduction of laparoscopy about 20 years ago revolutionized the treatment of gallbladder disease[22]. Since then the laparoscopic cholecystectomy has become the standard of care and one of the most common laparoscopic procedures performed today. It is thus no

surprise that the first robotic surgical procedure performed on a human was a laparoscopic cholecystectomy in 1997 by Himpens, Leman, and Cadiere[23].
Since that time, many clinical series have been published documenting experiences with robotic-assisted cholecystectomy[10, 24-28]. All of these studies have shown few intra- or post-operative complications confirming the feasibility and safety of using the da Vinci® robotic system to perform laparoscopic cholecystectomy[29, 30]. Studies comparing totally robotic to conventional laparoscopic cholecystectomy generally demonstrate significantly longer OR times with the robotic procedures[31-34]. No clinical outcome advantage is presently apparent for robotic cholecystectomy over laparoscopic cholecystectomy. Nonetheless, robotic cholecystectomy is an excellent procedure for teaching the basics of robotic surgery, and may be useful as a training procedure.

6.2 Fundoplication

Telerobotic fundoplication, like cholecystectomy, also has been used by many centers to initiate their clinical experience with telerobotic gastrointestinal surgery. There are several series in the literature demonstrating that robotic fundoplication is feasible and safe with a low conversion rate and an acceptable morbidity rate, however similar to robotic cholecystectomy, robotic fundoplications resulted in longer operating room times[30, 35-41]. Several randomized control trials of robot-assisted versus conventional laparoscopic fundoplications have been published. Most of these show similar results to the studies mentioned above, in that the procedure is feasible, and the outcomes are similar to conventional laparoscopy. Some argue that the small field of operation and the importance of suturing for repair of the hiatus and construction of the fundoplication makes this procedure an ideal application for telerobotic surgical systems[29]. The most recent randomized control trial by Müller and colleagues[42], did in fact demonstrate shorter operative times for robotic fundoplication when performed by an experienced team. However, given the higher costs and similar clinical outcomes, the advantages of robot-assisted fundoplication over standard laparoscopic techniques are yet to be proven.

6.3 Heller Myotomy

The role of robotic technology in assisting minimally invasive Heller myotomy is more apparent. Laparoscopic Heller myotomy is a difficult operation to perform, with a steady rate of esophageal perforation occurring (approximately 7%) even for very experienced surgeons[30, 43]. The published telerobotic Heller myotomy series, in comparison, have demonstrated extremely low rates of esophageal perforation[43-45]. It is felt that the performance enhancing features of the robot such as increased dexterity, 3D imaging, and tremor filtration permit greater precision during performance of the myotomy compared to traditional laparoscopic techniques. No randomized controlled trials have been published as of yet, to validate these claims.

6.4 Bariatric Surgery

Robotic surgical systems are being used to assist in a variety of bariatric surgical procedures. Cadiere and colleagues[46] were the first to enter this area, performing a gastric banding procedure in 1999. Since then telerobotic surgical techniques have also been reported for biliary pancreatic diversion with duodenal switch, as well as various elements of laparoscopic Roux-en-Y gastric bypass procedures[47-51]. All studies demonstrate the feasibility and safety of performing robotic bariatric procedures. Mohr and colleagues[52] developed a totally robotic Roux-en Y gastric bypass technique. They reported telerobotic operations were accomplished significantly faster than the laparoscopic operations and suggest that their results point to the potential superiority of telerobotic bariatric surgery. In general, authors suggest that the robotic surgical system may enhance performance particularly in superobese patients. The strength of the robotic arms, as well as the additional degrees of freedom in motion offered by the wristed instruments appears to overcome the problems generated in these patients by their thick abdominal walls.

7. Colorectal Surgery

Given that conventional laparoscopic colorectal surgery is still in its infancy, it is not surprising that telerobotic colorectal surgery remains in an early state of development. However, one would expect the benefits of robotic surgery in other deep pelvic procedures including prostatectomy[53] and hysterectomy to translate into benefits in low anterior colon procedures. The first reported robotic colectomy was performed by Weber end colleagues in 2002[54]. Several studies have since reported safety and feasibility of a variety of colorectal procedures[55-62]. Some difficulties have been encountered in obtaining adequate excursion with the robotic arms, primarily in procedures requiring dissection both up to the splenic flexure and down to the pelvis. As is the case for many of the other procedures discussed above, robotic colorectal operations have similar clinical outcomes to conventional laparoscopic techniques along with longer operating times, and higher overall costs, and thus no demonstrable patient benefit[30, 63]. Some suggest, however, that the true benefit of robotic surgery systems may be in enabling more surgeons in the future to perform minimally invasive colorectal surgery, where they would otherwise perform open procedures[64].

7.1 Endocrine Surgery

There are published reports on a variety of telerobotic endocrine procedures including adrenalectomy, parathyroidectomy as well as pancreatic procedures[29, 41, 65-70]. While very few telerobotic pancreatic procedures have been performed to date, some argue that complex gastrointestinal surgeries such as pancreatic resections, which require fine dissection and accuracy in a small operating field may prove to benefit most from robotic technology[30, 41].
The most documented robotic endocrine procedure is the adrenalectomy. The first reported fully robotic adrenalectomy was done in 2002 by Young and colleagues from the Brody School of Medicine[71]. Since then several other case series have reported feasibility and safety of robotic adrenalectomy. One randomized control trial has been published comparing robotic to standard laparoscopic adrenalectomy[72]. However, the study concluded that the telerobotic adrenalectomy is inferior to the conventional laparoscopic procedure due to longer OR times, higher conversion rates, and higher post-operative complications.

8. Robotics in General Surgery: The Future

8.1 Remote Telesurgery

The original vision for robotic surgery—to escape the confines of operating rooms, hospitals, and even the planet and provide skilled surgical care remotely, is becoming a reality. The separation of surgeon and patient inherent to telerobotic surgical systems has been leveraged to develop remote telesurgery, the use of robotics to perform surgery at a distant location. This was first accomplished in September, 2001 by Jacques Marescaux of Strasbourg, France, with the help of sophisticated asynchronous transfer mode telecommunications technology. While sitting at the surgical console in New York City, he performed a telerobotic cholecystectomy, dubbed "operation Lindbergh" on his patient in Strasbourg, who was 4000 km away[73, 74]. This was truly a technical tour de force that required an enormous amount of planning and execution to keep the latency, time from hand motion of surgeon at console to actual response of robot at the patient's side, within acceptable limits. While this certainly was not a procedure easily reproduced for daily use, Anvari and colleagues[59] have had remarkable success in establishing an actual telesurgery program using commercial fiberoptic networks. Dr. Anvari and his group have successfully performed 22 telerobotic laparoscopic surgeries including 13 fundoplications, 3 sigmoid resections, 3 right hemicolectomies, 1 anterior resection, and 2 inguinal hernia repairs, between Hamilton, Canada and a remote hospital in North Bay, Canada (a distance of 400 km).

8.2 Augmented Reality Surgery

Digital integration is another future domain for the surgical robot. In recent years, sophisticated imaging modalities have expanded beyond their role as mere diagnostic techniques, and are now the foundation of sophisticated interactive computer applications which directly guide surgical procedures (image guided therapy-IGT). The overlaying of radiologic imaging data onto the operative visualization system, known as augmented reality, can guide the surgeon's dissection path, by demonstrating vital anatomic structures beyond the visible surface[75-77]. The immediate future promises integration of preoperative and intraoperative imaging data with the robot-assisted platform into a unified surgical delivery system. This union of image-guided therapy and robotic surgery may eventually give rise to operative techniques that truly transcend human capability.

9. Miniaturization

Advances in Micro-Electro-Mechanical-Systems (MEMS) promise the future of robotics will see smaller and smaller embodiments. MEMS are devices measured in micrometers that are built using a variety of advanced fabrication methods including electromagnetic discharge and laser micromachining[78]. MEMS technology began as electro-mechanical sensors and actuators but has grown to integrate biologic, fluid, optical and magnetic systems[79]. Miniaturized sensors and actuators will soon address the limitations of current robotic surgery through haptic feedback and advanced tracking systems. In the long term, these devices will enable complex therapeutic manipulations inside increasing small structures such as the intestinal tract, the vasculature and beyond[80].

10. Automation

As noted earlier in the chapter, surgical robotics used in General Surgery today has not included significant automation. Analogous to the airline industry, computer control of surgical robots has zero tolerance for failure. Despite the ability to automate many basic surgical tasks, the safety bar will be set high. The FDA has yet to approve an automated device for General Surgery and will undoubtedly require significant pre-market testing prior to approval. Other surgical fields have seen small inroads into automation as with the ROBODOC®, a reaming system for the femoral component of hip implants used in orthopedic surgery. The system is programmed based on pre-operative imaging and intra-operative registration to cut a precise cavity in the femoral canal[81-84]. The FDA approved the system after significant pre-market testing for failure modes[85-87]. Many believe that a fully automated surgical robot is unattainable due to subtle variations in human anatomy that demands human skills beyond the capabilities of an algorithm[88]. Although not on the immediate horizon, automation may one day meet the safety challenges it faces and become reality.

11. Conclusion

In summary, robotics has made a significant contribution to General Surgery in the past 20 years. In its infancy, surgical robotics has seen a shift from early systems that assisted the surgeon to current teleoperator systems that can enhance surgical skills. Telepresence and augmented reality surgery are being realized, while research and development into miniaturization and automation is rapidly moving forward.

The future of surgical robotics is bright. Researchers are working to address the electro-mechanical limitations of current robotic systems. Increasing utilization and competition in the marketplace should drive the cost of robotic systems down, improving their cost-effective proposition. By ultimately enabling increasingly complex interventions through minimally invasive approaches, robotics will have a significant role in the future of surgery.

	Robot-Assisted Surgery	**Conventional Minimal Access Surgery**
Advantages	Tremor Filtration	Affordable, ubiquitous
	Stereoscopic Visualization	Some haptic feedback
	Seven degrees of freedom	Well-developed, established technology
	Improved dexterity	
	Elimination of fulcrum effect	
	Motion Scaling	
	Ergonomic Positioning	
	Tele-surgery	
	Improved hand-eye coordination	
Disadvantages	Minimal haptic feedback	Two-dimensional visualization
	Expensive	Compromised dexterity
	Longer set-up times	Limited degrees of motion
	Large footprint	
	New technology	Fulcrum effect (hand-instrument motion reversal)

Table 1. Advantages and Disadvantages of Robot-Assisted Surgery vs. Conventional Minimal Access Surgery

Robotic General Surgery Procedures
Cholecystectomy
Heller Myotomy
Anti-reflux surgery
Colon Resection
Bariatric surgery
Endocrine surgery
Esophageal resection
Small bowel surgery
Liver resection
Splenectomy
Gastric Surgery

Table 2. Applications of Robotics in General Surgery

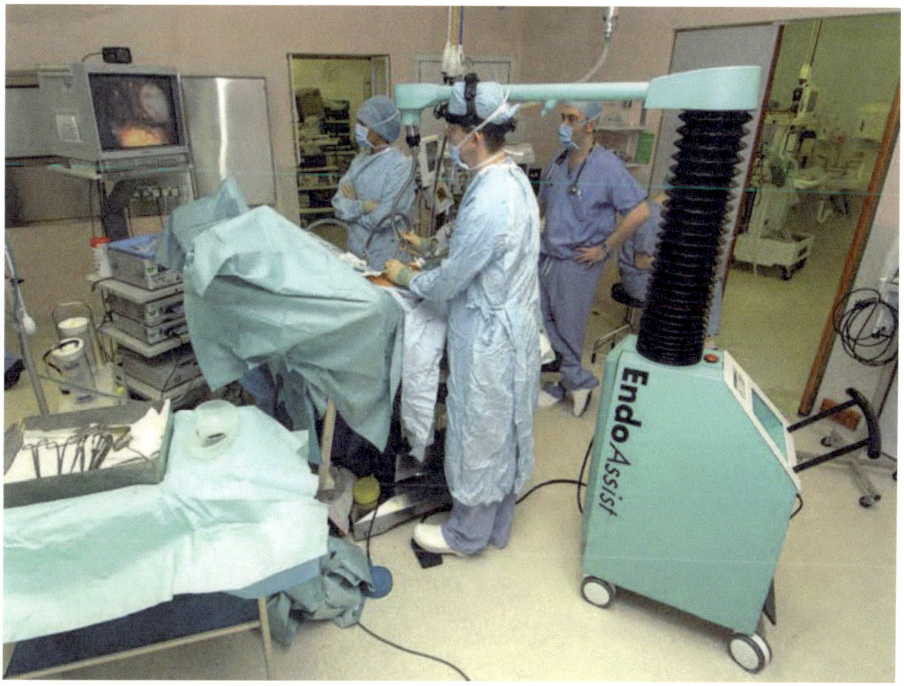

Figure 1. The EndoAssist manipulates a laparoscopic camera at the command of the surgeon. ©*[2006] Prosurgics, Limited*

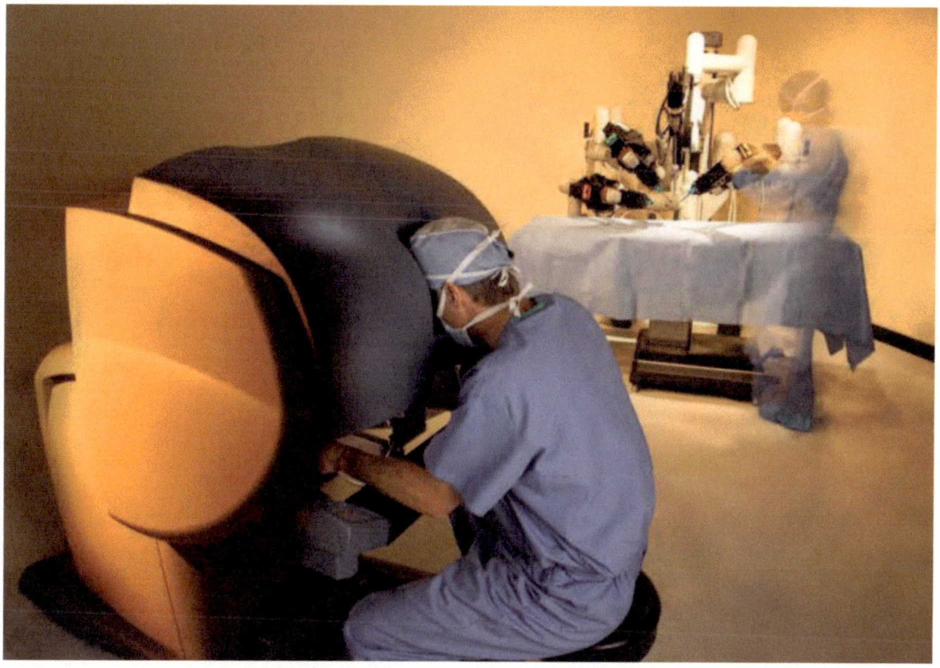

Figure 2. The da Vinci® robotic surgical system comprising of a surgeon's console and a patient side cart. ©*[2007] Intuitive Surgical, Inc*

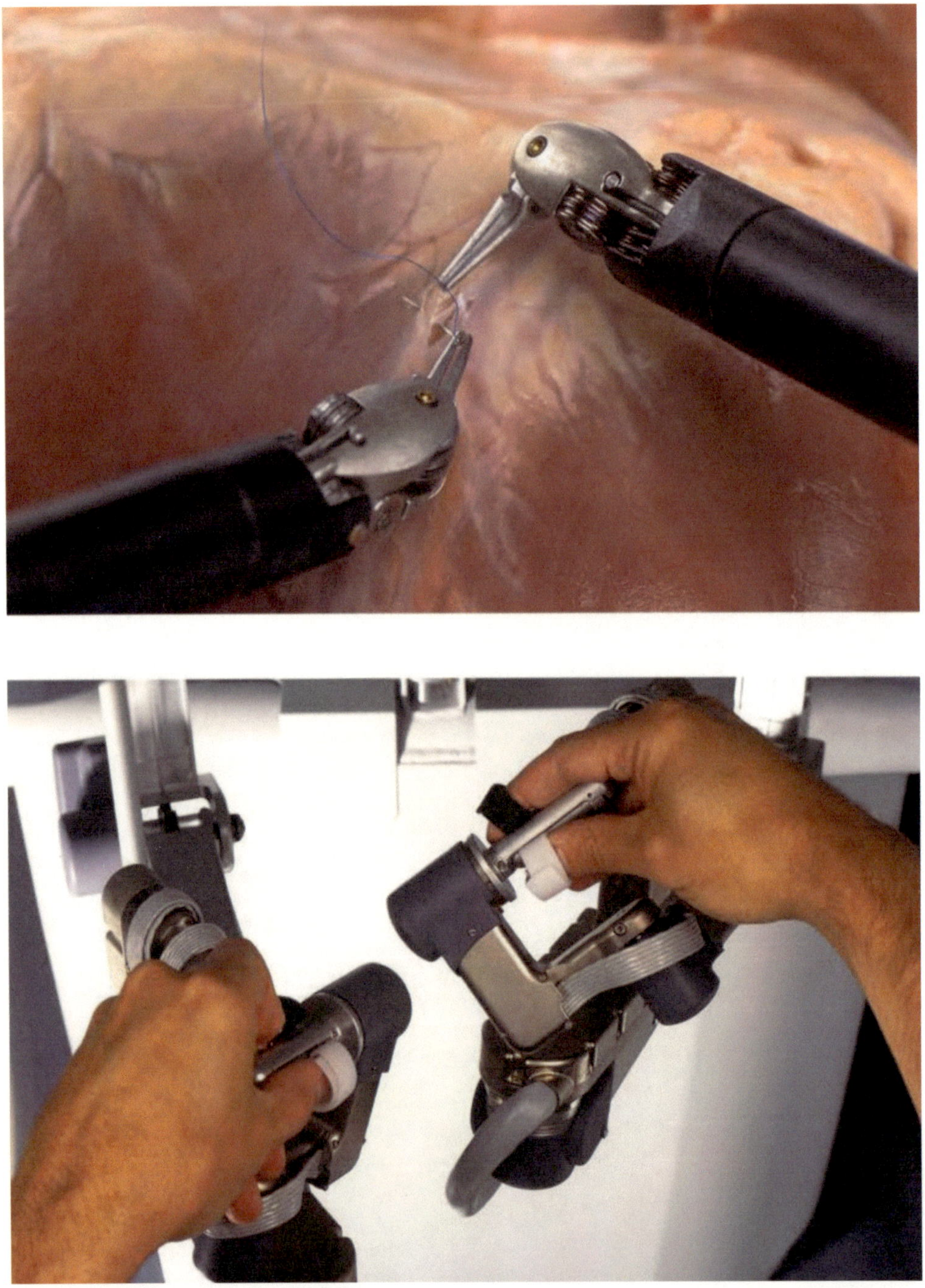

Figure 3. Surgeon's console including operative field view (above) and master controls (below). ©*[2007] Intuitive Surgical, Inc*

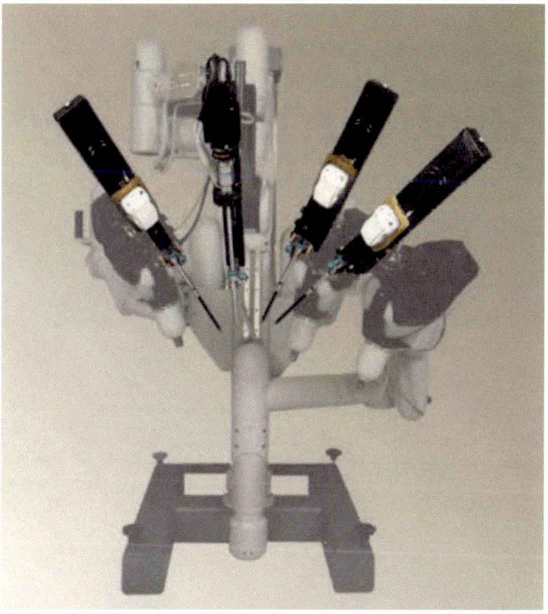

Figure 4. Patient side cart. ©*[2007] Intuitive Surgical, Inc*

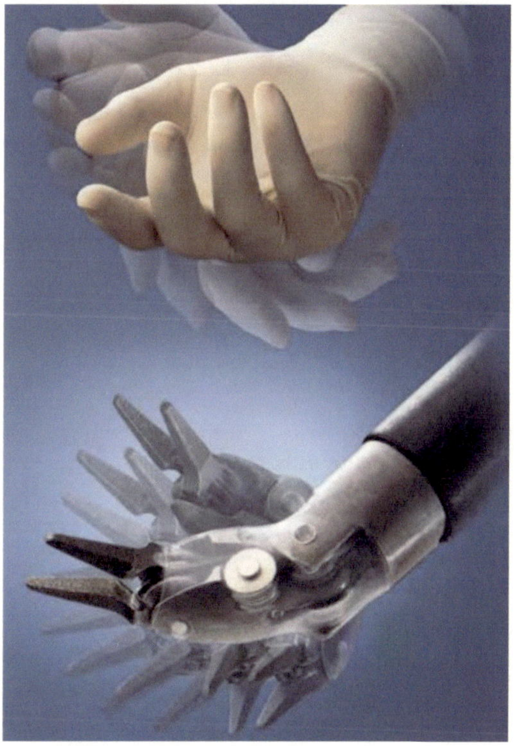

Figure 5. Demonstration of the 7 degrees of freedom with Endowrist® technology compared to surgeon hands. ©*[2007] Intuitive Surgical, Inc*

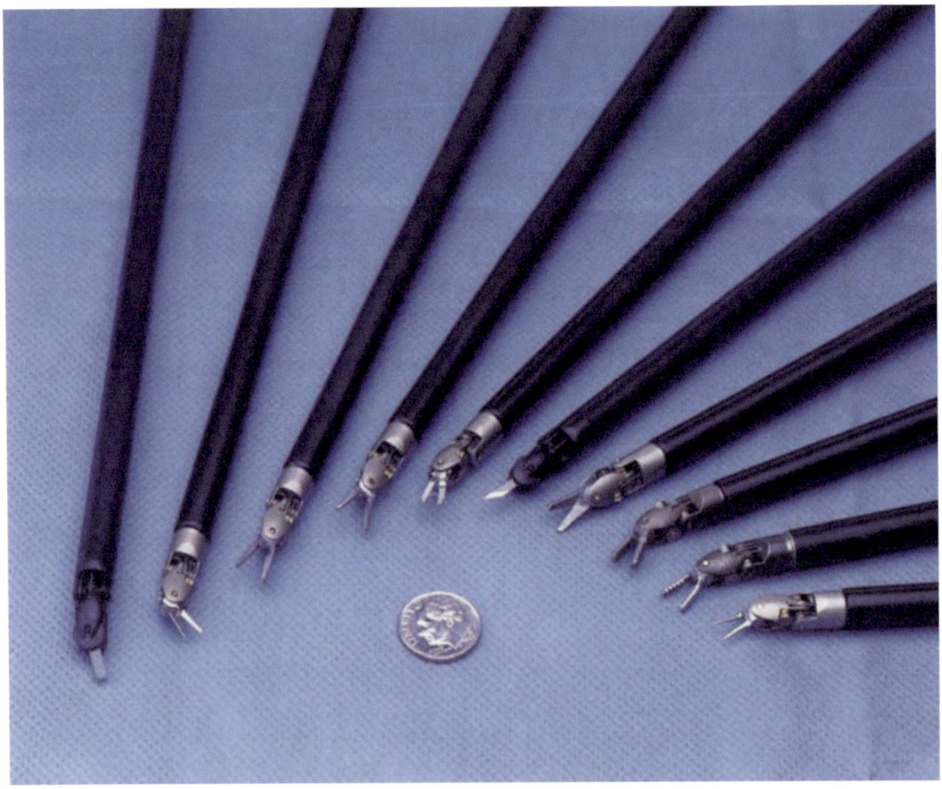

Figure 6. Range of available "wristed" instruments. *EndoWrist® ©[2007] Intuitive Surgical, Inc*

11. References

"robot", *Merian-Webster Online Dictonary*. 2007. http://m-w.com/dictionary/robot (16 Jul. 2007). [1]

Unger, S.W., H.M. Unger, and R.T. Bass, *AESOP robotic arm*. Surg Endosc, 1994. 8(9): p. 1131. [2]

Sackier, J.M. and Y. Wang, *Robotically assisted laparoscopic surgery. From concept to development*. Surg Endosc, 1994. 8(1): p. 63-6. [3]

Allaf, M.E., et al., *Laparoscopic visual field. Voice vs foot pedal interfaces for control of the AESOP robot*. Surg Endosc, 1998. 12(12): p. 1415-8. [4]

Omote, K., et al., *Self-guided robotic camera control for laparoscopic surgery compared with human camera control*. Am J Surg, 1999. 177(4): p. 321-4. [5]

Merola, S., et al., *Comparison of laparoscopic colectomy with and without the aid of a robotic camera holder*. Surg Laparosc Endosc Percutan Tech, 2002. 12(1): p. 46-51. [6]

Aiono, S., et al., *Controlled trial of the introduction of a robotic camera assistant (EndoAssist) for laparoscopic cholecystectomy*. Surg Endosc, 2002. 16(9): p. 1267-70. [7]

Wagner, A.A., et al., *Comparison of surgical performance during laparoscopic radical prostatectomy of two robotic camera holders, EndoAssist and AESOP: a pilot study*. Urology, 2006. 68(1): p. 70-4. [8]

Nebot, P.B., et al., *Comparison of task performance of the camera-holder robots EndoAssist and Aesop.* Surg Laparosc Endosc Percutan Tech, 2003. 13(5): p. 334-8. [9]

Kim, V.B., et al., *Early experience with telemanipulative robot-assisted laparoscopic cholecystectomy using da Vinci.* Surgical laparoscopy, endoscopy & percutaneous techniques, 2002. 12(1): p. 33-40. [10]

Lanfranco, A.R., et al., *Robotic surgery: a current perspective.* Ann Surg, 2004. 239(1): p. 14-21. [11]

Kant, A.J., M.D. Klein, and S.E. Langenburg, *Robotics in pediatric surgery: perspectives for imaging.* Pediatric radiology, 2004. 34(6): p. 454. [12]

Maniar, H.S., et al., *Comparison of skill training with robotic systems and traditional endoscopy: implications on training and adoption.* J Surg Res, 2005. 125(1): p. 23-9. [13]

Reyes, D.A., B. Tang, and A. Cuschieri, *Minimal access surgery (MAS)-related surgeon morbidity syndromes.* Surg Endosc, 2006. 20(1): p. 1-13. [14]

Uhrich, M.L., et al., *Assessment of fatigue, monitor placement, and surgical experience during simulated laparoscopic surgery.* Surg Endosc, 2002. 16(4): p. 635-9. [15]

Berguer, R., *Surgical technology and the ergonomics of laparoscopic instruments.* Surg Endosc, 1998. 12(5): p. 458-62. [16]

Woo, R., et al., *Robot-assisted pediatric surgery.* The American journal of surgery, 2004. 188(4A Suppl): p. 27S. [17]

Kitagawa, M., et al., *Effect of sensory substitution on suture-manipulation forces for robotic surgical systems.* J Thorac Cardiovasc Surg, 2005. 129(1): p. 151-8. [18]

Morgan, J.A., et al., *Does robotic technology make minimally invasive cardiac surgery too expensive? A hospital cost analysis of robotic and conventional techniques.* Journal of cardiac surgery, 2005. 20(3): p. 246-251. [19]

Lotan, Y., J.A. Cadeddu, and M.T. Gettman, *The new economics of radical prostatectomy: cost comparison of open, laparoscopic and robot assisted techniques.* The Journal of urology, 2004. 172(4 Pt 1): p. 1431-1435. [20]

Talamini, M., K. Campbell, and C. Stanfield, *Robotic gastrointestinal surgery: early experience and system description.* Journal of laparoendoscopic & advanced surgical techniques, 2002. 12(4): p. 225-232. [21]

Reynolds, W., Jr., *The first laparoscopic cholecystectomy.* Jsls, 2001. 5(1): p. 89-94. [22]

Himpens, J., G. Leman, and G.B. Cadiere, *Telesurgical laparoscopic cholecystectomy.* Surgical endoscopy, 1998. 12(8): p. 1091-1091. [23]

Ruurda, J.P., et al., *Feasibility of robot-assisted laparoscopic surgery: an evaluation of 35 robot-assisted laparoscopic cholecystectomies.* Surgical laparoscopy, endoscopy & percutaneous techniques, 2002. 12(1): p. 41-45. [24]

Marescaux, J., et al., *Telerobotic laparoscopic cholecystectomy: initial clinical experience with 25 patients.* Annals of surgery, 2001. 234(1): p. 1-7. [25]

Miller, D.W., R.T. Schlinkert, and D.K. Schlinkert, *Robot-assisted laparoscopic cholecystectomy: initial Mayo Clinic Scottsdale experience.* Mayo Clinic proceedings, 2004. 79(9): p. 1132-1136. [26]

Corcione, F., et al., *Advantages and limits of robot-assisted laparoscopic surgery: preliminary experience.* Surgical endoscopy, 2005. 19(1): p. 117-119. [27]

Cadière, G.B., et al., *Feasibility of robotic laparoscopic surgery: 146 cases.* World journal of surgery, 2001. 25(11): p. 1467-1477. [28]

Hazey, J.W. and W.S. Melvin, *Robot-assisted general surgery.* Seminars in laparoscopic surgery, 2004. 11(2): p. 107-112. [29]

Ballantyne, G.H., *Telerobotic gastrointestinal surgery: phase 2--safety and efficacy.* Surg Endosc, 2007. 21(7): p. 1054-62. [30]

Ruurda, J.P., P.L. Visser, and I.A.M.J. Broeders, *Analysis of procedure time in robot-assisted surgery: comparative study in laparoscopic cholecystectomy.* Computer aided surgery, 2003. 8(1): p. 24-29. [31]

Nio, D., et al., *Robot-assisted laparoscopic cholecystectomy versus conventional laparoscopic cholecystectomy: a comparative study.* Surgical endoscopy, 2004. 18(3): p. 379-382. [32]

Kornprat, P., et al., *Prospective study comparing standard and robotically assisted laparoscopic cholecystectomy.* Langenbecks Arch Surg, 2006. 391(3): p. 216-21. [33]

Vidovszky, T.J., et al., *Robotic cholecystectomy: learning curve, advantages, and limitations.* J Surg Res, 2006. 136(2): p. 172-8. [34]

Newlin, M.E., D.J. Mikami, and S.W. Melvin, *Initial experience with the four-arm computer-enhanced telesurgery device in foregut surgery.* Journal of laparoendoscopic & advanced surgical techniques, 2004. 14(3): p. 121-124. [35]

Melvin, W.S., et al., *Computer-enhanced vs. standard laparoscopic antireflux surgery.* Journal of gastrointestinal surgery, 2002. 6(1): p. 11-5; discussion 15. [36]

Melvin, W.S., et al., *Computer-enhanced robotic telesurgery. Initial experience in foregut surgery.* Surgical endoscopy, 2002. 16(12): p. 1790-1792. [37]

Wright, A.S., J.C. Gould, and W.S. Melvin, *Computer-assisted robotic antireflux surgery.* Minerva Gastroenterol Dietol, 2004. 50(3): p. 253-60. [38]

Ayav, A., et al., *Early results of one-year robotic surgery using the Da Vinci system to perform advanced laparoscopic procedures.* Journal of gastrointestinal surgery, 2004. 8(6): p. 720-726. [39]

Costi, R., et al., *Robotic fundoplication: from theoretic advantages to real problems.* J Am Coll Surg, 2003. 197(3): p. 500-7. [40]

Giulianotti, P.C., et al., *Robotics in general surgery: personal experience in a large community hospital.* Archives of surgery, 2003. 138(7): p. 777-784. [41]

Müller, S., et al., *Robot-assisted versus conventional laparoscopic fundoplication: short-term outcome of a pilot randomized controlled trial.* Surgical endoscopy, 2007. [42]

Galvani, C., et al., *Laparoscopic Heller myotomy for achalasia facilitated by robotic assistance.* Surg Endosc, 2006. 20(7): p. 1105-12. [43]

Melvin, W.S., et al., *Computer-enhanced robotic telesurgery minimizes esophageal perforation during Heller myotomy.* Surgery, 2005. 138(4): p. 553-8; discussion 558-9. [44]

Horgan, S., et al., *Robotic-assisted Heller myotomy versus laparoscopic Heller myotomy for the treatment of esophageal achalasia: multicenter study.* J Gastrointest Surg, 2005. 9(8): p. 1020-9; discussion 1029-30. [45]

Cadiere, G.B., et al., *The world's first obesity surgery performed by a surgeon at a distance.* Obes Surg, 1999. 9(2): p. 206-9.[46]

Sudan, R., V. Puri, and D. Sudan, *Robotically assisted biliary pancreatic diversion with a duodenal switch: a new technique.* Surg Endosc, 2007. 21(5): p. 729-33. [47]

Sanchez, B.R., et al., *Comparison of totally robotic laparoscopic Roux-en-Y gastric bypass and traditional laparoscopic Roux-en-Y gastric bypass.* Surg Obes Relat Dis, 2005. 1(6): p. 549-54. [48]

Mohr, C.J., et al., *Totally robotic laparoscopic Roux-en-Y Gastric bypass: results from 75 patients.* Obes Surg, 2006. 16(6): p. 690-6. [49]

Ali, M.R., B. Bhaskerrao, and B.M. Wolfe, *Robot-assisted laparoscopic Roux-en-Y gastric bypass.* Surgical endoscopy, 2005. 19(4): p. 468-472. [50]

Moser, F. and S. Horgan, *Robotically assisted bariatric surgery.* The American journal of surgery, 2004. 188(4A Suppl): p. 38S-44S. [51]

Mohr, C.J., G.S. Nadzam, and M.J. Curet, *Totally robotic Roux-en-Y gastric bypass.* Archives of surgery, 2005. 140(8): p. 779-786. [52]

Rigdon, J.L., *Robotic-assisted laparoscopic radical prostatectomy.* Aorn J, 2006. 84(5): p. 760-2, 764, 766-770; quiz 771-4. [53]

Weber, P.A., et al., *Telerobotic-assisted laparoscopic right and sigmoid colectomies for benign disease.* Diseases of the colon & rectum, 2002. 45(12): p. 1689-94; discussion 1695. [54]

D'Annibale, A., et al., *Robotic and laparoscopic surgery for treatment of colorectal diseases.* Diseases of the colon & rectum, 2004. 47(12): p. 2162-2168. [55]

Kariv, Y. and C.P. Delaney, *Robotics in colorectal surgery.* Minerva Chir, 2005. 60(5): p. 401-16. [56]

Delaney, C.P., et al., *Comparison of robotically performed and traditional laparoscopic colorectal surgery.* Diseases of the colon & rectum, 2003. 46(12): p. 1633-1639. [57]

Woeste, G., W.O. Bechstein, and C. Wullstein, *Does telerobotic assistance improve laparoscopic colorectal surgery?* International journal of colorectal disease, 2005. 20(3): p. 253-257. [58]

Anvari, M., *Remote telepresence surgery: the Canadian experience.* Surg Endosc, 2007. 21(4): p. 537-41. [59]

Satava, R.M., *Robotics in colorectal surgery: telemonitoring and telerobotics.* Surg Clin North Am, 2006. 86(4): p. 927-36. [60]

Pigazzi, A., et al., *Robotic-assisted laparoscopic low anterior resection with total mesorectal excision for rectal cancer.* Surgical endoscopy, 2006. 20(10): p. 1521-1525. [61]

Braumann, C., et al., *Computer-assisted laparoscopic colon resection with the Da Vinci system: our first experiences.* Dis Colon Rectum, 2005. 48(9): p. 1820-7. [62]

Gutt, C.N., et al., *Robot-assisted abdominal surgery.* The British journal of surgery, 2004. 91(11): p. 1390-1397. [63]

Hance, J., T. Rockall, and A. Darzi, *Robotics in colorectal surgery.* Digestive surgery, 2004. 21(5-6): p. 339-343. [64]

D'Annibale, A., et al., *The da Vinci robot in right adrenalectomy: considerations on technique.* Surgical laparoscopy, endoscopy & percutaneous techniques, 2004. 14(1): p. 38-41. [65]

Morino, M., et al., *Robot-assisted vs laparoscopic adrenalectomy: a prospective randomized controlled trial.* Surg Endosc, 2004. 18(12): p. 1742-6. [66]

Sung, G.T. and I.S. Gill, *Robotic renal and adrenal surgery.* The Surgical clinics of North America, 2003. 83(6): p. 1469-1482. [67]

Melvin, W.S., et al., *Robotic resection of pancreatic neuroendocrine tumor.* Journal of laparoendoscopic & advanced surgical techniques, 2003. 13(1): p. 33-36. [68]

Bodner, J., et al., *Mediastinal parathyroidectomy with the da Vinci robot: presentation of a new technique.* Journal of thoracic and cardiovascular surgery, 2004. 127(6): p. 1831-1832. [69]

Augustin, F., T. Schmid, and J. Bodner, *The robotic approach for mediastinal lesions.* The international journal of medical robotics and computer assisted surgery, 2006. 2(3): p. 262-270. [70]

Young, J.A., et al., *Robotic-assisted adrenalectomy for adrenal incidentaloma: case and review of the technique.* Surgical laparoscopy, endoscopy & percutaneous techniques, 2002. 12(2): p. 126-130. [71]

Morino, M., et al., *Robot-assisted vs laparoscopic adrenalectomy: a prospective randomized controlled trial.* Surgical endoscopy, 2004. 18(12): p. 1742-1746. [72]

Marescaux, J., et al., *Transatlantic robot-assisted telesurgery.* Nature, 2001. 413(6854): p. 379-380. [73]

Marescaux, J., et al., *Transcontinental robot-assisted remote telesurgery: feasibility and potential applications.* Annals of surgery, 2002. 235(4): p. 487-492. [74]

Marescaux, J. and L. Solerc, *Image-guided robotic surgery.* Seminars in laparoscopic surgery, 2004. 11(2): p. 113. [75]

Wagner, A., et al., *Virtual image guided navigation in tumor surgery--technical innovation.* J Craniomaxillofac Surg, 1995. 23(5): p. 217-3. [76]

Wagner, A., et al., *Image-guided surgery.* Int J Oral Maxillofac Surg, 1996. 25(2): p. 147-51. [77]

Cepolina, F. and R.C. Michelini, *Review of robotic fixtures for minimally invasive surgery.* Int J Med Robot, 2004. 1(1): p. 43-63. [78]

Menciassi, A., M. Quirini, and P. Dario, *Microrobotics for future gastrointestinal endoscopy.* Minim Invasive Ther Allied Technol, 2007. 16(2): p. 91-100. [79]

Rebello, K.J., *Surgical MEMS Research Activity.* Proceeding of the IEEE, 2004. 92(1): p. 43-55. [80]

Nishihara, S., et al., *Clinical accuracy evaluation of femoral canal preparation using the ROBODOC system.* J Orthop Sci, 2004. 9(5): p. 452-61. [81]

Sugano, N., *Computer-assisted orthopedic surgery.* J Orthop Sci, 2003. 8(3): p. 442-8. [82]

Bargar, W.L., A. Bauer, and M. Borner, *Primary and revision total hip replacement using the Robodoc system.* Clin Orthop Relat Res, 1998(354): p. 82-91. [83]

Cowley, G., *Introducing "Robodoc". A robot finds his calling--in the operating room.* Newsweek, 1992. 120(21): p. 86. [84]

Spencer, E.H., *The ROBODOC clinical trial: a robotic assistant for total hip arthroplasty.* Orthop Nurs, 1996. 15(1): p. 9-14. [85]

Taylor, K.S., *Robodoc: study tests robot's use in hip surgery.* Hospitals, 1993. 67(9): p. 46. [86]

Cain, P., et al., *Safety considerations in a surgical robot.* Biomed Sci Instrum, 1993. 29: p. 291-4. [87]

Korb, W., et al., *Robots in the operating theatre--chances and challenges.* Int J Oral Maxillofac Surg, 2004. 33(8): p. 721-32. [88]

37

Telemanipulated Long Bone Fracture Reduction

Ralf Westphal[1], Simon Winkelbach[1], Thomas Gösling[2], Markus Oszwald[2], Tobias Hüfner[2], Christian Krettek[2] and Friedrich Wahl[1]
[1]*Institute for Robotics and Process Control, Technical University of Braunschweig,*
[2]*Department of Trauma Surgery, Hannover Medical School*
Germany

1. Introduction

Fractures of the human thigh bone, the femur, are commonly caused by high-energy injury mechanisms, like traffic accidents, predominantly in young males or by low-energy mechanisms, like falling, in elderly females (Martinet et al., 2000; Zlowodzki et al., 2006). With approximately 37 per 100,000 persons per year this is an extremely frequently encountered injury (Arneson et al., 1988; Zlowodzki et al., 2006). In 1999 334,410 patients with fractures of the lower extremities have been counted in Germany[1]. 144,659 of which had fractures of the thigh bone. After subtracting fractures in the proximal (hip side) femur, 25,695 patients remain with fractures in the femoral shaft (the middle, diaphyseal) region to which this work is dedicated.
Today, the treatment of choice for femur shaft fractures preferred by many surgeons is the minimal invasive technique of intramedullary nailing, which has been established as a standard technique for a definite stabilizing treatment in diaphyseal fractures of the lower extremities (Kempf et al., 1985; Krettek et al., 1996; Krettek, 2001; Winquist et al., 1984).
The complete process of intramedullary nailing is shown as a sketch in figure 1. The process starts with the opening of the medullary cavity. A small soft tissue cut of about 5 cm has to be placed at the proximal end of the femur. In extension of the femoral shaft, the bone's cavity has to be opened. This is achieved with a surgical drill. Now the intramedullary nail is inserted into the bone's medullary cavity until it reaches the fracture region. Subsequently the two major bone fragments are aligned accordingly to their correct anatomical position. For this the distal (knee side) fracture segment is moved by the surgeon by means of a so-called Schanz' screw, whereas the proximal fracture segment is hold in its position by means of a second Schanz' screw. According to (Rüedi & Murphy, 2000), this form of manipulation is called "joystick" reduction. When the fracture segments are finally aligned correctly, the intramedullary nail is further inserted. Finally the nail is locked with the bone by means of lateral screws. During the final insertion and the locking of the nail, the correct retention, which means maintaining the correct segment positions, has to be ensured. The whole process is supervised by means of X-ray imaging. A detailed description of this surgical procedure can be found in (Rüedi & Murphy, 2000).

---

[1] Source: Statistisches Bundesamt Deutschland (German Federal Statistical Office)

Compared to open fracture reduction surgeries, in which the soft tissue around the fracture region is opened and the fracture segments are relocated and fixed with plates, this minimally invasive technique of intramedullary nailing has a number of advantages. It has proven high primary union rates of 90-99% while only having a very low incidence of surgery induced infection of <10% (Bhandari et al., 2000; Finkemeier et al., 2000; Kempf et al., 1985; Krettek et al., 1998; Winquist et al., 1984; Wolinsky et al., 1999).

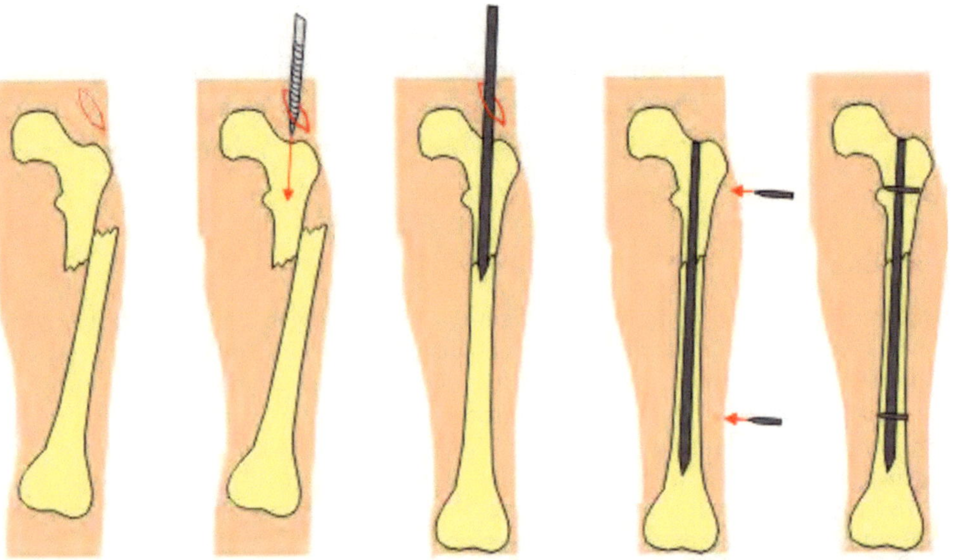

(a) (b) (c) (d) (e)

Figure 1. The process of closed intramedullary nailing (taken from (Winkelbach, 2006)) (a) Soft tissue cut at the hip. (b) Opening of the femur's medullary cavity. (c) Insertion of the intramedullary nail and reduction of the fracture. (d) Complete insertion of the nail which is locked by means of screws. (e) Result of the fracture reduction procedure

Besides its advantages, the closed intramedullary nailing also has a number of disadvantages, which are well-known in clinical practice and revealed in the open literature. Malalignment of the fracture segments is the most significant one which has a high impact on functional biomechanics. While being a personal tragedy for the patient, malalignment also has socio-economic effects as it leads to non-physiological conditions, which may result in a lengthened and costly rehabilitation during which the patient might be inhibited from working. In several cases even consecutive revision operations might become necessary.

A correct rotational alignment around the shaft axis is difficult to achieve, as intraoperatively only 2D fluoroscopy (X-ray imaging) is used for assessment. The limited visualization of structures on the bone surface and the limited display window are the main problems for achieving a correct rotational alignment. The frequent occurrence of rotational deviations of more than 10° is remarkable (Prevot et al., 1998; Winquist et al., 1984). Significant malalignment in the sagittal and frontal plane between 2% and 18% (Prevot et al., 1998; Winquist et al., 1984; Wolinsky et al., 1999)

and shortening of the femur by more than 2cm (Prevot et al., 1998; Winquist et al., 1984) are also reported.
The high radiation exposure to the patient and the operating staff is a second well-known problem. In open literature average X-ray image intensifier usage between 158 and 316 seconds is reported (Kempf et al., 1985; Sugarman et al., 1988). As the surgeon's hands are unprotected and close to the X-ray imaging field during the process of reduction, this is a particular point of criticism. Both problems, the malalignments and the high radiation exposure, are related to difficulties in achieving and maintaining the correct reduction. These problems are evidently specific for a long bone like the femur because of its tube-shaped anatomy and its counteracting muscle forces. Experiments performed during the course of our project revealed maximum forces of over 400 Newton during the reduction process (Gösling et al., 2006a; Gösling et al., 2006b; Gösling, 2007).
Accordingly, the aim of this interdisciplinary research project between the Hannover Medical School and the Technical University of Braunschweig is to support the described surgical procedure by developing and utilizing modern and emerging technologies like 3D imaging, surgical navigation, and robotics. The following objectives have been declared for the project:

- **Increased precision**: The overall precision of the fracture reductions should be increased. In particular, unacceptable reduction results with rotational deviations of 10 or more degrees, which might result in subsequent revision surgeries, should be averted.
- **Reduction of X-ray irradiation**: The number of X-ray images required to achieve the fracture reduction should be reduced. Especially for the operation staff, this point is highly desirable. Therefore not just simply reducing the number of X-ray images would be an advantage, but also the possibility to keep the operation staff away from the radiation during imaging.
- **Decreased operation time**: The possibility of decreasing the overall operation time would have two benefits. First, a shorter time of anesthesia means a reduction of the patient's stress. Second, from an economical point of view it would be desirable to shorten the operation times in order to reduce the overall costs. However, set-up time is often a crucial point for modern surgical procedures like navigation and especially robotics. So this point should be taken with care.

1.1 Related Work

Since its early beginnings in the mid 1980s, the research field of medical and in particular surgical robotics produced many different robotic systems for a wide variety of surgical applications. A complete review of this field will be beyond the scope of this paper, so we will just present research projects with a direct relation to the work presented in this paper. On the internet one can find an extensive database of surgical robotic systems (Pott, 2006). Further interesting reviews about research and development in this field can be found in (Cleary & Nguyen, 2003; Dario et al., 2003; Taylor & Joskowicz, 2002; Taylor & Stoianovici, 2003).
There is a world wide copious research in many different areas of surgical robotics, but only little work is done in the field of robotized fracture reduction. And so far, no commercially available robotic system exists, which supports fracture reduction procedures. Femoral

fracture reduction utilizing a robotic assistance system was first described by Bouazza-Marouf et al. in the year 1995 (Bouazza-Marouf et al., 1995). However, they just declared requirements for the reduction tool and did not publish anything about an implemented system or experimental results of fracture reductions performed by a robot.
The research group which worked on a project most similar to our group's work was the group of Nerlich, Monkman et al. from Regensburg, Germany (Füchtmeier et al., 2004). But as far as we know, their "RepoRobo" project has not been continued.
A second group which is working especially in the field of femur fracture reduction is the one headed by Warisawa from Tokyo, Japan. They follow the commendable approach of a non-invasive fracture reduction robot. Their robot system is attached to the patient's foot and performs respectively supports the reduction procedure in the femur via the knee joint. The only publication of this project we know from is from the year 2004 (Warisawa et al., 2004).
Seide et al. have been performing extensive research in developing a fracture reduction robotic system based on a parallel kinematic (a hexapod). Starting with purely manually actuated links (Seide & Wolter, 2000) where a software program computes the required link lengths, they have already performed successful clinical trials on patients with a completely automated actuated robotic system (Seide et al., 2004).
Another important research group is the one headed by Leo Joskowicz from The Hebrew University of Jerusalem, Israel. So far however, they haven't developed a robotic system for fracture reduction. Besides a robot for screw placement and distal locking their main contribution to CAS (Computer Assisted Surgery) in femoral fracture reduction is research on navigation (Hazan & Joskowicz, 2003; Joskowicz et al., 1998a; Joskowicz et al., 1998b; Yaniv et al., 1998).

1.2 Previous Work

Our first implementation of a surgical telemanipulator system for femur shaft fracture reduction, was a laboratory set-up in which artificial bones where used for the reduction process and CCD cameras where used to emulate intraoperative X-ray imaging. The good results of these tests, with very high reduction accuracies and short operation times, encouraged the further development of this telemanipulated fracture reduction concept. Furthermore, this pilot study revealed the importance of haptic and metric information to the surgeon during the reduction process (Gösling et al., 2005; Westphal et al., 2003; Westphal et al., 2004).
The next development step, was the telemanipulated reduction in a more realistic surgical environment. Using real X-ray images instead of CCD camera images and human specimens with intact soft tissues surrounding the broken femur bone, we were able to evaluate telemanipulated fracture reduction in an environment as close to clinical practice as possible. We could show, that telemanipulated fracture reduction in real human specimens is possible yielding overall satisfactory accuracies. It was shown that the required image intensifier usage could be reduced conspicuously, when compared with manually performed reductions. However, the accuracies obtained by the telemanipulator did not differ significantly from those obtained by the manual control group, so we couldn't show a definite benefit of the telemanipulated procedure in this set-up (Gösling, 2007; Westphal et al., 2006).

1.3 Contribution of this Work

As we have seen in our previous work, the telemanipulated reductions based on 2D X-ray imaging suffer from the same problems as the conventional manual reduction procedure: the limited view of the X-ray image and the low level of detail on the bone surface in the image. The way of interacting with the joystick has turned out to be a second weak point of the implemented telemanipulator system, as the operator had control over all three rotational degrees of freedom (DoFs) at the same time, while only having control over the two translational DoFs of the current X-ray viewing direction. Supporting all rotational DoFs at the same time using a joystick was shown to be not intuitively controllable by the operating surgeon. Therefore a more intuitive way of interaction is desirable.

The problems arising due to the low level of detail in the 2D X-ray images can be solved best by using high resolution 3D volume data, which can, for example, be obtained by computer tomography (CT) scanners or intraoperatively using motorized 3D C-arms. Therefore in this paper, a surgical telemanipulator system is presented, which uses a new and intuitive interaction principle based on a conventional joystick with force feedback capabilities and 3D imaging data. This telemanipulator system is evaluated extensively and successfully on human bones and complete human specimens.

The rest of the paper is organized as follows. In the next section, the telemanipulator system is described in detail, together with the experimental set-up, which was used for evaluation. Section 3 presents the results obtained by these experiments and section 4, finally gives a conclusion and an outlook on further research in the context of robotized fracture reductions.

2. Methods

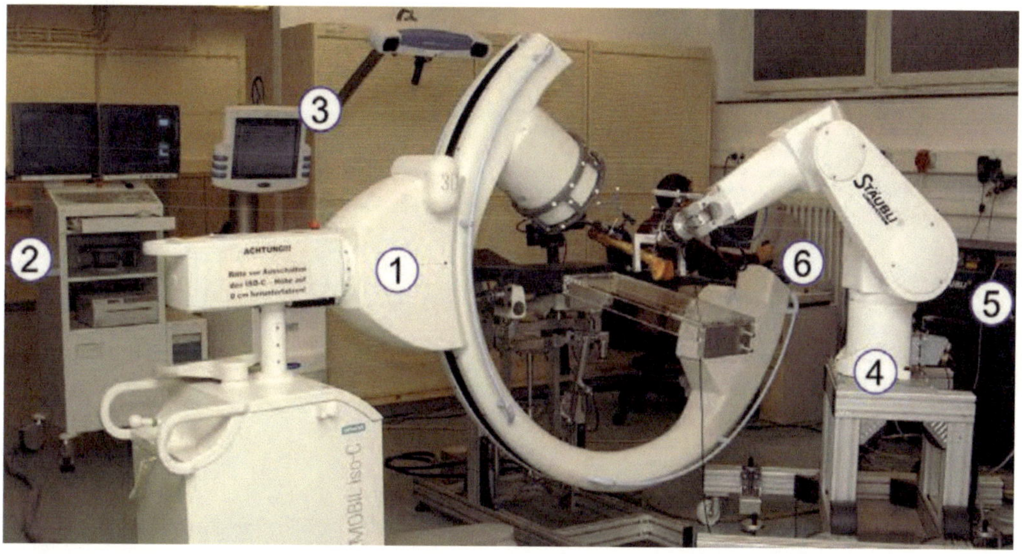

Figure 2. View of the 3D Telemanipulator set-up. 1: Fluoroscopy device. 2: Fluoroscopy workstation. 3: Surgical navigation system. 4: RX 90 robot. 5: Robot controller unit. 6: Controller PC

By using a telemanipulator system for supporting the fracture reduction process, the following benefits for the surgical procedure and for the surgeon can be expected.

- **Well-controlled motions**: A stable control of the fracture segment positions in all anatomical planes at the same time is difficult to achieve by the surgeon manually when using the conventional surgical method. But by ensuring a stable motion control, many control images and frequent reorientations of the fluoroscopic C-arm could be avoided, which would result in a reduction of X-ray exposure and a reduction of the risk of infection due to C-arm reorientations.
- **Fatigue-proof reduction and retention control**: In clinical pre-tests we measured forces and torques applied by the surgeon in order to achieve the fracture reduction (Gösling et al., 2006a; Gösling et al., 2006b; Gösling, 2007). These measurements revealed maximum peek forces of over 400 Newton. Obviously, under these conditions a human surgeon will have difficulties performing fine manipulations or keeping the retention over a longer period of time.
- **Keeping the surgeon distant to X-ray radiation**: In contrast to manually performed fracture reductions, the operation team can keep a distance from the X-ray device during imaging. Especially for the surgeon, who usually has his hands within or near the X-ray beam, this would result in a conspicuous reduction of the applied radiation dose.

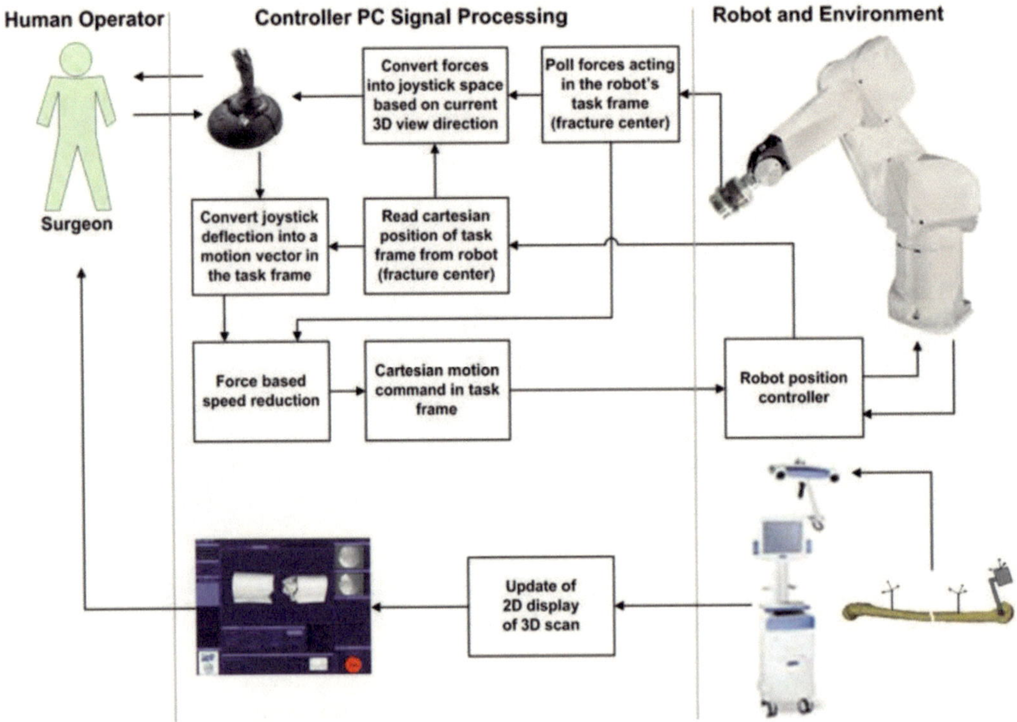

Figure 3. Signal flow diagram of the telemanipulator system during the fracture reduction process, illustrating interconnections between the surgeon, the controller PC, the robot, the force/torque sensor, and the navigation system

The telemanipulator set-up for robot assisted fracture reduction, developed by our work group, is shown in figure 2 and an overview of the system in figure 3. As can be seen in those images, our telemanipulator set-up uses an industrial robot, a Stäubli RX 90CR with its standard CS7B controller programmable in V+ (Stäubli Tec-Systems, Faverges, France). The robot is mounted on a wheeled platform so it can be placed besides the operation table. Furthermore, the robot is equipped with a force/torque sensor (FT Delta SI-660-60; Schunk, Lauffen, Germany) connected via an ISA card to a standard PC (Pentium® 4 2.8 GHz) running Microsoft® Windows® 2000. Intraoperative 3D imaging is achieved by the Siemens Siremobil Iso C 3D (Siemens AG, Medical Solutions, Erlangen, Germany) fluoroscopic C-arm. For the 3D tracking of the fracture segments and for the registration of the 3D image volume, we use an optical surgical navigation system (VectorVision, BrainLAB, Munich, Germany). The input device, a force feedback joystick (Microsoft®, SideWinder® ForceFeedback 2; Microsoft Corp., USA), is also connected to the PC. All four sub systems (PC, robot controller, navigation system, and fluoroscopic C-arm) are connected via a TCP/IP 100Mbit network.

2.1 Robotized Fracture Reduction

The process of fracture reduction is separated into two steps. The First step is the acquisition of a 3D DICOM data set and the reconstruction and registration of a 3D surface model, which is subsequently used for displaying a 3D scene on the PC. The second step is the reduction process itself.

At first, a 3D DICOM data set is acquired intraoperatively using the Siemens Iso C 3D C-arm. Within this 3D DICOM data set the bone has to be segmented from the surrounding soft tissue. This is performed simply by thresholding, with the threshold value being set manually by the surgeon. Next, 3D surface models are reconstructed from these segmented bone regions using the Marching Cube algorithm (Lorensen & Cline, 1987). This way surface geometries - meshes - are created for the two major fracture segments, the proximal and the distal part of the femur. For the smaller fragments, which in complex fractures may be located between the two major parts, no 3D meshes are generated, as they neither can be tracked nor manipulated by this telemanipulator approach. Both meshes have a local coordinate space in which the vertex positions are given. These coordinate spaces are defined in relation to the coordinate space of the DICOM data set. So we get the transformations ${}^{DICOM}\boldsymbol{T}_{PROX}$ and ${}^{DICOM}\boldsymbol{T}_{DIST}$ for the two meshes (table 1 summarizes all coordinate systems which are used in the following system description, as also illustrated in figure 4).

Having just these meshes of the fracture segments is not sufficient for being able to use them during navigated or telemanipulated surgeries. They need to be brought in relation to real world entities, i.e., to the current bone poses and to the robot. This process is called registration. The main application of registration algorithms in the field of computer assisted surgery is to bring preoperatively acquired data sets, like the ones from a CT scanner, in relation to an eventually changed intraoperative situation. In (Maintz, & Viergever, 1998; Zitova & Flusser, 2003) surveys on registration methods can be found. At this point it should just be noted, that the registration process can be simplified, if the data set is acquired intraoperatively, because then there is no need to deal with changes of the fracture segment poses between the preoperatively acquired data set and the intraoperative situation. Today, all major vendors of fluoroscopic C-arms have devices which are capable of acquiring such

3D data sets intraoperatively. The only prerequisite when using intraoperatively acquired 3D data sets is, that the objects which are represented in the data set can be set into relation with the coordinate space of the data set. Therefore, dynamic reference bases (DRBs) are rigidly mounted to the objects of interest, which are the proximal and distal fracture segments. These DRBs are visible to the navigation system during the acquisition of the 3D data set. The C-arm is equipped with infrared light reflecting elements as well; this way the 3D data set can be automatically set in relation to the DRBs by the navigation system. Figure 4 illustrates how the DRBs are mounted to the femur and which transformations are required in order to achieve the registration. The system uses three DRBs: the Y DRB, which is rigidly mounted to the proximal (hip side) fracture segment, the T DRB which is rigidly mounted to the distal (knee side) segment, and the SMS DRB which is mounted at the robot's hand. The surgical navigation system provides the robot controller program with the transformations between those three DRBs, namely ${}^{Y}T_{T}$ and ${}^{Y}T_{SMS}$. Additionally it obtains the pose of the 3D DICOM data set in relation to the DRBs at the time of the scan as transformation ${}^{Y}T_{DICOM}$ between the world DRB and the DICOM data set. With this transformation, the registration of the two fracture meshes can be finalized in the following way.

$$ {}^{Y}T_{PROX} = {}^{Y}T_{DICOM} \cdot {}^{DICOM}T_{PROX} \quad (1) $$

$$ {}^{T}T_{DIST} = {}^{Y}T_{T}^{-1} \cdot {}^{Y}T_{DICOM} \cdot {}^{DICOM}T_{DIST} \quad (2) $$

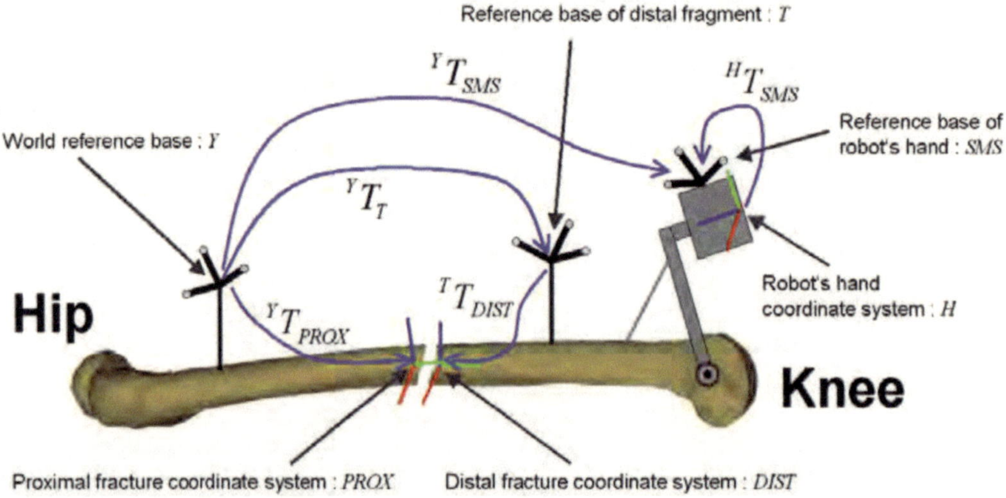

Figure 4. Registration of the intraoperative situation utilizing DRBs. The proximal DRB (left) is the world reference of the system, which is called the Y DRB. All other DRBs are given with respect to this DRB. The T DRB is the one rigidly mounted to the distal fracture segment. A third DRB, the SMS DRB, is mounted at the robot's hand with a fixed and known transformation ${}^{H}T_{SMS}$ between them

The third DRB, the SMS DRB, is used to register the robot to the DICOM coordinate space and the fracture segments. The SMS DRB is mounted at a fixed and known position to the robot's hand. The rigid transformation between the robot's hand and the SMS DRB is given as ${}^{H}T_{SMS}$. Using the data from the surgical navigation system and the robot's hand pose ${}^{R}T_{H}$, which can be obtained by the robot controller, the robot is registered to the surgical situs in the following way.

$$ {}^{Y}T_{R} = {}^{Y}T_{SMS} \cdot {}^{H}T_{SMS}^{-1} \cdot {}^{R}T_{H}^{-1} \quad (3) $$

We now describe the way the surgeon interacts with the robot by means of the joystick in order to perform the fracture reduction. The question is, how a 6D reduction problem (three translational and three rotational DoFs) can be solved efficiently by means of an input device with just two DoFs. The basic principle behind this is the reduction of the complex fracture reduction problem in 3D space to simpler reductions in 2D space. This is achieved by projecting the objects of the 3D world via standard computer graphics methods onto a 2D image plane. The reduction is now performed with respect to this 2D image with three DoFs. The interaction possibilities previously used for the 2D telemanipulator were simplified during the implementation of this 3D telemanipulator. While the translational way of interaction remains unchanged, the number of rotational DoFs controllable by the joystick was reduced. Only those rotational DoFs are controllable, which are "directly visible" from the current viewing direction: the rotation about an axis going through the fracture centre parallel to the viewing direction, and a rotation about the bone axis. In the translational motion mode the left/right and front/back deflections of the joystick are directly mapped to according translational motions of the distal fracture segment in the currently displayed viewing plane.

Y[2]	The world reference coordinate system, which is defined by the DRB rigidly attached to the proximal fracture segment.
T[2]	The coordinate system of the DRB, which is rigidly attached to the distal fracture segment.
SMS[2]	The coordinate system of the DRB, which is rigidly attached to the robot's hand.
H	The coordinate system of the robot's hand.
R	The robot's base coordinate system.
DICOM	The coordinate system of the DICOM data set.
PROX	The fracture centre of the proximal fracture segment.
DIST	The fracture centre of the distal fracture segment.
JOY	The joystick coordinate system.

Table 1. Coordinate systems used during robotized fracture reduction

In the rotational motion mode the front/back deflections are mapped to rotations about the bone axis, whereas the additional DoF of the joystick, the rotation about its own axis, is mapped to rotations of the distal fracture segment about an axis going through the fracture centre and resulting from the cross product of the view's up-vector and the bone axis. This vector is usually very close to an axis parallel to the current viewing direction, but facilitates a straight rotation path of the distal fracture segment in contrast to the curved path when rotating directly about the viewing direction. This is how the reduction can be performed in a 2D projection of the 3D scene. But how can the entire problem of a reduction in 3D space

[2] According to the DRB naming convention of the BrainLAB navigation system

be solved by this? This can be achieved by iteratively performing the 2D reduction described above from different viewing directions. Utilizing an additional switch on the joystick, the operator can pan the current viewing direction interactively to any arbitrary angle around the bone axis. Figure 5 illustrates this whole interaction principle.
When implementing this interaction mode, the coordinate space of the joystick has to be defined first, in which the two main DoFs of the stick (left/right and front/back deflection) are mapped to the X and Y axes. The additional DoF, the rotation about the stick's axis, is mapped to the Z axis. Therefore, a transformation matrix ${}^{DIST}\boldsymbol{T}_{JOY}$ has just to be found, which transforms the joystick's deflections into motions of the distal fracture segment. How can this transformation be obtained? Using the following notation for homogeneous transformation matrices,

$$\boldsymbol{T} = \begin{pmatrix} n_x & o_x & a_x & p_x \\ n_y & o_y & a_y & p_y \\ n_z & o_z & a_z & p_z \\ 0 & 0 & 0 & 1 \end{pmatrix} \tag{4}$$

the following equations have to be applied:

$$\vec{n} = (0,1,0)^T \tag{5}$$

$$\vec{o} = \vec{v} \times \vec{n} \tag{6}$$

$$\vec{a} = \vec{n} \times \vec{o} \tag{7}$$

Where $\vec{v}$ is the current viewing direction with respect to the distal fracture centre and the Y axis of the coordinate system corresponds with the bone axis. This results in the following homogeneous transformation matrix between the joystick coordinate system and the distal fracture centre:

$${}^{DIST}\boldsymbol{T}_{JOY} = \begin{pmatrix} 0 & -\vec{v}_z & \vec{v}_x & 0 \\ 1 & 0 & 0 & 0 \\ 0 & \vec{v}_x & \vec{v}_z & 0 \\ 0 & 0 & 0 & 1 \end{pmatrix} \tag{8}$$

Having this, a current joystick deflection $\vec{t} = (d_x, d_y, 0)^T$ for translational motions or $\vec{r} = (d_y, 0, dr_z)^T$ (cp. figure 5) for rotational motions can be transformed into a motion command which can be executed with respect to the distal fracture centre.

$$\vec{t}_{DIST} = s_t \cdot \left({}^{DIST}\boldsymbol{T}_{JOY} \cdot \vec{t}\right) \tag{9}$$

$$\vec{r}_{DIST} = s_r \cdot \left({}^{DIST}\boldsymbol{T}_{JOY} \cdot \vec{r}\right) \tag{10}$$

Where s_t and s_r are scaling factors to scale the deflection values in the range [-100; 100] used in $\vec{t}$ and $\vec{r}$ to an appropriate value in mm or radian. From this the final transformation can be computed, which has to be applied to the distal fracture segment.

$$T_{move} = T_{trans}(\vec{t}_{DIST}) \cdot T_{rot_{vectr}}(\bar{\vec{r}}_{DIST}, |\vec{r}_{DIST}|) \tag{11}$$

With

$$T_{trans}(\vec{t}) = \begin{pmatrix} 1 & 0 & 0 & \vec{t}_x \\ 0 & 1 & 0 & \vec{t}_y \\ 0 & 0 & 1 & \vec{t}_z \\ 0 & 0 & 0 & 1 \end{pmatrix} \tag{12}$$

$$T_{rot_{vctr}}(\vec{n}, \alpha) = \begin{pmatrix} \vec{n}_x^2 V\alpha + C\alpha & \vec{n}_x \vec{n}_y V\alpha - \vec{n}_z S\alpha & \vec{n}_x \vec{n}_z V\alpha + \vec{n}_y S\alpha & 0 \\ \vec{n}_x \vec{n}_y V\alpha + \vec{n}_z S\alpha & \vec{n}_y^2 V\alpha + C\alpha & \vec{n}_y \vec{n}_z V\alpha - \vec{n}_x S\alpha & 0 \\ \vec{n}_x \vec{n}_z V\alpha - \vec{n}_y S\alpha & \vec{n}_y \vec{n}_z V\alpha + \vec{n}_z S\alpha & \vec{n}_z^2 V\alpha + C\alpha & 0 \\ 0 & 0 & 0 & 1 \end{pmatrix} \tag{13}$$

Where $\bar{\vec{r}}_{DIST}$ is the normalized vector of $\vec{r}_{DIST}$, $C\alpha = \cos(\alpha)$, $S\alpha = \sin(\alpha)$, and $V\alpha = vers(\alpha) = 1 - \cos(\alpha)$.

The viewing direction, i.e. the position of the camera, can be changed by the following formula in which α is the angle by which the viewing direction should be rotated around the femur axis. This angle is controlled by an additional switch on the joystick.

$${}^{Y}T_{CAM}^{new} = {}^{Y}T_{CAM}^{-1\ old} \cdot {}^{Y}T_{PROX} \cdot T_{rot_y}(\alpha) \cdot {}^{Y}T_{PROX}^{-1} \cdot {}^{Y}T_{CAM}^{old} \tag{14}$$

With

$$T_{rot_y}(\theta) = \begin{pmatrix} \cos(\theta) & 0 & \sin(\theta) & 0 \\ 0 & 1 & 0 & 0 \\ -\sin(\theta) & 0 & \cos(\theta) & 0 \\ 0 & 0 & 0 & 1 \end{pmatrix} \tag{15}$$

One of the main points of criticism of current telemanipulator systems, like the da Vinci system, is the lack of haptic feedback. Haptic feedback is of particular interest during orthopaedic surgeries, because the forces caused by the surrounding soft tissue or due to interfragmental contacts can become quite high and play an important role for motion planning during the reduction process. Therefore, the feedback of acting forces was identified as an important aspect for the development of a telemanipulator system supporting this kind of surgeries. The force feedback can in this case be simply seen as the inverse problem to the control of the distal fracture segment by means of a joystick. So one can simply use ${}^{DIST}T_{JOY}^{-1}$ to convert the forces measured in the fracture centre of the distal fracture segment into the coordinate axes of the joystick, whereas only the forces in X and Y direction are fed back to the joystick axes.

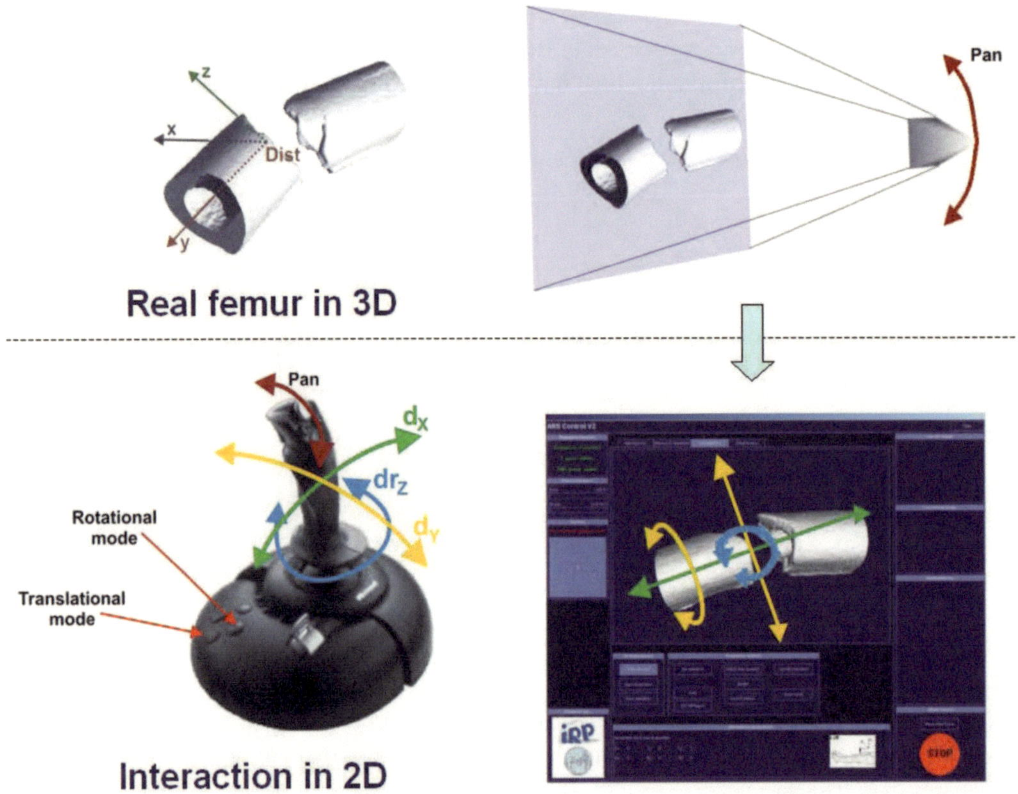

Figure 5. The interaction principle for telemanipulation based on 3D imaging data by means of a joystick with two DoFs. The surgeon can switch between rotational and translational manipulation mode. In every mode, he can control two DoFs with respect to the currently displayed viewing direction. The complete 3D reduction can be solved by performing the 2D reduction iteratively from different viewing directions. Therefore, the position from which the surgeon looks at the fracture site can be panned interactively around the bone axis to any arbitrary angle

2.2 Experiments

Figure 6 shows the process of the fracture reduction experiments carried out to evaluate the performance of telemanipulated fracture reductions based on 3D imaging data. The lower part of the procedure sequence presented in that figure could likewise be applied during real surgeries and can therefore be seen as a general procedure description for telemanipulated fracture reductions based on 3D imaging data.

First, two DRBs are mounted to the healthy bone in order to measure its unbroken reference transformation ${}^{Y}T_{T}^{ref}$. Next, the DRBs are removed, and a fracture is placed by means of a three-point-bending using a material testing machine. After remounting the DRBs to the broken bone parts, a 3D DICOM image data set is acquired with the IsoC 3D fluoroscopic C-arm. Resulting from the registration of this 3D data set, which is performed by the surgical navigation system, the transformations ${}^{T}T_{DIST}$ and ${}^{Y}T_{PROX}$ between the fracture segments and the attached DRBs are obtained. From these transformations, the reference transformation between the fracture centres ${}^{PROX}T_{DIST}^{ref}$ can be computed, utilizing ${}^{Y}T_{T}^{ref}$.

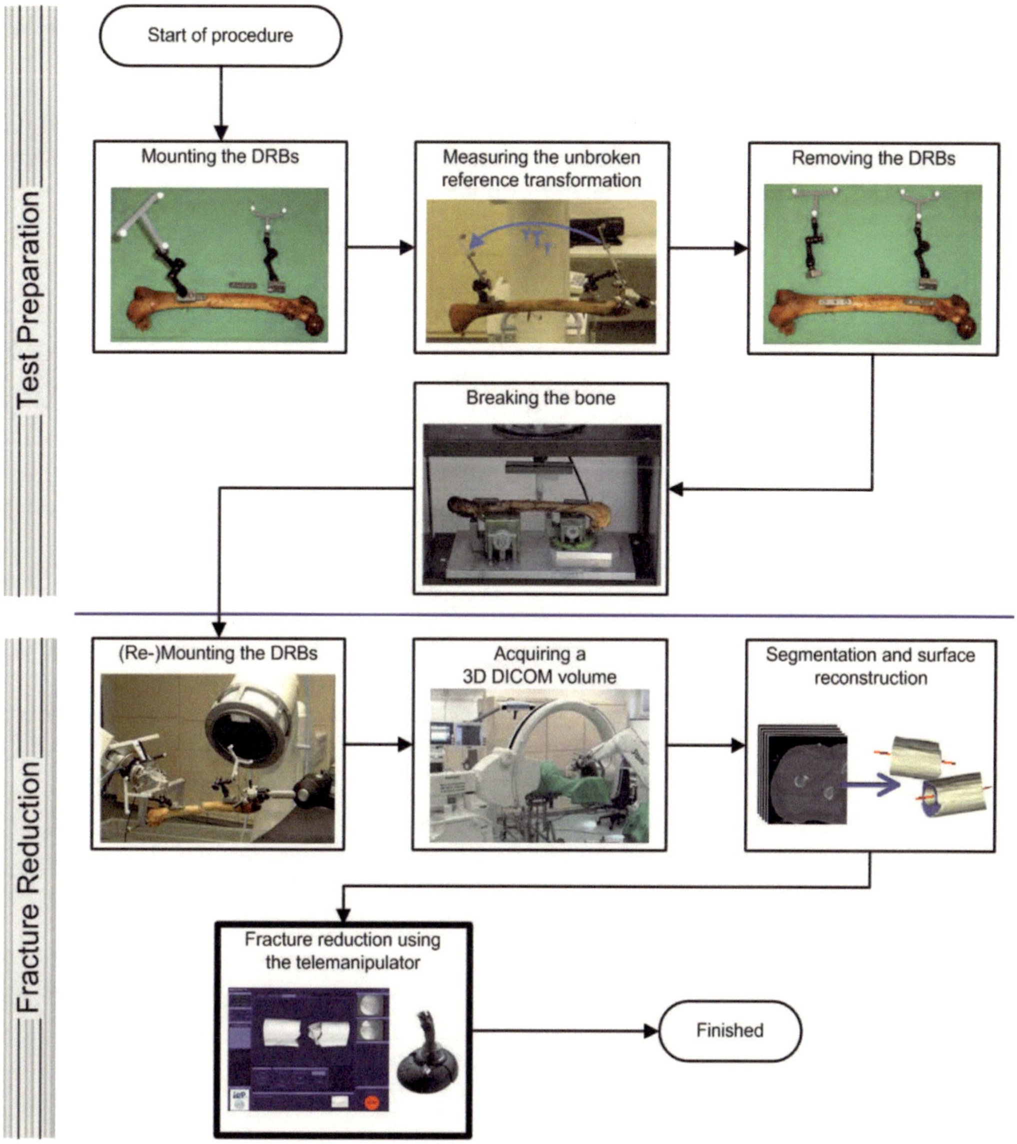

Figure 6. The process of telemanipulated reduction based on 3D imaging data. The upper "Test Preparation" part is only required for the test set-up. The lower part "Fracture Reduction" could likewise be used during real surgeries

Now the reduction is performed using the telemanipulator, controlled by means of the joystick as described before. As soon as the operator decides to finish the reduction process, the remaining deviations are computed based on the unbroken reference transformation and the current relative transformation between the two major fragments in the following way:

$$^{PROX}T_{DIST}^{dev} = {}^{PROX}T_{DIST}^{-1} \cdot {}^{ref}{}^{Y}T_{PROX}^{-1} \cdot {}^{Y}T_{T} \cdot {}^{T}T_{DIST} \qquad (16)$$

Using this set-up 144 fracture reductions on 14 exposed human femurs - which means real bones without surrounding soft tissue - were performed by four different operators in order to measure learning curves and achievable reduction accuracies. 96 fracture reductions on 12 femurs of complete human specimens with intact soft tissue were performed in a second test series by the same four operators. This time, the results were also compared to reductions on 10 of the same 12 femurs performed in the conventional manual way by an experienced surgeon using 2D X-ray imaging only.

3. Results

The experiments with exposed bones achieved very good results with mean deviations of less than 2° and 2mm for simple fractures (AO fracture type A). Compared to manually performed reductions, these values are very satisfactory. Table 2 summarizes the results in detail. However, the achievable reduction accuracy decreases with increasing fracture complexity (AO fracture types B and C) as displayed in table 3. Expectedly, avoiding axial displacements is very difficult in complex fractures (AO fracture type C) without a direct connection between the two major fragments. But even for complex fractures an accuracy with mean rotational deviations of less than 4° was achieved overall.

Parameter	Mean	Std. dev.	Min	Max
Reduction time (min:sec)	4:34	2:31	2:00	12:57
Lateral displacement (mm)	1.61	1.23	0.16	4.80
Axial displacement (mm)	1.08	0.63	0.05	3.20
Varus/valgus (left/right) (degrees)	1.09	0.73	0.03	2.66
Ante-/recurvature (front/back) (degrees)	1.42	0.84	0.19	4.04
Ex-/internal (axial) rotation (degrees)	1.37	1.39	0.02	5.82

Table 2. Results of the telemanipulated reductions based on 3D imaging for simple fractures of the AO fracture type A on exposed bones (bones without soft tissue) (N=64)

Parameter	Type A	Type B	Type C
Reduction time (min:sec)	4:34	4:18	2:48
Lateral displacement (mm)	1.61	2.03	0.96
Axial displacement (mm)	1.08	2.35	5.55
Varus/valgus (left/right) (degrees)	1.09	2.18	1.32
Ante-/recurvature (front/back) (degrees)	1.42	2.02	2.28
Ex-/internal (axial) rotation (degrees)	1.37	2.37	3.89

Table 3. Mean values of the remaining deviations after telemanipulated fracture reduction based on 3D imaging for all three AO fracture types on exposed bones

Experiments on human specimens with intact surrounding soft tissue revealed similar results regarding accuracy and operation time. When compared to conventional manual fracture reductions on the same human femurs, the results obtained by the telemanipulated fracture reductions were significantly better than the ones achieved in the manual control group as can be seen in table 4. However, the operation time was lengthened during our experiments when using the telemanipulator system, which will be discussed in the conclusion.

Parameter	Robot	Manual
Reduction time (min:sec)	6:14	2:16
Lateral displacement (mm)	1.98	3.37
Axial displacement (mm)	2.00	3.69
Varus/valgus (left/right) (degrees)	1.11	2.53
Ante-/recurvature (front/back) (degrees)	1.24	1.85
Ex-/internal (axial) rotation (degrees)	2.89	8.42

Table 4. Mean values of the remaining deviations after fracture reduction for the telemanipulated reductions based on 3D imaging compared to conventional manual reductions based on 2D X-ray imaging in complete human specimens with intact soft tissue

4. Conclusion

The results obtained by the extensive experiments with the telemanipulator system clearly revealed the potential of robotic systems supporting fracture reduction of the femur. Not only is it possible to achieve very high accuracies in the reductions, but also the exposure of the operation team to X-ray radiation can be reduced, utilizing a robotic system in the presented way. The direct and well controlled motions of the robotically moved fracture segments might support a gentle reduction, when compared with manually performed reductions, which generally suffer from repetitive motions under high forces, implying high stress to the soft tissue surrounding the fracture. However, whether or not this really has an impact on the healthy soft tissue, will have to be proven in the future.

One further point is remarkable here. The operation time could not be reduced utilizing a robot as telemanipulator when compared to the manual control groups. Keeping in mind the experience from clinical practice this is a surprising result, because from the possibility of a direct and well defined motion control utilizing the robot in combination with high resolution and detailed 3D imaging data we would have expected to shorten the operation time significantly. So far we haven't been able to determine the reasons for this, but the surgeon who performed the manual control groups observed, that the rigid soft tissue situation in the formalin conserved specimens eases the reduction considerably. How this circumstance influences the telemanipulated reductions and the results obtained by it too, can only be hypothesized at this time. Future experiments on fresh cadavers with soft tissue properties very close to the real life surgical situation will have to be done in order to clarify this point.

The implemented way of visualizing the fracture and interacting with the robotic system by means of a simple input device with two main and one supplementary DoF has proven to be very efficient and intuitive for the surgeons, who performed the experiments. However, this input device has its limitations, as torques can not be fed back intuitively via its force feedback interface. Future work will have to be done in order to evaluate whether input devices with six DoFs for input as well as force/torque feedback might have the potential of further improving this telemanipulated robotic approach. In this context the evaluation of how much of the benefit of the present method is due to the 3D fracture visualization and how much is due to the robotized fracture reduction would be of interest, too. Comparing the robotized reductions with reductions manually performed but supported by a navigation system with 3D visualization capabilities like (Hazan & Joskowicz, 2003; Joskowicz et al., 1998a) can answer this question.

In contrast to the system presented in this paper, the fracture reduction robot presented by Warisawa et al. in (Warisawa et al., 2004) is more like a robotized traction table. They described, how the robot can be used as a "power assistant" device. The question of how a precise fracture reduction might be achieved with that robot was not answered adequately in their publication. The main problem in our opinion being the fixation of the robot to the patient's foot, which doesn't allow the bone segment in the femur to be controlled directly and predictably, as the articulated knee joint is still between the robot and the bone segment. While having the great advantage of being completely noninvasive, it might yield a lot of problems regarding control and achievable accuracy. We are going to address the problem of invasiveness in a different way, by trying to combine a noninvasive robot attachment with precise and well controlled bone manipulations in the future. A second very promising fracture reduction robot was developed by Seide et al. (Seide et al., 2004) based on an external fixateur with a parallel kinematic. The fracture reduction is performed automatically by this robot based on a pre-planned trajectory. The reduction is performed over a longer period of time - up to several days - which has the advantage of being very gentle to the soft tissue, as stated by the authors. However, the applicability of the system is limited to long bones. Even the applicability for fractures close to the joints, like proximal femur fractures with a higher incidence rate, might be questionable. The usage of a standard robotic architecture, as used in this paper, might be advantageous, as it is theoretically applicable for all kinds of bone fractures and we already performed successful fracture reductions in the proximal femur.

But still the results achievable with our telemanipulator system revealed the limitations of such an approach. The reduction accuracy degrades conspicuously with the complexity of the fracture. Especially for fractures of the fracture type C, without a direct connection between the two major fragments, larger translational as well as rotational deviations after reduction have to be expected.

4.1 Outlook

In this paper, only the telemanipulated reduction was presented. We have shown, that very precise reductions are possible, with such a telemanipulated approach. However, the remaining accuracy problems in more complex fracture types can be solved best by an automatic planning and reduction procedure according to figure 7. In order to achieve this, we already developed methods to automatically compute the desired and precise target transformations between the fracture segments (Winkelbach et al., 2003; Winkelbach, 2006). The required path planning and robot motion planning in order to achieve this automated reduction are to be published in (Westphal, 2007).

The surgical fixation of femoral fractures with an intramedullary nail comprises two procedure steps, during which the surgeon has to drill accurate holes into the patient's bone. The first hole opens the bone's medullary cavity so that the intramedullary nail can be inserted. The second drilling task is the final fixation of the nail by interlocking it by means of screws with the bone at the end of the surgical operation (distal locking). For both procedure steps, we developed automated image analysis methods, which can compute precise drilling trajectories. The robot is used as drill guidance system during these procedure steps (Westphal, 2007). Whereas each of these surgical tasks has been evaluated separately so far, the evaluation of the complete surgical workflow starting with the robotized opening of the medullary cavity, following an automated reduction, finalized by a robotized distal locking is subject to our future work.

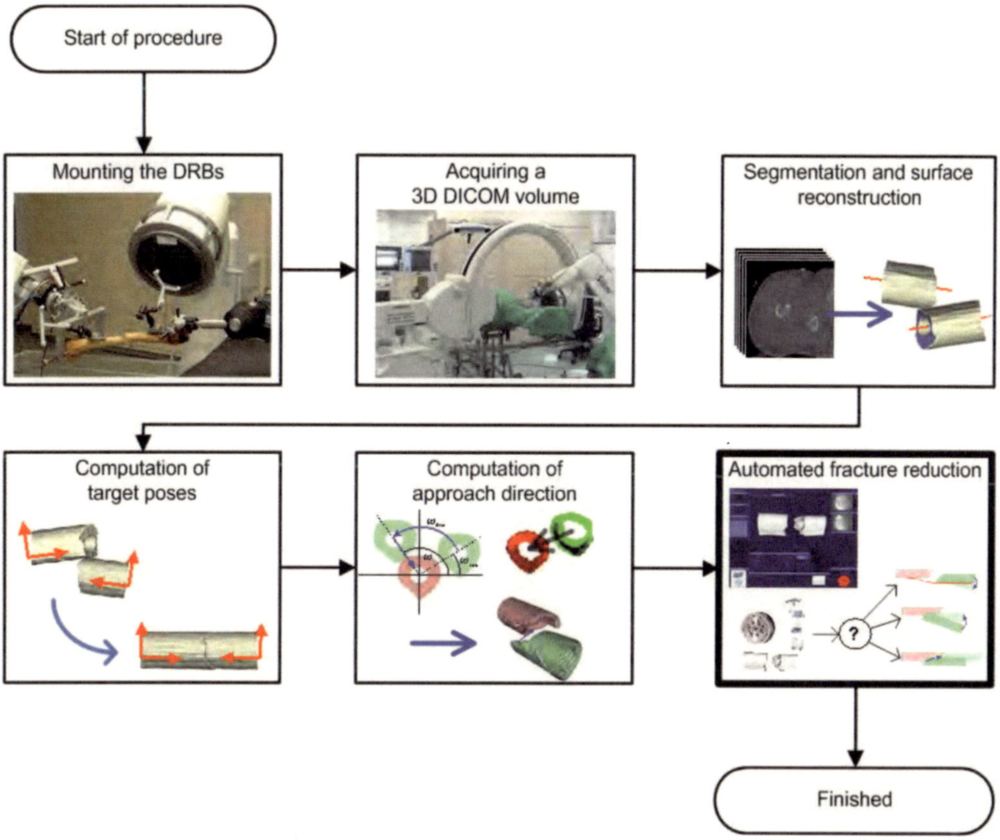

Figure 7. The process of automated fracture reduction based on 3D imaging data. After 3D data acquisition, segmentation, and surface reconstruction the desired target poses are computed automatically. A reduction motion plan is created, which is finally executed automatically under force/torque control by the robot

The generalization of the telemanipulation interaction principles presented herein for other fracture types is another topic, which is of interest both from a scientific and economic point of view. Basically the idea of reducing the complex 3D reduction problem to simple 2D reductions with intuitive and efficient visualization and interaction possibilities, is applicable for many fracture reduction problems, by simply extending the already proven conventional surgical procedures with the advantages of a robotized motion control. In order to evaluate this, our first laboratory set-up was adapted to perform reductions of hip fractures using plastic hips and again CCD cameras. The visualization and robot interaction was based on the three standardized 2D X-ray views, which are used by surgeons during conventional operations. As an extension to the femur fracture interaction principle we had to introduce a second centre of rotation, so the surgeon can decide interactively whether the dorsal or ventral fracture zone should be retained during rotations. Though the results of these tests have been very satisfactory (Hüfner et al., 2003), we have not extended research in this direction so far. However, we belief that further research would be worthwhile.

5. Acknowledgements

We would like to thank BrainLAB (Munich, Germany) for supporting us with an interface to their navigation system and the AO-Developing-Institute (ADI, Davos, Switzerland) for lending us their pneumatic fixation device. We thank the Department of Anatomy of the Hannover Medical School for making specimens available for our experiments. Finally, we thank the German Research Foundation (DFG) for funding this project under the grants WA 848/10-1/2 and KR 2161/1-1/2 "Roboterunterstützte Femurmarknagelung".

6. References

Arneson, T.; Melton, L. 3rd.; Lewallen, D. & O'Fallon, W. (1988). Epidemiology of diaphyseal and distal femoral fractures in Rochester, Minnesota, 1965-1984, In: *Clin Orthop Relat Res*, Vol. 234, pp. 188-94

Bhandari, M.; Guyatt, G.; Tong, D.; Adili, A. & Shaughnessy, S. (2000). Reamed versus nonreamed intramedullary nailing of lower extremity long bone fractures: a systematic overview and meta-analysis, In: *J Orthop Trauma*, Vol. 14, No. 1, pp. 2-9

Bouazza-Marouf, K.; Browbank, I. & Hewit, J. (1995). Robotic-assisted internal fixation of femoral fractures, In: *Proc.Inst.Mech.Eng*, pp. 51-58

Cleary, K. & Nguyen, C. (2003). Medical robotics. In: *Biomedical Technology and Devices Handbook*, Moore, J. & Zouridakis, G. (ed), CRC Press, chapter 32

Dario, P.; Hannaford, B. & Menciassi, A. (2003). Smart Surgical Tools and Augmenting Devices, In: *IEEE Transactions on Robotics and Automation*, Vol. 19, No. 5, October , pp. 782-792

Finkemeier, C.; Schmidt, A.; Kyle, R.; Templeman, D. & Varecka, T. (2000). A prospective, randomized study of intramedullary nails inserted with and without reaming for the treatment of open and closed fractures of the tibial shaft, In: *J Orthop Trauma*, Vol. 14, No. 3, pp. 187-93

Füchtmeier, B.; Egersdoerfer, S.; Mai, R.; Hente, R.; Dragoi, D.; Monkman, G. & Nerlich, M. (2004). Reduction of femoral shaft fractures in vitro by a new developed reduction robot system 'RepoRobo', In: *Injury, Int. J. Care Injured*, 35, pp. A113-A119

Gösling, T.; Westphal, R.; Hüfner, T.; Faulstich, J.; Kfuri, M.; Wahl, F. & Krettek, C. (2005). Robot-assisted fracture reduction: A preliminary study in the femur shaft. In: *Med. Biol. Eng. Comput.*, Vol. 43, pp. 115-120

Gösling, T.; Hüfner, T.; Westphal, R.; Faulstich, J.; Hankemeier, S.; Wahl, F. & Krettek, C. (2006). Overdistraction of the fracture eases reduction in delayed femoral nailing: results of intraoperative force measurements. In: *J Trauma*, Vol. 61, No. 4, October, pp. 900-4

Gösling, T.; Westphal, R.; Faulstich, J.; Sommer, K.; Wahl, F.; Krettek, C. & Hüfner, T. (2006). Forces and torques during fracture reduction: Intraoperative measurements in the femur, In: *J Orthop Res*, Vol. 24, No. 3, January, pp. 333-338

Gösling, T. (2007). *Die roboterassistierte Reposition von Schaftfrakturen - Grundlagenversuche am Femur*, Department of Trauma Surgery, Hannover Medical School, Habil.

Hazan, E. & Joskowicz, L. (2003). Computer-assisted image-guided intramedullary nailing of femoral shaft fractures, In: *Techniques in Orthopaedics*, Special Issue on Computer-Aided Orthopaedic Surgery, Vol. 18, No. 2, pp. 130-140

Hüfner, T.; Westphal, R.; Gösling, T.; Wahl, F.; Kfuri, M. Jr. & Krettek, C. (2003). Roboterassistierte Beckenreposition. In: *CURAC 2003, Computer und Roboter Assistierte Chirurgie*

Joskowicz, L.; Milgrom, C.; Simkin, A.; Tockus, L. & Yaniv, Z. (1998). FRACAS: a system for computer-aided image-guided long bone fracture surgery, In: *Computer-Aided Surgery*, Vol. 3, No. 6, May

Joskowicz, L.; Tockus, L.; Yaniv, Z.; Simkin, A. & Milgrom, C. (1998). Computer-aided image-guided bone fracture surgery: concept and implementation, In: *12th Int. Symp. on Computer Assisted Radiology and Surgery*, Lemke et al (Ed.), Elsevier

Kempf, I.; Grosse, A. & Beck, G. (1985). Closed locked intramedullary nailing. Its application to comminuted fractures of the femur. In: *J.Bone Joint Surg.Am.*, Vol. 67, pp. 709-720

Krettek, C.; Gluer, S.; Schandelmaier, P. & Tscherne, H. (1996). Marknagelung offener Frakturen. In: *Orthopade*, Vol. 25, pp. 223-233

Krettek, C.; Schandelmaier, P. & Tscherne, H. (1998). Treatment of femoral shaft fractures with an unreamed solid nail (UFN) and standard locking, In: *Operat.Orthop.Traumatol*, Vol. 6, pp. 179-192

Krettek, C. (2001). Prinzipien der intramedullären Knochenbruchstabilisierung. Teil 2: Operationstechnik. In: *Unfallchirurg*, Vol. 104, pp. 749-769

Lorensen, W. E. & Cline, H. E. (1987). Marching Cubes: A High Resolution 3D Surface Construction Algorithm. In: *Computer Graphics (Proceedings of SIGGRAPH '87)*, Vol. 21, pp. 163-169

Maintz, J. & Viergever, M. (1998). A survey of medical image registration. In: *Medical Image Analysis 2*, No. 1, pp. 1-36

Martinet, O.; Cordey, J.; Harder, Y.; Maier, A.; Buhler, M. & Barraud, G. (2000). The epidemiology of fractures of the distal femur, In: *Injury*, Vol. 31, Suppl 3, pp. C62-3

Pott, P. P. (2006). *MERODA, the MEdical RObotics DAtabase.* http://www.ma.uni-heidelberg.de/apps/ortho/meroda/, cited: 18. Jul. 2007

Prevot, N.; Charissoux, J.; Fiorenza, F.; Arnaud, J. & Pecout, C. (1998). Utilisation d'un clou non fendu de Russel-Taylor pour la stabilisation des fractures du femur. A propos de 57 fractures avec 30 etudes tomodensitometriques de la rotation. In: *Rev Chir Orthop Reparatrice Appar Mot*, Vol. 84, pp. 33-40

Rüedi, T. & Murphy, W. (2000). *AO Principles of Fracture Management*, Thieme

Seide, K. & Wolter, D. (2000). Korrekturen mit dem Hexapoden, In: *Orthopäde*, 29, pp. 39-46

Seide, K.; Faschingbauer, M.; Wenzl, M.; Weinrich, N. & Juergens, C. (2004). A hexapod robot external fixator for computer assisted fracture reduction and deformity correction, In: *Int. J. Medical Robotics and Computer Assisted Surgery*, Vol. 1, No. 1, pp. 64-69

Sugarman, I.; Adam, I. & Bunker, T. (1988). Radiation dosage during AO locking femoral nailing. In: *Injury*, Vol. 19, pp. 336-338

Taylor, R. & Joskowicz, L. (2002). Computer-integrated surgery and medical robotics. In: *Standard Handbook of Biomedical Engineering and Design*, Kutz, M. (ed), 1st Edition. McGraw-Hill Professional, pp. 325-353

Taylor, R. & Stoianovici, D. (2003). Medical robotics in computer-integrated surgery. In: *IEEE Transactions on Robotics and Automation*, Vol. 19, No. 5, Oct., pp. 765-781

Warisawa, S.; Ishizuka, T.; Mitsuishi, M.; Yonenobu, K.; Sugano, N. & Nakazawa, T. (2004). Development of a femur fracture reduction robot, In: *ICRA 2004 - IEEE International Conference on Robotics and Automation.*

Westphal, R.; Faulstich, J.; Gösling, T.; Winkelbach, S.; Hüfner, T.; Krettek, C. & Wahl, F. (2003). Fracture reduction using a telemanipulator with haptical feedback. *CARS 2003, Proceedings of the 17th International Congress and Exhibition, Computer Assisted Radiology and Surgery*, International Congress Series 1256, June 25-28, London, UK, Elsevier, Amsterdam, p. 1369

Westphal, R.; Winkelbach, S.; Finkemeyer, B.; Wahl, F.; Gösling, T.; Hüfner, T.; Faulstich, J. & Krettek, C. (2004). Progress in Robot Assisted Fracture Reduction. *Video-Proceedings - IEEE, International Conference on Robotics and Automation*, April 26-30, New Orleans, USA

Westphal, R.; Winkelbach, S.; Gösling, T.; Hüfner, T.; Faulstich, J.; Martin, P.; Krettek, C. & Wahl, F. (2006). A Surgical Telemanipulator for Femur Shaft Fracture Reduction, In: *Int. J. of of Medical Robotics and Computer Assisted Surgery*, Vol. 2, No. 3, pp. 238-50

Westphal, R. (2007). Fortschritte in der Robotik: Sensor-based Surgical Robotics: Contributions to Robot Assisted Fracture Reduction, (to be published), Shaker-Verlag, *Dissertation*

Winquist, R.; Hansen, S. Jr. & Clawson, D. (1984). Closed intramedullary nailing of femoral fractures. A report of five hundred and twenty cases, In: *J.Bone Joint Surg.Am.*, Vol. 66, pp. 529-539

Winkelbach, S. ; Westphal, R. & Gösling, T. (2003). Pose Estimation of Cylindrical Fragments for Semi-automatic Bone Fracture Reduction, In: *Pattern Recognition (DAGM 2003), Lecture Notes in Computer Science*, Michaelis, B. & Krell, G. (ed), Vol. 2781, Springer, September, pp. 566-573

Winkelbach, S. (2006). Fortschritte in der Robotik. vol. 10: Das 3d-Puzzle-Problem - Effiziente Methoden zum paarweisen Zusammensetzen von dreidimensionalen Fragmenten, Shaker-Verlag, *Dissertation*

Wolinsky, P.; McCarty, E.; Shyr, Y. & Johnson, K. (1999). Reamed intramedullary nailing of the femur: 551 cases. In: *J.Trauma*, Vol. 46, pp. 392-399

Yaniv, Z.; Joskowicz, L.; Simkin, A.; Garza-Jinich, M. & Milgrom, C. (1998). Fluoroscopic image processing for computer-aided orthopaedic surgery, In: *1st Int. Conf. on Medical Computing and Computer-Assisted Intervention*, Grimson et al. (Ed.), Lecture Notes in Computer Science, Springer

Zitova, B. & Flusser, J. (2003). Image registration methods: a survey. In: *Image and Vision Computing*, Vol. 21, No. 11, pp. 977-1000

Zlowodzki, M.; Bhandari, M.; Marek, D.; Cole, P. & Kregor, P. (2006). Operative treatment of acute distal femur fractures: systematic review of 2 comparative studies and 45 case series (1989 to 2005), In: *J Orthop Trauma*, Vol. 20, No. 5, pp. 366-71